Manual of Anesthesia Practice

Edited by

MANUEL PARDO, Jr., MD

Associate Professor
Department of Anesthesia and Perioperative Care
University of California at San Francisco
School of Medicine

JAMES M. SONNER, MD

Associate Professor
Department of Anesthesia and Perioperative Care
University of California at San Francisco
School of Medicine

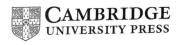

CAMBRIDGE
UNIVERSITY PRESS

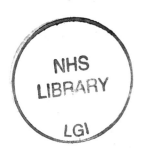

CAMBRIDGE UNIVERSITY PRESS
Cambridge, New York, Melbourne, Madrid, Cape Town, Singapore,
São Paulo, Delhi

Cambridge University Press
32 Avenue of the Americas, New York, NY 10013-2473, USA

www.cambridge.org
Information on this title: www.cambridge.org/9780521709354

First published 2007

Printed in the United States of America

A catalog record for this publication is available from the British Library.

Library of Congress Cataloging in Publication Data

Manual of anesthesia practice / [edited by] Manuel Pardo, James Sonner.
      p. ; cm.
ISBN-13: 978-0-521-70935-4 (pbk.)
ISBN-10: 0-521-70935-0 (pbk.)
1. Anesthesiology–Handbooks, manuals, etc. 2. Anesthesia–Handbooks,
manuals, etc. I. Pardo, Manuel, 1965- II. Sonner, James, 1959-
[DNLM: 1. Anesthesia–Handbooks. 2. Anesthetics–Handbooks.WO 231
M2937 2007]
RD82.2.M352   2007
617.9′6–dc22   2007016910

ISBN   978-0-521-70935-4 paperback

NOTICE

Because of the dynamic nature of medical practice and drug selection and dosage, users are advised that decisions regarding drug therapy must be based on the independent judgment of the clinician, changing information about a drug (e.g., as reflected in the literature and manufacturer's most current product information), and changing medical practices.

While great care has been taken to ensure the accuracy of the information presented, users are advised that the authors, editors, contributors, and publisher make no warranty, express or implied, with respect to, and are not responsible for, the currency, completeness, or accuracy of the information contained in this publication, nor for any errors, omissions, or the application of this information, nor for any consequences arising therefrom. Users are encouraged to confirm the information contained herein with other sources deemed authoritative. Ultimately, it is the responsibility of the treating physician, relying on experience and knowledge of the patient, to determine dosages and the best treatment for the patient. Therefore, the author(s), editors, contributors, and the publisher make no warranty, express or implied, and shall have no liability to any person or entity with regard to claims, loss, or damage caused, or alleged to be caused, directly or indirectly, by the use of information contained in this publication.

Further, the author(s), editors, contributors, and the publisher are not responsible for misuse of any of the information provided in this publication, for negligence by the user, or for any typographical errors.

NHS The Leeds Teaching Hospitals NHS Trust

This book must be returned by the date shown below or a fine will be charged.

The NHS Staff Library at the L.G.I.
☎ 0113 39 26445

Contents

PART TWO. PROCEDURES

Contents

PART THREE. CRITICAL EVENTS

PART FOUR. TECHNIQUES

PART FIVE. DRUGS

Preface

The aim of this work is to provide, in one convenient source, authoritative information to guide the anesthesia provider at the point of care. Its five sections arose from the clinician's perspective.

CO-EXISTING DISEASES

What medical problems does this patient have and how should I manage them?

PROCEDURES

What do I need to know about the proposed surgical procedure to safely care for the patient?

CRITICAL EVENTS

How do I diagnose and treat unexpected life-threatening perioperative problems?

TECHNIQUES

What are the important aspects of performing certain anesthetic techniques or procedures?

DRUGS

What information do I need to know about a medication I am about to give, or that the patient is receiving on a chronic basis?

We wish to acknowledge the 63 residents and 43 faculty who contributed to this project, as well as our department chair, Dr. Ronald D. Miller.

Manuel Pardo, Jr., and James M. Sonner

PART ONE

Co-Existing Diseases

ACHONDROPLASIA

GRETE H. PORTEOUS, MD

OVERVIEW
- Definition: Rare (4/100,000) genetic disorder characterized by abnormal endochondral bone formation.
- Achondroplasia is the major cause of dwarfism.
- Etiologies
  - Spontaneous mutation is the most common cause (80% of cases).
  - Autosomal dominant inheritance accounts for the remaining cases.
- Characterized by
  - Short stature
  - Shortened extremities
  - Enlarged head
  - Saddle nose
  - Trunk of relatively normal length
- In most cases there are no changes in intelligence, longevity, or reproductive ability.
- Usual Rx: None

PREOP

Issues/Evaluation
- Difficult airway. Pts w/ achondroplasia are traditionally considered to have difficult airways because of
  - Large tongue
  - Large mandible
  - Foramen magnum stenosis
  - Limited neck extension
  - Increased incidence of atlanto-axial instability
- Difficult spinal & epidural anesthetic. This is the result of several spine abnormalities:
  - Marked kyphoscoliosis & lumbar lordosis.
  - Bony landmarks are difficult to identify.
  - Prolapsed intervertebral discs, osteophytes, shortened pedicles, & a narrow epidural space increase the risk of dural puncture & decrease the chance of successful catheter placement.
  - Spinal stenosis may impair free flow of CSF, making dural puncture hard to identify.

- ➤ Anesthetic may spread unpredictably in the epidural space, leading to "patchy" block or higher-than-expected block.
- ➤ In the past, many considered regional anesthesia to be contraindicated in this pt population, but several recent studies have reported success w/ few complications from regional.
- ■ Pulmonary
  - ➤ May have decreased chest wall compliance & FRC because of thoracic kyphoscoliosis & rib deformities.
  - ➤ Frequent respiratory tract infections may (rarely) lead to cor pulmonale.
- ■ Pregnancy
  - ➤ High incidence of cesarean section for delivery due to cephalopelvic disproportion.
  - ➤ Airway management can become even more difficult because of the typical changes of the parturient superimposed on a preexisting difficult airway.

What To Do
- ■ Obtain careful surgical/anesthetic history & any available anesthetic records.
- ■ Inform pt of potential difficulty of airway management & possibility of awake fiberoptic intubation.
- ■ Document neurologic exam carefully if regional anesthesia planned, as preexisting neuropathies due to spinal abnormalities are not uncommon.

INTRAOP
- ■ Airway management. Prepare for difficult intubation:
  - ➤ Multiple laryngoscope blades
  - ➤ Smaller-than-usual endotracheal tubes
  - ➤ LMAs
  - ➤ Fiberscope readily available
  - ➤ Avoid vigorous cervical extension w/ intubation
- ■ Regional anesthesia
  - ➤ Spinal block: There is no consensus in the literature on type & dose of anesthetic; it is probably rarely performed.
  - ➤ Epidural block: There is more reported experience w/ this technique. Epidural catheters are placed in the usual manner, maintaining high suspicion for unrecognized subarachnoid catheter placement. Recommended test dose is the usual (1.5 cc of lidocaine 1.5% + epinephrine 1:200,000). The most appropriate type

& volume of epidural dose is unclear, but generally considered to be less than a usual dose. Successful examples in the literature for lumbar epidurals for C-section:

- 8 cc of 2% lidocaine + bicarb + epi (1:200,000)
- 12 cc of 2% lidocaine + bicarb + epi (1:200,000) + fentanyl 37.5 mcg
- 9 cc of 3% 2-chloroprocaine
- 5–12 cc of 0.5% bupivacaine (at 12 cc a C5 level achieved)
- 21 cc of 0.75% bupivacaine

POSTOP

- Standard management, w/ attention to airway patency & adequacy of ventilation.
- Document neurologic exam prior to discharge from PACU.

ACROMEGALY

BETTY LEE-HOANG, MD

OVERVIEW

- Definition
  - Acromegaly is a condition caused by overproduction of growth hormone from the anterior pituitary, usually by a pituitary tumor.
  - The condition results in overgrowth of skeletal, soft & connective tissues.
  - Pts usually have enlarged hands, feet, jaw & tongue.
  - Major organs including the heart, lungs, liver & kidney are also increased in size.
  - Airway anatomy is altered, including enlargement of the tongue & epiglottis, mandible hypertrophy & generalized soft tissue growth, which may make airway management difficult
- Usual Rx
  - Hypophysectomy (excision of the pituitary tumor)
  - The surgical approach usually taken is transsphenoidal; alternately, a bifrontal craniotomy approach can be taken.

PREOP

Issues/Evaluation

- A thorough history & airway exam are required.
- If pt complains of dyspnea, hoarseness or stridor or has been recently diagnosed w/ sleep apnea, indicating a risk of airway obstruction

w/ sedation or general anesthesia, consider an awake fiberoptic intubation.

- Pts w/ acromegaly may have glottic or subglottic stenosis, nasal turbinate enlargement, vocal cord thickening, or recurrent laryngeal nerve involvement.
- Evaluate pts for hypertension, hyperglycemia, congestive heart failure, peripheral nerve or artery entrapments, skeletal muscle weakness.

INTRAOP
- Be prepared for a difficult airway w/ several laryngoscope blades, laryngeal mask airways (LMA) & a fiberoptic bronchoscope as backup.
- Pts may need treatment of hypertension intraop, especially if a transsphenoidal procedure is performed, since the nasal septum is usually prepped w/ cocaine, epinephrine, or phenylephrine.

POSTOP
- Because pts are at risk of airway obstruction & may have difficult airways, make sure pt is fully awake & following commands before extubation.
- If pt has undergone a hypophysectomy as treatment for acromegaly, pituitary insufficiency may arise postop (eg, TSH, ACTH may be low).

ACUTE HEPATITIS

JOSEPH COTTEN, MD, PHD

OVERVIEW
- Definition: inflammation of hepatocytes
  - Multiple causes, including viral infection, toxin, fatty liver infiltration of pregnancy, sepsis, congestive heart failure.
- Viral hepatitis
  - Symptoms in order of incidence: dark urine, fatigue, anorexia, nausea, fever, emesis, headache, abdominal discomfort, light-colored stool, pruritus.
  - Hepatitis A
    - Fecal-oral transmission; blood transmission is rare.
    - Chronic disease or carrier state does not exist.
  - Hepatitis B
    - Parenteral, oral-oral, sexual transmission.

- HBsAg indicates infectivity.
- HBcAg indicates high infectivity.
- HBsAg presence for >6 mo suggests a chronic carrier state (1–10% become chronic).
- Chronic active disease often progresses to cirrhosis.
➤ Hepatitis C
- Causes most posttransfusion hepatitis.
- Chronic liver disease develops in 80% of infected pts & 20% of these will develop cirrhosis.
- Sexual & casual household contact w/ saliva is inefficient means of transmission.
➤ Hepatitis D
- Requires the presence of hepatitis B for its expression.
- Hepatitis B vaccination prevents hepatitis D.
➤ Epstein-Barr virus (EBV): usually produces mild hepatitis associated w/ infectious mononucleosis
➤ Cytomegalovirus (CMV): CMV is present in most adults; liver disease is mild & nonchronic
■ Drug-induced
➤ Toxins: alcohol, carbon tetrachloride, vinyl chloride
➤ Therapeutic drugs most frequently implicated: isoniazid, methyldopa, rifampin, acetylsalicylic acid, nonsteroidal anti-inflammatory drugs (NSAIDs)
➤ Halothane produces two types of hepatotoxicity:
- Mild self-limited postop toxicity due to changes in hepatic blood flow that affect hepatic oxygenation
- Halothane hepatitis, a life-threatening immune-mediated response after repeat exposure to halothane via trifluoroacetyl metabolite (less likely in pediatric pts)
➤ Isoflurane/enflurane/desflurane/sevoflurane, like halothane, can produce mild self-limited postop toxicity due to changes in hepatic blood flow. However, they all maintain blood flow similarly & better than halothane
- These compounds, w/ exception of sevoflurane, may be capable of producing a more severe immune-mediated hepatitis but undergo less extensive metabolism than halothane

PREOP

Issues/Evaluation
■ Elective surgery should be postponed for pts w/ acute hepatocellular injury due to increased morbidity & mortality.

- ➤ One study found a 31% mortality rate for pts undergoing exploratory laparotomy w/ unsuspected parenchymal liver disease.
- ➤ Another study noted a 9.5% mortality rate for pts w/ acute viral hepatitis undergoing laparotomy.
- ■ Severely jaundiced pts (>8 mg/dL) are more likely to develop postop renal failure & sepsis.
- ■ Decreased perfusion of the liver, which occurs during all anesthetics, neuraxial & general, may be responsible for poor outcomes in pts w/ parenchymal liver disease.
- ■ Liver perfusion is affected most greatly by procedures anatomically adjacent (eg, cholecystectomy).

What To Do
- ■ Rule out acute liver failure (as opposed to merely acute hepatitis).
  - ➤ Findings in acute liver failure can include encephalopathy, cerebral edema, coagulopathy, renal failure, infection, hypoglycemia, etc.
  - ➤ See also Coexisting Disease chapter "Acute Liver Failure."
- ■ Blood glucose may be low w/ severe liver injury & should be corrected.
- ■ Thrombocytopenia should be corrected if present.
- ■ Evaluate LFTs & viral serology if appropriate.
  - ➤ Prothrombin time: assesses current liver synthetic function
    - May be prolonged by vitamin K deficiency; consider vitamin K administration if this is suspected
  - ➤ Aspartate aminotransferase (AST), alanine aminotransferase (ALT):
    - Found in large quantity in the liver.
    - Levels >500 U/L occur w/ acute hepatocellular injury.
    - Modest injury <300 U/L occurs in a variety of conditions (eg, acute or chronic hepatocellular injury, infiltrative disease, biliary obstruction).
    - ALT is generally more sensitive than AST for viral hepatitis.
    - AST is elevated twofold in excess of ALT in alcoholic liver disease.
    - If transaminase levels are >3 times normal, nonelective procedures requiring general or regional anesthetic should be postponed & a gastroenterologist consulted.

- Lower elevations require repeat evaluation to assess for worsening levels, stable levels, or improvement in levels as well as viral hepatitis serologies.
- Surgery may proceed if moderately elevated transaminase levels are stable or trending down & viral serologies are negative; otherwise, seek gastroenterology consult.

➢ Albumin
- Synthesized by liver
- Half-life of 14–21 days, so is not beneficial for evaluation of acute disease

➢ Alkaline phosphatase (AP): present in bone, intestine, liver. AP is elevated in biliary obstruction, cholestasis, space-occupying lesions, infiltrative diseases.

➢ Gamma-glutamyl transpeptidase (GGT)
- Increases in GGT & AP tend to occur in similar diseases.
- GGT is elevated in pts ingesting certain agents (eg, alcohol, barbiturates, phenytoin).

➢ Lactate dehydrogenase (LDH): abundant in the liver but may arise from many sources, including red blood cells, as during hemolysis

➢ Total bilirubin (a byproduct of heme degradation) is either conjugated (direct-acting, water-soluble, renally excreted) or unconjugated (indirect-acting, protein-bound).
- Jaundice is apparent when levels exceed 3–4 mg/dL.
- Indirect bilirubin increases w/ hemolysis, Gilbert's or Crigler-Najjar syndrome, heart failure, or portosystemic shunting.
- Direct bilirubin increases w/ hepatocellular dysfunction or biliary tract obstruction.

INTRAOP

Management
- Drug disposition may be difficult to predict.
  - ➢ Isoflurane, desflurane, sevoflurane may be best for maintenance of hepatic blood flow; consider supplementation w/ nitrous oxide & IV agents (which may have delayed clearance).
  - ➢ Pseudocholinesterase deficiency is rare such that succinylcholine & mivacurium action should not be prolonged.
  - ➢ Atracurium & cis-atracurium are cleared independent of liver function.

➤ Vecuronium & rocuronium are unlikely to be prolonged unless large doses are used.
■ To optimize liver perfusion & prevent secondary ischemic injury, minimize hypotension & hypoxia & maintain normocarbia.
■ Administer fresh-frozen plasma for coagulopathy.
■ Consider monitoring of blood glucose, acid-base status, coagulation profile, urine output.

POSTOP
■ Be alert to worsening liver function after surgical stress.
■ Severe postop jaundice may be related to hypotension, hypoxia, multiple transfusions.
■ "Shock liver" is a condition caused by marked or prolonged hypotension.
  ➤ Typical findings include
    • Tenfold increase in transaminase levels
    • Coagulopathy
    • Possibly liver failure
  ➤ A milder form can be seen in pts after cardiopulmonary bypass.
■ Reversible, minor abnormalities in LFTs can be detected in up to 50% of all patients postop.
■ Postop jaundice is present in 20% of all patients after major surgery.
■ Causes of postop jaundice (can be distinguished by LFT evaluation).
  ➤ Increased bilirubin
    • Hemolysis
    • Hemolysis of transfused blood
    • Resorption of hematoma
  ➤ Hepatic damage
    • Intrahepatic cholestasis
    • Circulatory failure
    • Drug-induced
    • Pre-existing disease
  ➤ Obstructive
    • Common bile duct stone
    • Bile duct injury
    • Pancreatitis
  ➤ Other
    • Gilbert's disease (7–10% of patients) exacerbated by fasting state, cholecystitis

ACUTE LIVER FAILURE (FULMINANT HEPATIC FAILURE)

JOSEPH COTTEN, MD, PHD
MANUEL PARDO, JR., MD

OVERVIEW

- Definition: hepatic encephalopathy & coagulopathy in the setting of acute hepatic disease. Time from onset of jaundice until onset of encephalopathy distinguishes fulminant (within 8 wks) from subfulminant (within 26 wks) liver failure.
- Pts w/ fulminant hepatic failure (FHF) are usually critically ill & do not undergo elective procedures. Urgent procedures that may involve the anesthesia provider include central line placement, dialysis line placement, tracheal intubation for airway protection, GI endoscopy, ICP monitor placement, head CT scan, or liver transplantation.
- Causes
  - Viral hepatitis
    - Most commonly A or B
    - Occasionally cytomegalovirus, Epstein-Barr virus, herpes viruses are implicated
  - Drugs
    - Predictably toxic drugs (eg, acetaminophen; typically >12 g ingestion, less in the presence of alcohol or starvation)
    - Idiosyncratic reactions to inhaled anesthetics, sulfonamides, phenytoin, oral hypoglycemics (troglitazone), others
  - Toxins
    - Organic solvents: trichloroethylene, tetrachlorethane
    - Herbal remedies: kava kava
    - Toxins from the "death cap" mushroom (*Amanita phalloides*)
  - Vascular
    - Myocardial infarction, cardiac arrest, cardiomyopathy, pulmonary embolism, metastatic or infiltrative cancer, amyloidosis, veno-occlusive disease (Budd-Chiari, chemotherapy)
  - Miscellaneous causes
    - Fatty liver of pregnancy (third trimester; frequently w/ preeclampsia)
    - Reye's syndrome
    - Wilson's disease (acute liver failure can be first presentation)
- Important: Understand the multiple organ system complications of FHF. The most significant complications include

➤ CNS: cerebral edema, hepatic encephalopathy
➤ Hematologic: bleeding
➤ ID: infection, sepsis
➤ Renal: acute renal failure
➤ Cardiovascular: hypotension
➤ Metabolic: hypoglycemia, lactic acidosis, electrolyte abnormalities

CNS
■ Cerebral edema & hepatic encephalopathy are two different conditions that can occur together & have the same presenting symptoms in FHF.
  ➤ Signs & symptoms can include
    • Agitation, delusions, hyperkinesis, coma, pupillary abnormalities, increased muscle tone, decerebrate posturing, seizures, hypertension, bradycardia.
  ➤ Cerebral edema is rare in chronic liver failure but occurs in about 75% of pts w/ FHF & stage IV encephalopathy.
  ➤ Cerebral edema is the leading cause of death & is due to loss of cell membrane integrity & alterations in the blood-brain barrier.
  ➤ Cerebral herniation is associated w/ an untreated ICP >20 mm Hg & occurs in 25% of pts w/ grade 4 encephalopathy.
  ➤ Cerebral edema treatment
    • Mannitol 0.3–0.4 g/kg IV
    • Elevate head of bed 30 degrees to promote venous drainage.
    • Maintain cerebral perfusion pressure by balancing MAP, ICP & cerebral oxygen consumption (vasopressors, pentobarbital coma).
    • Unlike some other types of cerebral edema, dexamethasone & hyperventilation are of minimal value.
■ Grading scale for hepatic encephalopathy, based on level of consciousness
  ➤ Grade 1: restlessness, sleep abnormalities
  ➤ Grade 2: lethargy
  ➤ Grade 3: confused, somnolent but arousable
  ➤ Grade 4: coma
■ Conditions that can worsen encephalopathy
  ➤ Hypoxemia
  ➤ Hypoglycemia
  ➤ Infection

➤ Hypokalemia
➤ Hyponatremia
➤ GI bleeding

■ Pts w/ grade 3 or 4 coma are generally intubated for airway protection.
■ Subdural or epidural ICP monitor may be placed to follow ICP.

Hematologic

■ Decreased levels of factors II, V, VII, IX, X cause prolonged prothrombin time & partial thromboplastin time & predispose to bleeding complications.
■ Platelet counts are commonly $<100,000/mm^3$ & platelet function is altered.
■ Laboratory values are difficult to distinguish from DIC.
■ GI bleeding common
■ Routine correction of coagulopathy w/ FFP does not lead to improved outcome.
➤ FFP & platelets often administered for active bleeding, or immediately prior to invasive procedures to minimize bleeding risk.

ID

■ Up to 80% of pts develop bacterial infection (mostly gram-positive) & 30% develop fungal infection.
■ Pt may be receiving broad-spectrum antibiotics.

Renal

■ Renal failure may be due to acute tubular necrosis, hepatorenal syndrome, or intravascular dehydration.
➤ Can also be secondary to a toxin (eg, acetaminophen)
■ Conventional hemodialysis can be complicated by hypotension & bleeding & may worsen cerebral edema.
➤ Pt may receive continuous dialysis therapy, which has less impact on hemodynamics.

Cardiovascular

■ Hypotension is common & usually related to very low systemic vascular resistance (SVR).
➤ Low SVR may be resistant to alpha agents.
■ Cardiac index is increased secondary to decreased systemic vascular resistance (SVR) by A-V shunting & vasodilation.
■ Elevated ICP may cause cardiac dysfunction.
■ Arrhythmias may occur from electrolyte abnormalities or elevated ICP.

Pulmonary

- Pulmonary complications may occur in up to 50% of cases secondary to aspiration, infection, or noncardiogenic pulmonary edema (ARDS).
- Respiratory alkalosis is common, secondary to cerebral edema or encephalopathy.
- Ascites in subfulminant liver failure may affect ventilation & lung volumes.

Metabolic

- Hypoglycemia is very common. Pts require dextrose 10% infusion.
  - Occurs secondary to diminished gluconeogenesis & decreased insulin uptake
- Lactic acidosis can occur secondary to poor tissue perfusion/oxygen extraction & altered oxygen-hemoglobin dissociation characteristics.
- Hyponatremia occurs from water retention & intracellular sodium shift.
- Hypokalemia related to respiratory alkalosis may be profound.

PREOP

Issues/Evaluation

- ICU management is mandatory. Therapy is largely supportive & a bridge to transplant or recovery of native liver function.
- Prognosis should be determined quickly so that pt can be referred for liver transplant evaluation.
- Specific toxin antidotes may be administered.
  - Penicillin and silymarin are antidotes to *Amanita* mushroom poisoning.
  - N-acetyl cysteine improves acetaminophen toxicity & is beneficial up to 36 hours after toxin ingestion.

What To Do

- Evaluate pt carefully for the multiple organ system manifestations of FHF.
  - Recheck pertinent laboratory values, as they can change quickly.
  - Type & cross-match for PRBC & consider FFP or platelet transfusion to reduce bleeding risk of invasive procedures.
- Since pts are generally critically ill, consider the complexity & risks of transport.

INTRAOP

- Specific concerns depend on the nature of the procedure.

Management
- General issues
  - ➤ If pt not already intubated, consider rapid sequence intubation.
  - ➤ Obtain adequate IV access to manage bleeding.
  - ➤ Arterial access useful to facilitate BP monitoring & lab studies
  - ➤ Monitor labs frequently, including
    - Glucose: dextrose infusion may be required, or dose may need to be adjusted
    - Coagulation studies
    - Acid-base balance
    - Electrolytes: in particular, FFP transfusion may lead to hypocalcemia; PRBC transfusions may lead to hyperkalemia
- CNS issues
  - ➤ Maintain cerebral perfusion pressure (CPP) >50 mmHg.
    - Avoid excess elevation of head of bed. Although this may reduce ICP, it may further reduce MAP & CPP.
  - ➤ Anticipate prolonged or unpredictable drug effects because of liver & renal dysfunction.
  - ➤ For pt w/ cerebral edema, use precautions to minimize ICP rise during tracheal intubation.
- Renal issues
  - ➤ Consider intraop continuous dialysis therapy if fluid, acid-base, or electrolyte management becomes difficult.

POSTOP
- Plan for postop intubation.
- Continue ICU mgt.
- Re-evaluate fluid & electrolyte status & consider potential need for dialysis.

ACUTE RENAL FAILURE

ALICIA GRUBER, MD

OVERVIEW
- Definition: a rapid deterioration in renal function resulting in retention of nitrogenous waste products & inability to maintain fluid & electrolyte balance
  - ➤ There are numerous specific definitions, including

- 50% increase in baseline creatinine
- 0.5 mg/dL increase in baseline creatinine
- 50% decrease in creatinine clearance

- Usual Rx
  - Identify & treat underlying cause (prerenal, renal, postrenal)
  - Correct fluid & electrolyte imbalances
  - Dialysis for acidosis, hyperkalemia, fluid overload, or uremia

PREOP

Issues/Evaluation

- Fluid & electrolyte issues
  - Sodium & water retention can result in fluid overload, making pts prone to hypertension, CHF, pulmonary edema.
  - Failure to excrete nonvolatile acids can result in a high-gap metabolic acidosis & a compensatory increase in minute ventilation.
  - Multiple electrolyte abnormalities may be present
    - Hyperkalemia
    - Hypermagnesemia
    - Hyperphosphatemia
    - Hypocalcemia
    - Hyponatremia
    - Hypoalbuminemia
- Uremia-related issues
  - Signs/symptoms of uremia include nausea, vomiting, anorexia, lethargy, confusion, asterixis, seizure, qualitative platelet dysfunction, pruritus, pericarditis.
  - Pericarditis is most significant because it can lead to cardiac tamponade & hemodynamic instability.
  - Treatment of uremic bleeding may require desmopressin (DDAVP) or estrogen, since dialysis does not consistently improve the platelet function.
- Hemodialysis issues
  - Pts w/ acute renal failure can undergo intermittent or continuous hemodialysis.
  - Critically ill pt may benefit from improved cardiovascular stability of continuous dialysis.
    - Continuous dialysis can be maintained intraop but is complex to manage & usually requires ICU nurse to manage the dialysis machine.
  - Access line is typically a large-bore double-lumen catheter.

- If necessary, can use dialysis line for venous access
- Line is typically flushed w/ heparin solution. Remove this before using line.

What To Do
- Postpone elective surgery.
- Assess volume status & electrolytes.
  - Pts are susceptible to fluid overload.
  - Pt can also have hypovolemia from excess fluid removal w/ dialysis.
  - Consider preop ABG to supplement electrolyte evaluation of acid-base status.
  - Check ECG for signs of hyperkalemia or hypocalcemia.
- Decide whether preop dialysis is needed for procedure.
  - Despite appropriate medical mgt, pt may still have hyperkalemia, metabolic acidosis, or fluid overload.
  - Dialysis on the day of surgery or previous day may be necessary.
- Regional anesthesia considerations
  - Check coagulation tests & consider effects of uremic platelet dysfunction on risk of nerve block.

INTRAOP
- Drug therapy issues
  - Many drugs rely on at least partial excretion by the kidney for elimination.
  - The systemic effects of azotemia can alter the pharmacokinetics of many drugs administered during anesthesia. Mechanisms include
    - Decreased protein levels, leading to increased unbound drug
    - Decreased drug delivery to kidneys
    - Decreased excretion of renally cleared drugs or drug metabolites
  - Pt can also have altered pharmacodynamics, especially if pt is debilitated or cachexic
  - Pharmacokinetics of specific anesthetic drugs
    - Barbiturates: Pts w/ renal insufficiency are more sensitive to barbiturates, which may be a result of decreased protein binding as well as an increase in the nonionized fraction of the drug
    - Propofol, etomidate & ketamine pharmacokinetics are minimally changed by renal impairment.

- Succinylcholine can be used safely, provided the serum potassium level is known to be <5.0 mEq/L at the time of induction & the normal rise of 0.5–1.0 mEq/L of potassium is expected. Avoid muscle relaxants that depend primarily on the kidney for elimination (eg, pancuronium).
- Volatile agents are ideal for maintenance as they affect renal blood flow minimally, control hypertension & do not rely on the kidney for elimination; avoid sevoflurane as it is potentially nephrotoxic.
- Morphine may be used carefully, but one of its active metabolites, morphine-6-glucoronide, is renally excreted & can lead to respiratory depression.
- Meperidine should be avoided as its active metabolite, normeperidine, is renally eliminated & can cause seizures.

Management
■ General mgt
  ➤ Consider rapid sequence induction, as pts w/ uremia may be at risk for aspiration.
  ➤ Standard monitors for procedures w/ minimal fluid loss.
  ➤ Arterial & central lines can help to monitor intravascular volume for operations w/ significant blood loss or fluid shifts.
  ➤ Ensure adequate intravascular volume prior to induction to prevent hypotension & decreased renal perfusion.
    - Preserve renal perfusion to prevent further insult to the kidneys.
  ➤ Maintain controlled mechanical ventilation to avoid hypoventilation from spontaneous respiration if acidemia & hyperkalemia are of concern.
  ➤ If vasopressors are needed, avoid predominantly alpha antagonists in favor of dopamine to try to preserve renal blood flow & renal function.
■ Fluid & electrolyte management
  ➤ Replace fluids judiciously, but not at the expense of decreased renal perfusion.
    - Fluid mgt is most challenging for pts w/ oliguria or anuria.
  ➤ Minimize lactated Ringer's solution in pts w/ elevated potassium as it contains 4 mEq/L potassium.
  ➤ If pt has significant electrolyte or blood gas abnormalities preop, serial measurements of ABGs should be continued intraop.

POSTOP

- Pts will continue to require aggressive monitoring of volume status postop.
- Pts who received large volumes of fluid or experienced large volume shifts intraop may develop pulmonary edema & require continued mechanical ventilation.
- Consider whether postop dialysis is needed.
  - Indications can include fluid overload, pulmonary edema, hyperkalemia, or severe acidosis.
  - If PCA is used for postop pain control, consider using an agent that is not dependent on renal excretion for elimination (eg, Dilaudid or fentanyl).

ACUTE RESPIRATORY DISTRESS SYNDROME (ARDS)

LUNDY CAMPBELL, MD

OVERVIEW

- Definition: consists of the following criteria
  - Acute onset
  - Bilateral infiltrates on chest radiography
  - PCWP <18 mmHg or absence of left atrial hypertension by clinical signs
  - Poor oxygenation as determined by PaO_2/FiO_2 (P/F) ratio
    - Acute lung injury present if P/F <300
    - ARDS present if P/F <200
- Usual Rx
  - Supportive care
  - Low tidal volume ventilation strategies (6 mL/kg based on ideal body weight) shown to improve outcome, including reduced mortality
  - Ventilation strategy for most pts allows permissive hypercarbia, w/ acceptable pH of 7.32–7.45.
- Pts w/ ARDS usually do not undergo elective surgical procedures, except for tracheotomy or feeding tube placement to facilitate long-term care. Urgent or emergent procedures may include
  - Procedures related to ARDS or pulmonary disease
    - Bronchoscopy
    - Chest tube placement for pneumothorax
    - Drainage of pulmonary effusion

➤ Procedures related to sepsis or underlying critical illness
  • Exploratory laparotomy for abdominal catastrophe (eg, perforated bowel)
  • Drainage of abscess
  • Mgt of injuries related to trauma

PREOP

Issues/Evaluation
■ ARDS usually associated w/ direct or indirect source of lung injury to endothelial or epithelial cells. The resulting syndrome is the same. Some of the more common causes include
  ➤ Direct lung injury
    • Pneumonia
    • Aspiration
    • Pulmonary contusion
    • Fat emboli
    • Inhalational injury
    • Near-drowning
    • Reperfusion injury
  ➤ Indirect lung injury
    • Sepsis
    • Trauma
    • Acute pancreatitis
    • Massive transfusion
    • Cardiopulmonary bypass
    • Drug overdose
■ Important pathophysiologic findings
  ➤ Hypoxemia is prominent early, related to intrapulmonary shunt.
  ➤ Lung compliance is reduced. High peak airway pressures w/ mechanical ventilation are common.
  ➤ Pulmonary dead space is elevated, leading to increased minute ventilation requirement or hypercarbia.
  ➤ Incidence of barotrauma increases w/ duration of ARDS.
  ➤ ARDS may cause secondary sepsis syndrome.

What To Do
■ Evaluate pt thoroughly for common problems related to critical illness, which may include
  ➤ Hemodynamic instability requiring vasopressors
  ➤ High sedative requirement to tolerate mechanical ventilation

- ➤ Altered mental status
- ➤ Hyperglycemia
- ➤ Large number of IV infusion pumps & IV lines, which make transport more challenging
- ■ Check ABG & ventilator settings in ICU
  - ➤ If pt requires PEEP >10 or minute ventilation >15 L/m or has peak airway pressure >50 cm H_2O, an ICU ventilator may be required for satisfactory intraop gas exchange.
  - ➤ Pts requiring high PEEP, high minute ventilation & high FiO_2 are more likely to develop hypoxemia & hypercarbia w/ transport, especially if PEEP is discontinued.
    - • Prior to transport, ensure that pt will tolerate hand ventilation for transport. May require PEEP valve.
    - • Consider use of transport ventilator.
    - • Consider obtaining an ABG on the transport ventilator settings.
  - ➤ If using a non-ICU ventilator in the OR, ensure that pt will be able to be ventilated adequately. Perform a "trial run" on any different ventilator settings & obtain a new ABG to check for adequate ventilation.
- ■ Monitoring issues
  - ➤ Consider arterial line for blood gas monitoring.
  - ➤ Central line may be useful for managing volume status.
  - ➤ Arterial & central lines are commonly in place in these ICU pts.

INTRAOP
- ■ Anticipate worsening gas exchange for abdominal or intrathoracic procedures.
- ■ Sudden hypotension may indicate development of tension pneumothorax.
  - ➤ Consider obtaining intraop CXR.
  - ➤ May need to place chest tube urgently if pt has severe hypotension
- ■ Follow ABGs closely.
  - ➤ Normocarbia may be difficult to achieve.
  - ➤ Pt may already have hypercarbia as part of preop mechanical ventilation strategy.
- ■ Follow fluid status closely.
  - ➤ Administration of large fluid volumes can precipitate worsening pulmonary edema.
- ■ If possible, perform procedure in the ICU instead of OR.

➤ This is likely safer for the pt as transport carries a significant risk.
➤ Will depend on nature of procedure, equipment requirements & other factors

Management
■ Transport carefully, w/ full monitoring.
■ Ideally, continue ventilator settings used in ICU.
  ➤ Ventilate w/ low tidal volumes in 6–7 mL/kg range.
■ Allow elevations in $PaCO_2$ (permissive hypercarbia).
■ Monitor ABGs regularly.
■ Consider increasing PEEP if PaO_2 decreases.
■ Limit IV fluids if possible.

POSTOP
■ Transport to ICU will have same issues as preop.
■ Gas exchange may worsen, depending on nature of procedure, fluid administration, intraop course.
  ➤ Ventilator settings may need to be changed postop.

ADRENAL INSUFFCIENCY

ANNEMARIE THOMPSON, MD

OVERVIEW
■ Definition: Endocrine disorder resulting in deficient endogenous glucocorticoid production $+/-$ deficient mineralocorticoid production
■ Acute adrenal crisis is rare but life-threatening
■ Recommendation for treatment of acute adrenal crisis: hydrocortisone 100 mg IV bolus $+100–200$ mg IV over 24 h
■ "Stress dose" steroid replacement: hydrocortisone 50 mg IV q6h for 2–3 days

PREOP
Issues/Evaluation
■ Etiology of adrenal insufficiency:
  ➤ Primary: autoimmune, TB, AIDS, metastatic cancer, trauma/hemorrhage
  ➤ Secondary: long-term glucocorticoid therapy, brain disease

- Symptoms: fatigue, weakness, orthostasis (primary > secondary), weight loss, abdominal pain/nausea/vomiting/diarrhea, hyperpigmentation (seen in primary only)
- Lab abnormalities: hyperkalemia/acidosis (primary only), hyponatremia, lymphocytosis, eosinophilia
- Catecholamine-resistant hypotension in critically ill pts should raise suspicion of adrenal insufficiency

What To Do
- Determine if pt is taking exogenous corticosteroids.
- Have hydrocortisone available in OR.

INTRAOP
- Perioperative cardiovascular complications are rare in pts w/ adrenal insufficiency even if supplemental ("stress dose") steroids are not given.
- If decision is made to give stress-dose steroids, give hydrocortisone 50 mg IV q6h.
- If CV instability (acute adrenal crisis), give hydrocortisone 100 mg IV stat; then give 100–200 mg IV over 24 h.

POSTOP
- If stress dose steroids were given intraop, they are typically continued for 2–3 days.
- Endocrinologist should be consulted if diagnosis of adrenal insufficiency was made in the perioperative period.

ADULT CONGENITAL HEART DISEASE (CHD)

KATHRYN ROUINE-RAPP, MD

OVERVIEW
- Approx 85% of infants w/ CHD will survive to adulthood.
- Approx 10% of adults w/ CHD are diagnosed in a specialized clinic during adulthood.
- Classification of CHD:
  - Simple lesions tend to be isolated defects such as atrial & ventricular septal defects.
  - Complex pathology includes severe malformations of cardiovascular structures & the heart & visceral organs.

- Pts w/ with single-ventricle physiology are considered to have complex lesions.
- Another classification scheme assigns lesions to an acyanotic vs. cyanotic group.
- Except for those w/ simple lesions, recommendation is to refer pts to regional centers for noncardiac operations.

PREOP

Issues/Evaluation

- Characterize primary pathology.
- Determine how many chambers the heart has, how the blood enters & leaves the heart, how the atria are related to the ventricles, & how the ventricles are related to the great vessels.
  - Diagnostic modalities include echocardiography, cardiac catheterization, MRI.
  - Caveat: there is a 53% diagnosis error rate in community-based adult echocardiography lab.
- Determine if the pt has had palliation, surgical repair, or no operation.
  - Determine the presence of residual pathology or sequelae after surgical repair.
- Identify associated defects.
- Look for an increase in size of cardiac chambers.
- Evaluate biventricular function.
- Evaluate valvular function.
- Evaluate functional status at rest and w/ exercise.
- Look for presence of arrhythmias.
- Does the pt have too much or too little pulmonary blood flow?
  - Pts w/ too much pulmonary blood flow are at risk to develop pulmonary hypertension & Eisenmenger's syndrome (ie, obliteration of much of the pulmonary vascular bed & an increase in pulmonary vascular resistance).
  - Pts w/ too little pulmonary blood flow can have chronic cyanosis, erythrocytosis, & abnormal hemostasis.
  - Cyanotic pts who undergo placement of an arterial to pulmonary shunt can have too little or too much pulmonary blood flow following the procedure.
- Pts w/ erythrocytosis & hematocrit >55% can have a falsely elevated PT/PTT. Ask the lab for special tubes to assess PT/PTT in these pts.

- Symptoms of hyperviscosity in pts w/ erythrocytosis include headache, dizziness, blurred vision, fatigue, muscle weakness, depressed mentation, chest pain, abdominal discomfort.
- Some centers recommend preoperative isovolumic hemodilution in symptomatic cyanotic pts w/ hematocrit >60%.

■ Nearly all adults w/ CHD are at risk of infective endocarditis & require antibiotic prophylaxis.
- Most dental, respiratory, & GI procedures require prophylaxis.
- Pts w/ prosthetic material in place or cyanotic heart disease are in the high-risk category.

INTRAOP

■ Remove air from all IV tubing & syringes.
■ Use large-bore IV access & anticipate larger than usual blood loss in cyanotic pts.
■ Use arterial & central venous access & pulmonary artery pressure monitoring as dictated by planned procedure & functional status of pt.
■ Monitor ventricular function in pts w/ compromised functional status.
■ Pts w/ inadequate pulmonary blood flow may have a connection (shunt) between systemic & pulmonary arteries. This group of pts can experience a decrease in saturation caused by a decrease in arterial blood pressure or a decrease in hemoglobin.
■ Treatment of pulmonary hypertension includes
- Hyperventilation
- Hyperoxia
- Alkalinization of the blood; one formula to calculate the dose of $NaHCO_3$ to administer is (base deficit times weight in kg)/3.
- Keep pt warm.
- Provide adequate depth of anesthesia.
- Consider IV nitrates.
- Some pts may improve w/ inhalation of nitric oxide. The dose range is 5–80 ppm.
■ Most pts undergo general anesthesia for procedures.
- There is very little literature reporting the safely and efficacy of regional anesthesia in cyanotic pts w/ erythrocytosis.

POSTOP

■ Some pts need close monitoring in the ICU.

- The perioperative complication rate in pts w/ pulmonary hypertension is approximately 3 times greater than other pts w/ adult CHD. It seems highest in pts undergoing procedures performed on the respiratory or nervous systems.

AIDS

DON TAYLOR, MD, PHD

OVERVIEW
- Definition: Severe immunodeficiency syndrome caused by HIV infection
- Usual Rx
  - Nucleoside analog reverse transcriptase inhibitors (NRTIs)
  - Non-nucleoside reverse transcriptase inhibitors (NNRTIs)
  - Protease inhibitors (PIs)
  - CD4 count & viral load guide antiretroviral Rx.

PREOP

Issues/Evaluation
- Drug interactions (protease inhibitors inhibit cytochrome P450)
- Drug side effects
  - Bone marrow suppression
  - Peripheral neuropathy
  - Nephrolithiasis
  - Hyperlipidemia
  - Lipodystrophy
- Transmission risks to health care providers & other pts
- Preop risk determined by
  - ASA class
  - Surgical risk
  - CDC stage of infection (degree of immunosuppression)
  - Presence & severity of opportunistic infections
- Pneumocystis pneumonia is less common w/ CD4 counts >200.
  - CXR may be normal in its presence.
  - SpO_2 may be useful if suspected.

What To Do
- Universal Precautions for all pts.
- Adjust dosage of fentanyl, benzodiazepines, antiarrhythmics, cisapride, & other drugs metabolized via P450 in pts on PIs.

- Consider double gloves, heat & moisture exchange filters for anesthesia circuit.
- In the event of a needle stick, postexposure prophylaxis decreases transmission risks.

INTRAOP
- During anesthesia, tachycardia may be more common in pts w/ HIV.
- ZDV therapy & C-section are demonstrated to decrease vertical transmission from parturients to newborns.

POSTOP
- GA may have an immunosuppressive effect; implications are unclear.
- High fever, anemia, tachycardia more frequent in pts w/ HIV postop.
- Pain syndromes common in advanced disease, similar to pts w/ disseminated malignancy.

ALCOHOL ABUSE

BETTY LEE-HOANG, MD

OVERVIEW
- Alcohol abuse (according to American Psychiatric Association [APA])
  - ➤ Maladaptive pattern of alcohol use leading to clinically significant impairment or distress. Manifestations include at least one of the following:
    - Failure of role obligations (eg, work, home, school)
    - Recurrent use in hazardous situations
    - Alcohol-related legal problems
    - Continued use despite alcohol-related social or interpersonal problems
- Alcohol dependence (APA definition)
  - ➤ Maladaptive pattern of alcohol use leading to clinically significant impairment or distress. Manifestations include at least three of the following:
    - Tolerance
    - Withdrawal
    - Use of larger amount over longer-than-intended period
    - Persistent desire or unsuccessful attempt to decrease or control use

- Great deal of time spent obtaining, using, or recovering from use
- Reduction of important social, occupational, or recreational activities
- Use despite knowledge of alcohol-related physical or psychological problems

■ Usual Rx
  ➣ Attempts at behavioral change
  ➣ Some pts receive adjunct treatment for prevention of relapse w/
    - Disulfiram
    - Naltrexone

■ Alcohol abuse can have a wide range of presentations:
  ➣ Acute or chronic
  ➣ Mild to severe impairment
  ➣ Variable response to therapy

■ Alcohol withdrawal syndrome
  ➣ Pts w/ alcohol dependence are at high risk for withdrawal during the periop period.
  ➣ Postop alcohol withdrawal increases morbidity.
  ➣ Withdrawal scales (eg, Clinical Institute Withdrawal Assessment of Alcohol) can be used to quantify signs & symptoms & guide benzodiazepine therapy. Symptom assessment includes:
    - Agitation
    - Anxiety
    - Auditory disturbances
    - Clouding of sensorium
    - Headache
    - Nausea/vomiting
    - Paroxysmal sweating
    - Tactile disturbances
    - Tremor
    - Visual disturbances

■ CAGE questionnaire is useful for identifying pts at risk for withdrawal. Ask pt four questions:
  ➣ Have you felt you should cut down on your alcohol consumption?
  ➣ Have people annoyed you by criticizing your drinking?
  ➣ Have you felt guilty about your drinking?
  ➣ Have you ever had a drink first thing in the morning (eye-opener)?
  ➣ Patients who answer yes to any question should be monitored postop. If pt answers yes to 3 or more, pt is at high risk for withdrawal.

- Surgeon should be made aware of high potential for withdrawal. Consideration should be given to having pt abstain from drinking for 1 week to decrease chances of withdrawal.

PREOP

Issues/Evaluation

- Find out when the pt last drank to gauge the likelihood of withdrawal.
- Acutely intoxicated pts may be unable to give a medical history & may not cooperate.

INTRAOP

- Acute alcohol abuse depresses the CNS & decreases anesthetic requirements (MAC), while chronic alcohol abuse increases anesthetic requirement.
- Acute alcohol ingestion causes cutaneous vasodilation, increases heart rate via sympathetic reflex, hyperventilation, & decreases ventilatory response to carbon dioxide.
- Chronic alcohol abuse can cause cardiac dysfunction, including hypertension, cardiomyopathy, pulmonary hypertension, heart failure, arrhythmias.
- Chronic alcohol use can cause abnormalities of respiratory function, including dysfunction of the cilia, macrophage mobility & surfactant production, which may lead to higher risk of pulmonary infections.
- Effects of chronic alcohol abuse on the GI system include delayed gastric emptying & relaxation of the lower esophageal sphincter, which can increase the risk of aspiration.
- Chronic hepatobiliary changes include progressive cirrhosis, hepatitis & impaired synthetic function, including decreased production of albumin & coagulation factors.
- There may be deficiencies of folic acid & thiamine w/ chronic alcohol abuse, characterized by thrombocytopenia, leukopenia, anemia, Wernicke's encephalopathy, polyneuropathy, cardiac failure.

POSTOP

- Watch for acute alcohol withdrawal.
  - ➤ Presentation may be nonspecific & include tachycardia, diaphoresis, hyperthermia.
  - ➤ Seizures may occur as part of withdrawal.
    - 2–5% of alcoholics experience withdrawal seizures, usually within 48 hours of abstinence from alcohol.

- Consider benzodiazepine therapy to prevent withdrawal in pts w/ alcohol dependence.
- Delirium tremens (DTs): usually a 2- to 3-day onset time after alcohol abstinence; severe tachycardia, fever, confusion, convulsions
  - 10% mortality rate w/ DTs
- If pt develops alcohol withdrawal, consider mgt in a monitored or ICU setting.
  - Therapy may include
    - Benzodiazepines: lorazepam, diazepam, chlordiazepoxide
    - Beta-blockers: atenolol, metoprolol, propranolol
    - Alpha-agonists: clonidine
    - Antiepileptics: carbamazepine

ANEMIA

JOHN R. FEINER, MD
HARRIET W. HOPF, MD

OVERVIEW
- Definition: low hemoglobin level or low hematocrit
  - Assumes volume status is normal (ie, isovolemic anemia)
- Usual Rx
  - Transfusion of red blood cells, if sufficiently severe
  - Supplemental oxygen & volume as temporizing measure
  - Oral iron supplementation and/or erythropoietin if time permits
- Arterial oxygen content = $(1.34 \times SaO_2 \times Hb) + (0.003 \times PaO_2)$

PREOP

Issues/Evaluation
- Anemia may be a sign of other medical problems that may require evaluation.
- Preop anemia has implications for intraop mgt:
  - More units of red blood cells may need to be cross-matched.
  - Red cell transfusion may be required sooner.
  - Red cell salvage techniques may be used more aggressively.

What To Do
- If sufficient time is available, treatment of anemia w/ iron supplements is indicated; treatment w/ erythropoietin may be also be warranted.

■ In the Jehovah's Witness pt, treatment of anemia w/ both iron & erythropoietin is indicated, w/ possible delay of the surgical procedure to permit time for synthesis of sufficient red cell mass.

INTRAOP

■ Managing anemia requires understanding the physiology of isovolemic anemia & the normal cardiovascular response.

■ Understanding transfusion thresholds is essential; both transfusion & severe anemia have risks; transfusions should be given only when the benefits outweigh the risks.

■ Understanding the way hemoglobin levels change w/ blood loss helps to anticipate when transfusion will be required. This relationship is:

➤ Allowable blood loss (ABL) = estimated blood volume (EBV) $\times$ Ln(Hct1/Hct2)

➤ If no access to calculator w/ natural log function, can substitute (starting Hct minus lowest allowed Hct) divided by (average of starting and lowest allowed Hct)

■ Physiology of anemia

➤ The main compensatory cardiovascular responses to isovolemic anemia are
  • Increased HR
  • Increased stroke volume
  • Increased CO/cardiac index
  • Decreased systemic vascular resistance (decreased viscosity)
  • Decreased mean arterial pressure (mild)

➤ These responses help maintain oxygen delivery (CO $\times$ CaO$_2$).

➤ In young healthy subject at rest, increased cardiac output compensates almost completely down to Hb approximately 5 g/dL.

➤ Pts w/ cardiovascular disease & older pts do not tolerate profound anemia as well because of decreased capacity to increase CO; increased HR also puts them at risk for myocardial ischemia.

➤ HR does not increase reliably under GA, although w/o anesthesia, HR increases linearly w/ hemoglobin decrease & is poorly blunted w/ beta blockers.

➤ When blood is unavailable or is refused, temporizing measures include
  • FIO$_2$ = 1.0 (or hyperbaric oxygen for brief periods)
  • Volume infusion to maintain CO

- Decreasing oxygen consumption (eg, sedation, paralysis, mechanical ventilation)
- Transfusion thresholds
  - Transfusion of red blood cells should be started when a level of anemia is reached that cannot be tolerated physiologically, or that impairs oxygen delivery to tissues.
  - Signs of inadequate oxygen delivery include development of a metabolic acidosis, hypotension & hemodynamic instability.
  - Unfortunately, such a level is rarely clearly apparent on any single laboratory panel. Usually one must rely on clinical instinct, based on an understanding of the physiologic consequences.
  - Many professional societies have recommended transfusion triggers for red blood cells.
    - ASA task force: transfusion of red cells is rarely indicated for Hb >10 g/dL & almost always indicated for Hb <6 g/dL
    - JAMA consensus conference: target 7 g/dL (healthy), 10 g/dL (cardiovascular disease)
  - Trigger also depends on clinical circumstance: ongoing bleeding vs bleeding that has stopped

Management
- Mgt of anemia during surgical blood loss requires measurement of hemoglobin levels, either by sending CBCs or using point-of-care testing.
- Assess potential physiologic changes of anemia for pt.
- Decide on an appropriate transfusion trigger for pt, given the clinical situation.

POSTOP
- Consideration for appropriate hemoglobin levels postop may be different than intraop.
- Transfusion is not indicated for concerns of wound healing until transfusion is indicated for other reasons, since tissue perfusion & not hemoglobin level is of primary importance.
- Pts w/ significant anemia may be extremely fatigued & have lower exercise tolerance.
- Postop monitoring of hemoglobin may be somewhat more difficult but may need to be done frequently in cases where ongoing bleeding, such as wound drainage, is occurring.

ANKYLOSING SPONDYLITIS

JAMES BRANDES, MD

OVERVIEW

- Definition: A systemic disease characterized by ossification of ligaments, cartilage, & the disc space of the axial spine. An autosomal dominant disease seen mostly in males, it is associated w/ HLA B-27 & has an onset in the third to fourth decades of life.
- Usual Rx: Physical therapy to maintain mobility, potent nonsteroidal anti-inflammatory drugs.

PREOP

Issues/Evaluation

- Difficult airway: atlanto-axial instability, kyphosis, TMJ & cricoarytenoid involvement possible
- Cardiac conduction defects, cardiomyopathy, 1–4% w/ aortic valve/ root involvement
- Decreased pulmonary function from rigid rib cage, pleuritic involvement, apical cavitary lesion mimicking tuberculosis
- Assoc w/ ulcerative colitis via HLA B-27
- Radiculopathies/chronic back pain
- Possible cervical cord compression from atlanto-axial involvement
- Uveitis/conjunctivitis common
- Extra-articular involvement becomes more prominent w/ the duration of the disease. Renal involvement is possible also
- Osteoporosis common in these pts

What To Do

- Airway exam critical. Pt may have a "frozen neck" that will not extend at the atlanto-occipital joint. Mouth opening may be limited. Larynx may be affected if pt has a hoarse voice.
- Complete neurologic exam
- Evaluate ROM of extremities, which may be limited; implications for positioning during surgery
- CXR, EKG, possible cardiac echo, possible PFTs based on symptoms
- Examine back if neuraxial anesthetic technique is contemplated as these blocks may be challenging or impossible in these pts
- Side effects from potent NSAID use should be considered (platelet dysfunction, increased BUN/creatinine, bone marrow suppression from indomethacin)

INTRAOP

- If GETA planned, difficult airway cart should be available. Strongly consider awake fiberoptic intubation, as these pts may be difficult to ventilate w/ a bag & mask.
- Neuraxial anesthesia may be very difficult, especially the midline approach. The spread of local anesthetic in the epidural space is unpredictable in these pts. Consider caudal anesthesia if appropriate. Interscalene block for upper extremity operations may be difficult due to limited neck movement. Pt may have a preexisting neurologic deficit.
- If pt has aortic involvement, endocarditis prophylaxis may be indicated.
- Pt may have a pacemaker for cardiac conduction disease.
- Pay careful attention to positioning, especially of head & neck.
- Smaller tidal volumes may be needed during positive-pressure ventilation because of the restrictive component of the chest wall.
- Somatosensory evoked potentials for cervical spine osteotomy

POSTOP

- Extubate fully awake. Consider leaving intubated if pulmonary compromise present or if airway swelling is likely.
- Consider local infiltration/nerve block for pain relief if regional technique not used.
- Pt may be opioid tolerant from preop use for chronic back pain.

AORTIC STENOSIS (AS)

RICHARD PAULSEN, MD
MICHELLE PARAISO, MD

OVERVIEW

- Definition: narrowing of the aortic valve causing reduced & turbulent systolic blood flow
- Aortic valve area
  - Less than normal: 2.5–3.5 cm^2
  - Mild stenosis: 1.2–2.5 cm^2
  - Moderate stenosis: 0.7–1.2 cm^2
  - Severe stenosis: 0.5–0.7 cm^2
  - Critical stenosis: <0.5 cm^2

- Critical AS is defined clinically by presence of symptoms: CHF, angina, or syncope. Mean life expectancy with AS & these conditions is
  - CHF: 2 yr
  - Syncope: 3 yr
  - Angina: 5 yr
- Hemodynamically significant stenosis occurs at pressure gradients >50 mmHg.
- Common etiologies: calcification of a congenitally bicuspid valve, senile degeneration, rheumatic degeneration
- Usual Rx: Symptomatic pts or those w/ hemodynamically significant stenosis should have surgical correction. Percutaneous valvuloplasty may be considered in selected pts.
- Important: pts w/ AS have increased risk of periop cardiac complications.
  - This risk is greatest in major surgery associated w/ significant hemorrhage or fluid hifts.

PREOP

Issues/Evaluation
- Hemodynamic goals
  - Maintain preload.
    - Filling pressures must be maintained to maintain BP. Ventricle is thickened & poorly compliant, which leads to a compensatory increase in LV end-diastolic pressure, which maintains stroke volume.
  - Avoid decreases in SVR.
    - Because stroke volume is relatively fixed, need to maintain adequate SVR to maintain BP.
  - Maintain normal HR.
    - Avoid severe bradycardia (also related to relatively fixed stroke volume).
    - Avoid tachycardia (may cause myocardial ischemia & reduce LV filling).
- Increased myocardial work & oxygen demand create the potential for ischemia.
- Pts have a propensity for arrhythmias.
  - Risk includes sudden cardiac death.
- Crescendo-decrescendo systolic murmur of AS is heard best at second right intercostal space w/ radiation into the neck.

What To Do
- CXR
- ECG
- Echo
- Consider antibiotics for endocarditis prophylaxis

INTRAOP
- Maintain normal sinus rhythm, which is essential to maintaining cardiac output.
  - Treat atrial fibrillation & SVT aggressively.
  - Avoid tachycardia.
- A normal heart rate is preferred, but bradycardia should be avoided because it can decrease cardiac output.
- Avoid hypotension.
  - A decreased diastolic BP in the face of high ventricular filling pressures can lead to ischemia, which can lead to a hemodynamic spiral in which BP & myocardial perfusion are further impaired.
- Optimize intravascular fluid volume to maintain left ventricular filling.
- Minimize negative inotropes.

Management
- Consider arterial line, central line, PA line, or TEE based on severity of disease & procedure being performed.
- GA or regional anesthesia can be used if hemodynamic goals are met (eg, drop in preload & tachycardia are avoided).
  - Induction of GA is a time of particular risk. Closely monitor BP during this phase & prepare to administer phenylephrine for hypotension.
  - Narcotic-based anesthetic is usually well tolerated.
- Use caution in administration of vasodilators for ischemia because these may reduce preload.
- Treat ischemia by increasing coronary perfusion pressure & decreasing oxygen consumption (eg, increase afterload, decrease HR).
- Be prepared to treat arrhythmias rapidly.

POSTOP
- Obtain ECG to look for ischemic changes.
- Monitor for worsening signs & symptoms of aortic stenosis (eg, ischemia, CHF, syncope).

- Analgesia as dictated by procedure performed, which will help prevent tachycardia
- Consider whether ICU monitoring is warranted based on intraop course & type of surgery.

AORTIC VALVE REGURGITATION (AORTIC INSUFFCIENCY)

RICHARD PAULSEN, MD

OVERVIEW

- Definition: incompetent aortic valve causing blood flow into the left ventricle during diastole
- Etiologies include bacterial endocarditis, trauma, aortic dissection, rheumatic fever, syphilitic aortitis, various congenital diseases
- Usual Rx: surgical correction when symptomatic or when LV dysfunction is present

PREOP

Issues/Evaluation

- Acute regurgitation may require emergent surgical replacement.
- Chronic regurgitation may be asymptomatic for 20 yrs.
- Symptoms can include dyspnea, fatigue, palpitations, angina.
- Physical exam findings may include
  - ➤ Widened pulse pressure
  - ➤ Decreased diastolic pressure
  - ➤ Bounding peripheral pulses
  - ➤ Diastolic murmur is best auscultated at second right intercostal space.
- Pt w/ symptoms has ~5 yr survival.
- Ultimately, regurgitation leads to volume overload, LV hypertrophy, LV dilation, LV dysfunction, LV failure.
- Sudden death is rare.

What To Do

- CXR
- ECG
- Echocardiogram
- Consider antibiotics for endocarditis prophylaxis

INTRAOP
- Hemodynamic goals
  - Maintain HR approx 90.
  - Avoid drugs that decrease HR.
  - Avoid sudden increases in SVR.
    - This increases regurgitation & decreases forward cardiac output.
  - Minimize negative inotropes.
  - Augment preload.

Management
- Standard monitors
  - Consider arterial line, central line, TEE, or PA line based on severity of disease & stress of proposed surgery.
- GA or regional can be used, but avoid precipitous drops in SVR.
- Afterload reducing agents, beta-agonists, phosphodiesterase inhibitors can be used to improve cardiac output.
- Intra-aortic balloon pump is contraindicated.
- Treat atrial fibrillation & SVT aggressively–they will markedly decrease cardiac output in the presence of aortic regurgitation.

POSTOP
- ECG
- Maintain appropriate analgesia.

ARNOLD-CHIARI MALFORMATION

JAMES CALDWELL, MB, CHB

OVERVIEW
- Definition: Downward displacement of lower pons, medulla, & cerebellar tonsils through foramen magnum
- Usual Rx:
  - Surgical decompression by suboccipital craniectomy & cervical laminectomy
  - VP shunt if assoc hydrocephalus
  - Repair of myelomeningocele if present

PREOP

Issues/Evaluation
- Associated problems:
  - In infancy, myelomeningocele & hydrocephalus
  - In adults, syringomyelia
- Infants may present w/
  - Stridor
  - Episodic apnea
  - Bulbar palsy
  - Upper extremity weakness
- Adults present w/
  - Headache
  - Meningismus
  - Upper extremity weakness
  - Ataxia
  - Bulbar palsy
- ICP may be increased in both infants & adults

What To Do
- Document pre-existing neurologic deficits, including increased ICP.
- Determine range of movement of neck that does not exacerbate symptoms.
- Explain possible need for postop tracheal intubation & ventilatory support.

INTRAOP
- Surgery may be in the prone or sitting position.
- Avoid extreme flexion or extension of the neck.
- Rapid blood loss & air embolism are significant risks.

Management
- Venous access sufficient for rapid blood transfusion.
- Place intra-arterial catheter for pressure monitoring.
- Place central venous catheter & precordial Doppler if pt in sitting position to treat & monitor for air embolism.
- Avoid preop respiratory depressant drugs if ICP increased.
- Succinylcholine may be contraindicated if significant muscle weakness exists.
- Neuromonitoring of SEP, MEP, & lower cranial nerves possible but not routine

POSTOP
- Lower cranial nerve dysfunction may compromise airway protection.
- Tracheal intubation & ventilatory support may be required.

ASTHMA

IVAN ZEITZ, MD

OVERVIEW
- Definition: a chronic inflammatory disorder of the airways. Airway inflammation contributes to airway hyperresponsiveness.

PREOP

Issues/Evaluation
- Ask about historical features that may indicate severity of disease:
  - Current meds
  - Previous therapy (including ED visits, hospitalizations, intubations)
  - Precipitating factors
  - Patterns of asthma (eg, seasonal, exercise-induced)
  - Typical manifestations
- Highest-risk pts
  - Previous intubation for asthma exacerbation
  - Repeated hospitalization for asthma
  - Requirement for chronic systemic steroid therapy
- Pts w/o recent symptoms & off all meds may not require further evaluation, whereas pts w/ active wheezing or recurrent bronchospasm or on multiple meds may require further evaluation, including spirometry & ABG.
  - Findings such as FEV1 <50% of predicted, hypoxia, or hypercarbia are signs of severe disease.

What To Do
- Determine adequacy of current treatment regimen.
- Delay elective surgery if pt has evidence of bronchospasm due to inadequate therapy or a precipitating cause such as pneumonia or upper respiratory infection.

- Whenever possible, offer these pts regional anesthesia. However, certain surgeries require GA. In these circumstances, avoid meds that cause histamine release.
- If possible, avoid tracheal intubation.

INTRAOP

- Premedicate w/ an inhaled beta agonist.
- Pts w/ severe asthma should be premedicated w/ PO or IV corticosteroids (eg, methylprednisolone 60–120 mg IV) should tracheal intubation be anticipated.
- Consider effects of induction agent on bronchospasm.
  - ➤ Propofol is a favorable agent for induction because it blunts airway reflexes & has been shown to decrease airway resistance.
  - ➤ Ketamine causes bronchodilation secondary to sympathomimetic effect & possibly through direct inhibition of muscarinic receptors.
  - ➤ Lidocaine (used w/ other agents) decreases airway reactivity & also possibly causes bronchodilation.
  - ➤ Thiopental & etomidate are generally thought to be less effective for blunting airway reflexes.
- Consider effect of intraop opioid on bronchospasm.
  - ➤ Opioids may inhibit bronchoconstriction.
  - ➤ Morphine has been associated w/ histamine release, which could potentially cause bronchoconstriction. However, this histamine response is short-lived.
  - ➤ Fentanyl & the other potent synthetic narcotics do not cause histamine release.
- Some muscle relaxants may promote histamine release.
- Reversal agents such as neostigmine can cause increased airway secretions & may require higher doses of glycopyrrolate.
- All inhalational anesthetics (except N_2O) cause bronchodilation.

Management

- Monitor capnograph to assess for signs of obstructive lung physiology.
- Monitor peak airway pressures.
- Use low tidal volumes & slow respiratory rates to allow for increased expiratory time & minimize air trapping.
- For further mgt of bronchospasm see Critical Event chapter "Bronchospasm." Essentials of bronchospasm mgt include
  - ➤ Increase inhaled O_2 to 100%.

➤ Confirm diagnosis w/ auscultation & evaluation of airway pressures.
➤ Increase depth of anesthesia.
➤ Administer inhaled beta agonist (eg, metaproterenol, albuterol).
➤ Adjust ventilator settings.
  • Use a slow respiratory rate to allow adequate expiratory time.
  • If exhalation is incomplete, air trapping will occur, potentially leading to barotrauma or circulatory depression.
  • Allow hypercarbia if necessary to minimize air trapping.
➤ Administer IV steroids.
➤ Consider infusion of IV sympathomimetics (epinephrine or isoproterenol).

POSTOP
■ Pts w/ reactive airway disease are at increased risk of developing bronchospasm after extubation & should be monitored for symptoms.
  ➤ Treat w/ an inhaled beta agonist & steroids if necessary.
■ Consider postop ICU care for pt w/ severe or persistent bronchospasm.

ATRIAL FIBRILLATION (AF)

JOAN J. CHEN, MD

OVERVIEW
■ Definition: commonly occurring arrhythmia characterized on ECG by rapid, disorganized atrial activity & irregular ventricular response
  ➤ Typical ventricular rate of new-onset AF: 110–130
  ➤ Ventricular rate >150 may occur more commonly w/ increased sympathetic tone.
  ➤ Very high ventricular rate (>250) may occur in pt w/ Wolff-Parkinson-White syndrome.
■ Complications of AF
  ➤ Tachycardia, which can cause hypotension, pulmonary edema, angina
  ➤ Systemic embolization, typically related to atrial thrombi

Management
- Use techniques & agents that minimize sympathetic stimulation:
  - Adequate depth of anesthesia.
  - Adequate oxygenation & ventilation.
- Maintain adequate ventricular rate control.
  - IV beta blockers (eg, esmolol, metoprolol) are especially useful for increased sympathetic tone or elevated catecholamine states.

POSTOP
- AF may recur or worsen in the postop period because of fluid shifts, stress of surgery, increased catecholamine state related to anxiety, stress, pain.
  - AF is very common after cardiac surgery; some pts receive prophylactic antiarrhythmic therapy (eg, amiodarone).
  - Consider postop ECG monitoring depending on severity of disease & stress of surgery.
- Adequate postop analgesia will help reduce sympathetic tone.
- Continue medical therapy for AF, including adequate ventricular rate control.
- Resume anticoagulation therapy after risk for surgical bleeding is deemed appropriately low.

ATRIAL FLUTTER

DORRE NICHOLAU, PHD, MD

OVERVIEW
- Type I atrial flutter is recognized on EKG as a saw-toothed pattern of atrial activity at a rate of 250–350 beats/min. This pattern is best identified in lead V1 & the inferior leads (II, III, aVf). A true flutter pattern produces no isoelectric interval between A waves.
  - Typical atrial flutter rate is 300 beats/min w/ a ventricular response of 1:2 (150 beats/min).
  - 1:1 conduction w/ a ventricular rate of 300 beats/min can occur in children & pts w/ pre-excitation syndrome, hyperthyroidism & rapidly conducting AV nodes.
  - The ventricular rate in atrial flutter is most often regular due to a constant conduction ratio of 1:2 or 1:4 (conducted beats reflect

even numbers). Less commonly an irregular ventricular rate may result from a variable or alternating AV block. In these cases the ventricular response is usually consistent w/ a Wenckebach periodicity.

■ Type II atrial flutter is faster, with an atrial rate of 350–450 beats/min, while slower atrial rates in the range of 200 beats/min may result from pharmacologic treatment.

Usual Rx

■ The initial treatment of choice is conversion to sinus rhythm w/ electricity.

■ Synchronous DC cardioversion, if unsuccessful, is followed by rapid atrial pacing w/ a catheter in the right atrium or the esophagus.

■ Pts who fail attempts at electrical cardioversion are managed pharmacologically.

➤ Calcium channel blockers, beta blockers & digoxin are used to slow the ventricular response.

➤ Class IA or IC agents are used to chemically convert the pt to sinus rhythm.

• Because of their ability to speed conduction through the AV node & facilitate a 1:1 ventricular response, class IA agents are used only after the ventricular rate has been controlled pharmacologically.

• Amiodarone, a class IC agent, has inherent AV nodal blocking as well as beta-blocking activity & therefore does not require pretreatment w/ AV nodal blocking agents. Low-dose amiodarone at 200 mg/day is effective in maintaining sinus rhythm while minimizing adverse effects.

• Both procainamide & amiodarone are proarrhythmic. Amiodarone & the active metabolite of procainamide, N-acetyl-procainamide (NAPA), are class IC agents that can prolong the QT interval & precipitate torsades de pointes ventricular arrhythmia.

PREOP

Issues/Evaluation

■ Atrial flutter is less common than atrial fibrillation. It is typically an unstable rhythm that quickly degenerates into atrial fibrillation or spontaneously reverts to sinus rhythm. If it is chronic, it is predictably a reflection of a chronic underlying cardiac condition.

- Preop evaluation should focus on identifying the underlying cardiac condition. Common etiologies include
  - Rheumatic heart disease
  - Ischemic cardiomyopathy
  - Associated cardiac structural lesions include atrial septal defects, mitral stenosis, tricuspid stenosis and/or insufficiency, chronic pulmonary emboli. Atrial dilation is a common denominator of these precipitating structural lesions.
  - Associated toxic metabolic conditions include thyrotoxicosis, alcohol abuse, pericarditis.
- An echocardiogram may be the most useful test to simultaneously identify structural cardiac abnormalities, atrial size, LV size & function & wall motion abnormalities.
- Ps w/ atrial flutter are likely to be anticoagulated preop.
  - Coumadin anticoagulation should be discontinued 3–4 days prior to elective surgery. INR should be evaluated preop to document normalization.
  - Because the atrial contractions are organized in atrial flutter, the rhythm tends to result in fewer embolic complications than atrial fibrillation.
- The EKG of pts w/ a history of atrial flutter who are pharmacologically maintained on procainamide or amiodarone may show evidence of QT prolongation, a risk for torsades de pointes.

INTRAOP
- Diagnosis
  - A regular heart rate of 150 beats/min should alert the clinician to the possibility of A flutter.
  - An atrial rate of 300 beats/min w/ 1:2 conduction is the most common presentation.
  - 1:1 conduction w/ a ventricular rate of 300 beats/min may result from high catecholamine states or drugs that shorten AV conduction.
  - An irregular heart rate is the result of variable AV block or alternating fibrillation/flutter.
  - Flutter waves are best identified in inferior leads or V1.
- Adenosine can be used to transiently block the AV node & allow the atrial rhythm to be clearly identified if a definitive diagnosis cannot be made by EKG interpretation.
  - Incremental doses of 3, 6 & 12 mg can be given to achieve desired AV block.

➤ Inject adenosine rapidly, followed by 10 cc saline, both by rapid IV push.

➤ Central line injection is preferable.

Management

■ If atrial flutter results in hemodynamic instability, restore sinus rhythm immediately by electrical DC cardioversion. The initial dose is <50 joules; follow w/ 100, 200, 300, up to 360 joules.

■ If pt is hemodynamically stable, the ventricular rate can be controlled pharmacologically. A goal HR <100 beats/min should return the stroke volume towards normal, followed by chemical cardioversion.

➤ For rate control

• Esmolol: 0.5 mg/kg IV over 1 to 2 min; infuse 50–300 mcg/kg/min. This is a short-acting drug hydrolyzed by red blood cell esterase w/ a half-life of 8–9 min.

• Metoprolol: 5 mg over 2 min; repeat q5min to a total dose of 15 mg. Metoprolol is cardioselective but not as easily titrated as esmolol.

• Diltiazem: 0.25 mg/kg over 2 min, then 0.35 mg/kg in 15 min if needed. Infuse 10–15 mg/h. Diltiazem has less myocardial depression than verapamil.

• Verapamil: 0.075 mg/kg over 2 min; infuse at 5 mcg/kg if needed. Verapamil provides effective rate control but is often accompanied by myocardial depression and hypotension

• Digoxin: 0.75 mg over 5 min, then 0.25 mg in 4 hours. Digoxin is not useful for rapid rate control; the effect may take hours.

➤ For chemical cardioversion

• Amiodarone 1 g over 24 h in three phases: (1) Rapid: 15 mg/min × 10 min. (2) Slow: 1 mg/min × 6 h. (3) Maintenance: 0.5 mg/kg × 18 h. Watch for bradycardia (AV nodal blockade), hypotension (alpha and beta blockade), prolonged QT.

• Procainamide: 10 mg/kg over 30 min (max rate 25 mg/min), then infuse at 1–4 mg/min. Procainamide may speed AV conduction; dose it after giving an agent to block AV node. It can also prolong the QT interval.

POSTOP

■ New-onset atrial flutter will require cardiac evaluation to determine etiology.

■ Postop telemetry should be ordered for pts w/ a rapid ventricular response requiring rate control in the OR.

BLISTERING SKIN DISEASES (PEMPHIGUS, EPIDERMOLYSIS BULLOSA)

JAMES M. SONNER, MD

OVERVIEW
- Definition: conditions in which skin is easily sloughed or forms blisters. Includes pemphigus & epidermolysis bullosa.
- Usual Rx
  - ➤ Steroids are the primary treatment for pemphigus & epidermolysis bullosa.
  - ➤ Many adjuvants are used, including methotrexate, azathioprine, cyclosporine, dapsone.

PREOP

Issues/Evaluation
- Pt may have scarring limiting mouth opening or joint movement.
- Areas of skin or oral mucosa affected by blistering, denudation, or scarring should be noted.
- Electrolytes may be abnormal.
- Side effects of steroid use may be present.

What To Do
- Careful exam focusing on skin & mucosa
- May want to check electrolytes

INTRAOP

Management
- Avoid applying adhesives to skin; remove adhesive from ECG pads, oximeter.
- Do not use tape: attach monitors by wrapping w/ a loose bandage, secure ETT w/ sutures.
- Place padding (eg, Webril) under BP cuff.
- Do not use LMA (placement may erode oral mucosa).
- Do not use local infiltration as this may produce blisters.
- Lubricate facemask to reduce sloughing of skin from friction.
- Lubricate, do not tape, eyes.

POSTOP
- Be alert to development of new blisters, skin trauma, infection.

■ Trauma to airway may place pt at risk of airway obstruction or bleeding.

BURNS

JASON WIDRICH, MD

OVERVIEW

■ Definition: chemical, thermal, or electrical damage to the skin or deep tissues
■ Usual Rx
  ➤ Debridement of burn
  ➤ Aggressive support for each organ system affected
  ➤ Protection from infection at burn sites
■ Pt w/ burn injury may present at different times during hospital course:
  ➤ Debridement on initial presentation (typically within hours of injury)
  ➤ Subsequent debridement & skin grafting during initial hospitalization (days to weeks after initial injury)
  ➤ Later debridement, grafting, or other cosmetic repair (months to years after injury)
■ Burn injury leads to increased risk of sepsis w/ the potential for multiple organ system failure (eg, ARDS, cardiovascular instability)

PREOP

Issues/Evaluation
■ Depth of burn graded by level of injury
  ➤ First degree: epithelium
  ➤ Second degree: dermis
  ➤ Third degree: entire skin thickness
  ➤ Fourth degree: deeper than skin thickness
■ Agent of burn may have specific other concerns requiring evaluation:
  ➤ Fire
    • Can lead to carbon monoxide toxicity: interferes w/ hemoglobin binding to oxygen. Measured PaO_2 & oxygen saturation can be normal.
  ➤ Steam
  ➤ Immersion

➢ Chemical
  • Need to know if there was a toxic agent
➢ Electrical burns
  • Higher likelihood of causing deep tissue damage, myoglobinuria, renal failure
■ Time since the burn occurred can affect mgt or likelihood of certain problems.
■ Hyperkalemia may occur as a result of tissue destruction or reperfusion.

What To Do
■ Classify burns by % BSA affected.
  ➢ Rule of Nines: upper anterior torso, lower anterior torso, upper posterior torso, lower posterior torso, entire arm, posterior leg, anterior leg, entire head and neck each count toward 9% of BSA affected (perineum is 1%).
■ Determine hemodynamic & respiratory stability.
  ➢ Pts may have already developed hypotension requiring vasopressors or respiratory failure requiring tracheal intubation.
  ➢ May need to be transported from ICU w/ ventilator & full hemodynamic monitoring & support
■ Resuscitation by Parkland formula, supplemented by clinical evaluation of volume status, CVP, urine output evaluation
  ➢ Lactated Ringer's 4 mL/kg × %Burn (up to 50%) over the first 24 h
  ➢ Half given in the first 8 h and half given in the next 16 h
■ Co-oximetry should be used to identify carbon monoxide levels.
  ➢ Normally 2% for nonsmokers, 10% for smokers
  ➢ Treatment is 100% oxygen & hyberbaric oxygen therapy if available.
■ Initial labs: ABG/co-oximetry, CBC, BUN, creatinine, electrolytes
■ Inhalation injury may result in airway obstruction or respiratory failure several hours after the initial injury.
  ➢ Assess airway for signs of inhalation injury.
    • Respiratory distress or upper airway obstruction occurring early after burn.
    • Burns around face or neck.
    • Edema or inflammation of face, lips, oropharynx
    • Oropharyngeal carbon deposits or carbon in sputum.
    • Singed facial hair.
  ➢ Early airway intervention can be lifesaving.

➤ If there is facial contracture or facial trauma, consider awake fiberoptic intubation.

INTRAOP

- For major burns, consider additional monitors & lines:
  - ➤ Arterial line
  - ➤ Two large-bore peripheral IVs
  - ➤ Central line or PA catheter may be required for major debridements that have major blood loss & fluid shifts.
  - ➤ Foley catheter
    - Urine output used as a measure of renal perfusion
    - Goal is to maintain urine output >0.5 cc/kg/h
- Tape & electrodes may not stick to burned skin; monitors or ETT may have to be sutured in place.
- The acute phase of a burn will alter vascular permeability, causing a large drop in intravascular volume. High-output cardiac failure may require massive resuscitation w/ IV fluids & inotropic agents.
- IV fluids are often administered at 4 cc/kg per % BSA affected.
- Warm all fluids, humidify airway gases, maintain core temp as close to normal as possible.
- Keep at least 2–4 units PRBC typed & crossed.
- Muscle relaxant issues in burn pts.
  - ➤ In the acute phase of a burn injury, succinylcholine may be used if indicated.
  - ➤ Avoid succinylcholine beginning 72 h postburn.
    - After 72 h upregulation of Ach receptors can cause hyperkalemic cardiac arrest after succinylcholine.
  - ➤ Higher doses of nondepolarizing relaxants may be required.
- Metabolism is increased in burn pts & they will require higher minute ventilation.

POSTOP

- Pt w/ major burn is typically managed in ICU or specialized burn unit.
- Follow ABGs, electrolytes, BUN, creatinine, urine output, glucose, ionized Ca++, PT, PTT.
  - ➤ Diuresis & gastric fluid loss may alter intravascular status or cause hypokalemia.
- Massive fluid requirements in these pts often lead to coagulopathy, fluid overload, pulmonary edema.
- Pts remain at high risk of sepsis & multiple organ failure.

- Pain mgt for debridement will require IV narcotics. Ketamine has been used for these pts as well.

CARCINOID SYNDROME

JAMES BRANDES, MD

OVERVIEW
- Definition: syndrome caused by overproduction of vasoactive substances by a carcinoid tumor
  - Best-characterized substance is serotonin, but others include histamine, corticotropin, dopamine, kallikrein, neurotensin, prostaglandins, substance P.
  - Carcinoid tumors presumed to arise from neuroendocrine cells. Usually occur in the GI tract, but may also occur in lungs, bronchi.
  - Manifestations of carcinoid syndrome include
    - Episodic flushing
    - Wheezing
    - Diarrhea
    - Right-sided valvular disease

PREOP

Issues/Evaluation
- Present in approx 2–5% of pts w/ carcinoid tumors
- Signs/symptoms usually present only in pt w/ liver mets, or if tumor releases vasoactive substances outside of portal circulation
- Cardiac valve lesions include
  - Tricuspid regurgitation & stenosis
  - Pulmonic regurgitation & stenosis
  - Left-sided valve disease less common
- Pt w/ carcinoid syndrome will likely be receiving the somatostatin analog octreotide
  - Octreotide is highly effective in reducing symptoms. Mechanism involves binding to somatostatin receptor on tumor
  - Typical dose: 150 mcg SC TID

What To Do
- Evaluate for symptoms of carcinoid syndrome.
  - Consider echo to evaluate for tricuspid regurgitation & pulmonic stenosis.
- In pts w/ diarrhea, check electrolytes & fluid status.

■ If pt is presenting for tumor resection, check abdominal CT scan for tumor location/multiplicity.
■ Continue preop treatment w/ octreotide.

INTRAOP
■ Give octreotide IV (50 mcg) & SQ (50 mcg) prior to tumor manipulation to help block hemodynamic effects.
■ Pts are at risk for carcinoid "crisis": flushing associated w/ bronchospasm, severe hypotension, cardiovascular collapse.
    ➤ Additional IV bolus of 50 mcg may be helpful to manage carcinoid crisis.
■ Avoid drugs that may cause histamine release.
■ Catecholamines may increase release of substances from tumor & worsen symptoms.
■ Rarely, a hypertensive carcinoid crisis may occur (eg, from tumor manipulation) & may respond to IV octreotide as well as vasodilator therapy.

POSTOP
■ Watch for continued signs of carcinoid syndrome or crisis.
■ Surgical resection of carcinoid tumor may not eliminate all metastatic lesions, so hemodynamic changes may persist.
    ➤ Consider continuation of octreotide therapy.

CHRONIC LIVER DISEASE & LIVER CIRRHOSIS

PERRY LEE, MD
JASON WIDRICH, MD
MANUEL PARDO, JR., MD

OVERVIEW
■ Definitions
    ➤ Chronic liver failure: hepatic encephalopathy in setting of chronic liver disease
    ➤ Liver cirrhosis is a histologic diagnosis characterized by
        • Diffuse disease of liver parenchyma
        • Hepatic fibrosis
        • Nodules replacing normal liver architecture
■ Cirrhosis is caused by chronic liver disease from a variety of causes. Mechanisms of disease causing cirrhosis include
    ➤ Hepatocellular disease

- Viral hepatitis (B, C)
- Alcohol
- Autoimmune hepatitis
- Metabolic disease
- Hemochromatosis
- Nonalcoholic steatohepatitis
- Wilson's disease
- Alpha-1 antitrypsin deficiency
- Drugs/toxins
➤ Cholestasis
  - Primary biliary cirrhosis
  - Primary sclerosing cholangitis
  - Secondary biliary cirrhosis
  - Drugs/toxins
➤ Hepatic venous outflow obstruction
  - Veno-occlusive disease
  - Budd-Chiari syndrome
  - Congestive heart failure
  - Constrictive pericarditis
  - Drugs/toxins
■ Most common causes of cirrhosis in US
  ➤ Chronic hepatitis C infection
  ➤ Alcohol
  ➤ Primary biliary cirrhosis
  ➤ Primary sclerosing cholangitis
  ➤ Nonalcoholic steatohepatitis
■ Usual Rx
  ➤ Depends on cause of liver disease
  ➤ Supportive care of complications
  ➤ Liver transplant for pt w/ end-stage liver disease
    - Some diseases (eg, alcoholic liver disease) may take decades to cause end-stage liver disease.
■ Contrast chronic liver disease w/ acute liver failure:
  ➤ Acute liver failure: hepatic encephalopathy & coagulopathy in the setting of acute hepatic disease
    - Fulminant liver failure: hepatic encephalopathy develops within 8 wks of onset
    - Subfulminant failure: encephalopathy develops within 26 wks of onset
  ➤ See also Coexisting Disease chapter "Acute Hepatitis."
  ➤ See also Coexisting Disease chapter "Acute Liver Failure."

PREOP

Issues/Evaluation

■ Staging of liver disease can be done by a variety of means, including liver biopsy or clinical staging. The modified Child-Pugh classification is commonly used to assess prognosis in cirrhosis & predict complications & periop risk. Grade is determined by adding points from 5 factors:

➤ Bilirubin (mg/dL)
  • One point: <2
  • Two points: 2 or 3
  • Three points: >3
  • For pt w/ sclerosing cholangitis or primary biliary cirrhosis, bilirubin <4 = one point, bilirubin 4–10 = two points, bilirubin >10 = three points

➤ Albumin (g/dL)
  • One point: >3.5
  • Two points: 3–3.5
  • Three points: <3

➤ Ascites
  • One point: none
  • Two points: easily controlled
  • Three points: poorly controlled

➤ Hepatic encephalopathy
  • One point: none
  • Two points: mild (stage I, II)
  • Three points: moderate to severe (stage III, IV)

➤ Prothrombin time: seconds prolonged (INR)
  • One point: 0–4 (<1.7)
  • Two points: 4–6 (1.7–2.3)
  • Three points: >6 (>2.3)

➤ Child's class A: 5 or 6 points

➤ Child's class B: 7–9 points

➤ Child's class C: 10–15 points

■ Studies of operative risk for portosystemic shunt or nonshunt procedures, based on Child's classification, suggest approximate periop mortality ranges of

➤ Child's A: 0–10%

➤ Child's B: 5–30%

➤ Child's C: 20–80%

➤ Risk is higher for emergency surgery, especially intra-abdominal surgery.

- Complications of cirrhosis occur from portal hypertension & decreased hepatic synthetic function.
  - Coagulation abnormalities occur from a variety of factors & predispose to bleeding.
    - Decreased synthesis of procoagulant proteins (fibrinogen, prothrombin, factors V, VII, IX, X, XI)
    - Decreased synthesis of coagulation inhibitors (proteins C, S, antithrombin III)
    - Decreased vitamin K absorption & metabolism
    - DIC or systemic fibrinolysis
    - Thrombocytopenia from splenic sequestration
  - Cardiovascular abnormalities
    - Vasodilated state characterized by high cardiac output, low SVR, normal blood pressure
    - Reduced sensitivity to vasoconstrictors
    - Rarely, pts develop pulmonary hypertension (unclear etiology)
  - Respiratory abnormalities
    - Hypoxemia can occur from usual causes, but also from intrapulmonary shunt related to intrapulmonary vascular dilations (hepatopulmonary syndrome).
  - Bleeding from esophageal or gastric varices
  - Hepatic encephalopathy. Grading scale based on level of consciousness:
    - Grade 1: inverted sleep pattern, restlessness
    - Grade 2: lethargy
    - Grade 3: confusion, somnolence, but still arousable
    - Grade 4: coma
  - Ascites
    - If severe, can lead to decreased FRC, hypoxemia, respiratory difficulty
  - Hepatorenal syndrome
    - "Functional" oliguric renal failure characterized by intense renal vasoconstriction
    - A diagnosis of exclusion
  - Predisposition to infection
    - Including spontaneous bacterial peritonitis, sepsis
  - Hepatocellular cancer
- General mgt of cirrhosis complications
  - Coagulation abnormalities
    - Supportive vitamin K, FFP or platelet transfusion for bleeding or invasive procedures, as guided by PT, PTT, platelet count

➤ Bleeding from esophageal or gastric varices
  • Nonspecific beta blockade for prevention (propranolol, nadolol)
  • Appropriate blood & fluid resuscitation
  • Octreotide (preferred over vasopressin) to reduce splanchnic blood flow
  • Endoscopic sclerotherapy or banding
  • Balloon tube tamponade (eg, Minnesota, Blakemore tube)
  • Transjugular intrahepatic portosystemic shunt (TIPS)
  • Surgical shunt procedure
➤ Hepatic encephalopathy
  • Treat any precipitating factor (eg, infection, CNS active drug, GI bleeding, electrolyte abnormality)
  • Low-protein diet
  • Lactulose
  • Supportive tracheal intubation for airway protection in stage 4 coma
➤ Ascites
  • Sodium restriction
  • Diuretics
  • Serial paracentesis
  • Peritoneal-venous shunt
  • TIPS
➤ Hepatorenal syndrome
  • Treat potentially reversible causes: nephrotoxic drugs, sepsis, diuretics, excess paracentesis.
➤ Hepatocellular cancer
  • Resection or ablation
  • Adjunct chemotherapy
■ Manifestations of cirrhosis
➤ Physical exam findings can vary by etiology & stage of disease:
  • General: muscle wasting, cachexia
  • Neurologic: asterixis, confusion, coma
  • Skin & extremities: warm extremities, palmar erythema, petechiae, ecchymosis, spider angioma, digit clubbing, peripheral edema, jaundice
  • Abdominal: hepatomegaly, splenomegaly, ascites, dilated abdominal veins (including caput medusae), umbilical hernia
➤ Common lab findings
  • CBC: anemia, thrombocytopenia

- Electrolytes: sodium, potassium abnormalities, acid-base disturbances (eg, lactic acidosis, diuretic-induced metabolic alkalosis)
- BUN, creatinine: elevations from volume depletion, renal failure or hepatorenal syndrome
- PT/PTT: elevated (reflection of reduced synthetic function)
- AST, ALT, bilirubin, alkaline phosphatase: elevations depending on etiology & stage of disease
- Albumin: decreased (reflection of reduced synthetic function)
- Fibrinogen: decreased (from DIC or fibrinolysis)
➤ Specialized lab tests for certain causes of liver disease
- Viral serologies
- Drug or ethanol levels
- Autoimmune disease: ANA, anti-smooth muscle antibodies (ASMA)
- Hemochromatosis: iron saturation
- Wilson's disease: ceruloplasmin

What To Do
- Determine etiology & chronicity of liver disease.
- Determine severity of liver disease & presence of cirrhosis.
- Determine complications of cirrhosis & adequacy of treatment.
- For elective surgery, consider postponing surgery for poorly controlled manifestations of cirrhosis.
  ➤ For chronic active hepatitis, consider consultation w/ hepatologist to determine adequacy of therapy.
- For pts w/ cirrhosis, Child's class may provide estimate of operative risk.
  ➤ Child's C class pts are at high risk of morbidity & mortality. In general, elective surgery should be deferred.
- Obtain lab tests & studies.
  ➤ CBC
  ➤ PT/PTT
  ➤ Electrolytes, BUN, creatinine
  ➤ ECG
  ➤ AST, ALT, alkaline phosphatase, albumin
  ➤ ECG
  ➤ CXR
- Correct coagulopathy & anemia prior to surgery.
  ➤ Give vitamin K, since vitamin K deficiency is common in pts w/ cirrhosis.
  ➤ FFP or platelets as indicated by lab testing.

- Regional anesthesia considerations.
  - Regional block options often limited due to coagulopathy, ascites w/ respiratory insufficiency, or hepatic encephalopathy.
- Premed issues.
  - Minimize sedatives or narcotics, which could precipitate hepatic encephalopathy & contribute to postop altered mental status.

INTRAOP
- Consider important drug therapy issues w/ liver failure.
  - Liver failure can alter the pharmacokinetics of many drugs administered during anesthesia. Mechanisms include
    - Decreased hepatic drug metabolism (eg, benzodiazepines, opioids)
    - Decreased protein levels, leading to increased unbound drug (eg, thiopental)
    - Decreased biliary excretion of drugs or drug metabolites
  - Pt can also have altered pharmacodynamics, especially if debilitated or cachexic (eg, sensitivity to CNS-acting drugs).
  - Pts w/ cirrhosis may display resistance to usual doses of vasopressor drugs.
  - Drugs not dependent on hepatic (or renal) metabolism include
    - Succinylcholine
    - Cisatracurium
    - Atracurium
    - Esmolol
    - Remifentanil
  - Sedatives, narcotics can precipitate hepatic encephalopathy.
  - Avoid halothane administration in pt w/ known liver disease due to reduction in hepatic blood flow & association w/ acute hepatitis ("halothane hepatitis").
- Blood product mgt
  - Coagulopathy is common & may predispose to bleeding.
  - Monitor hematocrit, platelets, PT, PTT, fibrinogen regularly during surgery.
  - Anticipate need for FFP, since 45 minutes typically needed for preparation.
  - Citrate-containing blood products such as FFP can lead to ionized hypocalcemia, especially when given rapidly.
- Abdominal surgery is particularly risky in pts w/ advanced cirrhosis.
  - Risk of intraop bleeding related to adhesions or portosystemic collaterals

➤ Abdominal surgery is associated w/ a large reduction in hepatic blood flow.

Management
- Perform rapid sequence induction.
  - ➤ Risk of aspiration is increased by ascites, increased abdominal pressure, decreased GI motility, encephalopathy.
- Minimize sedative & narcotic drugs, which can precipitate hepatic encephalopathy.
- Monitor labs & coagulation status. Correct as necessary.
  - ➤ FFP
  - ➤ Platelets
  - ➤ Vitamin K
- Consider invasive monitoring.
  - ➤ Depending on stress of surgery, anticipated fluid shifts & blood loss, arterial line & CVP or PA catheter may be useful to assess volume status & hemodynamics.
  - ➤ Maintain hemodynamics & fluid status closely to maintain liver perfusion & prevent ischemic liver injury.
  - ➤ Deliberate or controlled hypotension is contraindicated.

POSTOP
- Consider postop ICU care depending on severity of liver disease, intraop course, stress of proposed surgery.
- Watch for new complications of liver disease or worsening of existing complications.
- Postop complications include
  - ➤ Renal failure
  - ➤ Sepsis
  - ➤ Precipitation or worsening of hepatic encephalopathy
  - ➤ Hemorrhage
  - ➤ Worsening liver function, including coagulopathy

CHRONIC OBSTRUCTIVE PULMONARY DISEASE (COPD)

STEVEN YOUNGER, MD

OVERVIEW
- COPD is the most common respiratory disease encountered in adult anesthesia practice.

- Risk factors include
  - Cigarette smoking (including second-hand smoke)
  - Male gender
  - Urban living
  - Other chronic respiratory disease (eg, chronic asthma)
  - Other
    - Alpha-1 antitrypsin deficiency
- Two commonly recognized clinical pictures
  - Chronic bronchitis ("blue bloaters")
    - Develop chronic bronchitis, hypersecretory airway tissues, airflow obstruction.
    - There is sometimes a reversible component to outflow obstruction, probably from bronchospasm.
    - Over time, intrapulmonary shunt increases, leading to chronic hypoxia.
    - Hypoxia leads to pulmonary hypertension & eventually right heart failure (cor pulmonale) as well as erythrocytosis.
    - Outflow obstruction leads to chronic CO_2 retention. Theoretically, respiratory drive becomes dependent on PaO_2 rather than $PaCO_2$ and pH. However, only in a minority of patients does supplemental oxygen depress respiratory drive.
  - Emphysema ("pink puffers")
    - Loss of pulmonary parenchymal elasticity leads to distal small airway enlargement & alveolar septal destruction, sometimes leading to bulla formation.
    - Small airways, lacking elasticity, collapse prematurely during exhalation, leading to air trapping & increased residual volume (RV), FRC, TLV.
    - As alveoli are destroyed, alveolar capillaries are destroyed, leading to pulmonary hypertension & eventually right heart failure
    - Dead space fraction increases.
    - In contrast to chronic bronchitis, $PaCO_2$ & PaO_2 are often normal.
    - Respiratory rate is chronically increased to blow off CO_2 in the face of increased dead space.
    - Pts often exhale through pursed lips, stenting small airways open, generating "auto-PEEP."
- Usual Rx: may include low-flow nasal cannula oxygen, beta-2 agonist inhalers, ipratropium (Atrovent) inhaler.

PREOP

Issues/Evaluation

- Pt's clinical status should be optimized prior to surgery.
- Continue low-flow supplemental O_2 for chronic hypoxemia.
  - All hypercarbic pts will need supplemental oxygen to maintain an adequate oxygen saturation (90%).
  - Do not stop oxygen in pts who are severely hypercarbic as this can precipitate right heart failure.
- Right heart failure/peripheral edema may improve w/ oxygen therapy, diuretics, digoxin, afterload reduction.
- Pts have high chance of coexisting coronary artery disease (CAD).
  - Consider whether perioperative beta blockade will decrease risk of cardiac complications.
  - Only a minority of these patients develop bronchospasm w/ beta blockers.

What To Do

- Pts w/ component of reversible bronchospasm should be treated w/ bronchodilators & inhaled steroids.
- Advise smokers to quit smoking.
  - Benefits of stopping 6–8 wks prior to surgery
    - Decreases airway secretions
    - Improves O_2 carrying capacity
  - Quitting as late as 24 hours prior to surgery has theoretical benefits.
    - Improved O_2 carrying capacity
  - Periop pts may be more receptive to discussions about smoking cessation & may be more likely to quit.
  - Can consider nicotine patch or Wellbutrin (bupropion SR) to facilitate smoking cessation.
- Pts should be screened for evidence of impending exacerbations (worsening cough, purulent sputum, wheezing). In such pts:
  - Consider antibiotics.
  - Increase bronchodilators.
  - Postpone surgery until optimized symptomatically & objectively (see testing, below).
- Preop testing
  - Consider preop room-air O_2 saturation, ABGs, electrolytes.
    - Consider supplemental O_2 therapy for hypoxemia.
    - Screen for CO_2 retention: serum bicarbonate may be elevated; follow-up ABG will likely show increased $PaCO_2$

- If pt's oxygen saturation is normal & electrolytes are normal, no further testing is indicated unless pt is having pulmonary surgery.
- ➤ Pulmonary function testing
  - There is controversy about whether routine PFTs can predict intraop & postop complications.
  - PFTs are most useful when lung surgery is contemplated.
- ➤ CXR/chest CT can identify pts w/ bullous disease.
- ➤ Screen for coexisting cardiac disease.
- ■ Discuss the possibility of postop ventilation w/ high-risk pts. This will also depend on the nature of surgery.

INTRAOP

Management

- ■ For suitable procedure, consider regional technique w/ the following cautions:
  - ➤ High neuraxial block (SAB, epidural) may impair pulmonary function, especially expiratory function.
  - ➤ Operative positioning may make spontaneous ventilation difficult (ie, lithotomy).
  - ➤ Opiates may decrease respiratory drive & lead to respiratory failure.
- ■ General anesthesia
  - ➤ Access: guided by specific procedure
  - ➤ Monitors
    - Standard ASA monitors
    - Consider arterial line for blood gasses (see below).
    - Consider CVP in pts w/ evidence of heart failure.
    - Consider PA catheter for pts w/ (suspected) pulmonary hypertension.
    - Decision to use invasive monitoring must be guided by the type of procedure being performed & pt comorbidities.
  - ➤ Judicious preoxygenation before induction.
  - ➤ Ventilate w/ long expiratory times to prevent excess air-trapping & the risk of pulmonary barotrauma.
    - Use small tidal volumes to avoid barotrauma & auto-PEEP.
    - Bronchodilators may be useful if auto-PEEP becomes a problem.
  - ➤ Inhaled anesthetics may not reverse airflow obstruction, in contrast to asthmatic pts.

➤ For the small group of pts w/ reactive airways disease, steroids might be of use if there are problems in ventilation.

➤ Avoid N_2O in pts w/ bullous emphysema or pulmonary hypertension. N_2O may increase PA pressure & enlarge a pneumothorax.

➤ Consider ABG monitoring:
- To sensitively detect worsening hypoxia due to intrapulmonary shunting
- To judge adequacy of ventilation

■ Ventilate to normalize pH, not $PaCO_2$.

■ Normalizing $PaCO_2$ in CO_2 retainers results in alkalosis & possibly decreased ventilatory drive.

POSTOP

■ Concerns regarding extubation
➤ Smokers may have irritable airways, making awake extubation difficult due to risk of bronchospasm.
➤ Deep extubation carries the risk of inadequate ventilation & CO_2 retention.
➤ High-risk pts may require postop mechanical ventilation.

■ Postop analgesia concerns
➤ Postop narcotics must be used judiciously as pt's respiratory drive may be easily depressed.
➤ Consider starting with half (or less) the normal dose & titrating to effect.
➤ Regional nerve blockade, including epidural, may allow reduction in systemic narcotic requirement.
➤ Analgesia is important to allow pt to tolerate respiratory care regimen.

■ Take steps to optimize postop respiratory function.
➤ Aggressive pulmonary toilet.
➤ Incentive spirometry.
➤ Early mobilization when possible.

CHRONIC RENAL FAILURE (CRF) AND END-STAGE RENAL DISEASE (ESRD)

JASON WIDRICH, MD
MANUEL PARDO, JR., MD

OVERVIEW

■ Definition

➤ Chronic renal failure: progressive, permanent loss of renal function over a period >3 months

■ ESRD requires renal replacement therapy for survival.

■ Common causes include DM, HTN, glomerulonephritis, polycystic kidney disease.

■ Usual Rx
  ➤ Dialysis or kidney transplant

■ Dialysis access procedures or complications related to access (eg, infection, dysfunction) are common reasons for surgery in pts w/ ESRD.

PREOP

■ Major complications of CRF & symptoms of uremia include
  ➤ Fluid and electrolyte disorders
    • Metabolic acidosis
    • Sodium disorders
    • Potassium disorders (hyperkalemia can cause life-threatening arrhythmias)
  ➤ Cardiac (cardiac disease is the major cause of death in pts w/ ESRD)
    • Accelerated atherosclerosis & coronary artery disease
    • HTN
    • Congestive heart failure
    • Pulmonary edema
    • Pericarditis (can lead to tamponade)
  ➤ Neuromuscular
    • Lethargy
    • Peripheral neuropathy
    • Fatigue
    • Seizures
    • Coma
    • Gastropathy
  ➤ Hematologic
    • Anemia (some treated w/ erythropoietin)
    • Uremic platelet dysfunction
  ➤ Other
    • Increased susceptibility to infection & sepsis
    • Malnutrition (pts have decreased lean body mass, although fluid retention may mask weight loss)
    • GI bleeding

■ In pts w/ CRF not yet requiring dialysis, periop renal hypoperfusion (eg, from prolonged hypotension) may lead to worsening renal function & acute on chronic renal failure.

What To Do
■ Determine etiology of CRF.
  ➤ Certain causes of CRF have anesthetic implications (eg, DM, HTN).
■ Determine urine output.
  ➤ Lack of urine output increases challenges of periop fluid mgt.
■ Determine type & schedule of dialysis, including most recent treatment.
  ➤ Method of dialysis: peritoneal vs hemodialysis
    • Peritoneal typically involves multiple daily exchanges.
    • Hemodialysis typically 3 times/wk
■ Assess volume status & electrolytes.
  ➤ Pts are susceptible to fluid overload.
  ➤ Pt can also have hypovolemia from excess fluid removal w/ hemodialysis.
  ➤ Check ECG for signs of hyperkalemia or hypocalcemia.
  ➤ Knowledge of pt's "dry" weight may help determine volume status.
■ Determine site of dialysis access: peritoneal, AV fistula, central dialysis access catheter (tunneled or percutaneous).
  ➤ Check for patency of AV fistula.
  ➤ Do not put IV in extremity w/ AV fistula.
■ Determine presence of uremic symptoms described above.
■ Because of increased likelihood of cardiac disease, decide whether to pursue additional workup. This will depend on symptoms & the stress of proposed surgery.
■ Hyperkalemia can be life-threatening: obtain ECG to look for manifestations & postpone elective surgery for pt w/ cardiac manifestations of hyperkalemia. (See also Critical Event chapter "Hyperkalemia.")
■ Treatment of uremic bleeding may require desmopressin (DDAVP 0.3 mcg/kg) or estrogen, since dialysis does not consistently improve platelet function.
■ Obtain labs & other tests:
  ➤ CBC
  ➤ Electrolytes, BUN, creatinine

➤ ECG
➤ CXR

INTRAOP

■ Avoid BP cuffs, IV lines or arterial lines in extremities w/ AV fistulas.
■ Need for invasive monitoring (arterial line, central line) depends on presence of cardiac disease, risk of proposed surgery & anticipated fluid shifts or blood loss.
  ➤ Central line may permit closer evaluation of volume status & may help prevent volume overload.
■ Regional anesthesia can be used but must consider risk in pt w/ uremic coagulopathy or peripheral neuropathy.
■ Drug therapy issues
  ➤ Many drugs rely on at least partial excretion by the kidney for elimination.
  ➤ The systemic effects of azotemia can alter the pharmacokinetics of many drugs administered during anesthesia. Mechanisms include.
    • Decreased protein levels, leading to increased unbound drug.
    • Decreased drug delivery to kidneys.
    • Decreased excretion of renally cleared drugs or drug metabolites.
  ➤ Pt can also have altered pharmacodynamics, especially if pt is debilitated or cachexic.
  ➤ Pharmacokinetics of specific anesthetic drugs
    • Barbiturates: pts w/ CRF are more sensitive to barbiturates; this may be a result of decreased protein binding as well as an increase in the nonionized fraction of the drug
    • Propofol, etomidate, ketamine pharmacokinetics are minimally changed by renal impairment.
    • Succinylcholine can be used safely provided the serum potassium level is known to be <5.0 mEq/L at the time of induction & the normal rise of 0.5–1.0 mEq/L of potassium is expected; avoid muscle relaxants that depend primarily on the kidney for elimination (eg, pancuronium).
    • Volatile agents are ideal for maintenance as they affect renal blood flow minimally, control hypertension & do not rely on the kidney for elimination; avoid sevoflurane as its metabolite Compound A is potentially nephrotoxic.

- Morphine may be used carefully but one of its active metabolites, morphine-6-glucoronide, is renally excreted and can lead to respiratory depression.
- Meperidine should be avoided as its active metabolite normeperidine is renally eliminated & can cause seizures.
➤ Drugs not dependent on renal (or hepatic) metabolism include
  - Succinylcholine
  - Cisatracurium
  - Atracurium
  - Esmolol
  - Remifentanil

Management
■ Consider rapid sequence induction, as pts w/ uremia may be at risk for aspiration.
■ Fluid & electrolyte mgt
  ➤ Maintain adequate volume status.
  ➤ Fluid overload may lead to acute pulmonary edema. Limitation in urine output may require postop dialysis.
  ➤ Minimize lactated Ringer's solution in pts w/ elevated potassium as it contains 4 mEq/L potassium.
  ➤ If pt has significant electrolyte abnormalities preop, check electrolytes periodically during surgery, depending on blood loss & anticipated fluid shifts.
  ➤ Treat electrolyte disturbances accordingly.
■ Maintain controlled mechanical ventilation to avoid hypoventilation from spontaneous respiration if acidemia & hyperkalemia are of concern.

POSTOP
■ Evaluate for fluid & electrolyte disorders that may have developed during surgery.
■ Pts will continue to require aggressive monitoring of volume status postop.
■ Pts who received large volumes of fluid or experienced large fluid shifts may develop pulmonary edema & require continued mechanical ventilation.
■ Consider whether postop dialysis is needed.
  ➤ Indications can include fluid overload, pulmonary edema, hyperkalemia, severe acidosis.

■ If PCA is used for postop pain control, consider using an agent that is not dependent on renal excretion for elimination (eg, hydromorphone, fentanyl).

CONGENITAL HEART DISEASE, PEDIATRIC

PATRICK ROSS, MD

OVERVIEW
■ Congenital heart disease (CHD) includes a wide variety of anatomically different structural heart lesions.
■ Incidence is <1% of all live births in the US.
■ 25% of pts with CHD have other congenital anomalies
■ Most common lesions presenting in infancy are ventricular septal defect (VSD; 28%), patent ductus arteriosus (PDA; 12%), atrial septal defect (ASD; 10%), coarctation of aorta (9%).
■ Common CHD lesions in which the pt may survive into adulthood w/o any surgical correction include bicuspid aortic valve, coarctation of aorta, pulmonary valve stenosis, ASD, PDA.
■ The number of pts w/ CHD surviving into adulthood is steadily increasing. Patients are
  ➤ Awaiting surgery
  ➤ Status post corrective surgery requiring no further surgical treatment
  ➤ Status post palliative surgery w/ possible further surgical treatment
  ➤ Awaiting heart transplantation
■ Usual Rx: Varies w/ lesion in both timing & surgical center

PREOP

Issues/Evaluation
The anatomically diverse lesions can be classified as follows:
■ Lesions that cause outflow obstruction:
  ➤ Coarctation of the aorta
  ➤ Aortic stenosis (AS)
  ➤ Pulmonic stenosis (PS)
■ Lesions causing left to right shunting:
  ➤ VSD
  ➤ PDA

- ➤ ASD
- ➤ Endocardial cushion defect (AKA atrioventricular canal defect)
- ➤ Partial anomalous pulmonary venous return (PAPVR)
- ■ Lesions causing right to left shunting w/ decreased pulmonary blood flow (PBF):
  - ➤ Tetralogy of Fallot (TOF)
  - ➤ Pulmonary atresia
  - ➤ Tricuspid atresia
- ■ Lesion causing right to left shunting w/ increased pulmonary blood flow:
  - ➤ Transposition of the great arteries (TGA)
  - ➤ Truncus arteriosus
  - ➤ Single ventricle
  - ➤ Double-outlet right ventricle
  - ➤ Total anomalous pulmonary venous return (TAPVR)
  - ➤ Hypoplastic left heart syndrome (HLHS)
- ■ Preop evaluation includes
  - ➤ Thorough history, including past & present medications as well as prior surgical procedures
  - ➤ Physical exam w/ attention to signs of congestive heart failure
  - ➤ Laboratory data, including CXR, ECG, electrolytes, glucose, Hb (pts w/ chronic cyanosis require elevated hemoglobin compared to normal pts; in some pts increased Hb can place them at risk for hyperviscosity)
  - ➤ A consult note from pt's pediatric cardiologist
  - ➤ Further details vary w/ the noncardiac surgery to be undertaken.

What To Do

- ■ Infants & children requiring adequate preload to maintain cardiac output should not be made NPO for a prolonged period of time w/o maintenance IV fluid.
- ■ In preparing fluid lines for the case all air bubbles must be removed as any lesion has the potential for right to left shunting w/ air embolism to the cerebral or coronary circulations.
- ■ Antibiotic prophylaxis for endocarditis needs to be started before the surgery has begun.
- ■ Premedication should be considered in almost every child as tachycardia & excessive crying can alter the pt's hemodynamics. However, they must remain closely monitored after it is given as this pt population does not tolerate hypercapnia or hypoxemia.

INTRAOP

General Precautions

- Infants & children increase cardiac output by increasing heart rate as stroke volume is relatively fixed. Bradycardia is a grave warning sign of hypoxemia, hypercarbia, metabolic acidosis, hypotension, or other insults. Cardiac arrest may follow bradycardia if the underlying condition is not corrected.
- Blood should be administered via a warming device as cold blood or fluids can cause bradycardia. Blood should be fresh because older blood is more acidotic & hyperkalemic.
- For any shunting lesion air bubbles & blood clots must be removed as they can be a source of embolism.
- Follow Hb level intraop to avoid relative anemia (decreased oxygen delivery) or possible hyperviscosity if too elevated.
- ABGs (acid-base status) are helpful as an indicator of adequacy of oxygen delivery.

Management

- Obstructive lesions
  - Inhaled anesthetics may benefit pts w/ dynamic outflow obstruction such as TOF as a slightly decreased myocardial contractility may increase flow through the obstruction.
  - Avoid hypovolemia, light anesthesia, direct-acting inotropes, & decreasing systemic vascular resistance (SVR) as these may worsen the obstruction.
- Left to right shunting
  - Avoid conditions that will increase left to right shunting, such as
    - Low Hgb
    - Decreased pulmonary vascular resistance (PVR)
    - Increased SVR, hyperoxemia
    - Hyperventilation
  - Avoid air bubbles because shunting may reverse during anesthesia.
  - Onset of IV induction may be slightly prolonged.
- Right to left shunting w/ decreased PBF
  - Avoid conditions that will increase PVR, such as
    - Hypoxemia
    - Hypercarbia
    - Acidosis
    - High mean airway pressure
    - Hypervolemia

- Raised intra-abdominal pressure
- Light anesthesia
- Cold

➤ It may be necessary to increase FiO_2, hyperventilate, & start vasodilators such as nitroglycerin or nitroprusside to increase PBF & oxygenation.

➤ Avoid embolization of air or blood clots.

➤ Inhaled induction of anesthesia may be slightly prolonged & IV induction slightly delayed.

■ Right to left shunting w/ increased PBF

➤ Similar to left to right shunting in that lowering PVR will increase PBF & can lead to significant pulmonary congestion & CHF symptoms.

➤ Therefore, avoid hyperoxemia & hyperventilation.

➤ Avoid embolization of air or blood clots.

➤ IV induction of anesthesia may be slightly delayed.

POSTOP

■ ➤ Maintain close cardiorespiratory monitoring as hypoventilation will severely affect hemodynamic status.

➤ Monitoring in a pediatric ICU may be appropriate.

➤ Continue maintenance IV fluids until adequate PO intake.

CONGESTIVE HEART FAILURE (CHF)

GIAC VU, MD

OVERVIEW

■ Definition: inability of the heart to meet the body's metabolic demands

➤ Typically occurs from systolic or diastolic failure of cardiac contraction

➤ May be related to congenital heart disease, congenital or acquired valvular disease, coronary artery disease, or hypertensive cardiovascular disease

➤ Clinical descriptors sometimes include systolic vs diastolic failure, high- vs low-output failure, right- or left-sided failure, acute vs chronic failure.

➤ This chapter focuses on pts w/ CHF from LV systolic dysfunction.

■ Symptoms include dyspnea on exertion or at rest, orthopnea, paroxysmal nocturnal dyspnea, decreased exercise tolerance, fatigue.

- Rx for CHF w/ decreased LV systolic function may include
  - Nonpharmacologic therapy
    - Dietary restrictions (eg, sodium)
    - Exercise
  - Pharmacologic therapy demonstrated to improve outcome in large clinical trials
    - ACE inhibitors
    - Beta blockers
    - Spironolactone
  - Pharmacologic therapy for symptom control
    - Loop diuretics
    - Digoxin
  - Other pharmacologic therapy
    - Antiarrhythmics
    - Anticoagulants (esp in pt w/ atrial fibrillation)
    - Vasodilators for treatment of hypertension or angina
    - Inotropes
  - Other therapy, some under investigation
    - Biventricular pacing
    - Implantable cardioverter-defibrillator (ICD)
    - Ventricular assist device
    - Heart surgery for specific conditions (eg, CAD, valvular disease)
    - Heart transplantation

PREOP

Issues/Evaluation
- CHF is an important risk factor for periop cardiac morbidity.
- Periop fluid mgt is more challenging w/ decreasing LV ejection fraction <40%.
- Underlying causes of heart failure include
  - Ischemic heart disease
  - Valvular heart disease
  - Cardiomyopathy
  - Systemic HTN
  - Pulmonary HTN
  - Congenital heart disease
  - High-output states
- Manifestations of heart failure include
  - Dyspnea
  - Dyspnea on exertion

- Orthopnea
- Paroxysmal nocturnal dyspnea
- Pulmonary crackles
- Cardiac S3 gallop
- Jugular venous distention
- Hepatosplenomegaly
- Ascites
- Peripheral edema

■ Pt w/ arrhythmias may have pacemaker or ICD or may be taking antiarrhythmic therapy.

■ Functional capacity may be assessed by NYHA functional capacity classification:

- Class I: No limitation of physical activity. Ordinary physical activity does not cause symptoms.
- Class II: Slight limitation of physical activity. Ordinary physical activity results in symptoms.
- Class III: Marked limitation of physical activity. Pt comfortable at rest. Less than ordinary activity causes symptoms.
- Class IV: Severe limitation of physical activity. All physical activity causes discomfort. Symptoms may be present at rest.

What To Do

■ Determine treatment regimen for CHF & determine adequacy of treatment.

- Consider whether further medical therapy is necessary before surgery.
- Postpone elective surgery in pt w/ decompensated heart failure.
- Consider cardiology consult to determine adequacy of treatment & recommendations for further mgt. This may be more important for pt w/ class III or IV CHF.

■ Continue cardiac medications.

- Consider withholding digoxin in pts undergoing cardiopulmonary bypass as hypokalemia during CPB may induce digitalis toxicity.

■ Studies to consider in all pts

- CBC
- ECG
- CXR
- Electrolytes, BUN, creatinine
- Recent echocardiogram

> Reports of prior cardiac evaluation (echocardiogram, cardiac cath, etc.)

INTRAOP

■ Monitoring requirements (arterial line, central line, PA catheter, TEE) depend on severity of disease & stress of proposed surgery.

■ Fluid mgt can pose significant challenge.

> Hypotension from anesthesia-induced vasodilation often treated w/ IV fluid administration.

> Vasodilation may decrease w/ discontinuation of anesthesia, leading to increased preload & risk of pulmonary edema.

> This becomes more significant as LV ejection fraction decreases.

■ Determine hemodynamic goals.

> Preload: pt w/ CHF will require adequate preload for optimal cardiac function but is susceptible to pulmonary edema w/ excess preload.

> Afterload: afterload reduction is beneficial; increases in afterload may worsen cardiac function.

> Contractility: since LV systolic function is typically depressed, minimize further decreases.

■ Consider effects of anesthetics on hemodynamic goals.

> Most IV induction agents reduce contractility.
  • Consider decreased or incremental dosing, or choose induction agent w/ minimal effect on contractility (eg, etomidate).
  • Anticipate hypotension w/ anesthesia induction.

> Inhaled agents vary in the degree of vasodilation & reduction of contractility.

> Opiates have minimal effects on cardiac contractility.

> Vasodilation from anesthesia may cause hypotension.

Management

■ Optimize preload.

■ Preserve contractility. Avoid cardiac depressant drugs.

> Consider temporary inotropic agent (eg, dobutamine) to offset effects of anesthetic agents.

■ Continue afterload reduction as necessary.

> Vasodilators such as nitroglycerin or nitroprusside are effective for afterload reduction & increasing venous capacitance.

■ Monitor electrolytes closely, especially in pt receiving digoxin.

POSTOP

■ Pt is at high risk of cardiac complications.

- Consider postop care in monitored or ICU setting, depending on severity of disease, stress of surgery, intraop course.
- Monitor for development of pulmonary edema; consider need for postop mechanical ventilation.

CORONARY ARTERY DISEASE (CAD)

JIENY M. HAN, MD

OVERVIEW

Definitions

- Atherosclerosis: a process of damage to the vessels supplying the heart. Damage can include flow-limiting obstructive deposits or plaques, which can rupture & lead to thrombosis
- Infarction: death of myocardial cells
- Ischemia: myocardial oxygen demand exceeds supply
    - Can lead to angina, arrhythmias, myocardial infarction (MI)
    - Thrombosis of coronary artery limits myocardial oxygen supply & may cause infarction
- Predisposing factors
    - Increased age
    - Male sex (menopause increases risk in women)
    - Hypertension
    - Cigarette smoking
    - Hyperlipidemia
    - Genetics
    - Obesity
    - Diabetes mellitus
- CAD affects 11 million people in U.S.
    - 1.5 million of these will have MI, & 1/3 of those will die
    - Single largest cause of death in men & women
- Perioperative cardiac events, including MI, unstable angina, congestive heart failure, & serious dysrhythmias, are the leading cause of perioperative deaths (25–50% of deaths following noncardiac surgery).

Usual Rx: Treatment usually fivefold:

- Correction of risk factors (smoking cessation, cholesterol-lowering agents)
- Lifestyle modification: diet, weight loss, exercise
- Correction of medical comorbidities that can exacerbate ischemia:

- ➤ Hypertension
- ➤ Anemia
- ➤ Hypoxemia
- ➤ Thyrotoxicosis
- ➤ Fever
- ➤ Infection
- ➤ Adverse drug effects

- ■ Pharmacologic manipulation of the myocardial oxygen supply/demand relationship. The most commonly used pharmacologic agents are:
  - ➤ Beta-adrenergic blocking agents: Decrease myocardial oxygen demand by decreasing heart rate & contractility. Optimal blockade results in a resting HR 50–60 bpm. Care should be exercised in pts w/ significant ventricular dysfunction, conduction abnormalities, or bronchospastic disease.
  - ➤ Angiotensin-converting enzyme inhibitors: Reduce afterload & improve survival in pts w/ MI or CHF. May reduce or reverse ventricular remodeling.
  - ➤ Lipid modifiers: Improve long-term survival by modifying coronary plaque.
  - ➤ Nitrates: Vasodilator (venous > arterial) that dilates all vessels. Lowering of blood pressure reduces myocardial oxygen demand while maintaining coronary blood flow constant. Improves demand/supply balance. May improve symptoms in CHF. No negative inotropic effect.
  - ➤ Calcium channel blockers: Reduction of myocardial oxygen demand by decreasing cardiac afterload & increasing blood flow to the heart (coronary vasodilation). Verapamil & diltiazem also reduce demand by slowing HR. All agents potentiate the circulatory effects of volatile agents. No improvement in long-term survival.
  - ➤ Antiplatelet agents: Aspirin & super-aspirins. May prevent thrombosis. May cause profound bleeding after surgery.
  - ➤ Diuretics: Lower total blood volume to reduce myocardial demand. May affect electrolyte balance.
- ■ PTCA
  - ➤ Catheter-based intervention for correction of coronary lesions
  - ➤ Technique & indications for use constantly evolving
  - ➤ Stent & treated stent placement reduces re-stenosis rate.
  - ➤ PTCA in last 3 months increases risk of myocardial events.
- ■ CABG

➤ Indicated in significant 3-vessel disease, significant left main lesion, or in pts w/ significant disease & CHF
➤ Can be performed w/ or w/o extracorporeal circulatory support
➤ Risk is high: mortality 3.2%, stroke 3%, global encephalopathy 3%.

PREOP

Preop risk factors of cardiac morbidity:
■ Primary risk factors
➤ CHF
  • Risk of perioperative cardiac complications is increased in pts w/ CHF.
  • Many die suddenly, presumably of dysrhythmias.
  • CHF progresses w/ time.
  • Beta blockers, ACE inhibitors, & implantable cardioverter/defibrillator (ICD) improve survival.
➤ Previous MI
  • Along with CHF, one of two most important preoperative risk factors is a history of recent MI (within 6 mo).
  • Risk of perioperative MI in the surgical population is 0.7%; with CAD, risk is 3%; prior MI (6 mo) risk is 6–37%.
➤ Angina
  • Stable angina is induced by exercise or stress, resolves with rest, can be controlled with medication. No change in pattern, frequency, or causes.
  • Unstable angina occurs at rest or is characterized by increasing severity or number of anginal episodes. Unstable angina may be difficult to control medically & reflects severe underlying coronary disease. It frequently precedes MI. Diabetics have a relatively high incidence of silent ischemia. Women often present w/ atypical chest pain.
➤ Hypertension
  • A risk factor for CAD & perioperative MI
➤ Dysrhythmias
  • Ventricular dysrhythmias & supraventricular dysrhythmias are often assoc w/ underlying myocardial disease (CAD, dilated CM) & are assoc w/ increased risk.
  • There is no increase in risk assoc w/ isolated premature ventricular contractions w/o evidence of underlying cardiac disease.
➤ Prior cardiac surgery

- Review old records to determine the nature of surgery, adequacy of repair, cardiac anatomy, need for anticoagulation therapy and/or antibiotic prophylaxis.
- CABG has been shown to decrease future risk, but PTCA has not been proven to have the same result.
- Graft patency after CABG varies with time & type. LIMA grafts have 95% 10-year patency. Most saphenous grafts occlude by 10 years.

■ Secondary risk factors
➤ Diabetes mellitus
- Morbidity & mortality are greater in diabetic pts.
- Duration of disease increases risk.
- Pts on oral hypoglycemic agents have equal risk to those on insulin.
➤ Age
- The incidence of CAD & perioperative MI increases w/ age.
- By age 65, the incidence of CAD is close to 37% for men, 18% for women.
➤ Cigarette smoking
- Smoking may double the risk of CAD.
➤ Hypercholesterolemia
➤ Obesity
➤ Genetics
- Cardiac morbidity & mortality in a first-degree relative is significant.
➤ Vascular disease
- All pts undergoing vascular surgery or w/ prior vascular surgery should be assumed to have CAD.
- Vascular surgery pts have an increased incidence of perioperative MI.
- Peripheral vascular disease has higher risk than aortic disease.
■ Surgical procedures carrying the highest risk of perioperative MI:
➤ Major abdominal, thoracic, & emergency surgery.
➤ Highest-risk procedures are vascular since all pts have CAD.

Preop Evaluation
■ History
➤ Questions should encompass symptoms, current & past treatment, complications, results of previous evaluations.

➣ The most important symptoms to elicit are chest pain, dyspnea, orthopnea, paroxysmal nocturnal dyspnea, poor exercise tolerance, syncope, or near-syncope.

➣ Relate symptoms to activity level.

➣ Cardiac function is the best predictor of outcome in surgery.

■ Physical exam: Routine PE w/ particular attention to the following:

➣ Evidence of jugular venous distention and/or carotid bruits.

➣ Pulmonary evidence of rhonchi, rales, wheezing, or effusion.

➣ Cardiac exam documenting evidence of heaves, thrills, murmurs, rubs, or gallops.

➣ Abdominal exam for evidence of aortic aneurysm or cardiac dysfunction (hepatomegaly).

➣ Examination of extremities & peripheral pulses. Note cyanosis, clubbing, or edema.

■ Routine laboratory evaluation

➣ Tailor to pt & specifics of surgery.

➣ Pts w/ known CAD should have BUN & creatinine studies, CXR, ECG.

➣ Obtain a hemoglobin level if significant blood loss is expected.

➣ For pts who have a history compatible w/ recent unstable angina or MI, enzyme release (Troponin-I) will demonstrate increased risk.

■ Specialized studies: No current recommendations for prophylactic testing. Tests should be obtained only if there will be a modification of technique or procedure. Indications for periop testing are identical to those for pt's medical condition w/o regard for planned operation.

➣ Preop ECG: Useful for comparison to postop ECG in face of clinical event. Low-risk screen in pts w/ risk for CAD.

➣ Preop CXR: Useful in cases of pulmonary disease or CHF

■ None of the following tests are indicated prior to noncardiac surgery:

➣ Holter monitoring: Used to evaluate arrhythmias, antiarrhythmic drug therapy, severity & frequency of ischemic episodes

➣ Exercise stress testing: Gives estimate of functional capacity. Highly predictive when ST-segment changes are characteristic of ischemia. Usefulness of test limited in those w/ baseline ST-segment abnormalities and those who are unable to raise heart rate. 65% sensitivity, 90% sensitivity.

➣ Thallium imaging: Thallium is a radioactive tracer injected IV & avidly extracted as a potassium analog by cardiac muscle. Best for detecting 3-vessel disease. High sensitivity but only fairly good specificity. A dipyridamole-thallium study may be useful in pts who are unable to exercise.

> 2-D echocardiography: Provides information about both regional & global ventricular function. Transesophageal views provide better visualization of valvular function, mural or atrial thrombi, aortic atheroma, aortic aneurysms. Dobutamine stress echocardiography indicates presence of reversible ischemia.

> Radionuclide angiography: Evaluates left ventricular ejection fraction both at rest & following exercise. Failure of ejection fraction to rise w/ exercise AND evidence of new wall motion abnormalities has a 90% specificity & sensitivity for CAD.

> Coronary angiography: Gold standard in evaluating CAD. Should be performed only to determine if pt would benefit from CABG or PTCA. Presence of left main disease w/ high degree of stenosis is life-threatening. Ventriculography & measurement of intracardiac pressures can also be performed.

Preop Management

■ Periop beta blockade

> All pts w/ known coronary artery disease, peripheral vascular disease, or two risk factors for coronary artery disease (age >=65, hypertension, diabetes, smoking, cholesterol >=240 mg/dL) should be on a beta blocker unless absolute contraindications exist.

> In cases of beta blocker intolerance alpha-2 agonist therapy (clonidine #2 TTS Patch + 0.2 mg PO tablet) reduces risk of mortality.

■ Maintain all cardiac medications throughout the periop period. Stopping beta blockers, nitrates, calcium channel blockers, alpha-2 agonists, or ACE inhibitors increases risk of death & significant morbidity (stroke, renal failure, CHF).

■ Supportive preop interview may reduce fears, anxiety, pain. Anxiolytic premedication may blunt rises in sympathetic tone. Pain mgt is critical to reduce stress of surgery.

■ Supplemental oxygen preop to all w/ significant ischemia.

INTRAOP

■ Regional vs. general anesthesia: There are no outcome data showing the superiority of a form of anesthesia

■ Monitoring

- ➤ Use standard monitoring in all cases
- ➤ Intra-arterial pressure monitoring
  - Useful in pts w/ known coronary artery disease, CHF, or cardiac risk factors
- ➤ Transesophageal echocardiography
  - Useful in cardiac surgery to evaluate aortic atherosclerosis, valve function, ventricular function, volume status, ventricular dysfunction
  - No benefit in routine use in noncardiac surgery
- ➤ CVP/PA catheter
  - No proven benefit to CVP or PA catheter monitoring
  - Controversial: PA catheter monitoring may increase risk of death in pts w/ acute MI or in ICU pts.
- ■ Induction
  - ➤ Avoid precipitous changes in perfusion pressure. Initiation of vasoactive therapy prior to induction may stabilize pt.
- ■ Maintenance
  - ➤ No demonstrated benefits to a particular anesthetic agent
    - Desflurane can increase the risk of myocardial ischemia, MI, & pulmonary hypertension. Consider another agent or use w/ caution in pts w/ known CAD.
  - ➤ Hemodynamic management
    - Avoid tachycardia.
    - Maintain diastolic blood pressure.
    - Transient hypertension is well tolerated.
    - Prolonged periods of hypotension, tachycardia, & anemia are not well tolerated.
  - ➤ Drug therapy
    - Beta blockers by bolus or infusion decrease HR & can be used to treat ischemia & prevent MI infarction & death.
    - Nitroglycerin by continuous infusion (0.5–4.0 mcg/kg/min) can be used to treat ischemia.

POSTOP

- ■ Decide postop disposition (ward, ICU, telemetry) based on severity of CAD, stress of surgery, intraop course.
- ■ In immediate postop period, pt should receive supplemental oxygen until adequate oxygenation established.
- ■ Maintain good analgesia to blunt stress response.
- ■ If there is a suspicion of fluid overload, or if pt has history of poor ventricular function, obtain postop CXR. Important: Maintain all

cardiac medications, including beta blockers, calcium channel blockers, nitrates, ACE inhibitors, alpha-2 agonists.

- Issues related to postop MI
  - Most common cause of postop MI is tachycardia. Emergence, pain, & nondepolarizing neuromuscular blockade reversal can exacerbate tachycardia.
  - Atrial fibrillation on postop days 1–3 from fluid mobilization is a risk factor for MI.
  - Postop days 0–3 is the most common time for MI in noncardiac surgical pts.
  - A single 1-min episode of myocardial ischemia increases risk of MI 10-fold and death 2-fold.
  - A common presentation is unexplained hypotension or confusion.

CUSHING'S SYNDROME

ANNEMARIE THOMPSON, MD

OVERVIEW

- Definition: Cushing's syndrome is a term used to describe the manifestations of excessive corticosteroids. Usually due to exogenous steroid administration but can also be caused by adrenal cortical tumors.
- Cushing's disease refers to hypercortisolism due to ACTH secretion by a pituitary adenoma.
- Ectopic ACTH production by small-cell lung cancer or carcinoid tumor, for example, can stimulate adrenal hyperfunction.
- Clinical manifestations of hypercortisolism
  - Central obesity
  - "Moon face"
  - "Buffalo hump"
  - Supraclavicular fat pad
  - Abdominal striae
  - Thin extremities
  - Easy bruising
  - Poor wound healing
  - Hyperglycemia/diabetes
  - Hypertension
  - Mood instability

PREOP

Issues/Evaluation

- May be difficult IV access due to easy bruising & thin skin/tissue over extremities
- Increased risk of infection
- Need to consider glucose control perioperatively to improve wound healing & maintain hydration (hyperglycemia can lead to polyuria)

What To Do

- As per pt's comorbid conditions

INTRAOP

Management

- If taking oral corticosteroids, pt may need stress-dose steroids perioperatively.
- Glucose control w/ insulin to facilitate wound healing & to prevent polyuria from hyperglycemia.
- Consider minimal use of tape/adhesive on skin (especially eyelids) to avoid injuring skin w/ tape removal.
- Pt may need intraop management of HTN.

POSTOP

- Continued glycemic control

DEEP VENOUS THROMBOSIS (DVT)

MANUEL PARDO, JR., MD

OVERVIEW

- Definition: thrombosis of the deep venous system. The most serious complication is subsequent pulmonary embolism (PE). Greatest risk is for thrombosis in pelvic & thigh veins.
- Classic risk factors for venous thrombosis: venous stasis, hypercoagulability, endothelial damage
- Postop DVT is common in certain settings (eg, hip & joint replacement surgery, multiple trauma, major surgery in cancer pt).
- Usual Rx: anticoagulation w/ unfractionated heparin, low-molecular-weight heparin (LMWH), or warfarin

PREOP

Issues/Evaluation

- Pt w/ superficial venous thrombosis may have tender, erythematous cord along path of vein. These pts may have coexisting DVT.
- DVT may be asymptomatic.
- Physical exam is notoriously unreliable in detecting DVT, but findings may include edema, pain on extremity palpation.
- Diagnostic tests may include Doppler ultrasound, plethysmography, or venography.

What To Do

- Important: If pt is on anticoagulants, or if postop DVT prophylaxis includes LMWH, risk of epidural hematoma w/ central neuraxial block is increased. Discuss risk/benefit ratio w/ pt & surgeon, & consider following guidelines in Spinal & Epidural complications chapter.
- If pt is on anticoagulants, determine previous history of thrombosis & assess risk of DVT/PE if anticoagulants are stopped. May need to consult hematology to define this risk, especially for thrombotic disorders.
- Important: Decide, in conjunction w/ surgeon and/or hematologist, whether to stop anticoagulant, & when to stop.
- Obtain PT if pt on warfarin & PTT if pt on unfractionated heparin. PTT not useful in assessing anticoagulation w/ LMWH.
- If pt suspected of having preop DVT, obtain diagnostic test & postpone elective surgery if positive for DVT.
- Assess risk for postop DVT & discuss DVT prophylaxis plan w/ surgeon and/or hematologist.
  - ➤ Most significant risk factors
    - Inherited or acquired thrombotic disorder: activated protein C resistance (factor V Leiden), antiphospholipid antibody syndrome, lupus anticoagulant, protein C or S deficiency, antithrombin III deficiency, prothrombin variant 20210A, heparin-induced thrombocytopenia, hyperhomocystinemia, myeloproliferative disorders
    - Prior DVT or PE
    - Age >60
  - ➤ Other risk factors: MI/CHF, stroke, spinal cord injury, multiple trauma, malignancy, hip fracture or joint replacement surgery, major surgery, morbid obesity, prolonged operative time, oral contraceptive use, varicose veins, pregnancy

INTRAOP

■ If pt has known DVT, watch for signs of PE during surgery (eg, impaired oxygenation, decreased end-tidal CO_2, increased end-tidal CO_2 to PCO_2 gradient, unexplained hypotension). TEE may be useful intraop diagnostic test.

■ For pts at high risk of developing DVT, consider intermittent pneumatic compression (IPC) device & elastic stockings. Place at start of case or preop.

POSTOP

■ Appropriate DVT prophylaxis

■ For high-risk pts, options include LMWH, warfarin, heparin + IPC devices & elastic stockings.

■ Other options: low-dose unfractionated heparin or LMWH alone, IPC or elastic stockings, early ambulation

■ Appropriate vigilance for DVT or PE

DEMENTIA AND DEVELOPMENTAL DELAY

JASON WIDRICH, MD

OVERVIEW

■ Developmental delay: refers to a child who does not reach expected milestones.
  ➤ This can be related to congenital or other genetic disorders (eg, inborn errors of metabolism), or it may result from infectious or environmental insult (eg, birth trauma).
  ➤ Many people w/ developmental delay survive to adulthood.

■ Dementia: refers to a decline from a former level of cognitive function, usually w/ a normal level of consciousness.
  ➤ Often associated w/ deficits in memory, orientation, judgment, concentration.
  ➤ Most common causes: Alzheimer's disease, metabolic/endocrine disorders, infection (bacterial, viral, prion), cerebrovascular disease

PREOP

Issues/Evaluation

■ Determine the etiology of the dementia or developmental delay. If this has not been diagnosed, then an evaluation prior to proceeding w/ surgery may be in the pt's best interest (eg, diagnosis of treatable causes of dementia).

■ Determine if pt is at his/her baseline physical condition.

■ Pt may not have the capacity to communicate well.
  ➤ Include medical history, periop problems.
  ➤ Informed consent from the pt may not be possible.
  ➤ Interview the person who is legally responsible for making medical decisions & check for documentation re: advance directives or requests.

■ Many pts w/ dementia are from the geriatric population & have physiologic changes w/ aging that may affect anesthetic mgt.
  ➤ Diminished cardiac reserve can cause BP drop w/ anesthetic induction.
  ➤ Decreasing maximal HR w/ age.
  ➤ Decreased baroreceptor reflex.
  ➤ Closing capacity begins to exceed functional residual capacity.
  ➤ Decreased PaO_2, cough, muscle strength, peak flow
  ➤ Blunting of response to hypoxia & hypercapnia
  ➤ Decreased GFR, renal blood flow, tubular function
  ➤ Hepatic blood flow, liver function, biotransformation decrease.
  ➤ Arthritic joints & decreased bone density (may have implications for positioning during surgery)
  ➤ Skin more friable & likely to bruise

■ Many pts w/ developmental delay exhibit signs or symptoms as part of a known syndrome. Pay particular attention to cardiovascular (cyanotic heart disease), musculoskeletal (scoliosis, tethered cord, atlantoaxial subluxation w/ Down's syndrome), or airway (micrognathia, microcephaly) anomalies.

What To Do

■ Prepare pt for surgery in a quiet area w/ caregiver present.

■ Try to establish rapport w/ pt. Do not be disturbed by the pt's behavior, even if others are. Try to work at the pt's tempo. Avoid rushing pt.

■ Pt may be uncooperative for physical exam & lab studies, but these should be performed if needed.

■ Pt may be reluctant to go to the OR. Mgt depends on whether pt will permit an IV to be placed.
  ➤ Place an IV if possible.
  ➤ Be prepared to give IV premedication. Pt may permit IV placement but nonetheless be reluctant to go to the OR.

- If pt will not permit IV placement
  - For children, consider oral premedication w/ midazolam 0.5–1.0 mg/kg or ketamine 10 mg/kg.
  - If child will not take PO, can give midazolam intranasally, 0.3 mg/kg.
- For pt who will not take IV or PO
  - Consider IM ketamine 2–5 mg/kg (use a ketamine concentration of 100 mg/mL to minimize the injected volume).
    - Pt should be prone or facing a wall so he/she has fewer escape options during injection.
    - Syringe & needle should be hidden until the last minute so pt doesn't know he/she is receiving an injection.
    - Once the injection is performed, monitor pt until appropriately sedated, then take to OR.
    - Keep an oxygen supply source nearby & apply pulse oximetry as soon as possible.

INTRAOP
- General anesthesia is preferred because it may not be possible to obtain pt cooperation for regional anesthesia.
- If pt has an IV line, anesthesia may be induced IV.
- If pt does not have an IV placed preop, an inhaled induction may be performed.
  - Look for relative contraindications (eg, symptomatic gastroesophageal reflux disease).
- If pt w/o IV received ketamine (either PO or IM), it is often possible to place an IV in the OR prior to induction.
- A simple anesthetic is often the best choice, because pts w/ developmental delay or dementia may be more sedated than expected postop.
  - Assessment of postop altered mental status may be easier if a simple anesthetic with few drugs is used.
  - Developmentally delayed pts who are otherwise healthy may present for dental work requiring general anesthesia. A volatile anesthetic, w/ or w/o premed, is often all that is required.

Management
- In elderly pts w/ dementia, pay close attention to positioning secondary to "stiff joints." Risks of neurologic & dermatologic (tape/Bovie pads/pinching) injury is higher in these pts.

■ Pts w/ comorbid conditions (cardiac/respiratory/renal/hepatic) should be treated according to recommendations for their specific conditions.

POSTOP
■ Pt may require restraints or padding of gurney to prevent injury from excessive movement or thrashing during emergence from anesthesia.
■ Emergence & return to baseline mental status after anesthesia may be delayed.
■ Any measures to assist in reorientation should be employed (eg, window view, presence of family or caregiver).
■ Assess ability of family or caretaker to bring pt home after outpt surgery.
■ Investigation into other causes of altered mental status should be considered for pts who do not return to baseline mental status or are exhibiting new deficits after the initial recovery period.

DIABETES INSIPIDUS

LISA SWOR-YIM, MD

OVERVIEW
■ Definition: disorder characterized by polyuria & polydipsia
  ➣ Can lead to hypernatremia if thirst mechanism defective or if no access to water
  ➣ Two types: central (also called neurogenic) & nephrogenic
■ Central diabetes insipidus: a condition associated w/ inadequate secretion of antidiuretic hormone (ADH)
  ➣ Causes
    • Idiopathic (approx 50%)
    • Disease of the hypothalamus or pituitary, including trauma, tumor, cysts, granuloma, aneurysm, meningitis, encephalitis
  ➣ Usual Rx: DDAVP (desmopressin), vasopressin, or drug that promotes release of ADH (eg, chlorpropamide)
■ Nephrogenic diabetes insipidus: a condition associated w/ decreased renal sensitivity to ADH
  ➣ Variety of etiologies: congenital, drug-induced, hypokalemia, hypercalcemia, sickle cell disease, myeloma, renal disease

- Microvascular disease
  - Neuropathy (peripheral & autonomic)
  - Nephropathy
  - Retinopathy
- Macrovascular disease
  - Coronary artery disease
  - Cerebrovascular disease
  - Peripheral vascular disease
- Nonvascular complications include
  - Gastropathy, gastroparesis
  - Altered large & small bowel motility (both constipation & diarrhea)
  - Sexual dysfunction
- Complications of therapy
  - Hypoglycemia related to excess insulin, oral agent or inadequate carbohydrate intake
  - Side effect of oral agent
    - Metformin is associated w/ lactic acidosis in type II DM w/ renal failure or other condition predisposing to decreased tissue perfusion.
    - Stop metformin at least 1 day prior to surgery & before any procedure involving iodinated contrast dye.
- DM & cardiovascular disease
  - DM is a major risk factor for CAD.
  - Pts may have silent ischemia related to neuropathy.
  - Periop beta blockade (eg, metoprolol, atenolol) can reduce risk of cardiac complications.
  - Increased risk of CAD w/ DM plus HTN supports long-term control of BP to <130/80 mmHg.
- Anesthetic implications of DM complications include
  - CAD concerns mentioned above.
  - Peripheral neuropathy: pt may be more vulnerable to positioning injury.
  - Hyperglycemia worsens injury from CNS ischemia, which is a risk of certain surgical procedures (eg, carotid surgery, neurosurgery, cardiac surgery).
  - Hyperglycemic pts may be hypovolemic from osmotic diuresis.
  - Pts are at increased risk of IV contrast-induced nephropathy.
    - Treatment w/ oral Mucomyst (acetylcysteine) plus IV hydration may prevent this.

- Dose for renal protection is acetylcysteine 600 mg PO BID for 2 days, starting day before IV contrast procedure.

What To Do
■ Evaluate for the presence of acute or chronic complications of DM.
 ➤ Consider specialized workup for CAD, given common occurrence of silent ischemia.
 ➤ Consider administration of periop beta blockers (eg, metoprolol, atenolol) to reduce risk of cardiac complications.
 ➤ Electrolytes, BUN, creatinine to assess renal function.
■ Determine drug therapy for DM & assess glycemic control.
 ➤ Tight glycemic control has been shown to prevent or reduce neuropathy, retinopathy, nephropathy for both type I and type II DM.
■ Correct ketoacidosis or hyperosmolarity before surgery if possible.
 ➤ Surgery may need to be performed to bring hyperglycemia or ketoacidosis under control (eg, in pts w/ an abscess or uncontrolled infection).
■ Correct hypoglycemia before surgery if possible.
■ For pt w/ gastroparesis.
 ➤ Give metoclopramide & nonparticulate antacid.
 ➤ Plan for rapid sequence induction.
■ For type I DM: strongly consider tight control of glucose, which may lead to improved periop outcomes.
 ➤ Tight control involves insulin & glucose infusion to target glucose 80–120 mg/dL, although upper glucose limit of 150 is probably acceptable.
 ➤ Would certainly maintain glucose <200 mg/dL, as this has been demonstrated to reduce infection rate
 ➤ Best option is for pt to withhold insulin on morning of surgery & have insulin drip started on arrival to the hospital.
 ➤ Ideally, pt should be scheduled as first case of the day. Alternatively, pt can be admitted to preop area or PACU prior to surgery for IV start & insulin drip.
■ For type II DM
 ➤ Withhold oral agent on the day of surgery (to minimize risk of hypoglycemia).
 ➤ Monitor blood glucose w/ IV start, or at start of surgery.
 ➤ Decide threshold for insulin administration. 200 mg/dL may be reasonable, depending on pt, procedure, length of surgery (see below).

- One suggested adult insulin drip regimen
  - ➤ Add 25 units regular insulin to 250 mL NS (concentration 0.1 units/mL).
  - ➤ Flush IV tubing w/ at least 50 mL solution (due to insulin adsorption to tubing).
  - ➤ Start infusion of D5NS or D5 1/2 NS at 100 mL/h (provides insulin substrate & reduces risk of hypoglycemia).
  - ➤ Start insulin drip using an infusion pump at 1 unit/h if pt taking >30 units insulin/day.
    - Start insulin drip at 1.5 unit/h if taking >30 units insulin/day.
  - ➤ Check glucose prior to starting drip & continue hourly. Adjust insulin drip accordingly:
    - Glucose <60: stop insulin, administer 50 mL D50. Check glucose q15min until >100. Resume drip at reduced rate when glucose >100.
    - Glucose 60–80: stop insulin, check glucose q15min until >100. Resume drip at reduced rate when glucose >100.
    - Glucose >250: bolus 5 units IV regular insulin, increase drip by 0.5 units/h.
    - Glucose within target range: continue infusion at current rate.
    - Glucose above target range but <250: increase infusion by 0.5 units/h.
    - Glucose below target range but >80: decrease infusion by 0.5 units/h.

INTRAOP

- In type I DM, tight glycemic control is desirable. Priorities also include
  - ➤ Avoiding ketoacidosis from inadequate insulin.
  - ➤ Avoiding hypoglycemia from overaggressive treatment.
- For type II DM, pts undergoing long or stressful surgery (eg, cardiac surgery, major vascular surgery) may benefit from tight glycemic control, although the evidence is not as strong as for type I DM.
  - ➤ Tight glucose control is required if CNS ischemia is anticipated.
- Monitor for myocardial ischemia. If severe CAD, CHF, or autonomic dysfunction is present, invasive monitoring may be needed.
- Pt w/ peripheral neuropathy may be at increased risk of positioning injury & hence should be positioned carefully.

Management

- Rapid sequence induction if gastroparesis present

■ Anticipate lability in BP (eg, from hypovolemia secondary to osmotic diuresis, or autonomic dysfunction).
■ Monitor glucose regularly (eg, hourly).
  ➤ For type I DM, goal is blood glucose 80–150 mg/dL.
  ➤ For type II DM, would consider insulin therapy to maintain glucose <200 mg/dL.
■ Rx w/ regular insulin IV
  ➤ IV infusion (discussed above) is preferable given short half-life of IV insulin.
  ➤ Do not give SQ owing to irregular absorption in vasoconstricted pt (eg, from hypothermia or pressors). Do not give long-acting insulin formulations.

POSTOP
■ Continue glucose monitoring postop.
  ➤ Avoid SQ regular insulin sliding scale, as this can create periods of insulin deficiency.
■ For pts requiring postop ICU care
  ➤ One large randomized study demonstrated improved outcome in hyperglycemic surgical pts requiring postop ICU care (both type I and II DM) w/ tight glycemic control (insulin drip to maintain blood glucose 80–110 mg/dL).
■ Evaluate for postop myocardial ischemia or infarction.
  ➤ Check ECG.
  ➤ Consider cardiac enzyme evaluation (eg, troponin) depending on risks of surgery & intraop course.

DISSEMINATED INTRAVASCULAR COAGULATION (DIC)

ANNE NOONEY, MD

OVERVIEW
■ Definition: widespread activation of clotting system
  ➤ Leads to IV fibrin deposition & thrombosis of small & medium-sized blood vessels
    • Can lead to multiple organ failure
  ➤ Leads to consumption of coagulation factors & platelets, leading to coagulopathy & bleeding
■ Causes: high-risk situations for development of DIC include
  ➤ Sepsis, especially w/ bacterial infection
  ➤ Trauma, especially w/ head trauma

➤ Malignancy, both solid organ & hematologic
➤ Obstetric complications (eg, preeclampsia, placental abruption)
➤ Vascular causes: giant hemangioma, large aortic aneurysms
➤ Other
  • Severe allergic reaction
  • Hemolytic transfusion reaction
  • Transplant rejection
  • Toxins
■ Usual Rx
  ➤ Treatment of underlying disease is most important & effective.
  ➤ Supportive therapy depends on major complication: thrombosis (eg, acrocyanosis or multiorgan failure) or hemorrhage.
    • PRBC, FFP, platelets, coagulation inhibitors
  ➤ Heparin therapy is controversial & has not shown consistent effectiveness.
    • Typical dose: 300–500 units/h

PREOP

Issues/Evaluation
■ DIC requires urgent evaluation & mgt.
  ➤ DIC is a risk factor for morbidity & mortality.
■ Diagnosis: no single test is definitive
■ Typical findings
  ➤ Underlying disorder w/ increased risk of DIC
  ➤ Elevated PT, PTT
  ➤ Platelet count <100, or decreasing on serial measurements
  ➤ Increase in fibrin degradation products (eg, D-dimers)
  ➤ Decreased level of plasma coagulation inhibitors (eg, antithrombin III)
  ➤ Decreased fibrinogen (not reliable since fibrinogen is an acute-phase reactant)
■ Pt may be presenting for surgery to correct underlying disease, or for complication of disease (eg, severe trauma & brain injury; abscess in pt w/ sepsis).

What To Do
■ Treat underlying disease.
■ Postpone elective surgery in pt w/ treatable cause of DIC.
■ If pt w/ DIC requires surgery, discuss risks of thrombosis & hemorrhage w/ pt & surgeon.

> Correct abnormalities in PT, PTT, platelets w/ appropriate blood products.
> Avoid regional nerve blocks.

INTRAOP

■ Arterial line may be useful to facilitate multiple blood draws, though bleeding risk of invasive lines may be increased.
■ Check CBC & coagulation panel regularly during surgery. Administer blood products as necessary.
■ Anticipate increased surgical blood loss due to coagulopathy.
> Place adequate IV access.
> Order FFP early, as time to thaw may be 45 min or greater.

POSTOP

■ Continue close evaluation of lab values & appropriate blood transfusion.
■ Consider whether pt will benefit from postop care in the ICU.

ELEVATED INTRACRANIAL PRESSURE

KURT DITTMAR, MD
DHANESH K. GUPTA, MD

OVERVIEW

■ Definition: although normal intracranial pressure (ICP) is <10 mm Hg, elevated ICP is usually defined as >20 mmHg. This chapter deals w/ the pt w/ a known elevation in ICP. See also Critical Event chapter "Elevated ICP" for pt who acutely develops elevated ICP.
■ Increased ICP places the brain at risk for ischemia & herniation.
> Ischemia may result since adequate cerebral perfusion pressure (CPP) relies upon the difference between mean arterial pressure (MAP) & ICP.
> Herniation can occur when pressure increase is enough to force brain contents through the foramen magnum. Other types of herniation are also possible.
■ Since the cranial vault size is fixed, initial compensatory mechanisms (CSF & venous blood translocation) to maintain a normal ICP in the presence of a volume-increasing lesion (tumor, edema, hematoma, hydrocephalus) will eventually fail.
■ Cardiovascular manifestations

> Tachyarrhythmias
> Bradyarrhythmias
> Hypertension
- Pulmonary manifestations
  > Irregular respirations
  > Respiratory arrest
- Other manifestations: neurologic deficit, coma, death
- Procedures or conditions w/ increased risk
  > Any intracranial procedure
  > Blunt trauma (eg, motor vehicle accident)
  > Head trauma
  > Recent stroke

PREOP
- Evaluate carefully if pt at risk for intracranial process.
- Early signs
  > Headache
  > Nausea
  > Vomiting
  > Somnolence
  > Blurred vision
  > Papilledema
- Late signs
  > Hypertension
  > Irregular respiration
  > Third cranial nerve palsy (pupillary dilation)
  > Contralateral hemiplegia/paresis
- Very late signs
  > Coma
  > Respiratory arrest
- Cushing's triad: increased ICP, leading to
  > Hypertension
  > Bradycardia
  > Respiratory irregularities
- CT scan findings
  > Midline shift
  > Loss of sulci
  > Edema
  > Ventricular effacement
  > Basal cistern obliteration
- ICP monitors

➤ Pt w/ known or suspected elevation in ICP may have an ICP monitor in place. The monitors differ in their monitoring method & ability to drain CSF.
  • Epidural or subdural fiberoptic monitor (eg, Camino bolt): no CSF drainage possible
  • Ventriculostomy (AKA external ventricular drain [EVD]): CSF drainage possible. Drain connected to pressure transducer & reservoir system. Height of reservoir w/ respect to brain determines CSF pressure required for CSF to drain.

INTRAOP

■ Providing anesthesia care for a pt w/ a known elevation of ICP requires knowledge of the specific intracranial process (eg, stroke vs trauma vs tumor, etc.) & therapy already administered. It is important to reduce ICP to prevent herniation & minimize secondary brain injury that can worsen neurologic outcome.
■ Reduction of ICP revolves around decreasing volume of the intracranial vault & treating the underlying process if possible.
  ➤ Intracranial volume consists of normal brain, CSF, blood vessels, plus abnormal masses or collections (eg, tumor, edema, hematoma).
  ➤ Specific treatment depends on exact intracranial process.
■ General measures to consider
  ➤ Elevate head of bed to 30 degrees & avoid extreme head rotation or neck flexion to encourage cerebral venous drainage.
  ➤ Prevent straining & coughing, which may precipitously worsen ICP from elevated intrathoracic pressure & reduced cerebral venous drainage.
    • In mechanically ventilated pt, consider administration of opiates or neuromuscular blockade.
    • Risk of these drugs is that neurologic exam is altered.
    • Discuss risk/benefit ratio w/ neurosurgeon or neurologist (eg, if ICP monitor in place, exam may be less important).
  ➤ Control airway w/ tracheal intubation.
    • Hyperventilation to $PaCO_2$ of 25–30 mmHg reduces ICP within 5 min.
    • Avoid excessive hyperventilation, since cerebral ischemia may result from decreased cerebral blood flow (CBF).
    • If ICP returns to normal, consider allowing CO_2 to rise to 30–35 mmHg (mild hyperventilation).

- If pt has received hyperventilation for >12–16 h, do not allow CO_2 to rise rapidly, as this can cause rebound increase in CBF & increased ICP.
➤ Mannitol, 0.5–2.0 g/kg IV, & Lasix, 10 mg, to reduce cerebral edema (works within 30 min)
➤ Reduction of CSF volume through a ventriculostomy
  - This leads to an immediate reduction in ICP.
➤ Steroids not useful for acute treatment of elevated ICP
  - Longer-term therapy may reduce cerebral edema associated w/ tumors.
➤ Consider barbiturate therapy (eg, pentobarbital, thiopental).
  - Barbiturates decrease cerebral blood volume secondary to cerebral vasoconstriction & decrease $CMRO_2$.
  - Net result is reduction in ICP w/ a less metabolically active brain.
  - Main risk is hypotension & hemodynamic instability, which could worsen CPP & lead to secondary brain injury.
➤ Arterial line monitoring is useful to follow ABGs, MAP, CPP.
■ Procedural considerations
➤ Pts w/ elevated ICP may require anesthesia care for a variety of procedures.
➤ Procedures to treat the intracranial process such as
  - Bur hole
  - Craniotomy
  - Endovascular surgery
➤ Diagnostic procedures
  - Head CT scan
  - Angiography
➤ Procedures unrelated to intracranial process such as
  - Exploratory laparotomy in blunt trauma pt w/ intra-abdominal hemorrhage
➤ Transport issues
  - Transport of a critically ill pt w/ elevated ICP can be challenging.
  - Maintain all ongoing therapies during transport, including hyperventilation, if appropriate.
  - Minimize episodes of hypoxemia or hypercarbia, which could result from the switch from mechanical ventilation to hand ventilation.

- If ventriculostomy is in place to measure ICP, ensure that reservoir height does not change during transport & that drain is not inadvertently clamped. This could result in rapid rise in ICP.
- Anesthetic considerations: basic principle is to choose drugs that avoid increases in CBF.
  - Volatile anesthetics: all tend to increase CBF & decrease $CMRO_2$.
    - Halothane > isoflurane, desflurane, sevoflurane
    - N_2O can increase ICP, but not as much as other volatile agents.
    - Effect increases w/ dose.
    - If volatile anesthetics used, keep dose <0.5 MAC.
  - Intravenous anesthetics: all tend to either reduce ICP due to decrease in $CMRO_2$ and CBF or have little effect, except ketamine, which increases ICP.
    - Barbiturates & etomidate have the greatest relative fall in ICP; narcotics have little decrease or no effect.
  - Muscle relaxants: goal is to minimize cardiovascular & intracranial effects by choosing agents that have little or no histamine release.
    - Histamine will cause cerebrovascular dilation.
    - Vecuronium & rocuronium are examples of relaxants w/ minimal histamine release.
    - Succinylcholine has been associated w/ mild ICP elevations; can be prevented with defasciculation; has been safely used in STP-succinylcholine-hyperventilation inductions.
  - Vasoactive drugs: vasopressor-induced increases in arterial blood pressure can elevate ICP if MAP is greater than the upper limit of pressure autoregulation (150 mmHg in normotensive pts)
    - If MAP is maintained within the limits of pressure autoregulation (50–150 mmHg in normotensive pts), higher MAP will result in reflexive vasoconstriction that decreases cerebral blood volume & therefore decreases ICP.
    - Vasodilators elevate ICP by increasing cerebral blood volume secondary to decreased cerebrovascular resistance.
- Induction
  - Pt w/ elevated ICP may already be intubated.
  - Otherwise goal is to have a smooth induction, w/ minimal response to laryngoscopy & other noxious stimuli.
  - Begin hyperventilation as soon as possible.
  - Use cricoid pressure to reduce risk of aspiration.
  - Use IV induction agents that reduce ICP.

- Etomidate may be less likely to cause hypotension compared to thiopental or propofol.
- Opioids usually have no effect on ICP as long as ventilation is controlled.

➤ Lidocaine IV 1.5 mg/kg may decrease response to laryngoscopy.

■ Maintenance
  ➤ Use constant neuromuscular blockade to prevent pt movements that can increase ICP (eg, coughing, bucking).
  ➤ Limit volatile anesthetics to <0.5 MAC or use propofol in 100% oxygen for maintenance.

POSTOP
■ Smooth emergence helps decrease the incidence of postop complications caused by hypertension & elevated CVP.
■ Depending on the procedure performed, pt will likely require continued tracheal intubation, mechanical ventilation & ICU monitoring.

ELEVATED PT, aPTT

JULIE HAMBLETON, MD

OVERVIEW
■ Definition: elevated PT, aPTT
■ Usual Rx: depends on underlying cause

PREOP

Issues/Evaluation
■ Approach to the isolated elevation of aPTT
  ➤ Disorders w/ high risk for bleeding
    - Heparin
    - Inherited coagulation factor: factor VIII, IX, XI
    - von Willebrand disease (VWD)
    - Acquired coagulation factor inhibitor. Pts w/ acquired inhibitors to factor VIII or VWD are at very high risk of bleeding & require subspecialty mgt. Standard factor replacement is ineffective
  ➤ Disorders w/ low risk for bleeding
    - Lupus anticoagulant
    - Factor XII, prekallikrein, or contact factor deficiency

> Pt evaluation
  • Personal history of excessive bleeding: surgery, tooth extractions, menses, postpartum, trauma
  • Family history
  • Drugs
> Labs
  • Repeat aPTT
  • Factor VIII, IX, XI levels
  • Anticardiolipin antibody
  • Russell viper venom test

Approach to isolated elevation of PT

■ Differential diagnosis
> Warfarin therapy
> Vitamin K deficiency: nutritional, antibiotic, malabsorption
> Decreased hepatic synthetic function
> Cirrhosis
> Liver disease
> Increased consumption of clotting factors–DIC
> Rare: factor VII deficiency (inherited)
■ Pt evaluation
> Personal history
> Diet, medications
> Surgery
> Alcohol intake
■ Labs
> Repeat PT
> CBC, platelets
> Fibrinogen
> Repeat PT after vitamin K therapy

Approach to combined elevation of PT, aPTT

■ Differential diagnosis
> Advanced liver disease
> Supratherapeutic heparin or warfarin therapy
> Advanced DIC
> Common pathway factor deficiency or inhibitor: factor I (fibrinogen), II (prothrombin), factor V, factor X
> Dysfibrinogenemia (inherited: rare): may be seen in pts w/ advanced liver disease
> Inhibitors to factors II & V seen in pts who receive topical thrombin (eg, Gelfoam). Acquired deficiency of factor X seen in pts w/ amyloid.

> ➤ Rarely, lupus anticoagulant antibodies cause acquired factor II deficiency

- Labs
  - ➤ Repeat PT/aPTT
  - ➤ Consider Hepasorb
  - ➤ Consider empiric vitamin K therapy & recheck values
  - ➤ CBC, platelets, fibrinogen
  - ➤ Reptilase time to evaluate dysfibrinogenemia

What To Do

- Perform clinical & lab evaluation.
- Consider hematology consult for further evaluation.
- Depending on cause & risk of bleeding, consider whether to postpone surgery for further evaluation or treatment.
- Specific mgt will depend on cause of elevated PT or aPTT.
- For pts w/ hemophilia or VWD, see Coexisting Disease chapter "Inherited Coagulation Disorders (Hemophilia, Von Willebrand Disease)."

INTRAOP

- Obtain coagulation studies as needed.
- Administer factor or blood products as required by underlying bleeding disorder.

POSTOP

- Watch for signs of hemorrhage.
- Continue factor replacement or blood product therapy as needed.
- Depending on cause of coagulation disorder, consider involvement of hematologist in postop care to better assess adequacy of replacement therapy.

EPILEPSY

MIMI C. LEE, MD, PHD
DHANESH K. GUPTA, MD

OVERVIEW

- Epilepsy is a chronic condition characterized by recurrent seizures.
- There are many classes of seizures, including partial (simple or complex) vs generalized.
- Causes of seizures include intrinsic parenchymal pathology (mass lesions, necrosis, maldevelopment), trauma, & other medical

conditions (electrolyte abnormalities, chemical toxicities & psychosis [non-epileptic seizures]).

■ Usual Rx: anticonvulsants, surgical resection of epileptic focus

PREOP

Issues/Evaluation

■ Useful to know aura (to help determine when seizure occurring) & typical seizure events (to anticipate required intervention) especially for "MAC" cases

What To Do

■ Continue anticonvulsants preop.
■ Plan for treatment of intraop seizure (airway support & protection from physical harm for short procedure; use of short-acting anticonvulsants–benzodiazepines; or even endotracheal intubation for protection from aspiration during prolonged postictal state)

INTRAOP

■ Increase seizure threshold w/ benzodiazepines, barbiturates, propofol, or vapor anesthetics.
■ Avoid decreasing seizure threshold (hypercarbia, large doses of local anesthetics).

Management

■ Airway support–mask ventilation
■ Protection from aspiration–ETT if needed
■ Protection from physical injury during generalized seizure activity (physical restraint & padding)
■ Treatment of recurrent seizures or prolonged seizure activity (benzodiazepine vs STP/propofol)

POSTOP

■ If typical seizure w/ good recovery, no additional care needed.
■ Confirm that adequate plasma levels of antiepileptics are present.

ESSENTIAL HYPERTENSION (HTN)

EDWIN CHENG, MD

OVERVIEW

■ Definition: consistent elevation of blood pressure >140/90
  ➤ For pt w/ diabetes mellitus or renal disease & proteinuria, HTN defined as BP >130/80.

➤ Essential HTN diagnosed if pt does not have a secondary cause of HTN; eg:
  • Pheochromocytoma
  • Hyperaldosteronism
  • Cushing's syndrome
  • Renovascular HTN
  • Aortic coarctation
■ Usual Rx
  ➤ Lifestyle changes suggested
    • Weight loss for obese pts
    • Moderation of alcohol use
    • Limitation of sodium intake
  ➤ Antihypertensive medication may include more than one agent:
    • ACE inhibitors
    • Beta blockers
    • Thiazide diuretics
    • Calcium channel blockers
    • Angiotensin receptor blocker

PREOP

Issues/Evaluation

■ Pts w/ uncontrolled or poorly controlled HTN are at increased risk of labile BP & periop myocardial ischemia.
  ➤ Uncontrolled HTN typically defined as diastolic blood pressure >110 mmHg.
■ End-organ damage from HTN includes
  ➤ Atherosclerotic cardiovascular disease
    • Coronary artery disease
    • Cerebral vascular disease (TIA, ischemic stroke)
    • Peripheral vascular disease
  ➤ CNS disease
    • Hemorrhagic stroke
    • Hypertensive encephalopathy
  ➤ Hypertensive cardiac disease
    • LVH, diastolic dysfunction, ultimately LV dilation & congestive heart failure (CHF)
    • Renal failure
    • Retinopathy
■ Antihypertensive medication issues
  ➤ Therapy w/ ACE inhibitors & angiotensin receptor blockers has been associated w/ severe hypotension during GA.

➤ Cessation of long-term beta blockade may result in myocardial ischemia.

➤ Abrupt cessation of clonidine may result in hypertensive crisis.

What To Do

■ Determine current antihypertensive regimen & adequacy of BP control.

➤ Continue antihypertensive meds until time of surgery.

■ Look for evidence of hypertensive cardiac disease.

➤ Obtain ECG, which may show signs of LVH.

➤ Ask for history of CHF symptoms.

• Pt w/ CHF may need further cardiac evaluation (eg, CXR, echocardiogram).

■ Evaluate risk factors for coronary artery disease.

➤ Consider additional workup depending on symptoms & risk of proposed surgery.

➤ See also Coexisting Disease chapter "Coronary Artery Disease."

■ Other evaluation for end-organ damage from HTN

➤ BUN, creatinine to assess renal function

➤ Auscultation for carotid bruit

■ For pt w/ untreated or poorly treated HTN (systolic BP >180 or diastolic BP >110)

➤ Consider delaying elective surgery until antihypertensive therapy optimized.

➤ For pt on no therapy, discuss w/ primary care provider & consider starting beta blocker therapy.

➤ For noncompliant pt, emphasize importance of BP control to periop risk.

➤ For pt on inadequate therapy, consider adding beta blocker or increasing dose of current drug therapy. Consider consultation w/ primary care provider.

➤ For urgent or emergency surgery

• In addition to starting antihypertensive therapy, mgt may require use of invasive monitors (arterial line, possible central line) to follow periop hemodynamics closely.

INTRAOP

■ Monitor for cardiac ischemia w/ 5-lead ECG.

■ Anxiolytic premed (eg, midazolam) may help decrease BP.

■ Anticipate exaggerated BP decrease upon induction of anesthesia.

■ Direct laryngoscopy & intubation.

➤ Achieve adequate depth of anesthesia prior to intubation.
➤ Expect exaggerated BP increase.
  • HTN & tachycardia w/ laryngoscopy & intubation can lead to myocardial ischemia.
➤ To control hemodynamic response to intubation, consider
  • Additional anesthetic agents
  • IV opioid
  • IV esmolol (titrate 10-mg doses to effect) prior to laryngoscopy
  • Laryngotracheal lidocaine prior to intubation
■ Maintenance of anesthesia
  ➤ Monitor closely for large BP swings.
  ➤ Anticipate key operative events that may stimulate HTN (eg, skin incision).
  ➤ Most IV & inhaled agents (except ketamine) are appropriate for maintenance.
  ➤ Use of beta blockers may provide additional BP control after adequate depth of anesthesia is achieved.
  ➤ Support hypotension w/ fluids, decreased depth of anesthesia & vasopressors, as appropriate.

POSTOP
■ Monitor postop BP closely.
  ➤ Untreated postop HTN can contribute to myocardial ischemia & disruption of surgical wound hemostasis.
  ➤ Additional antihypertensive therapy may be necessary.
  ➤ See also Critical Event chapter "Hypertension."
■ Adequate postop analgesia will help maintain normal BP.
■ Monitor for myocardial ischemia.
■ PACU vs ICU postop care will depend on severity of disease, intraop course, stress of surgery.

EX-PREMATURE INFANT

CLAIRE M. BRETT, MD

OVERVIEW
■ Definition: "term infant" is defined as >37 weeks gestation. For risk stratification, consider both gestational age & birth weight.
  ➤ Low birth weight <2,500 g
  ➤ Very low birth weight (VLBW) <1,500 g

- This group of pts is diverse, unpredictable, & complicated. There can be no periop protocol for the "generic ex-preemie." Evaluate pts based on their own medical status as well as published data. Pay attention to events of previous surgeries, recent evaluations, current status, & proposed surgical intervention.
- Although "ex-premature infant" is not a specific diagnosis, implications of premature birth for the anesthesia provider extend into the first 5–10 years of life.
- Decisions concerning specific anesthetic agents are less important than appreciation for the "surprises" & "hidden risks" these pts may present in the periop setting.
- The parents of the ex-premature infant are often
  - Medically sophisticated
  - Extremely protective of their child
  - More specific in their questions & analysis of information
  - More demanding in outlining what they desire for their child
- Parents are often the best source for obtaining a concise summary of the medical history & may have an encyclopedic memory of hospitalizations, recent illnesses, current meds, referring physician phone numbers, etc. Prepare to discuss the anesthetic plan in depth.

PREOP

Issues/Evaluation

- Common diseases in this population include neurologic (major and minor), GI (gastroesophageal reflux), pulmonary (respiratory distress syndrome, chronic lung disease, apnea of prematurity), hematologic (anemia).
- During pt evaluation, consider whether to reserve an ICU bed prior to starting case.

Neurologic

- Neurologic morbidity assoc w/ preterm birth can be divided into major & minor dysfunctions.
- Major: "cerebral palsy," mental retardation, spastic motor dysfunction, sensorineural hearing loss, visual abnormalities. Hydrocephalus or seizures often accompany serious neurologic dysfunction. Many infants who had intraventricular hemorrhage will be status post VP shunt.
- Cerebral palsy
  - Cerebral palsy is not a specific diagnosis & not a single disease entity.

➤ It refers to a nonprogressive motor impairment that may change over time. Can be secondary to a wide spectrum of prenatal brain disorders, such as CNS structural or migrational abnormalities that may be part of a systemic global disorder (eg, chromosomal).

➤ Look for an underlying but unidentified medical problem that has anesthetic implications. For instance, certain myopathies may be assoc w/ a higher incidence of malignant hyperthermia. Pharmacology of muscle relaxants may be abnormal in pt w/ primary muscular abnormalities.

■ Minor neurologic dysfunction. 25–50% of low-birth-weight infants may have less significant developmental abnormalities, such as isolated intellectual or cognition problems, speech & language disorders, learning disabilities, difficulties w/ balance & coordination, perceptual problems, emotional instability, social competence, selective attention deficits.

GI (gastroesophageal reflux)

■ Gastroesophageal reflux is a common event in infants but usually resolves by 4 mo to 1 y of age.

■ Neurologically impaired children are at high risk for symptomatic gastroesophageal reflux & delayed gastric emptying. Reflux risk is increased w/ nasogastric or gastrostomy feedings.

■ Important: Review history for symptoms of reflux.

■ Treat gastroesophageal reflux aggressively to minimize upper & lower respiratory complications, especially since ex-premature infant is already predisposed to pulmonary dysfunction. Usual Rx: H_2 blockers or proton pump inhibitors.

Pulmonary

■ The most significant problems w/ the respiratory system in ex-premature infants include:

■ Chronic lung disease

■ Bronchospasm & chronic airways obstruction

■ Apnea of prematurity

Chronic Lung Disease Secondary to Prematurity

■ Usual definition: requirement for oxygen at 36 weeks post-conceptual age w/ an abnormal respiratory exam & an abnormal CXR.

■ Disorder most commonly results from lung injury & repair in premature infants w/ respiratory distress syndrome. Most infants

who develop sequelae were born <32 weeks gestation & required mechanical ventilatory support during the first week of life.
- Pulmonary function changes include decreased functional residual capacity, obstruction of small airways, & hyperinflation. Lung volume abnormalities gradually normalize but the process continues well into adolescence.
- Reactive airway disease is common.
- Borderline oxygenation is common. Oxygen therapy may be necessary for months to years to maintain oxygen saturation 90–95%.
- Usual Rx: bronchodilators & diuretics are common in outpatient medical regimens.
- Respiratory infections can lead to worsening reactive airway disease & oxygenation. This may require hospital admission for readjustment of medications, oxygen, & nutritional support. Increased airways reactivity can persist long beyond symptoms of the acute upper respiratory infection.

Bronchospasm & Chronic Airways Obstruction
- Develop a plan for treatment of periop bronchospasm. Seek advice from family & pediatric pulmonologist regarding the most effective therapies for pt. Drug regimens may include inhaled steroids, IV steroids, bronchodilators, theophylline.
- Ex-premature infant may have obstructive airflow at school age despite lack of symptoms, even w/o history of chronic lung disease.

Apnea of Prematurity
- Problem: ex-premature infants have an increased risk of perioperative apnea.
- Age at which the ex-premature infant is considered free from the risk of perioperative apnea is not definitively known. Some experts say 44–46 weeks post-conceptual age, but others recommend 60 weeks.
- Risk factors for periop apnea include gestational age, post-conceptual age, apnea at home, anemia. Anemia is most significant in pt <43 weeks post-conceptual age. Ask parents if they use home apnea monitoring.
- No relationship between perioperative apnea & necrotizing enterocolitis (NEC), neonatal apnea, RDS, BPD, or intraop use of opioids or muscle relaxants.

Hematologic: Anemia of Prematurity
- Anemia of prematurity is a normocytic, normochromic anemia w/ low reticulocyte count & low erythropoietin level.

■ Usual Rx: recombinant human erythropoietin (rhEPO) decreases need for blood transfusions.
■ Interpret normal hemoglobin values for the ex-premature infant during the first year of life based on overall physiologic status, surgical procedure, current status, & attitude of family.
■ Consider sending a type & crossmatch for these pts.
■ Acceptable hematocrit prior to surgery: varies with pt & surgery type.
■ Prototypical case & options: ex-premature infant w/ chronic lung disease or heart disease, scheduled for elective surgery, low hemoglobin (7–8 g/dL)
  ➤ Option if blood loss likely (eg, laparotomy) or if pt at risk for perioperative apnea: begin rhEPO & iron, wait for Hgb to increase before doing surgery.
  ➤ Option if blood loss not likely (endoscopy, hernia): proceed w/ surgery.

INTRAOP

Neurologic

■ Anticipate unpredictable response to sedatives, narcotics, & inhaled agents. Consider reduced doses & more careful titration to effect.
■ Anticipate psychological implications in child w/ developmental issues.
  ➤ Separation from parents may be more difficult. Consider need for premedication or inhaled induction prior to IV, even in older child.

GI

■ Address risk of gastroesophageal reflux & delayed gastric emptying.
  ➤ Consider longer NPO time.
  ➤ Consider cricoid pressure during induction.

Pulmonary

■ Mechanical ventilator: pt may require ICU-type ventilator. Consider input from neonatologists, critical care physicians, or respiratory therapy staff.
■ Bronchospasm: develop logical approach toward treatment knowing the specific response patterns for pt.
  ➤ Anticipate bronchospasm & propensity for periop hypoxemia even in seemingly low-risk pts (eg, the ex-premature infant who was "healthy" as a newborn, & the older, school-age

ex-premature infant who is now asymptomatic & no longer needs aggressive therapy).

■ If pt at risk for retinopathy of prematurity (<44 weeks post-conceptual age), consider titrating oxygen to saturation 93–98% instead of 98–100%.

Apnea of Prematurity

■ Consider caffeine to decrease incidence of apnea. Loading dose is 20 mg/kg IV (over 30 min) caffeine citrate w/ maintenance dose of 5 mg/kg caffeine citrate IV or PO q24h. Caffeine citrate 10 mg is equivalent to caffeine base 5 mg.

■ Regional anesthesia may have lower risk of apnea than general anesthesia. Consider an exclusively regional technique w/o sedation, such as a spinal block for lower body surgery.

Hematologic

■ Decide transfusion threshold based on pt's overall physiologic status, surgery, & family attitude.

■ Hemoglobin >15 g/dL often recommended by pulmonologist or cardiologist for highest-risk pts w/ oxygen-dependent chronic lung disease, cyanotic heart disease, or heart disease assoc w/ a large left to right shunt & CHF.

■ Essential: estimate "allowable red blood cell loss" so that the parents, surgeon, & blood bank can plan for possible transfusion. If anticipated loss >1 blood volume, plan for FFP or platelet transfusion.

POSTOP

Neurologic

■ Anticipate unpredictable response to sedatives & narcotics given in PACU.

■ Postop pain control: PCA may not be appropriate.

GI

■ Plan for IV or enteral nutritional intake, depending on surgery. Infants w/ chronic lung disease have high caloric needs due to increased work of breathing.

Pulmonary

■ Strongly consider postop monitoring & supportive care in a PICU.

■ Pt w/ intraop bronchospasm: consider PICU admission for postop mgt.

Apnea of Prematurity

■ Most important postop consideration is whether to monitor for apnea in ICU. Decision is based on pt, surgery, & practice setting.

■ Monitor:
➤ Pts w/ risk factors: <44–60 weeks post-conceptual age, apnea at home, anemia
➤ Other pts to monitor: infants >60 weeks post-conceptual age w/ significant risk factors despite simple surgery (eg, cataract). For example, 1-year-old ex-26-week gestation infant who is oxygen-dependent, w/ cerebral palsy and seizures, fed via a gastrostomy tube.

■ No monitoring needed
➤ Pt w/o risk factors
➤ Other pts may need no monitoring assuming uncomplicated surgery & anesthetic. Prototypical examples:
  • Ex-36-week gestation infant now 50 weeks post-conceptual age, never had respiratory problems or apnea as newborn, was discharged home at 4 days after phototherapy for mild hyperbilirubinemia, is growing well & has no acute or chronic medical problems who required minor surgery (eg, hypospadias repair).
  • Term infant who at 2 weeks of age is scheduled for a cataract extraction.

Hematologic

■ Continue to follow previously defined transfusion trigger.

GLAUCOMA

JESSICA SAMPAT, MD

OVERVIEW

■ Definition: two different forms of glaucoma
➤ Primary open angle glaucoma, the more common form
➤ Closed angle glaucoma, one-tenth as common.

■ Open angle glaucoma
➤ Increased resistance to outflow of aqueous humor at vitreo-corneal angle, near canal of Schlemm.

- Chronic gradual disease. Untreated, it leads to progressive optic nerve damage & blindness (4% of glaucoma pts in US become blind).
- Risk factors for developing optic nerve damage: family history, age, African American race, diabetes, CV disease.
- Symptoms include dull eye pain, visual changes.
- On physical exam, pt is noted to have asymmetric optic cups, firm pale eyeball. Intraocular pressure (IOP) >23 mmHg.

■ Angle-closure glaucoma
  - Angle closure occurs when peripheral iris comes to rest against trabecular meshwork & covers it, preventing outflow of aqueous humor.
  - Less common than primary open angle; unlike primary open angle glaucoma, there is no hereditary pattern.
  - Development is multifactorial, as it is usually associated w/ small eyes w/ flat anterior chambers but normal trabecular meshwork.
  - Attacks can be sudden & severe, w/ IOP reaching 60–70 mmHg within 1 h.
    • Attack can be precipitated by a mydriatic agent.
  - Symptoms include visual blurring, eye pain, nausea/vomiting, visual halos.
  - On physical exam, pt may have red eye, corneal edema, dilated fixed pupil, optic nerve edema, shallow anterior angle; IOP >30 mmHg.

■ Usual therapy
  - Medical: topical beta blocker (eg, timolol), mild miotic (eg, pilocarpine, carbachol), carbonic anhydrase inhibitor.
  - Surgery may be indicated.

PREOP

Issues/Evaluation
■ Periop risk of optic nerve ischemia.
■ Topical eye drops may have systemic effects.
  - The topical beta blocker timolol may have systemic effects such as bradycardia or exacerbation of asthma.
  - The topical cholinesterase inhibitor echothiophate may also decrease plasma cholinesterase & prolong the action of succinylcholine.
■ Chronic acetazolamide therapy can cause Na & bicarb diuresis & metabolic acidosis.

What To Do

- Continue preop glaucoma meds.
- Discontinue echothiopate 2–3 wks before surgery (pts on this med have decreased plasma cholinesterase activity).
- Check electrolytes if pt is on acetazolamide.

INTRAOP

- Anesthetic agents tend to decrease IOP.
- Laryngoscopy & intubation may cause temporary increase in IOP.
- LMA disturbs IOP less than endotracheal intubation.

Management

- At extubation, minimize coughing & bucking.

POSTOP

- Watch for acute glaucoma attack.
  - May present as dull periorbital headache
  - Eye will appear pale, dry, firm.
  - Consider consultation w/ ophthalmologist.
  - Treatment may include acetazolamide IV 250 mg.

HEAD TRAUMA

MIMI C. LEE, MD, PHD

OVERVIEW

- Definition: Traumatic brain injury including brain concussion or contusion, diffuse axonal injury, & subdural, epidural, intra-parenchymal, or intraventricular hematoma
- Goal: Maximize functional outcome, minimize secondary brain insult

PREOP

Issues/Evaluation

- Glasgow Coma Scale (GCS): Score based on eye opening, verbal, & motor responsiveness stratifies risk:
  - 13–15 Mild
  - 9–12 Moderate
  - <=8 Severe: assoc w/ highest morbidity & mortality
  - Score consists of best pt response in 3 areas: eye opening, motor, verbal

- Eye opening: spontaneous (4), to speech (3), to pain (2), no response (1)
- Motor: obeys (6), localizes painful stimulus (5), flexion-withdrawal to pain (4), flexion-abnormal to pain (3), extension w/ pain (2), no response (1)
- Verbal: oriented & converses (5), disoriented & converses (4), inappropriate words (3), incomprehensible sounds (2), no response (1)

■ Airway management (C-spine stabilization)
■ Cardiovascular dysregulation (eg, hypotension, tachycardia)
  ➤ Pt may have Cushing's reflex: hypertension w/ compensatory bradycardia occurring w/ acutely raised ICP.
■ Respiratory dysfunction (ie, hypoxemia, hypercapnia)
■ Elevated ICP (>20 mm Hg) secondary to mass effect or cerebral edema
■ Adequate CPP (>70 mm Hg)
■ Temperature regulation: keep temp <37.5 C

What To Do
■ Examine pt.
  ➤ Assess GCS, vital signs, overall injuries.
■ Assess airway.
  ➤ Decide whether emergent intubation is indicated.
  ➤ Nearly all pts w/ GCS <8 should be intubated for airway protection.
■ Assume C-spine instability.
  ➤ Use in-line stabilization for laryngoscopy & intubation.
  ➤ Alternatively, use a blind nasal approach, unless pt is apneic or may have sustained basilar skull or extensive facial fractures.
■ Assume a full stomach.
  ➤ Use rapid sequence induction (RSI) & cricoid pressure.
  ➤ Etomidate may have less hypotension than other commonly used induction agents, including thiopental & propofol.
■ Resuscitate pt.
  ➤ Be aggressive in preventing or correcting systemic hypotension.
  ➤ Use isotonic or hypertonic, glucose-free crystalloids (eg, 0.9% NS, 3% NS, 7% NS, or Plasmalyte).
    - Hypertonic saline solutions are assoc w/ improved outcome in pediatric pts w/ severe head injury.
  ➤ Pt may also need blood component therapy, inotropes, or vasopressors.

➤ Correct hypoxemia.
➤ Consider whether hyperventilation is appropriate.
  • Hyperventilation is effective in reducing ICP, but reduced cerebral blood flow.
  • Consider hyperventilation for pt w/ signs of elevated ICP.
  • Initially hyperventilate to $PaCO_2$ of 25–30 mm Hg.
  • Allow $PaCO_2$ to normalize when ICP controlled. For craniotomy, surgeon can evaluate cerebral pressure on dura w/ skull opening.
  • For pt in ICU, prophylactic hyperventilation in head injury has not been shown to improve outcome.
■ Reduce ICP if elevated.
  ➤ Elevate head of bed up to 30 degrees to facilitate cerebral venous drainage.
  ➤ Hyperventilation.
  ➤ Osmotic diuresis.
    • Mannitol 0.25–1 mg/kg IV bolus over 20–30 min q4–6h
    • Monitor Na, osmolality.
  ➤ Corticosteroid therapy is not indicated in head trauma but does have benefit for spinal cord injuries if given early.
■ Maintain temperature <37.5 C.

INTRAOP
■ Use GA with two large-bore peripheral IV catheters.
■ Standard monitors plus arterial line to closely follow BP.
■ CVP line useful to follow intraop fluid status.
  ➤ Avoid hypovolemia, hypotension, secondary brain injury.
  ➤ Can also use for inotrope & vasopressor administration.
■ Intubate trachea using RSI.
  ➤ Consider etomidate if induction drug given.
  ➤ Consider lidocaine or fentanyl to blunt response to laryngoscopy.
■ Insert a large-bore orogastric tube.
■ Avoid ICP elevation.
■ Maintain CPP >70 mm Hg; use inotropes or pressors if necessary.
■ Continue to maintain temperature <37.5 C.

POSTOP
■ Pts who were conscious, adequately ventilating, & hemodynamically stable preop may be considered for extubation in the OR to permit immediate neurologic exam.

■ Pts who presented w/ decreased levels of consciousness, massive brain injury, marked cerebral edema, or other compromising injury should remain intubated until stable.

HEART BLOCK

MICHAEL H. FAHMY, MD
WILLIAM A. SHAPIRO, MD

OVERVIEW

■ Definition: prolonged or intermittent conduction from the SA node to the ventricles; 3 types of heart block
  ➤ First-degree block:
    • PR interval >0.20 ms
  ➤ Second-degree block
    • Mobitz type 1 (Wenckebach) block is intermittent block generally within the AV node: progressively lengthening PR interval until there is a dropped QRS complex. The shortest PR interval is the first conducted beat after the pause; the longest PR interval is the last conducted beat before the pause.
    • Mobitz type 2 is intermittent block caused by conduction disease below the AV node: fixed PR interval, w/ intermittent dropped QRS complexes. The PR interval is the same for every conducted beat.
  ➤ Third-degree heart block (also known as complete heart block)
    • Most problematic for anesthesia mgt.
    • Manifests as P waves not causing a QRS complex, resulting in a different PR interval w/ every QRS complex.
    • Typically there are more P waves than QRS complexes.
    • The QRS rhythm is either junctional (narrow complexes) at rate of 40–60 or ventricular (wide complexes) at rate of 25–40.
■ Usual treatment
  ➤ First-degree block
    • No definitive therapy
  ➤ Second-degree block
    • Mobitz type 1: ephedrine, atropine, glycopyrrolate, isoproterenol.
    • Mobitz type 2 block: pacing.
  ➤ Third-degree block

- For congenital complete heart block, no treatment unless pt is symptomatic; otherwise, ventricular pacing.
- For all others, ventricular pacing is indicated.

PREOP

Issues/Evaluation
- Pre-existing heart block will be seen on preop 12-lead ECG.
- Evaluate overall heart function.

What To Do
- Pts w/ symptoms & type 2 second-degree block or third-degree (complete) heart block should have a pacemaker inserted prior to surgery.
- First-degree block: consider avoiding beta blocker administration, especially if ventricular rate is already slow.
- Second-degree type 1 block: increase HR if slow.

INTRAOP

Management
- First-degree block
  - No treatment required.
- Second-degree type 1 (Wenckebach) block
  - Ephedrine, atropine, glycopyrrolate, & isoproterenol will increase the rate of SA node firing, thereby increasing the heart rate, & enhance conduction through the AV node, resulting in more conducted beats.
- Second-degree type 2 and third-degree block
  - Atropine & isoproterenol can be tried but often don't work.
  - Ventricular pacing is indicated.
    - Transcutaneous pacing: relatively quick & widely available
    - Transvenous pacing: harder to get in an emergency, requires central venous access, possibly fluoro, but more reliable & allows the surgeons to work.

POSTOP

- Consider postop care in monitored setting.
- Newly recognized type 2 second-degree or third-degree block requires cardiology consult for further evaluation & possible permanent pacemaker placement.

HERBAL REMEDY USE

LINDA LIU, MD

- Definition
  - ➤ Herbal remedies or phytotherapeutics are plant-derived products used for medicinal purposes.
  - ➤ Classification of herbal remedies as dietary supplements means that they can be marketed w/o proven safety or efficacy.
- Usual Rx
  - ➤ Remember to inquire about herbal remedy use: <40% of pts disclose their use of alternative medicine to their physicians.
  - ➤ Herbal remedy use is increasing: 22% of preop pts reported using herbal remedies in a recent survey.

PREOP

Issues/Evaluation

- Use references to keep abreast of a rapidly changing field, such as
  - ➤ PDR for Herbal Medicine
  - ➤ Rational Phytotherapy: A Physician's Guide to Herbal Medicine
  - ➤ Complete German Commission E Monographs
  - ➤ Websites are available as well. Remember that not all are peer-reviewed, so be wary of the information.
    - nccam.nih.gov
    - www.cfsan.fda.gov/~dms/aems.html
- Some common herbal medicines & their possible side effects
  - ➤ Ginseng: tachycardia, hypertension, decreases warfarin's effectiveness
  - ➤ Feverfew: decreased platelet activity
  - ➤ Garlic: interactions w/ platelet activity
  - ➤ Valerian: potentiates barbiturates
  - ➤ Kava kava: potentiates barbiturates, benzodiazepines, alcohol; reports of liver failure requiring transplant
  - ➤ Ginkgo: inhibits platelet activating factor, potentiates aspirin or warfarin
  - ➤ St. John's wort: induces cytochrome P450 system, possible serotonin syndrome
  - ➤ Echinacea: may cause hepatotoxicity
  - ➤ Ginger: may increase bleeding time
  - ➤ Saw palmetto: additive effect w/ other hormone therapies (birth control pills or estrogen replacement therapy)

What To Do

- Lack of well-designed, placebo-controlled trials to prove efficacy, but pts are often staunch believers.
- Only case reports of adverse interactions have been reported in pts, no controlled studies.
- No definitive data on pharmacodynamics & pharmacokinetics, but try to have pt discontinue the herbal remedy as soon as possible preop.
- If pt is taking a remedy associated w/ bleeding, discuss case w/ surgeon if possible higher risk of bleeding will be a problem intraop.

INTRAOP

- Many herbal remedies can be associated w/ platelet dysfunction, liver toxicity, interactions w/ prescription meds, CNS depression.
- Watch for hemodynamic disturbances.
- Watch for signs of unusual clotting.

Management

- Transfuse if coagulation parameters are abnormal or no signs of clotting in field.
- If unusual response to indirect-acting vasopressors (ie, ephedrine), consider changing to direct-acting agents (ie, phenylephrine).
- Supportive care.

POSTOP

- Continue vigilance for abnormal events.
- Maintain open communication with pts so they don't feel their beliefs in herbal remedies are being dismissed.
- Website to report adverse effects of herbal products: www.fda.gov/medwatch

HIATAL HERNIA AND GASTROESOPHAGEAL REFUX DISEASE

GERALD DUBOWITZ, MB, CHB

OVERVIEW

- Definition: Gastroesophageal reflux disease (GERD) is the reflux of gastric contents into the esophagus
- GERD suggests incompetence of the lower esophageal sphincter, allowing caustic gastric contents to irritate the lower esophagus.

■ Definition: Hiatal hernia is the protrusion of the stomach above the diaphragm. Etiology is unclear but may be congenital or acquired.

■ Both hiatal hernia & GERD lead to passive reflux of gastric contents, which may be aspirated during the course of anesthesia.

■ Increased risk in obese pts.

■ Regurgitation is generally a silent process but can have potentially severe consequences:
  ➤ Minor pulmonary sequelae (eg, cough)
  ➤ Exacerbation of bronchospasm
  ➤ Aspiration pneumonitis & ARDS
  ➤ Aspiration is most severe w/ high-volume, particulate, acid aspirate

■ Usual Rx: Reduce gastric acidity & therefore the potential damage caused by reflux/aspiration of gastric contents.
  ➤ Histamine (H_2) blockers (eg, ranitidine)
  ➤ Proton pump inhibitors (eg, omeprazole)
  ➤ Antacids (eg, sodium bicitrate)
  ➤ Promotility agents to reduce gastric volume (eg, metoclopramide)

PREOP

■ Preop evaluation
  ➤ Obtain history of reflux:
    • Severity of reflux
    • Frequency
    • Assoc w/ eating or all the time
    • Worse lying down
    • Requires sleeping on many pillows

■ Preop mgt
  ➤ Major goal is to promote low gastric volume, high gastric pH, nonparticulate gastric contents.
  ➤ Fast at least 8 hours before surgery to reduce risk of aspiration of particulate matter.
  ➤ Continue preop medications for reflux.
  ➤ Consider adding promotility agents.
  ➤ Important: Administer nonparticulate antacid (eg, Bicitra 30 cc po) within 30 min of induction.
    • This is a low-risk medication that is very effective in raising gastric pH.

INTRAOP

- Plan rapid-sequence induction w/ cricoid pressure.
  - Minimize time from unconsciousness to tracheal intubation w/ cuffed ETT.
  - Apply cricoid pressure properly.
  - Succinylcholine has fastest onset of neuromuscular blockade.
  - Rocuronium has most rapid onset of nondepolarizing muscle relaxant but has much longer duration than succinylcholine. Consider this if airway exam suggests difficult intubation.
- Strategies to minimize risk of aspiration.
  - Avoid inhaled induction.
  - Consider regional techniques.
  - Protect airway w/ cuffed ETT if using general anesthesia.
  - Consider NG tube when asleep, though this does not guarantee empty stomach.
- Extubate when pt is awake, w/ intact airway reflexes. Generally, this occurs when pt is able to clearly follow a command.

POSTOP

- Monitor mental status closely on emergence. If pt develops altered mental status, consider tracheal intubation for airway protection.
- Maintain head-up position in PACU, as this may reduce passive reflux.

HYPERALDOSTERONISM

LUDWIG H. LIN, MD

OVERVIEW

- Definition: hypersecretion of the mineralocorticoid aldosterone; may be primary (adrenal cause of excessive production) or secondary (extra-adrenal stimulus for production)

Pathophysiology

- Primary
  - Usually caused by an aldosterone-producing adrenal adenoma (Conn's syndrome)
  - Sometimes by adrenal carcinoma or bilateral cortical nodular hyperplasia
  - Can be mimicked by inherited disorders involving corticosteroid synthesis, as well as ingestion of licorice
- Secondary

- Usually a result of hypoperfusion to the kidneys (eg, renal arterial atherosclerosis or fibromuscular hyperplasia), resulting in increased secretion of renin as a compensatory response
- Renin-producing tumors are rarely the cause of secondary aldosteronism.
- Bartter's syndrome, characterized by renal juxtaglomerular hyperplasia, is assoc w/ severe hyperaldosteronism because the defect in renal conservation of sodium stimulates renin & aldosterone production.
- Other diseases producing intravascular volume depletion can lead to increased renin & aldosterone production: cirrhosis, nephrotic syndrome, congestive heart failure.

- Aldosterone is responsible for sodium & water reabsorption in the distal renal tubule as well as secretion of potassium.
- Excessive aldosterone results in hypokalemia, hypernatremia, & hypervolemia, usually presenting as diastolic hypertension.
- Fatigue & muscle weakness may occur as result of hypokalemia; polyuria results from impairment of the urinary concentrating ability.

Abnormal Findings

- Abnormal overnight urinary concentration test
- Neutral to alkaline urine pH (excessive secretion of ammonium & bicarbonate ions to compensate for the metabolic alkalosis)
- Hypokalemia
- Hypernatremia

PREOP

Issues/Evaluation

- Diagnostic criteria for primary hyperaldosteronism
  - Diastolic hypertension w/o edema
  - Hyposecretion of renin
  - Hypersecretion of aldosterone that does not suppress appropriately in response to salt loading
- Diagnostic criteria for secondary hyperaldosteronism
  - High renin levels

What To Do

- Usual therapy for primary hyperaldosteronism
  - Surgical excision of adenoma.
  - Dietary restriction of sodium.
  - Use of aldosterone antagonist (spironolactone) also effective.

➤ Other anti-mineralocorticoids used include triamterene & amiloride.

➤ With inherited disorders, replacement w/ dexamethasone, a potent glucocorticoid that suppresses ACTH & endogenous cortisol production yet has only weak mineralocorticoid activity, could be the approach.

■ Preop mgt

➤ Obtain electrolytes & an ECG to look for signs of hypokalemia.

➤ Elective cases should be delayed if the plasma potassium concentration is <3 mEq/L.

INTRAOP

■ Issues include pre-existent hypervolemia & electrolyte imbalances, such as hypernatremia & hypokalemia. With secondary hyperaldosteronism, the cause of the intravascular volume depletion (eg, cirrhosis, CHF) may predispose the pt to intraop complications.

■ Hypokalemia can lead to myocardial dysfunction, conduction & rhythm abnormalities. A U wave characteristically appears, along w/ prolonged PR interval. Eventually, a terminal ventricular fibrillation pattern results.

■ Respiratory alkalosis, beta-agonist administration (even as additive to local anesthetics in a regional block), & hyperglycemia can lead to worsening hypokalemia.

■ Nondepolarizing muscle relaxants have an increased effect in pts w/ hypokalemia.

Management

■ Potassium chloride can be given as 0.5–1.0 mEq bolus injections in the event of ECG abnormalities seen w/ hypokalemia. With less urgent replacement, 10–20 mEq of KCl per hour in an IV infusion can be used.

POSTOP

■ Continued telemetry monitoring for pt w/ severe hypokalemia

---

HYPERCALCEMIA

LUDWIG H. LIN, MD

OVERVIEW

■ Causes

➤ Parathyroid related (primary, lithium therapy, familial)

➤ Malignancy-related

➤ Vitamin D-related (vitamin D intoxication, sarcoidosis, idiopathic hypercalcemia of infancy)

➤ Increased bone turnover (hyperthyroidism, immobilization, thiazides, vitamin A intoxication)

➤ Renal failure (secondary hyperparathyroidism, aluminum intoxication, milk-alkali syndrome)

■ Diagnosis: measurement of calcium, albumin, PTH, or ionized calcium

■ Usual Rx: Depends on specific cause, but general measures include hydration w/ saline, w/ or w/o diuresis w/ loop diuretics (furosemide or ethacrynic acid). Other treatments include:

➤ Bisphosphonates (etidronate, pamidronate)

➤ Calcitonin

➤ Glucocorticoids, in dosages of 40–100 mg QD in four divided doses, increase urinary calcium excretion & decrease intestinal calcium absorption; effective antitumor agent in certain malignancies

➤ Dialysis

➤ Gallium nitrate: inhibits bone resorption; nephrotoxin

➤ Mithramycin: inhibits bone resorption. Can lead to thrombocytopenia & hepatocellular necrosis

➤ PO, IV phosphates (can lead to ectopic calcification)

➤ Parathyroid surgery for primary hyperparathyroidism

PREOP

Issues/Evaluation

■ For severe symptomatic hypercalcemia, consider postponing elective surgery to determine cause & appropriate therapy.

■ Although most pts have only mild symptoms, hypercalcemia can cause multisystem abnormalities:

➤ Neuromuscular: generalized weakness, fatigue, mild depression, proximal muscle weakness, confusion

➤ Renal: renal stones w/ renal colic, polyuria, dehydration, renal insufficiency

➤ Cardiovascular: shortened QT interval, increased sensitivity to digoxin

➤ GI: anorexia, constipation, nausea/vomiting

➤ Other: bone demineralization, arthralgias, bone pain, pruritus

■ Get ECG to assess for prolonged PR or shortened QT intervals & cardiac arrhythmias.

- Serum calcium >13 mg/dL leads to calcification in tissue & renal insufficiency.
- Serum calcium >15 mg/dL is a medical emergency because of the risk of coma & cardiac arrest.

What To Do
- IV hydration w/ normal saline (2.5–4 L/day).
- Consider IV furosemide diuresis once hydration is adequate.
  - Follow other electrolytes closely during this process.

INTRAOP
- Maintain normocarbia. (Hyperventilation may be deleterious by decreasing plasma potassium, which can counterbalance the effects of calcium, but may be beneficial because it decreases the ionized calcium fraction.)
- Preop muscle weakness should be considered when dosing muscle relaxants.

Management
- Avoid thiazide diuretics (they enhance renal tubular resorption of calcium).
- Avoid prolonged immobilization (calcium release from resorbed bone increases).

POSTOP
- Treatment options such as calcitonin & mithramycin take hours for onset & hence are not helpful intraop but may be beneficial postop.

HYPERPARATHYROIDISM

BETTY LEE-HOANG, MD

OVERVIEW
- Definition: elevated level of parathyroid hormone (PTH)
  - Primary hyperparathyroidism
    - Elevated level of PTH is inappropriate in pt w/ normal or elevated serum calcium level.
    - Most commonly caused by parathyroid adenoma (75–85%) or parathyroid hyperplasia
  - Secondary hyperparathyroidism
    - Related to hypocalcemia

- Occurs most commonly w/ chronic renal failure & intestinal malabsorption
  - ➤ Tertiary hyperparathyroidism
    - Refers to pt w/ secondary hyperparathyroidism who subsequently develops "autonomous" function of hyperplastic parathyroid glands
- PTH increases the serum calcium level by stimulating vitamin D production & absorption of Ca, increasing renal tubular reabsorption of Ca & decreasing reabsorption of phosphate, & promoting movement of Ca from bone.
- Usual Rx: Depends on the cause of hyperparathyroidism & pt symptoms
  - ➤ Most symptomatic pts are referred for surgery
- May occur as part of multiple endocrine neoplasia syndromes (MEN)

PREOP
- Presents as hypercalcemia w/ serum calcium >5.5 mEq/L (10.5 mg/dL)
- Many pts are asymptomatic, but symptoms can include
  - ➤ Hypertension
  - ➤ Pain from renal stones
  - ➤ Lethargy
  - ➤ Muscle weakness, myalgias, arthralgias
  - ➤ (See also Coexisting Disease: Hypercalcemia)
- Continue medical mgt, which may include IV hydration, mithramycin, glucocorticoids, calcitonin.

INTRAOP
- Monitor for dysrhythmias since the QT interval is short, PR interval is prolonged, & QRS complex is wide.
- Monitor volume status closely to maintain hydration.

POSTOP
- Pts who have significant muscle weakness may require ventilatory support.

HYPERTHYROIDISM

JEREMY NUSSBAUMER, MD

OVERVIEW
- Definition: excessive levels of circulating T3 and/or T4 hormone

- Causes
  - Graves' disease is the most common cause (thyroid-stimulating autoantibodies)
    - Other features: exophthalmos, dermopathy
  - Excess administration of thyroid replacement hormone
  - Toxic nodular goiter
  - Thyroiditis
  - TSH-secreting tumors (rare)
- Signs/symptoms
  - Tremor
  - Weight loss w/ increased appetite
  - Heat intolerance
  - Muscle weakness
  - Hyperreflexia
  - Sinus tachycardia
  - CHF (typically high-output)
  - Atrial fibrillation
  - Possible cardiomyopathy
  - Increased cardiac output
- Usual Rx
  - Antithyroid drugs (eg, propylthiouracil, methimazole, carbimazole)
    - Decrease thyroid hormone synthesis
  - Iodine compounds (eg, potassium iodide, Lugol's solution)
    - Decrease hormone release
  - Beta blockers
    - Adjunctive therapy to decrease sympathetic activity
    - May reduce peripheral conversion of T4 to T3
  - Surgical removal of tumors

PREOP

Issues/Evaluation
- Postpone elective cases until pt is euthyroid.
- Thyroid storm can be life-threatening.
  - Check thyroid function tests.
  - Resting HR should be <85.
- Consider beta blockade for emergent cases.

What To Do
- Check T3, T4 levels.
- Render pt euthyroid before elective surgery.

INTRAOP
- Avoid meds that stimulate sympathetic nervous system (eg, pancuronium, ephedrine, epinephrine, ketamine).
- Consider thiopental for induction (decreases T4 to T3 conversion).
- Carefully protect the eyes of pts w/ exophthalmos.
- Watch for thyroid storm (see below).

Management
- Phenylephrine should be used for hypotension.
- Adequate anesthetic depth should be established to avoid exaggerated sympathetic response.

POSTOP
- The most serious complication in the hyperthyroid pt is thyroid storm.
- Thyroid storm may be precipitated by a variety of conditions.
  - Thyroid surgery
  - Other surgery
  - Acute medical illness (eg, sepsis, stroke, diabetic ketoacidosis)
- Signs/symptoms of thyroid storm
  - Fever
  - Hypotension
  - Tachycardia
  - Heart failure
  - Muscle weakness
  - Altered mental status including delirium, coma
- Thyroid storm can occur intraop or up to 24 h postop. Differential diagnosis includes
  - Malignant hyperthermia (characterized by fever, muscle rigidity, increased CK, or severe metabolic acidosis)
  - Drug or transfusion reaction
  - Sepsis
  - Pheochromocytoma
- Mgt of thyroid storm should occur in an ICU setting. Therapy includes
  - Propylthiouracil (PTU) (250 mg q6h PO, NG, or PR)
  - Beta blockade (eg, propranolol 2–4 mg IV q4h)
  - Potassium iodide 1 h after PTU (5 drops SSKI PO q6h)
  - Glucocorticoid therapy (eg, dexamethasone 2 mg IV q6h)
  - IV hydration

HYPERTROPHIC CARDIOMYOPATHY

LEI WANG, MD

OVERVIEW

- Definition: heterogeneous left ventricular hypertrophy w/o other cardiac or systemic causes
  - Septum is usually disproportionately affected.
  - Left ventricular outflow tract (LVOT) is obstructed during systole by anterior motion of the anterior leaflet of mitral valve against the hypertrophied septum.
  - The obstruction is dynamic & peaks at mid to late systole.
- Risk: rare. Inherited as autosomal dominant w/ variable penetrance, or occurs sporadically.
- About 25% of affected pts present w/ LVOT obstruction.
- Usual Rx: medical therapy w/ beta blockers, calcium blockers
  - Less commonly, more invasive therapy such as cardiac myomectomy

PREOP

Issues/Evaluation

- Most pts are asymptomatic, but symptomatic pts usually complain of
  - Dyspnea on exertion
  - Fatigue
  - Syncope, near syncope
  - Angina
  - Sudden death is often the first manifestation in young pts.
- Key clinical features
  - Severe diastolic dysfunction
  - Increased risk for myocardial ischemia
  - Supraventricular & ventricular arrhythmia common
  - Pts w/ obstruction present w/ harsh systolic murmur, which is increased w/ Valsalva & decreased w/ squatting or handgrip
  - EKG shows LVH.
  - Echocardiography or cardiac catheterization confirms the diagnosis

What To Do

- Place pt on beta blocker or calcium channel blocker preop to decrease contractility.
- Replace preop fluid deficit.
- Adequate sedation to avoid anxiety-induced sympathetic discharge.
- Amiodarone is generally effective in controlling arrhythmias.
- Avoid diuretics, digoxin, or nitrates.

INTRAOP

- Potential issues
  - Profound hypotension due to worsening obstruction w/ increases in sympathetic discharge, or decrease in preload or afterload
  - Myocardial ischemia
  - Arrhythmia

Management

- Consider arterial line, CVP, PAC; TEE when large fluid shift is anticipated.
- Take efforts to blunt sympathetic stimulation during induction.
  - Avoid prolonged laryngoscopy.
- Use volatile anesthetics that decrease ventricular contractility, such as halothane.
- Avoid tachycardia.
  - Give beta blocker or calcium channel blocker to treat worsening obstruction.
  - Avoid agents that can increase heart rate or contractility, such as ephedrine, pancuronium, or epinephrine.
- Avoid decreases in preload or afterload.
  - Provide adequate fluid replacement from the very start of procedure.
  - Avoid agents that decrease preload or afterload, such as nitroglycerin or nitroprusside.
- Treat hypotension w/ volume expansion & phenylephrine.

POSTOP

- Aggressive pain control to avoid sympathetic stimulation.
- Maintain adequate preload & afterload.
- Continue medical therapy (usually beta blockers, calcium blockers).

HYPOCALCEMIA

LUDWIG H. LIN, MD

OVERVIEW

- Definition: serum calcium <8 mg/dL, or ionized calcium <1 mmol/L
- Causes: acute hypocalcemia
  - Blood transfusions: owing to citrate in banked blood
  - Critically ill pts: associated w/ sepsis, burns, ARF, pancreatitis
  - Hypoalbuminemia: reduced total calcium concentration (but normal ionized calcium concentration)
  - Metabolic alkalosis: increases calcium's binding to protein, so will decrease ionized calcium concentration
  - Postop pts following parathyroidectomy or thyroidectomy
- Causes: chronic hypocalcemia due to parathyroid hormone (PTH) abnormalities
  - Hypoparathyroidism
    - Congenital
    - Hypomagnesemia
    - Surgical removal of parathyroids
  - Ineffective PTH (eg, pseudohypoparathyroidism, vitamin D deficiency)
  - Overwhelmed PTH (eg, hyperphosphatemia from tumor lysis or rhabdomyolysis)
- Usual Rx
  - Hypoparathyroidism: vitamin D or calcitriol; calcium supplement
  - Hypomagnesemia: IV magnesium administration

PREOP

Issues/Evaluation

- Look for systemic effects of hypocalcemia.
  - CNS: numbness & circumoral paresthesia, confusion, seizures
  - Hypotension, increased left ventricular filling pressures
  - Prolonged QT interval
  - Weakness & fatigue, skeletal muscle spasm, laryngospasm
    - Chvostek & Trousseau signs indicate neuromuscular irritability.
    - Chvostek sign: tapping on facial nerve anterior to ear results in ipsilateral facial muscle twitching

- Trousseau sign: inflating BP cuff above systolic pressure for several minutes results in muscular contraction of the hand

What To Do

■ Confirm hypocalcemia w/ an ionized calcium measurement (to exclude the contribution of the albumin level to the total calcium level).

■ Obtain ECG.

INTRAOP

■ Administer 500 mg to 1 g calcium chloride or calcium gluconate IV, check ionized calcium, & repeat IV calcium administration as needed to correct hypocalcemia.

■ Avoid hyperventilation, as respiratory alkalosis can increase calcium binding to serum proteins.

■ Consider checking phosphate & magnesium levels.

POSTOP

■ Continue to follow serum & ionized calcium levels; continue replacement as necessary.

HYPOPARATHYROIDISM

BETTY LEE-HOANG, MD

OVERVIEW

■ Definition: lack of parathyroid hormone (PTH).

■ Usual Rx: calcium supplement.

■ Hypoparathyroidism usually follows parathyroidectomy or occurs inadvertently after thyroidectomy; idiopathic forms are rare & will not be considered here.

PREOP

Issues/Evaluation

■ Presents as hypocalcemia: (total serum calcium) <4.5 mEq/L, or ionized calcium <1 mmol/L

■ Chvostek sign is painful facial twitching after tapping on the facial nerve.

■ Trousseau sign is carpal spasm after inflation of a tourniquet.

INTRAOP

- Treatment is w/ calcium IV in the form of calcium gluconate or calcium chloride.
- Intraop anesthetic agents that depress the myocardium may cause hypotension.
- Laryngospasm is more likely w/ hypocalcemia.
- Consider avoiding products that may lower Ca even further if possible, such as citrate-containing blood products & 5% albumin.

POSTOP

- Continue to follow Ca levels & treat appropriately.
- After parathyroidectomy, signs of hypocalcemia do not typically appear until after 24–72 h.

HYPOTHYROIDISM

JEREMY NUSSBAUMER, MD
BETTY LEE-HOANG, MD

OVERVIEW

- Definition: inadequate levels of circulating T3 & T4 hormone
- Primary hypothyroidism (95% of all cases) may be caused by
  - Hashimoto's thyroiditis (autoimmune)
  - Thyroidectomy
  - Radioactive iodine treatment
  - Iodine deficiency
  - Antithyroid medication
  - Neck irradiation
- Diagnosis of primary hypothyroidism: low levels of free thyroxine & increased TSH
- Secondary hypothyroidism is caused by failure of the hypothalamic-pituitary axis.
- Signs/symptoms of hypothyroidism may include
  - Fatigue, weakness
  - Weight gain despite poor appetite
  - Cold intolerance
  - Hair loss
  - Constipation
  - Dry skin w/ cool extremities
  - Delayed relaxation of deep tendon reflexes
  - Bradycardia

- ➤ Peripheral edema
- ➤ Myxedema (skin thickening w/o pitting edema)
- ■ Cardiovascular manifestations of hypothyroidism can include
  - ➤ Decreased myocardial contractility
  - ➤ Bradycardia
  - ➤ Decreased stroke volume
  - ➤ Decreased cardiac output
  - ➤ Increased systemic vascular resistance
  - ➤ Pericardial effusion
  - ➤ Despite these changes, cardiomyopathy & CHF are rarely seen.
- ■ Usual Rx: thyroid hormone replacement w/ levothyroxine

PREOP

Issues/Evaluation
- ■ Periop risks due to hypothyroidism are minimal if pt is on appropriate therapy & is clinically & biochemically euthyroid.
- ■ Onset of symptoms is usually gradual.
- ■ Possible alteration in physiologic responses
  - ➤ May have blunted responses to hypoxia & hypercarbia
  - ➤ May have blunted baroreceptor response
  - ➤ Impaired drug metabolism
- ■ Goiter, macroglossia & edematous vocal cords may be present.
- ■ The hypothyroid pt w/ coronary artery disease may develop angina when starting levothyroxine.
  - ➤ Pts usually require more careful escalation of dose.
- ■ Subclinical hypothyroidism is increasingly recognized due to increased screening of TSH.
  - ➤ Pt has minimal or no symptoms.
  - ➤ T3, T4 levels usually normal
  - ➤ TSH slightly elevated
- ■ Myxedema coma from severe hypothyroidism is a rare medical emergency that usually occurs in elderly pts.
  - ➤ Key findings (in addition to other signs/symptoms of hypothyroidism)
    - • Impaired mentation
    - • Possible seizures
    - • Hypothermia
  - ➤ Precipitating events may include
    - • Hypoventilation (potentially from anesthetic drugs, opiates, sedative-hypnotics)
    - • Hyponatremia

- Cold exposure
- Acute medical illness (eg, sepsis, stroke, CHF, pneumonia, GI bleeding)

What To Do

■ Pt w/ hypothyroidism who is on thyroid replacement should be euthyroid by clinical & laboratory evaluation.
  ➤ Confirm that pt is appropriately taking thyroid replacement therapy.
  ➤ Check T3, T4, TSH levels.
■ Postpone elective surgery for severe symptomatic hypothyroidism & myxedema coma.
■ Mild or subclinical hypothyroidism has not been shown to increase periop complications.
  ➤ Discuss w/ pt & surgeon the potential risks of surgery & potential benefits of thyroid replacement therapy.
■ Treatment of myxedema coma
  ➤ Treat precipitating cause (if present).
  ➤ Levothyroxine 300–500 mcg IV bolus plus maintenance dose of 25–100 mcg/day
  ➤ Passive warming w/ forced air warmer
  ➤ Correction of electrolyte imbalances
  ➤ Hydrocortisone 25–50 mg IV q6h

INTRAOP

■ Hypothyroid pts may not need premeds.
■ Pts may be more sensitive to hypotensive effect of anesthetic agents.
■ For refractory hypotension, particularly w/ severe hypothyroidism, consider glucocorticoid administration for adrenal insufficiency (eg, hydrocortisone 50–100 mg IV).
■ Hypothyroidism can blunt the response of the adrenal gland to stress.
■ Hypothyroidism does not significantly reduce MAC but may speed the rate of inhalational induction due to decreased cardiac output.
■ Potential intraop problems
  ➤ Hypothermia
  ➤ Hypoglycemia
  ➤ Hyponatremia
  ➤ Hypotension

Management

■ Keep pt warm
■ Check & correct electrolyte abnormalities

POSTOP
- Recovery from GA may be delayed.
- Pt may need postop ventilatory support.
  - ➤ Do not extubate until awake & near normothermic.
- Continue levothyroxine therapy postop.
  - ➤ Drug has half-life of 7 days.

IMMUNE THROMBOCYTOPENIC PURPURA (ITP)

ANNE NOONEY, MD

OVERVIEW
- Definition: primary immune thrombocytopenia
  - ➤ Acute: most common in children 2–6 y
  - ➤ Chronic: more common in young women
- Usual Rx
  - ➤ Steroids
  - ➤ IV immunoglobulin
  - ➤ Splenectomy
  - ➤ Immune suppression (eg, azathioprine)
- Diagnosis
  - ➤ Decreased platelets, increased bleeding time
  - ➤ Antiplatelet antibodies are present in the majority of cases.
- Intracranial hemorrhage is the most common cause of fatal bleeding.

PREOP
- For elective surgery, pt may benefit from a hematology consult to optimize treatment of ITP & platelet count.
- IV immune globulin and/or methylprednisolone 1 g may be recommended prior to platelet transfusion.
- Pt may require 2 to 3 times the usual volume of platelets to maintain satisfactory platelet count.
- Administer stress-dose steroids for pts on chronic glucocorticoid therapy.

INTRAOP
- Goal is to keep platelets >50,000–100,000, depending on the likelihood of blood loss intraop.
- Platelet transfusion may increase counts transiently.

- Nasal intubation should be avoided.
- Carefully weigh risk-benefit ratio of nerve blocks in thrombocy-topenic pts.

POSTOP
- Close monitoring for bleeding from surgical wound & other hemor-rhagic complications (eg, CNS bleed)
- Neonate can be transiently thrombocytopenic following delivery from a parturient w/ ITP.

INFECTIVE ENDOCARDITIS

KATHRYN ROUINE-RAPP, MD

OVERVIEW
- Definition: infection on the endothelium of the heart
  - Appears as a vegetation
  - Most common on the heart valves
  - Can occur on prosthetic material, at a cardiac defect site, or where an abnormal jet of blood strikes the endothelium
- Usual treatment: determined by organism
- Disease can be acute or subacute.

PREOP

Issues/Evaluation
- American Heart Association recommends antibiotic prophylaxis in pts at high or moderate risk for endocarditis.
- Pts at high risk include those w/
  - Prosthetic heart valves
  - Prior bacterial endocarditis
  - Cyanotic congenital heart disease (CHD) before & after surgical palliation or repair, patent ductus arteriosus (PDA), coarctation of the aorta, pts w/ surgically constructed systemic to pulmonary connections
- Pts at moderate risk include
  - Most other pts w/ repaired or unrepaired CHD
  - Those w/ acquired aortic & mitral valve disease
  - Mitral valve prolapse w/ regurgitation and/or valve leaflet thickening
  - Asymmetric septal hypertrophy

- No prophylaxis is required in pts w/
  - ➤ An isolated secundum atrial septal defect (ASD)
  - ➤ Totally repaired PDA
  - ➤ Totally repaired ventricular septal defect
  - ➤ Totally repaired secundum ASD
- Endocarditis prophylaxis is recommended for
  - ➤ Dental procedures (extractions, periodontal procedures, cleaning where bleeding is anticipated, implant placement, reimplantation of native teeth, endodontic procedures [eg, root canal], subgingival placement of antibiotic fibers or strips, placement of orthodontic bands, not brackets, intraligamentary injections)
  - ➤ Respiratory procedures (mucosal disruption, rigid bronchoscopy, flex bronchoscopy with biopsy, T&A)
  - ➤ GI procedures (esophageal sclerotherapy or dilation, biliary surgery or manipulation, intestinal surgery causing mucosal disruption)
  - ➤ GU procedures (urethral dilation, prostate or urethral surgery, cystoscopy)
- Prophylaxis is optional for
  - ➤ Bronchoscopy
  - ➤ GI endoscopy w/ or w/o biopsy
  - ➤ Vaginal delivery
  - ➤ Hysterectomy
  - ➤ TEE
  - ➤ Urinary catheterization w/o infection
  - ➤ Circumcision
- TEE can be very helpful for preop assessment of intracardiac masses, valvular regurgitation or abscess, cardiac function.
- If pt currently has endocarditis, morbidity & mortality are most often related to intracardiac or CNS complications of the disease, such as
  - ➤ Valvular regurgitation
  - ➤ Abscess
  - ➤ CHF
  - ➤ Pericarditis
  - ➤ Heart block
  - ➤ Embolic stroke (hemorrhagic or nonhemorrhagic)
    - • If possible, cardiac surgery should be delayed for 2–3 wks after a nonhemorrhagic & 4 weeks after a hemorrhagic embolic stroke.
  - ➤ In addition, pts can develop visceral ischemia & splenic abscess or mycotic aneurysms.

What To Do

- Antibiotic prophylaxis is as follows.
- PO doses are given 1 h before procedure, IV/IM doses within 30 min of procedure & vancomycin is given over 1–2 h & completed within 30 min of procedure.
- Cephalosporins are not recommended for penicillin-allergic pts who have urticaria, angioedema or anaphylaxis to penicillin.
- Oral cavity, respiratory tract or esophageal procedures
  - Amoxicillin 2.0 g PO, or
  - Ampicillin 2.0 g IV, or
  - In penicillin-allergic pts
    - Clarithromycin 500 mg PO, or
    - Cephalexin or cefadroxil 2.0 g PO, or
    - Clindamycin 600 mg PO, or
    - Cefazolin 1.0 g IV or IM. Administer half dose 6 h after the initial dose for pt at high risk.
- GU, GI tract procedures
  - High-risk pts: ampicillin 2.0 g IV/IM + gentamicin 1.5 mg/kg (120 mg max), repeat ampicillin 1.0 g IV/IM or amoxicillin 1.0 g PO 6 h later
  - High-risk penicillin-allergic pts: vancomycin 1.0 g IV + gentamicin 1.5 mg/kg (120 mg max) IV/IM; no second dose
  - Moderate-risk pts: amoxicillin 2.0 g PO or ampicillin 2.0 g IV/IM
  - Moderate-risk penicillin-allergic patients: vancomycin 1.0 g IV
- Pediatric dosing is as follows:
  - Amoxicillin, ampicillin, cephalexin, or cefadroxil, use 50 mg/kg PO
  - Cefazolin 25 mg/kg
  - Clindamycin 20 mg/kg PO, 25 mg/kg IV
  - Clarithromycin 15 mg/kg PO
  - Gentamicin 1.5 mg/kg IV/IM
  - Vancomycin 20 mg/kg

INTRAOP

- Continue antibiotics as above
- Mgt dictated by preop status of pt

POSTOP

- Continue antibiotics as above
- Mgt dictated by status of pt

INHERITED COAGULATION DISORDERS
(HEMOPHILIA, von WILLEBRAND DISEASE)

JONATHAN CHOW, MD
JULIE HAMBLETON, MD
MANUEL PARDO, JR., MD

OVERVIEW

- Definition
  - ➤ The hemophilias are bleeding disorders due to an inherited deficiency of a coagulation factor.
  - ➤ Von Willebrand disease (VWD) is an inherited bleeding disorder due to deficiency or dysfunction of the glycoprotein von Willebrand factor (VWF).
- Hemophilia A & hemophilia B are X-linked recessive disorders affecting males. Females may be asymptomatic carriers or may have significant factor deficiency due to extreme lyonization & behave as a pt w/ mild hemophilia.
  - ➤ Hemophilia A
    - Deficiency of factor VIII coagulant protein
    - Most common of the hemophilias (incidence 1:5,000 live male births)
  - ➤ Hemophilia B (Christmas disease)
    - Deficiency of factor IX coagulant protein
    - Second most common of the hemophilias (incidence 1:30,000)
  - ➤ Other: hemophilia C (factor XI deficiency) & deficiency of factors II, V, VII, X, XIII are uncommon or rare & will not be discussed.
- VWD
  - ➤ Most common inherited bleeding disorder.
  - ➤ Transmitted primarily in an autosomal dominant fashion; affects both men & women.
  - ➤ Incidence 1:1,000 or greater.
  - ➤ Functions of VWF.
    - Mediates platelet adhesion to vascular endothelium.
    - Stabilizes factor VIII in plasma.
  - ➤ Types of VWD
    - Type 1: partial quantitative deficiency of VWF (75% of pts). Clinically heterogeneous. Some pts have little to no bleeding history; others have a significant history.
    - Type 2: qualitative deficiency of VWF (subtypes A, B, M, N)

- Type 3: complete deficiency of VWF. Clinical features similar to mild hemophilia, as the residual factor VIII level is typically about 4%.
- Usual Rx
  - Hemophilia A
    - High-purity plasma-derived concentrates of coagulation factor VIII
    - Recombinant factor VIII concentrate.
    - DDAVP for mild hemophilia (factor VIII >10%), but must have documented a good response to DDAVP prior to using it therapeutically.
    - Cryoprecipitate contains factor VIII, but it is not virally attenuated as are the plasma & recombinant products.
    - Amicar (antifibrinolytic) for oral bleeding.
  - Hemophilia B
    - High-purity plasma-derived concentrates of coagulation factor IX.
    - Recombinant factor IX concentrate.
    - Amicar (antifibrinolytic) for oral bleeding.
  - VWD
    - DDAVP (may be contraindicated or ineffective in certain type 2 & 3 pts).
    - Amicar (antifibrinolytic) for oral bleeding.
    - VWF-containing concentrates ("Intermediate" pure factor VIII products).
    - Cryoprecipitate is rich in factor VIII & VWF (contains 5–10 times more factor VIII & VWF than an equivalent volume of fresh frozen plasma but is not virally attenuated).
  - There is no role for the administration of fresh frozen plasma in the treatment of hemophilia A & B or VWD unless purified products are unavailable. The recovery of coagulation factors is only about 20–30%.

PREOP

Issues/Evaluation
- Hemophilia A & B categorized as
  - Severe: <1% coagulation factor activity. Spontaneous bleeding into joints, soft tissue, muscles.
  - Moderate: 1–5% coagulation factor activity. Less frequent bleeding.
  - Mild: 5–30% coagulation factor activity. Bleeding infrequent, usually due to trauma or surgery.

- All pts w/ hemophilia A & B are susceptible to severe, persistent bleeding w/ surgery.
- Most pts w/ hemophilia A & B are diagnosed at birth or during childhood. Many are followed as outpts by hematologists.
  - Platelet count & bleeding time are normal. The aPTT may be prolonged, depending on pt's residual factor activity (eg, factor VIII activity <30%, factor IX activity <10%).
  - Specific factor assay reveals deficiency.
- Hemophilia pts who received plasma concentrates before the era of virus inactivation had a very high chance of developing.
  - Hepatitis B & C, w/ chronic liver disease.
  - HIV, AIDS.
- VWD pts usually suffer from prolonged oozing after surgery or mucosal bleeding (eg, epistaxis, menorrhagia, or postpartum bleeding).
  - Typically diagnosed by measuring
    - VWF antigen (<45% of normal)
    - Ristocetin cofactor activity. Measures the ristocetin-induced interaction of VWF w/ platelet receptor glycoprotein Ib/IX. <45% of normal.
    - Prolonged bleeding time. The bleeding time has a sensitivity of only 50–60% in detecting VWD type 1, the most common type of VWD.

What To Do
- For both hemophilia & VWD, strongly consider a hematology consult, if available, to better assess the severity of the disease & optimize coagulation factor replacement therapy perioperatively.
  - This is most important for the pt w/ acquired inhibitors to coagulation factors. Mgt may be quite complex & standard usage of factor products is ineffective.
  - Some subtypes of VWD will not respond to DDAVP.
- VWD
  - DDAVP effective for type I VWD
    - Raises factor VIII & VWF 3–5 times above pt's baseline.
    - Typical dose for surgery: 0.3 mcg/kg IV in 50 mL NS over 30–40 min.
    - Stored VWF will get depleted with frequent dosing. Can give QD × 3, then QOD. Restrict fluids & monitor sodium levels.
    - Consider following w/ ristocetin cofactor levels.
  - Transfusion therapy
    - VIII:VWF-containing concentrates: HumateP or Alphanate

- Cryoprecipitate (1 bag contains 80–100 IU) is generally contraindicated because it is not virally attenuated.

■ Hemophilia A
➤ DDAVP may be effective in mild cases for minor surgery, as factor VIII may increase 2–4 times in pts w/ a factor VIII level >10%. Must document DDAVP response before using it perioperatively. For major surgery, initial goal is 80–120% of normal factor level (80–120 IU/dL). Factor VIII dose is 50 IU/kg in someone with a normal hematocrit. Increased dosing is required for pts w/ a depressed hematocrit.
  - Factor level >50% may be needed for 2 weeks, depending on clinical course.
  - Monitor peak & trough factor VIII activities.
  - May require twice-daily dosing or continuous infusion
➤ Avoid cryoprecipitate due to lack of viral inactivation.

■ Hemophilia B
➤ High-purity plasma concentrate or recombinant factor IX.
➤ Dose of plasma-derived factor IX is 100 U/kg to raise the level 100%. Increased dosing is required in pts w/ a depressed hematocrit.
➤ Dose of recombinant factor IX is >=120 U/kg because of poor recovery.
➤ Monitor peak & trough factor IX activities.
➤ Subsequent factor IX dosing is q12–24h.

■ Because of coagulopathy
➤ Avoid unnecessary IM injections.
➤ Consider risks of invasive monitoring.
➤ Consider risk of bleeding w/ regional blockade, esp central neuraxial blockade.
➤ Avoid postop pharmacologic DVT prophylaxis.

INTRAOP
■ Administer factor products as discussed above.

POSTOP
■ Watch for signs of hemorrhage.
■ Continue factor replacement or blood product therapy as needed.
■ Consider involvement of hematologist in postop care to better assess adequacy of replacement therapy.
■ Monitor trough factor levels to maintain factor levels >=50–60% in early postop period.

INTRACEREBRAL HEMORRHAGE (ICH)

MIMI C. LEE, MD, PHD

OVERVIEW

- Definition: hemorrhage within the brain parenchyma; accounts for about 10% of all strokes
- Also called "hypertensive hemorrhage"
- Previous CVA of any type increases the risk of ICH to 23:1.
- Different types
  - Lobar
  - Cerebellar
  - Thalamic
  - Putaminal
- Possible etiologies
  - Hypertension
  - Increased CBF, especially to areas previously rendered ischemic
  - Vascular abnormalities (ie, aneurysms, AVMs, angiopathies)
  - Arteriopathies
  - Brain tumors
  - Coagulopathies
  - Thrombocytopenia
  - CNS infection
  - Venous or dural sinus thrombosis
  - Recreational drugs (cocaine, amphetamine)
  - Post-trauma
  - Eclampsia
  - Postop (after CEA or craniotomy)

PREOP

Issues/Evaluation

- Important to understand the degree of hemorrhage.
- CT scan w/o contrast enhancement will demonstrate acute hemorrhage.
- MRI is not ideal as the appearance of blood clot varies with time.
- Evaluate the pt. Stabilize & resuscitate as necessary.

What To Do

- Evaluate the need for tracheal intubation & mechanical ventilation.
- Correct possible etiologies

➤ Treat hypertension: untreated hypertension may contribute to rebleeding within the first hour. The goal is to return systemic blood pressure to baseline or to reduce by about 20% if baseline pressures are unknown.

➤ Correct coagulopathies: PT, PTT, platelet count w/ blood products, FFP, platelets. Some clinicians recommend keeping platelet counts >75K. Bleeding times may be a useful indicator of coag status. Beware of DIC in cases of massive hemorrhage.

■ Administer phenytoin (anticonvulsant) by loading 17 mg/kg slow IV over 1 h, then follow with 100 mg q8h or 300 PO qhs. Blood & its breakdown products are cortical irritants & may promote seizure activity.

■ Consider steroid administration (dexamethasone 10 mg IVP).

■ Treat increased ICP w/ diuretics (mannitol 0.5–1 mg/kg) or furosemide.

■ Be aware of SIADH.

INTRAOP

■ Use GA w/ two large-bore peripheral IV catheters, routine & invasive arterial monitoring. Use CVP monitoring if necessary.

■ Intubate the trachea using rapid sequence induction (see above) or "modified" rapid sequence induction in more stable pts, using rocuronium (0.6–1.0 mg/kg), lidocaine (1.5 mg/kg), and/or fentanyl (1–4 mcg/kg) prior to laryngoscopy.

■ Insert a large-bore orogastric tube.

■ Avoid ICP elevation.

■ Maintain CPP; use inotropes or pressors if volume resuscitation is inadequate.

Management

■ Continue resuscitation, hyperventilation & diuresis as above.

■ Strive for slight hypothermia.

POSTOP

■ Pts who were conscious, adequately ventilating & hemodynamically stable preop may be considered for extubation in the OR for immediate neurologic exam. Ensure airway protection & reversal of muscle relaxant.

■ Pts who presented w/ decreased levels of consciousness, massive brain injury, marked cerebral edema or other compromising injury should remain intubated until stable.

KYPHOSCOLIOSIS (SCOLIOSIS)

JOHN R. FEINER, MD

OVERVIEW

- Definition: curvature of the spine; deformity of the spinal column that includes lateral curvatures & anteroposterior displacements.
- Major causes of kyphoscoliosis include idiopathic, congenital & neuromuscular disorders.
- Usual Rx: may be managed conservatively w/ symptomatic treatment. Low degrees of curvature are usually monitored for progression. Ultimately, surgical intervention may be necessary to prevent progression to restrictive lung disease, which can ultimately be life-threatening.
- Severity determined primarily by x-rays.

PREOP

Issues/Evaluation

- Pulmonary: Severe kyphoscoliosis is associated w/ restrictive lung disease.
  - ➤ The severity of lung disease may be suspected on clinical grounds, such as exercise tolerance, & on physical exam.
  - ➤ CXR may also indicate probable restrictive disease.
  - ➤ PFTs may be useful in assessing the severity of restrictive disease, although their predictive value is not clear.
  - ➤ In severe cases, CO_2 retention may occur.
  - ➤ Planning for postop care is important in assessing the pt's preop pulmonary status.
- Neurological: Neuromuscular diseases are a significant cause of kyphoscoliosis & may entail additional considerations.
- Cardiac: Cor pulmonale is expected in only the most severe cases.
- Chronic pain: may be associated w/ significant preop pain.
- Other diseases/abnormalities may be associated w/ kyphoscoliosis, particularly in children w/ congenital abnormalities.

What To Do

- Pulmonary status should be optimized prior to any surgery, although few interventions may be possible.

INTRAOP

■ Intraop mgt depends on the type of surgery. Avoiding GA might be useful, but spinal or epidural anesthesia could be extremely difficult anatomically (if attempted, the lowest degree of curvature & anatomic problems would be expected at the L5-S1 interspace).

■ Significant C-spine abnormities do not necessarily occur w/ kyphoscoliosis but should be considered in some cases.

■ More rapid oxyhemoglobin desaturation due to lower functional residual capacity would be expected in the case of restrictive lung disease.

■ Gas exchange abnormalities such as V/Q mismatch & intrapulmonary shunting would be expected to parallel the severity of lung disease.

■ Lower pulmonary compliance should be noted during mechanical ventilation. Lower tidal volumes w/ higher respiratory rate may be necessary.

■ A lower threshold for monitoring w/ an arterial line may be indicated, but still depends on the specific surgery.

■ Mgt of other congenital diseases associated w/ kyphoscoliosis is considered elsewhere (refer to Procedures chapter "Spine Fusion").

POSTOP

■ The main postop considerations relate to the pt's pulmonary status.
  ➤ Any surgery having a significant impact on pulmonary function, such as upper abdominal or thoracic surgery, may lead to significant pulmonary deterioration.
  ➤ A patient with borderline CO_2 retention or very low vital capacity (<50% predicted) may be at risk of postop ventilatory failure. ICU mgt w/ postop ventilation may be indicated.

■ Pain mgt may be more difficult in pts taking opioids preop.

■ Remember the greater propensity for oxyhemoglobin desaturation, particularly in the face of postop pain meds.

■ A lower postop threshold for supplemental O_2 is warranted.

MAGNESIUM DISORDERS

ALISON G. CAMERON, MD

OVERVIEW

■ Definition: normal serum Mg is 1.7–2.1 mg/dL (1.5–2.5 mEq/L)

- Magnesium is the second most prevalent cation in the body. 99% of Mg is stored in bone & soft tissues, w/ only 1% in the serum.
- Mg has a role in many cellular processes & in cellular electrochemical balance.
  - Cofactor for many enzymatic reactions
  - Acts on renal tubule to maintain calcium & potassium levels
  - Multiple cardiac effects, including antiarrhythmic properties
- Usual Rx of hypomagnesemia
  - If asymptomatic, PO administration of Mg sulfate or Mg oxide.
  - If serious manifestations are present, IV administration of up to 4 g over 15–60 min.
- Usual Rx of hypermagnesemia
  - Limit Mg intake.
  - Enhance renal excretion (eg, loop diuretics or dialysis).
  - Calcium may be given to antagonize the effects of Mg.

PREOP

Issues/Evaluation

- Hypomagnesemia
  - Commonly causes low levels of calcium, potassium, phosphate
  - Manifestations
    - Muscle weakness
    - Neuromuscular excitability
    - ECG: prolonged PR & QT interval
    - Cardiac arrhythmias
    - Potentiation of digitalis toxicity
  - Causes include
    - Drugs (including ethanol, diuretics, aminoglycosides, theophylline, amphotericin B, cisplatin)
    - Increased renal excretion (eg, volume expansion, diuretics, hypercalcemia)
    - GI losses
    - Other causes: critical illness, decreased intake, alcoholism
- Hypermagnesemia
  - Potentiates effects of neuromuscular blocking drugs
  - Impairs the release of acetylcholine (ACH) from the neuromuscular junction & decreases motor end-plate sensitivity to ACH
  - Manifestations vary by Mg level:
    - 3 mEq/L: nausea/vomiting
    - 4 mEq/L: drowsiness, sweating, unsteady gait
    - 5 mEq/L: ECG shows widened QRS & PR intervals

- 6–7 mEq/L: bradycardia, hypotension
- >10 mEq/L: heart block & cardiac arrest; muscle weakness including respiratory muscles; respiratory arrest
- ➤ Causes include
  - Renal failure plus increased Mg intake
  - Hypothyroidism

What To Do

■ Correct all electrolyte abnormalities present (often more than just elevated or decreased Mg).

INTRAOP

■ Assess cardiac status carefully given effects of electrolytes on cardiac function.

■ Monitor neuromuscular function w/ peripheral nerve stimulator.
  - ➤ For hypermagnesemia, consider reducing muscle relaxant dose by 25–50%.

Management

■ Follow serum Mg levels, cardiac & neuromuscular function.

POSTOP

■ Continue cardiac monitoring & monitoring of Mg & electrolyte levels, especially in pts w/ pre-existing cardiac disease.

MARFAN'S SYNDROME

ALEX KAO, MD

OVERVIEW

■ Definition: congenital (autosomal dominant) disorder of connective tissue; mean survival 32 y

PREOP

Issues/Evaluation

■ Pt can have multisystem manifestations of connective tissue disease.

■ Cardiovascular
  - ➤ Cystic medial necrosis of large arteries (including coronary arteries, which may lead to angina)
  - ➤ Increased incidence of aortic aneurysms (usually ascending)
  - ➤ Increased risk of mitral valve prolapse (MVP) w/ possible mitral regurgitation

➤ Conduction abnormalities
■ Respiratory
  ➤ Kyphoscoliosis may be present, leading to restrictive lung disease.
  ➤ Increased risk for spontaneous pneumothorax, emphysema.
■ Ocular: risk of lens dislocation, retinal detachment
■ Skeletal: risk of jaw dislocation w/ extreme head positioning during intubation

What To Do
■ If pt has MVP, give prophylactic antibiotics.
■ Preop EKG to detect conduction disease or ischemia.
■ Consider echo for workup of valvular disease & aneurysm.
■ Consider workup for pulmonary disease if symptomatic.
■ If aortic aneurysm present, consider preop beta blockade.

INTRAOP
■ If aortic aneurysm present, dissection can occur. Extension to aortic valve can lead to acute aortic regurgitation. Extension to sinus of Valsalva can lead to tamponade.
■ Be aware of increased risk of pneumothorax.

Management
■ If aortic aneurysm present, avoid HTN & maintain slow heart rate (eg, w/ beta blocker).

POSTOP
■ Inadequate pain control can lead to HTN & increased risk of aortic dissection.

MEDIASTINAL MASS

RICHARD PAULSEN, MD

OVERVIEW
■ Definition: Rapidly growing tumor involving the mediastinum. Examples:
  ➤ Thymoma
  ➤ Teratoma
  ➤ Lymphoma
  ➤ Cystic hygroma

➤ Bronchogenic cyst

➤ Thyroid cancer

■ Because of potential for airway compromise, anterior mediastinal tumors are of most concern in anesthesia care.

■ Usual Rx: Palliative radiation, chemo, and/or surgical resection. Pt may also require therapy for comorbid conditions such as myasthenia gravis.

■ Pts w/ mediastinal mass may present for a number of different types of surgery, including:

➤ Diagnostic or biopsy procedures: bronchoscopy, mediastinoscopy.

➤ Definitive surgery: removal of mass via median sternotomy, thoracotomy, w/ or w/o cardiopulmonary bypass.

PREOP

Issues/Evaluation

■ Most tumors are asymptomatic or present w/ vague complaints (CP, dyspnea, cough).

■ Mass may cause life-threatening obstruction of major airways, main pulmonary arteries, atria, & superior vena cava.

■ Airway obstruction is most common complication during induction of GA, followed by cardiovascular collapse.

➤ Other airway problems can include tracheomalacia, which may cause lower airway obstruction.

■ History of dyspnea or inability to lie flat suggests potential airway compromise during induction.

■ Life-threatening events may occur in the absence of these symptoms.

■ Check for signs of SVC syndrome & right heart or pulmonary vascular compression.

■ Tumor Rx w/ radiation or chemotherapy may change risk profile.

■ Comorbid conditions: myasthenia gravis, thyrotoxicosis, hyperparathyroidism, recurrent laryngeal nerve damage, Horner's syndrome, paroxysmal HTN

What To Do

■ History

➤ Identify symptoms of airway or vascular obstruction.

➤ Evaluate response to any previous therapy.

■ Physical

➤ Evaluate airway carefully.

➤ Look for signs of SVC syndrome.

- Look at imaging studies to identify size & location of tumor, w/ special attention to proximity to tracheobronchial tree & great vessels.
    - CXR: Identifies 97% of mediastinal tumors (size, location, characteristics)
    - CT scan: Locate mass, define margins, define relationship to other structures, determine extent of tracheal/vascular compression
    - MRI: Same as CT scan but better for soft tissue vs vascular structures
- Consider other diagnostic studies:
    - Spirometry: may suggest intra- vs extrathoracic obstruction but is not a sensitive test
    - Cardiac echo: may suggest vascular compromise w/ changes in body position but is not a proven outcome predictor
- Consider alternate approach to planned surgery
    - For moderate, severe, or distal lesions, consider awake bronchoscopy for anesthesia/surgical inspection.
    - Consider tracheal stenting for severe distal lesions.

INTRAOP

- Specifics of mgt will vary w/ planned procedure.
- For biopsy procedures:
    - Tissue biopsy is usual first procedure.
    - Consider peripheral node biopsy: may avoid more invasive procedure.
        - Axillary or neck nodes may be possible biopsy sites.
    - If possible, perform biopsy under local anesthesia.
- In all cases be prepared to quickly change to prone/lateral positions to relieve airway or vascular obstruction.
- Have rigid bronchoscope readily available to bypass distal airway lesion.

Management

- Consider elective cardiopulmonary bypass in symptomatic pts or those w/ severe lesions.
    - Emergent CPB is rarely successful.
- Premedicate to prevent hyperventilation or tachycardia.
- Monitors
    - Standard ASA monitors w/ large-bore IV, A-line for all cases
    - Consider CVP if indicated (may require femoral placement if SVC syndrome present).

- Issues regarding induction
  - Consider intravascular volume loading preinduction.
  - Maintain spontaneous vent & avoid paralysis if possible.
  - Consider awake fiberoptic intubation, especially for moderate to severe, or distal lesions.
  - Consider inhaled induction maintaining spont vent.
  - Place ETT distal to obstructing lesion.
  - If controlled vent required, gradually take over ventilation as tolerated.
- Potential difficulties w/ mgt
  - Lower airway obstruction
    - Try assisted expiration w/ manual compression of chest wall.
    - Return pt to spontaneous respiration (if possible).
- Cardiovascular collapse
  - Inotropes or vasoconstrictors
  - Change of position

POSTOP
- Postop course will vary w/ severity of preop presentation, as well as type & success of surgery performed.
- If pt still has significant mediastinal mass (eg, only had biopsy or unsuccessful attempt at resection), will need to observe closely for signs of vascular or airway obstruction.
  - Consider whether patient would benefit from ICU care.
- Analgesia via PCA or epidural as indicated.

METABOLIC ACIDOSIS

DORRE NICHOLAU, PHD, MD

OVERVIEW
- Definition
  - Decreased plasma bicarbonate (HCO_3)
  - Disorder primary if pH <7.36 w/ normal or low pCO_2
- Three categories
  - Anion gap (accumulation of organic acids)
    - Anion gap $(AG) = Na^+ - (Cl^- + HCO_3^-)$
  - Non-gap (loss of bicarbonate anions)
  - Mixed (combined gap & non-gap acidosis)
- Etiologies of different types of acidosis
- Anion gap acidosis (AG >12)

- Ketoacidosis
  - Diabetic
  - Alcoholic
- Lactic acidosis
  - Septic shock
  - Cardiogenic shock
  - Ischemic bowel
- Renal failure
  - Uremia
- Toxins
  - Methanol (wood alcohol)
  - Ethylene glycol (antifreeze)
  - Paraldehyde
  - Salicylate
- Non-gap, hyperchloremic acidosis (AG <12)
  - Loss of bicarbonate
    - GI tract
    - Diarrhea
    - Ureteral diversions
    - Ileal loop conduit
    - Anion exchange resins (cholestyramine)
  - Renal
    - Proximal RTA
    - Early renal failure
    - Carbonic anhydrase inhibitors
    - Aldosterone inhibitors
    - Posthypocapnea
  - Acid retention
    - Distal RTA
    - Deficient ammonia synthesis
  - Administration of HCl
  - Large-volume saline infusion

Usual Rx
- Anion gap acidosis
  - Treat underlying cause; almost never requires bicarbonate therapy.
  - Bicarbonate no longer part of the ACLS protocol.
  - Treating the pH w/ sodium bicarbonate worsens the lactic acidosis of cardiogenic shock by decreasing intracardiac pH & further decreasing cardiac output.

➤ Hemodialysis may be required for the refractory acidosis of renal failure or to remove the toxic metabolites of methanol & ethylene glycol.

■ Non-gap hyperchloremic acidosis
➤ Bicarbonate replacement is indicated to replete bicarbonate losses.
➤ Calculate the bicarbonate deficit. Replace in increments, beginning with half the deficit.
➤ Total HCO_3 deficit = weight (kg) × 0.2 × (HCO_3 desired – HCO_3 measured [mmol/L])

PREOP

Issues/Evaluation
■ Determine if the metabolic acidosis is gap or non-gap.
■ If a gap acidosis is identified, treat the underlying cause prior to elective surgery. Bicarbonate replacement is rarely indicated. If pH <7.2 some would advocate partial bicarbonate repletion to 7.2.
■ Bicarbonate deficit should be replaced in hyperchloremic non-gap acidosis.
■ In either case it is not necessary to correct the pH to normal range.

INTRAOP
■ Determine if pt has a gap acidosis.
➤ AG is a measure of the relative abundance of unmeasured anions (unmeasured anions minus unmeasured cations).
➤ $AG = Na - (Cl + HCO_3)$
➤ Normal AG is 12 +/− 2.
➤ Unmeasured anions (UA) = 23 mEq/L
  • Proteins 15 mEq/L
  • Organic acids 5 mEq/L
  • Phosphates 2 mEq/L
  • Sulfates 1 mEq/L
➤ Unmeasured cations (UC) = 11 mEq/L
  • Calcium 5 mEq/L
  • Potassium 4.5 mEq/L
  • Magnesium 1.5 mEq/L
■ Determine if pt has a mixed disorder (gap + non-gap).
➤ Measured pH < 7.4 indicates a primary acidosis.
➤ Calculate the delta gap.
  • Delta gap = Measured AG – normal AG (12)
  • Add the delta gap to the serum bicarbonate concentration.

- Delta gap + bicarbonate <23 = underlying non-gap acidosis
- Delta gap + bicarbonate >30 = underlying metabolic alkalosis

➤ Correct the measured AG for a low albumin.
- A low serum albumin can mask an elevated AG.
- Adjusted AG = measured AG + 2.5 (normal alb — measured alb)
- Albumin is in g/dL.

■ Gap acidosis: AG >12 reflects the accumulation of organic acids (see above).
➤ Likely intraop causes
- Hypovolemic, cardiogenic or septic shock
- Ischemic bowel
- Diabetic ketoacidosis

■ Non-gap acidosis: AG <12 reflects loss of bicarbonate (see above).
➤ Likely intraop causes
- Loss of bicarbonate from the GI tract
- Ongoing renal tubular acidosis
- Posthypercapnea
- Dilution of bicarbonate w/ large-volume saline

Management
■ Gap acidosis
➤ Identify & treat the underlying cause.
➤ Bicarbonate is almost never indicated as it may worsen the myocardial function.
➤ Toxins may require dialysis; CVVHD may be the most practical way to proceed intraop.
➤ Refractory acidosis in renal failure is an indication for dialysis.
■ Non-gap acidosis
➤ Calculate the bicarbonate deficit & replace conservatively (see formula above).

POSTOP
■ Causes of metabolic acidosis are likely to persist or recur in the postop period.
■ Continue to monitor serum electrolytes & ABG in PACU or ICU setting.
■ Ongoing treatment of the underlying cause is necessary.
■ Severe metabolic acidosis may require ongoing mechanical ventilation to appropriately compensate.

METABOLIC ALKALOSIS

DORRE NICHOLAU, PHD, MD

OVERVIEW

- Definition
  - Elevated plasma bicarbonate (HCO_3)
- Primary disorder if pH >7.44 w/ normal or elevated PCO_2
- Due to loss of H^+ by kidneys or GI tract or the administration of base
- Frequent association w/ hypokalemia: decreased K^+ is both cause & effect
- Often iatrogenic: NG suction, diuretics, massive transfusion, acetate-rich TPN
- Causes of metabolic alkalosis
  - Chloride-responsive
    - GI losses
    - Vomiting
    - NG suction
    - Villous adenoma of colon
    - Volume depletion (contraction alkalosis)
    - In contraction alkalosis the kidneys will maintain extracellular volume at the expense of acid-base balance. Na is exchanged for H^+ or K^+ in the distal tubules w/o passive Cl reabsorption. As H^+ ions become scarce even more K^+ is lost as a result of the alkalosis. The result is hypochloremic hypokalemic alkalosis.
    - Diuretic therapy
    - Posthypercapnea
  - Chloride-resistant
    - Adrenal disorders
    - Hyperaldosteronism
    - Cushing syndrome
    - Exogenous steroid replacement
    - Gluco- or mineralocorticoid
    - Licorice ingestion
    - Exogenous base administration
    - Lactate, acetate (TPN)
    - Citrate (banked blood, FFP)
    - Bicarbonate administration
    - Bartter syndrome
    - Extreme hypokalemia

- Usual Rx
  - Chloride-responsive
    - Search for an iatrogenic or underlying cause that can be corrected.
    - Correct hypochloremia w/ NaCl infusion.
    - Correct hypokalemia w/ KCl infusion (10–40 mEq/h).
  - Chloride-resistant
    - Large-volume NaCl may exacerbate hypokalemia & perpetuate alkalosis.
    - May respond to aggressive KCl replacement.
    - Resolution requires correction of underlying etiology.
    - Extreme cases may require infusion of dilute HCl 0.1 mmol/L in saline or D5W.
- Compensatory metabolic alkalosis
  - Do not correct the elevated serum bicarbonate in pts w/ chronic respiratory acidosis in whom metabolic alkalosis is an appropriate compensation (pH <7.36).

PREOP

Issues/Evaluation

- Evaluate pt for intravascular volume depletion & hypokalemia.
- Correct volume & potassium preop if time allows.
- An elevated serum bicarbonate in a pt w/ COPD or restrictive lung disease may be appropriate compensation for chronic CO_2 retention.

INTRAOP

- Infuse NaCl to correct Cl-responsive alkalosis if desired.
- Consider arterial line for frequent ABG & electrolyte monitoring.
  - Especially useful for severely volume-depleted pts.
- Replete potassium at 10–20 mEq/h as indicated.
- Do not overventilate pt w/ chronic CO_2 retention due to lung disease.
- Metabolic alkalosis may be exacerbated by transfusion with citrate-containing banked blood products.

POSTOP

- Overventilation of pts w/ chronic CO_2 retention will acutely result in difficulty weaning from mechanical ventilation due to a decreased respiratory drive.
  - With time, overventilation will cause serum bicarbonate to decrease; the resulting increased minute ventilation requirement may produce respiratory distress.

➤ Extubated pts will have decreased drive to breathe & low minute ventilation.
- Ongoing chloride & potassium replacement may be needed.
- Continue efforts to identify & correct the underlying cause.

METHADONE MAINTENANCE THERAPY

J. W. BEARD, MD

OVERVIEW
- Definition: pt w/ history of opioid dependence placed on methadone to prevent withdrawal syndrome
- Usual Rx: once-daily oral methadone
  ➤ Dose varies by pt & clinic:
    - Low dose: 30 mg or less
    - Moderate dose: 30–50 mg
    - High dose: 80–100 mg

PREOP

Issues/Evaluation
- Opioid-dependent pts have tolerance to opioids & may be more sensitive to noxious stimuli.
  ➤ They require larger & more frequent doses of opioids for analgesia.
- 30–80% of substance abuse pts have coexisting psychiatric illness.
- Pts often fear ineffective treatment of pain, loss of maintenance therapy, disrespectful treatment by health care personnel.
- Methadone maintenance therapy does not provide analgesia.
- Pts w/ IV drug abuse are at increased risk of HIV, hepatitis B & C infection.

What To Do
- Determine if pt still takes opiates or other drugs of abuse in addition to methadone maintenance therapy.
- Reassure pt that postop pain mgt is a high priority. Address concerns regarding postop withdrawal.
- Continue outpt maintenance therapy perioperatively to prevent withdrawal.
- Consider regional anesthesia techniques.
- Avoid all medication w/ opioid antagonist properties. Administration could cause acute withdrawal.

INTRAOP

- Pts will require larger & more frequent opiate dosing to blunt reaction to surgical stimulation.

POSTOP

- Continue outpt methadone dose while using alternative narcotics for pain control.
- Fixed-schedule dosing of pain medication is preferable to PRN to avoid the misinterpretation of requests for analgesia as drug-seeking behavior.
- PCA narcotics are effective in pts secure in addiction recovery.
  - ➤ Use caution in pts who may abuse PCA or pts w/ visitors who may abuse PCA.
  - ➤ Pt will require higher-than-usual opiate dose because of tolerance.
- Although pts are tolerant to opiates, they will develop significant respiratory depression if opiate dose is high enough.
- Because high doses of opiates may be required, do not use meperidine (Demerol), because its metabolite normeperidine can cause seizures.
- Use nonnarcotic modes of analgesia if possible.
  - ➤ Regional block, when appropriate
  - ➤ Adjunct therapy w/ NSAIDs, tricyclic antidepressants or anticonvulsants may be of benefit.

MITRAL VALVE PROLAPSE

RICHARD PAULSEN, MD

OVERVIEW

- Definition: prolapse of the mitral valve leaflets into the left atrium during systole.
- Usual Rx: usually no treatment necessary. Some pts are treated w/ antidysrhythmic agents (beta blockers). Few pts are anticoagulated.
- Most common valvular disease (5–10% of population).

PREOP

Issues/Evaluation

- Most pts asymptomatic
- Symptoms may include atypical CP, palp, anxiety, dyspnea. Diagnosis confirmed by echocardiography

- Midsystolic click heard at apex +/– late systolic blowing murmur
- Pts at risk for mitral regurgitation, dysrhythmias, TIAs, infective endocarditis, ruptured chordae tendineae, AV block, nonspecific EKG changes, & rarely sudden death
- Higher incidence w/ Marfan's & von Willebrand syndromes
- Increasing left ventricular emptying will accentuate prolapse

What To Do
- ECG
- Antibiotics for endocarditis prophylaxis
- Echocardiography
- CXR

INTRAOP
- Minimize stimulation of sympathetic nervous system.
- Maintain normal HR, avoiding sudden changes.
- Maintain normal SVR, avoiding sudden changes.
- Minimize negative inotropes.
- Augment preload if tolerated.

Management
- Anxiolytic premed.
- Standard ASA monitors.
  - Additional monitors depend on severity of disease as well as stress of proposed surgery.
- With GA or regional, avoid drop in SVR.
- Use agents to attenuate sympathetic response.
- Avoid agents that promote dysrhythmias.

POSTOP
- ECG
- Continued risk for dysrhythmias
- Maintain appropriate analgesia

MITRAL VALVE REGURGITATION

RICHARD PAULSEN, MD
JASON WIDRICH, MD

OVERVIEW
- Definition: incompetent mitral valve causing systolic reverse blood flow

➤ Causes include
- Infective endocarditis
- Myxomatous degeneration of valve
- Chordae rupture
- Rheumatic disease
- Collagen-vascular disease

➤ Also associated w/ dilated cardiomyopathy

➤ Acute mitral regurgitation (MR) can result from papillary muscle dysfunction from myocardial ischemia or infarct, infective endocarditis.

■ Usual Rx: surgical valve replacement or repair. Repair may better preserve LV function.

■ Blood flow regurgitates across incompetent mitral valve during diastole.

➤ Leads to LA overload, pulmonary edema

➤ Compensatory tachycardia, LA enlargement, eccentric hypertrophy.

➤ Reduced EF & clinical deterioration indicate severe disease.

PREOP

Issues/Evaluation

■ Signs/symptoms include fatigue, dyspnea, orthopnea.

■ Physical exam findings include blowing pansystolic murmur, best at apex.

■ Indications for valve replacement/repair

➤ Acute MR w/ pulmonary HTN & right heart failure

➤ Chronic regurgitation w/ (regurgitant fraction/EF) >0.60

■ EF <60% is a sign of deterioration due to the altered loading conditions.

■ Acute MR can rapidly lead to LV dysfunction & failure.

■ Chronic MR can be present for 20–40 yrs w/o symptoms.

➤ Stage 1 (mild): asymptomatic w/ physiologic compensation (regurgitation <30% of stroke volume). Stage 2 (moderate): symptomatic impairment (regurgitation 30–60% of stroke volume).

➤ Stage 3 (severe): terminal failure (regurgitation >60% of stroke volume).

■ Left atrial volume overload leads to increased LVEDP & LVEDV in attempt to preserve stroke volume.

■ LVH, atrial fibrillation, left atrial enlargement, pulmonary HTN & recent MI are all associated w/ MR.

■ Mitral valve disease is an independent risk factor in CABG surgery.

What To Do

- ECG
- CXR
  - ➤ May show enlarged LA, prominent pulmonary system
- Echo
  - ➤ To evaluate location of mitral leaflet disease
  - ➤ May be useful to determine repair vs replacement of valve
  - ➤ Evaluate EF & regurgitant fraction
  - ➤ Direction & strength of regurgitant jet may give indication of severity
- Preop EF may be misleading in MR because force is against LA & not aortic outflow tract
- Antibiotics for endocarditis prophylaxis
- Consider evaluation for underlying CAD & dysfunctional myocardium

INTRAOP

- Standard monitors
  - ➤ Arterial line, CVP, PA line depend on severity of disease & risks of surgery.
  - ➤ Giant V wave may be seen w/ PA line but not appreciated w/ central line.
- Hemodynamic goals
  - ➤ Maintain HR & avoid bradycardia.
  - ➤ Maintain an appropriate preload.
  - ➤ Avoid decreases in cardiac contractility.
  - ➤ Avoid sudden increases in SVR.
    - Afterload reduction improves forward flow.

Management

- Regional or general anesthesia is usually well tolerated. Considerations include:
  - ➤ Maintain normal or slightly elevated HR & avoid sudden bradycardia.
  - ➤ Minimize drugs w/ negative inotropy.
  - ➤ Augment preload if tolerated.
  - ➤ Do not exacerbate pulmonary HTN if present.
- Avoid increases in pulmonary vascular resistance (PVR), including acidosis, hypoxia, hypercarbia, pain, cold, nitrous oxide.
- If necessary, positive inotropes & afterload reducing agents may improve cardiac function.

POSTOP
- ECG
- Watch for pulmonary edema & LV failure.
- Provide adequate analgesia.
- After surgical repair of MR, ventricular dysfunction may be unmasked.
  - ➤ Inotropic support & afterload reduction may be necessary.

MITRAL VALVE STENOSIS

RICHARD PAULSEN, MD
JASON WIDRICH, MD

OVERVIEW
- Definition: narrowing of the mitral valve causing reduced & turbulent diastolic blood flow
  - ➤ Mitral stenosis (MS) most often caused by rheumatic heart disease
- Usual Rx: surgical intervention prior to development of severe symptoms. Balloon dilation, commissurotomy, or valve replacement.

PREOP

Issues/Evaluation
- Normal mitral valve area 4–6 cm^2
- Progressive stenosis over 20 yrs prior to symptoms, then 7 yrs to incapacity
- Stage 1: mild
  - ➤ Valve area 1.5–2.0 cm^2 (mitral valve index >1–2 cm^2/m^2)
  - ➤ May be asymptomatic w/ physiologic compensation
  - ➤ May have increased filling pressures & may see dyspnea on exertion, hemoptysis
- Stage 2: moderate
  - ➤ Valve area 1.0–1.5 cm^2 (mitral valve index 0.6–1.0 cm^2/m^2)
  - ➤ Symptomatic w/ light exertion, may develop dilation of LA inducing AFIB & CHF
- Stage 3: severe
  - ➤ Valve area <1.0 cm^2 (mitral valve index <0.6 cm^2/m^2)
  - ➤ Terminal failure
  - ➤ Pulmonary HTN leading to RV dilation & failure; reduced LVEDP & LVEDV w/ preserved LV function

- Common signs/symptoms: dyspnea, paroxysmal nocturnal dyspnea, fatigue, chest pains, palp, hemoptysis
- Physical exam: diastolic murmur w/ opening snap, best at apex
- Atrial fibrillation common, related to left atrial enlargement
  - Anticoagulation required because of risk of embolism
  - Drug therapy for rate control is required to prevent rapid HR that impairs LV filling.
- Indications for mitral valve replacement include
  - New York Heart Association class III or IV heart failure (symptoms w/ minimal exertion or at rest)
  - Valvular area <1.0 cm^2
  - Systemic emboli
  - Pulmonary HTN

What To Do

- Antibiotics for endocarditis prophylaxis
- Document coexisting CAD or myocardial dysfunction.
- Assess exercise tolerance & functional status.
- ECG
- CXR
- Echo to evaluate
  - Valve area & flow
  - Pulmonary HTN
  - Ejection fraction
  - Diastolic pressure gradient across valve.
- HR control should be achieved prior to surgery if possible.
- For pt on anticoagulation.
  - Warfarin & aspirin will need to be stopped in advance.
  - May need heparin or low-molecular-weight heparin until a few hours prior to surgery.
  - Recognize that anticoagulation increases risk of central neuraxial block.

INTRAOP

- Hemodynamic goals
  - Maintain sinus rhythm; avoid tachycardia or rapid atrial fibrillation.
    - Atrial kick contributes 20–35% of cardiac output in MS.
  - Avoid sudden decreases in SVR.
  - Avoid large increases in central blood volume.

> Avoid increases in pulmonary vascular resistance (eg, avoid acidosis, hypoxia, hypercarbia, pain, hypothermia, nitrous oxide).

■ Use caution w/ regional anesthesia because of anticoagulation issues.

■ With neuraxial anesthesia, pts may be unable to compensate for an acute drop in SVR.

Management

■ Arterial line

■ Central access & PA line (depending on severity of disease & type of surgery)

■ CVP useful to monitor preload/overload to right heart

■ Consider TEE for major surgery or open heart surgery

■ For both general & regional anesthesia, maintain hemodynamic goals.

■ Treat tachycardia & dysrhythmias rapidly.

■ For worsening pulmonary HTN & RV failure, treat with inotropes & pulmonary vasodilators.

■ Watch for pulmonary edema, as pts are susceptible to volume overload.

■ If atrial fibrillation develops, provide rate control w/ esmolol, diltiazem, or other beta or calcium blocker.

> Consider cardioversion.

> Pts w/ chronic atrial clot are at risk of embolization.

POSTOP

■ ECG

■ Monitor pt for pulmonary edema & RV failure.

■ Given pt disease or stress of surgery, consider if ICU admission is warranted.

■ Provide adequate analgesia, which will help to prevent tachycardia.

> Analgesic plan must take into account limiting increases in PVR that can occur from hypoxemia or hypercarbia.

■ Optimize mgt of CHF, if present.

> If regional was used, fluid overload may occur as vasodilation from local anesthetic recedes.

■ Continue to maintain hemodynamic goals discussed above.

■ Know plan for restarting anticoagulants, especially if central neuraxial block was used.

MORBID OBESITY

JASON WIDRICH, MD
RICHARD PAULSEN, MD

OVERVIEW

- Definition: Twice ideal body wt. BMI $>40 \text{ kg/m}^2$
- Usual Rx: various attempts at wt loss, diet, exercise, behavior modification, bariatric surgery
- Patient may require Rx for comorbid conditions
  - HTN
  - CAD
  - Obstructive sleep apnea
  - Pulmonary HTN
  - Gastroesophageal reflux

PREOP

Issues/Evaluation

- Pts w/ morbid obesity are more likely to have:
  - Cardiac: CAD, HTN, LV/RV dysfunction, cor pulmonale, pulmonary HTN, increased cardiac output
  - Respiratory: restrictive lung disease w/ reduced FRC, obstructive sleep apnea, hypoventilation, Pickwickian (obesity hypoventilation) syndrome
  - GI: increased gastric volume, gastric acidity, intra-abdominal pressure w/ high incidence of hiatal hernia
  - Endocrine: DM, insulinoma, acromegaly
  - Hematologic: high risk for DVT/PE

What To Do

- History & physical: search for evidence of previously mentioned disorders
- Labs
  - CBC, lytes, BUN/Cr, glucose, LFTs, EKG
  - If indicated by symptoms or type of surgery, consider ABG (resting CO_2), echo (RV strain & pulmonary HTN), PFT, CXR.
- Premedication
  - Treat for GE reflux: give Bicitra, H2 antagonist, metoclopramide.
  - Consider effects of respiratory depressant premeds that could cause worsening obstructive sleep apnea.
- Anticipate difficulty w/ peripheral IV access.

➤ Consider central line for postop IV access or blood draws, depending on surgery & anticipated postop course.

INTRAOP
- Positioning issues
  - ➤ Get extra help w/ moving pt to OR table.
  - ➤ Confirm that OR table can support pt's weight.
  - ➤ Consider larger OR table.
  - ➤ Pad extremities carefully to minimize risk of nerve injury.
- Monitoring
  - ➤ Use appropriately sized BP cuff (small cuffs give artifactually high BP readings).
  - ➤ Noninvasive BP cuff may not detect BP adequately due to conical shape of arm.
  - ➤ May need arterial line for more reliable BP monitoring.
  - ➤ Consider central line if poor peripheral IV access.
- Airway issues
  - ➤ Anticipate difficult airway.
    - May have difficult mask ventilation because of excess pharyngeal soft tissue & decreased chest wall compliance.
    - May have difficult laryngoscopy for similar reasons.
    - Consider awake laryngoscopy or awake fiberoptic intubation.
    - Consider using short-acting muscle relaxant (eg, succinylcholine) to facilitate intubation.
  - ➤ Position pt properly for optimum airway mgt.
    - Elevate pt's shoulders by putting towels under the back for improved direct laryngoscopy.
    - May take 4–6 blankets to obtain best position.
  - ➤ Preoxygenate thoroughly.
    - Rapid desaturation w/ apnea, related to reduced FRC, relatively high O_2 consumption.
  - ➤ Use cricoid pressure & extubate when awake to minimize risk of aspiration.
- Drug metabolism concerns
  - ➤ Altered liver function & pharmacokinetics lead to possible prolonged drug elimination.
  - ➤ Lipid soluble drugs have larger Vd & longer T1/2, also leading to prolonged drug effect.
  - ➤ Volatile anesthetics are metabolized more; consider avoiding halothane & enflurane.
- Regional anesthesia issues

- ➤ Regional anesthesia difficult because of excess subcutaneous & adipose tissue
- ➤ Consider extra-long needles depending on block.
- ➤ For epidural, consider careful titration of local anesthetic because of possible exaggerated spread.
- DVT prophylaxis
  - ➤ Compression stockings.
  - ➤ Sequential compression device.
  - ➤ Discuss anticoagulation w/ surgeon.
    - Realize implications of anticoagulation for neuraxial blockade.

POSTOP
- Optimize conditions for extubation:
  - ➤ Hemodynamically stable
  - ➤ Normothermic
  - ➤ Alert & cooperative mental status
  - ➤ Full reversal of neuromuscular blockade
  - ➤ Adequate analgesia
- Watch respiratory status closely & consider monitoring in ICU setting
  - ➤ Hypoxemia & low FRC possible for next 3–7 days postop
  - ➤ Morbidly obese pt at higher risk for:
    - Atelectasis, PNA, DVT/PE
    - Respiratory depression from narcotics
    - Worsening obstructive sleep apnea
  - ➤ Recover in sitting position if possible.
  - ➤ Encourage pulmonary toilet (eg, incentive spirometry).
  - ➤ Have CPAP available, especially if pt on home CPAP for sleep apnea.
  - ➤ Continue DVT/PE prophylaxis.
- Pain mgt
  - ➤ Especially important because of pulmonary changes of morbid obesity.
  - ➤ Pts more susceptible to respiratory depressant effects of narcotics.
  - ➤ Pts may have worsening sleep apnea from narcotics.
  - ➤ Consider non-narcotic analgesic (eg, acetaminophen, NSAID).
  - ➤ If appropriate, regional anesthesia may decrease narcotic requirement.
  - ➤ Anticipate joint pain, back pain, or tissue damage from lying flat on OR table.

MUSCULAR DYSTROPHIES

PATRICK ROSS, MD

OVERVIEW

- Definition: A group of diseases of primary muscular atrophy of unknown cause. There is degeneration of muscle fibers & an increase in content of fat & fibrous tissue. The group includes Duchenne's, Becker's, facioscapulohumeral, limb-girdle, congenital, others.
- Duchenne's: 1 in 3,300 male births. Most common & severe. X-linked recessive but female "carriers" w/ severe disease have been reported. Onset of weakness 2–6 y, starting in pelvic girdle & then proximal muscle groups. The earlier the onset, the more rapid the downhill course. Disease leads to wheelchair dependence in 3–10 y & to death after 5–20 y, usually from respiratory illness.
- Becker's dystrophy: 1 in 18,000–33,000 male births. X-linked recessive. Onset mean age 12 y. Much more benign course than Duchenne's. Death occurs at an average age of 42 y, usually from pneumonia.
- Facioscapulohumeral (FSH) dystrophy: 1 in 20,000. Autosomal dominant (boys = girls). Weak pectoral & facial muscles. Present in teens w/ weak shoulders & winging of the scapula. May have slight decrease in vital capacity & some cardiac involvement. Life span is reduced minimally.
- Limb-girdle: "wastebasket" classification of 5 predominantly autosomal recessive diseases. Severity is midway between Duchenne's & FSH.
- Congenital: "wastebasket" used to classify onset of the disease at birth.
- Usual Rx: None, although some pts may be receiving steroids.

PREOP

Issues/Evaluation

- Respiratory: seen by reductions in inspiratory & expiratory effort as well as decreased vital capacity & total lung capacity. Obtain baseline room air saturation & consider PFTs. Pts who appear to be doing well may be severely limited after anesthesia. Pts have decreased cough & are more prone to pneumonia.

- Kyphoscoliosis occurs as result of muscular weakness & compounds decreased respiratory compromise.
- Cardiac abnormalities: severity of cardiac & skeletal disease does not correlate. May range from EKG abnormalities, arrhythmias, mitral valve prolapse, & cardiomyopathies. Atrial arrest or sudden death reported w/ some disease states. Obtain baseline EKG & rhythm strip. Consider echo. CK-MB fraction is present in skeletal muscle myopathies & thus cannot be used as a marker of cardiac injury.
- Malignant hyperthermia has been associated w/ this group of diseases. Speculated that inherent membrane defect renders the muscle more susceptible to injury induced by anesthesia.
- Gastric hypomotility: a feature for some pts

What To Do
- Consider regional anesthesia where appropriate.
- Avoid succinylcholine as it increases potassium & can trigger MH.
- Avoid premedication when possible as pts at increased risk for aspiration.
- Treat as if a full stomach.
- Teach pulmonary toilet & prepare pt for postop CPAP or mechanical ventilation.

INTRAOP
- Dose anesthesia to pt response rather than age/weight, trying to "minimize" anesthesia.
- Pts may be more "sensitive" to nondepolarizing neuromuscular blockers. Complete reversal seen by peripheral neuromuscular monitoring does not predict adequate respiratory muscle recovery.
- Anticipate & be prepared to treat arrhythmias.
- Place NG or OG tube to evacuate stomach contents for gastroparesis.

Management
- Avoid succinylcholine as above.
- Consider modified rapid-sequence induction for gastroparesis.
- Anticipate arrhythmias.

POSTOP
- Provide close cardiorespiratory monitoring.
- Anticipate need for further respiratory support, including adequate pulmonary toilet, CPAP or mechanical ventilation.

MYASTHENIA GRAVIS

EMILY REINYS, MD
WILLIAM A. SHAPIRO, MD

OVERVIEW

- Definition: chronic autoimmune disease characterized by weakness/fatigue of voluntary skeletal muscles w/ progressive use
- Disease results from antibody-mediated impairment of neuromuscular transmission at nicotinic acetylcholine receptors
- Usual Rx
  - Anticholinesterase agents (typically, pyridostigmine), which inhibit the enzyme responsible for the hydrolysis of acetylcholine
  - Thymectomy for pts refractory to anticholinesterase therapy
  - Occasionally, immunosuppressants and/or corticosteroids
  - Less commonly, plasmapheresis

PREOP

Issues/Evaluation

- Great variability in severity of disease, ranging from limited extraocular muscle involvement to generalized weakness w/ respiratory impairment
- Determine whether pt has been taking anticholinesterase meds in the periop period. These agents will markedly decrease sensitivity to nondepolarizing neuromuscular blockers & markedly prolong duration of succinylcholine.
- Consider type/location of surgery & whether neuromuscular blockers will be required.
- Other medications such as local anesthetics (esters) & aminoglycosides can exacerbate muscular weakness.

What To Do

- Obtain prior anesthetic records (if available) to determine previous response to general anesthesia, neuromuscular blockers & any postop complications.
- Perform preop testing w/ peripheral nerve stimulator to assess a baseline train-of-four; this helps predict pts w/ increased sensitivity to nondepolarizing neuromuscular blockers (T4/T1 <0.9 will have increased sensitivity).
- Inform pt of possible need for postop ventilatory support.
- Preop PFTs in pts w/ existing respiratory impairment may be helpful.

■ Administer very little, if any, sedative premed to avoid respiratory depression.

INTRAOP

■ Dose of neuromuscular blocker varies widely among pts & should be titrated individually.
■ Inherent muscle relaxant effects of halogenated volatile anesthetics may eliminate or decrease need for neuromuscular blockers.
■ Prolonged effects of opioids, especially in causing respiratory depression, detract from the use of these meds for maintenance of anesthesia.

Management

■ Use peripheral nerve stimulator to determine dose & dosing interval of neuromuscular blockers (if needed). Document peripheral nerve stimulator response before using any neuromuscular blocking agent.
■ If neuromuscular blockers are required for intubation, administer 1/3–1/2 usual dose of nondepolarizing agent & assess response w/ peripheral nerve stimulator. If depolarizing agent is used for intubation, dose required may be up to twice the usual dose.
■ Neuromuscular blockade reversal w/ anticholinesterase agents (neostigmine, edrophonium) is recommended at end of case; may not be effective if pt has been taking pyridostigmine in periop period.
■ Prior to extubation, ensure adequate muscle strength: check for sustained head lift >5 sec, regular respiratory pattern, adequate tidal volumes, return of 4/4 train-of-four ratio.

POSTOP

■ Close observation in PACU/ICU for respiratory distress.
■ Pts too weak to be extubated may require prolonged ventilatory support and/or pyridostigmine infusion.

MYOCARDIAL INFARCTION

ART WALLACE, PHD, MD

OVERVIEW

■ Definitions:
   ➤ Coronary artery disease (CAD): coronary artery atherosclerosis
   ➤ Myocardial infarction (MI): acute ischemic necrosis of an area of myocardium from inadequate blood supply for demand

- Angina pectoris: referred pain to chest, arm, or jaw from inadequate blood supply for demand to myocardium. No cellular death associated w/ episode. 95% of ischemic episodes occur w/o angina pectoris.
- Heart failure (CHF or HF): inadequate ventricular systolic or diastolic function leading to elevated filling pressures and/or low cardiac output
- Cardiogenic pulmonary edema: fluid accumulation in lungs from elevated pulmonary vascular pressures
- Unstable angina: new onset of angina or increased frequency or intensity of angina
- Stable angina: no change in pattern of angina or level of exertion that elicits angina
- Myocardial stunning: diminution in myocardial function from brief period of ischemia w/ no evidence of cellular necrosis
■ Usual Rx
  - Antianginal: beta blocker, calcium channel blocker, nitrates
  - Antihypertensive: beta blockers, calcium channel blockers, vasodilators, diuretics
  - Lipid-lowering drugs: statins
  - Antiplatelet & anticoagulants: aspirin, heparin, Coumadin, platelet inhibitors
  - Revascularization: PTCA w/ or w/o stenting, CABG

PREOP

Issues/Evaluation
■ Careful H&P w/ specific attention to cardiac history: MI, CHF, anginal pattern, change in anginal pattern, level of exercise tolerance, previous work-ups.
■ Prior CABG, prior PTCA, date of prior revascularization: the longer the time from previous revascularization the more likely pt will have return of ischemia. Recent PTCA (<2 mo) increases risk of periop MI.
■ Presence of devices: pacemaker, defibrillator.

What To Do
■ Evaluate if pt is stable.
■ If pt is stable but not on beta blockade, start beta blocker therapy: atenolol 25 mg PO QD or equivalent – increase dose as tolerated to maintain heart rate >50 bpm & systolic blood pressure >100 mm Hg.

- If pt is stable on medical therapy including beta blockers, maintain this therapy throughout periop period, increasing dose as needed to maintain heart rate at 50–75 bpm.
- If pt is unstable, risk stratify for possible revascularization and/or medical therapy. Tests may include exercise thallium, Persantine thallium, or cardiac cath.
- All pts w/ CAD, prior MI, angina, peripheral vascular disease, or two risk factors for CAD (hypertension, age >=65, diabetes, cigarettes, cholesterol >=240) must be on periop anti-ischemia therapy (beta blockers) unless absolutely contraindicated.
- If absolute contraindication for beta blockade, consider alpha-2 agonist therapy with clonidine (0.2 mg PO night before surgery & #2-TTS patch for 4 d placed night before surgery).

INTRAOP
- Monitor as needed – arterial line, 5-lead ECG.
- Long-acting beta blockers (atenolol, metoprolol) to maintain heart rate at 50–75 bpm.
- Avoid tachycardia.

POSTOP
- Maintain beta blockade for at least 1 week postop & for 30 d in high-risk pts.

OBSTRUCTIVE SLEEP APNEA

MADELEINE BIBAT, MD

OVERVIEW
- Definition: >10 episodes per hour of sleep involving cessation of airflow for at least 10 sec despite respiratory effort
- Usual treatment: continuous positive airway pressure (CPAP) during sleep

PREOP
Issues/Evaluation
- Occurs in obese pts due to increased fat deposition in pharyngeal tissues; may also be present in children w/ tonsillar hypertrophy

- Ascertain presence by inquiring about daytime somnolence, nocturnal snoring, witnessed apnea while sleeping, or feeling of fatigue upon awakening.
- Refer pts for a sleep study for definitive diagnosis & to distinguish severity of sleep apnea.
- Pts often have coexisting hypertension, diabetes, coronary artery disease, cor pulmonale.
- Evaluate airway for Mallampati class, tongue size, neck range of motion, tissue redundancy. Devise plan for pts w/ potentially difficult & easily obstructed airways.
- Focus physical exam on signs of right heart failure & evidence of pulmonary hypertension or cor pulmonale.
  - Obtain preop CXR, EKG.
    - Consider echocardiogram & pertinent cardiac workup based on history & proposed surgery.

What To Do
- Avoid preop sedation because of high risk for airway obstruction.
- Provide antiemetics, gastric acid neutralizers, and/or promotility agents to obese pts who are at risk for aspiration.
- Perform regional anesthesia when pt is amenable & airway is readily accessible.

INTRAOP
Management
- Consider awake fiberoptic intubation in these pts because their obesity, neck anatomy, & excess pharyngeal tissue make them potentially difficult to intubate.
- Ensure adequate preoxygenation prior to attempts at endotracheal intubation because obese pts desaturate more quickly due to their low FRC & high oxygen consumption.
- Invasive monitoring is dictated by severity of cardiac & pulmonary disease.
- Manage hypertension, diabetes, & pulmonary hypertension if present.
- Reverse neuromuscular blockade & avoid CNS & respiratory depressants prior to awakening & extubation.
- Extubate pt only when fully awake; consider extubation in semi-upright or reverse Trendelenburg position to decrease pressure of abdomen on diaphragm.

- Residual anesthesia may exacerbate the severity or frequency of apneic episodes postop.

POSTOP

- Keep pt intubated if anesthetics & narcotics have continued CNS & respiratory effects or if surgery further compromised the upper airway.
- Closely monitor extubated pts for airway obstruction, desaturation, & development of negative-pressure pulmonary edema; may require reintubation or establishment of an emergency airway.
- Avoid narcotics & sedatives; use acetaminophen, ketorolac, and/or regional anesthetic blocks when possible as alternatives for pain relief.
- Provide CPAP by nasal or full face mask.
- Consider ICU monitoring for apnea, airway obstruction, cardiac arrhythmias.

PARKINSON'S DISEASE (PD)

SUSAN RYAN, PHD, MD

OVERVIEW

- Definition: neurodegenerative disease primarily of the dopamine-containing neurons of the substantia nigra. This results in extrapyramidal motor dysfunction characterized by
  - Tremor ("pill-rolling")
  - Rigidity (cogwheel)
  - Hypokinesis
- Select nondopamine cell groups also degenerate, resulting in
  - Bulbar dysfunction
  - Gastroparesis
  - Autonomic instability from sympathetic fiber loss
  - Dementia & depression are often present
- Usual Rx
- Most common treatments until recently
  - Sinemet (L-dopa + carbidopa)
  - Anticholinergics
- Newer treatments now used prior to & in combination w/ Sinemet
  - Dopamine agonists (ropinirole, pramipexole)
  - Newer MAO inhibitors (selegiline)

➤ COMT enzyme inhibitors (tolcapone, entacapone)
➤ Amantadine
➤ Atypical neuroleptics (risperidone, olanzapine)

PREOP

Issues/Evaluation

■ Aspiration risk
  ➤ Evaluate history of aspiration or "choking."
  ➤ Examine pt for inability to handle secretions.
  ➤ Pt may have bulbar dysfunction.
  ➤ Also evaluate history of reflux, since gastroparesis may be present.
■ Tremor/rigidity/hypokinesis
  ➤ Obtaining IV access can be challenging.
  ➤ Evaluate pt's ability to cooperate w/ a procedure under sedation.
  ➤ Tremor & rigidity can worsen acutely when medications are held or stopped for surgery.
  ➤ Rigidity & hypokinesis can lead to decreased neck extension or mouth opening.
■ Pulmonary function
  ➤ Advanced PD pts may have pulmonary dysfunction from rigidity, a restrictive pattern.
  ➤ They may also have a history of aspiration pneumonia.
■ Autonomic dysfunction: PD pts can have high, low or variable blood pressure as a result of meds & autonomic degeneration.
■ Dementia
  ➤ Can pt provide informed consent to surgery & to anesthesia?
  ➤ Can pt cooperate w/ a procedure under sedation or regional anesthesia?
■ Meds: Many new meds are available to PD pts. Be familiar w/ side effects & toxicities. Some meds require surveillance of specific lab tests such as platelets or LFTs.

What To Do

■ Aspiration risk
  ➤ Provide antacid preop.
■ Tremor/rigidity
  ➤ Continue medications up to am of surgery.

➤ Plan to restart them ASAP postop & coordinate this w/ surgeons.
- Pulmonary function
  - ➤ Check preop O_2 saturation.
  - ➤ Consider obtaining CXR, ABGs, PFTs. ABGs & PFTs may be useful intraop & for prognostication when the planned operation will impair pulmonary function (ie, upper abdominal or thoracic surgery).
- Dementia: Obtain proper consent from relative or durable power of attorney if dementia present.

INTRAOP
- GA, MAC, regional anesthesia have all been used successfully in PD pts. For GA, both inhalation agents & propofol have been used.
- Avoid the following meds:
  - ➤ Dopamine antagonists, such as droperidol or haloperidol
  - ➤ Meperidine if pt is taking an MAO inhibitor

Management
- Aspiration risk
  - ➤ Consider a rapid sequence intubation if reflux/gastroparesis is present. Succinylcholine did not lead to hyperkalemia in one small study.
  - ➤ Avoid use of LMA for GA in pts w/ gastroparesis.
- Tremor/rigidity
  - ➤ Avoid meds that could worsen the condition, such as dopamine antagonists (droperidol or haloperidol).
- Pulmonary function
  - ➤ Monitor ABGs if preop concerns indicate it.
  - ➤ Evaluate ventilation in particular prior to extubation.
- Hypotension
  - ➤ Use direct-acting agents, such as phenylephrine, for BP support.
  - ➤ Indirect agents, such as ephedrine, may be more unpredictable.
- Hypertension: labetalol, hydralazine, nitrates all acceptable
- Extubation: Do not extubate deep if at risk for aspiration or bulbar dysfunction. PD pts may have further impaired bulbar function secondary to missing medications & could have trouble protecting the airway, even if not evident preop.

POSTOP
- Resume meds ASAP.
- If pt requires postop intubation, restart PO PD meds by NG or feeding tube ASAP.

PATIENT STATUS POST CARDIAC TRANSPLANT

KURT DITTMAR, MD

OVERVIEW

- Definition: pt who has undergone heart transplant
- Noncardiac surgery is common in heart transplant recipients.
- Recipient has a higher incidence of pancreatitis & cholecystitis than the general population.
- Malignancy & infection rates are increased secondary to immuno-suppression.

PREOP

Issues/Evaluation

- Electrophysiology changes
  - ➤ Two P waves might be present due to atrial cuff remnant.
  - ➤ ST-segment depression can be present w/o coronary disease.
  - ➤ Conduction disturbances such as right bundle branch block are common.
  - ➤ ECG signs may accompany rejection episodes: atrial arrhythmias, bradycardia, low voltage, ST-segment depression, PVCs.
  - ➤ Some pts may be pacemaker-dependent.
- Cardiac physiology changes (discussed further in Intraop section)
  - ➤ Ejection fraction (EF) & cardiac output (CO) are usually normal.
  - ➤ Cardiac allograft vasculopathy, a form of accelerated atherosclerosis, occurs frequently.
    - CHF, acute MI, sudden death are the most common clinical findings. Angina is unlikely secondary to denervation of the transplanted heart.
- Immunosuppression
  - ➤ Pts will be immunocompromised & susceptible to infections.
  - ➤ Immunosuppression must be continued perioperatively. Typical agents & associated problems are listed below.
    - Cyclosporine: may cause renal failure w/ secondary hypertension. BUN/Cr frequently elevated.
    - Steroids: must continue intraop. Adrenal suppression & glucose intolerance are possible.
    - Azathioprine: thrombocytopenia & anemia may result.

What To Do

- Clinical evaluation should include

➤ History & physical
- Medications, especially immunosuppression drugs & doses
- Pacemaker information
- Functional status changes that could be attributed to rejection

➤ ECG
- Look for signs of rejection described above

➤ Echocardiogram

➤ Recent cardiac cath report

➤ CBC

➤ Electrolytes, BUN, creatinine, glucose

■ Continue all immunosuppressant medications perioperatively

■ MAC & regional & general anesthesia have all been used successfully

INTRAOP

■ Most important intraop concerns relate to cardiac physiology changes & the immunocompromised state.

■ Cardiac physiology changes
➤ Resting HR usually 90–100.
➤ Since both sympathetic & parasympathetic innervation is lost in the transplanted heart, many of the reflex arcs are lost (eg, carotid sinus massage).
➤ Laryngoscopy, light anesthesia, hypoxia, hypotension & hypovolemia usually do not promote tachycardia.
➤ CO is dependent on preload since the reflex tachycardia found w/ hypotension & hypovolemia is severely blunted.
- Therefore, it is important to avoid dehydration & positions that compromise preload.
- Pay particular attention to intraop volume status.

■ Important drug pharmacology issues
➤ Certain agents will not produce their expected hemodynamic response because of the altered cardiac physiology (especially denervation).
➤ Agents that have their usual effects include isoproterenol, epinephrine, dopamine, dobutamine, beta blockers.
➤ The usual changes in HR associated w/ atropine, glycopyrrolate, edrophonium, neostigmine, pancuronium, succinylcholine & phenylephrine will not be seen.
➤ Nitroglycerin & nitroprusside will demonstrate an exaggerated BP decrease since reflex tachycardia will be absent.
➤ Ephedrine & alpha-1 agonists show decreased effectiveness.

■ Immunosuppression

➤ Sterile technique is crucial.

➤ Antibiotic prophylaxis is mandatory.

➤ >Staphylococcus> coverage should be implemented prior to invasive line placement.

➤ Nasal intubation is generally avoided due to higher incidence of bacteremia.

➤ Continue corticosteroids perioperatively.

■ If central line required, do not use the right IJ, as most cardiologists prefer this access site for cardiac biopsies.

POSTOP

■ Recovery & discharge criteria are similar to other pts.

■ Outpt surgery is not contraindicated.

■ As in the intraop phase, PACU interventions should take into account the altered HR response to various pharmacologic therapies, preload dependence of the denervated heart & the immunocompromised state.

PATIENT WITH IMPLANTABLE CARDIOVERTER-DEFIBRILLATOR (ICD)

HSIUPEI CHEN, MD
WILLIAM A. SHAPIRO, MD

OVERVIEW

■ Definition: Implantable (internal) cardioverter-defibrillator (ICD)

■ Possible indications (indications are evolving & may become broader)

➤ Cardiac arrest from VT/VF not due to reversible cause

➤ History of spontaneous sustained VT

➤ Syncope of undetermined origin w/ hemodynamic instability & VT/VF inducible at electrophysiologic testing (EPS) & not pharmacologically treatable

➤ Symptomatic nonsustained VT assoc w/ CAD, previous MI, or LV dysfunction

➤ Inducible VT/VF at EPS not pharmacologically treatable

PREOP

Issues/Evaluation

■ Obtain old EPS & any other cardiac test results.

■ High likelihood of CAD, CHF, depressed LV function, HTN, DM, PVD

- Continue all perioperative cardiac meds, including beta blockers & antiarrhythmics.
- Correct any electrolyte abnormality, especially if pt taking digoxin or diuretics.

What To Do

- Identify the ICD make & model number, date of insertion, indication for implantation.
  - ➤ Ask patient for device ID card.
  - ➤ Check medical record.
  - ➤ Obtain CXR of the pulse generator; may reveal the unique radiopaque company code.
  - ➤ Contact cardiologist or hospital ICD clinic or service.
  - ➤ Contact ICD company representative.
  - ➤ Contact numbers: Biotronik® 1-800-547–9001, Guidant® 1-800-227–3422, Medtronic® 1-800-328–2518, Saint Jude Medical® 1-800- 777–2237
- Check ICD function, intrinsic rhythm, magnet response.
- Deactivate the ICD: tachycardia sensing should be programmed off (consider doing only after fully monitored).
- If rhythm is 100% paced (ICD with antibradycardia pacing), magnet will not produce asynchronous pacing. This can be done only by reprogramming the ICD generator.
- Have external defibrillator available in OR if the ICD is programmed off.

In an Emergency

- Emergent surgery that poses risk of activating ICD: consider a magnet during cautery
- Truly emergent surgery that poses little risk to pulse generator or leads (surgery on extremity, eye cases, bipolar cautery cases) may not require ICD reprogramming.

INTRAOP

Management

- Place grounding pad as far as possible from the ICD & in a way that a line drawn between the grounding pad & the cautery does not cross the ICD. If the ICD is still activated during cautery, cautery should be <5 sec.
- Intraop external defibrillation should be done with anterior-posterior paddle configuration & when possible w/ the paddles at

least 10 cm from the pulse generator. Use the lowest possible energy for cardioversion or defibrillation.

■ Removing the magnet will reactivate the ICD sensing.

Special Situations
■ MRI will inhibit the pulse generator.
■ Lithotripsy may damage the pulse generator; the ICD should be deactivated & the beam should not be focused on the pulse generator site.

POSTOP
■ Immediately after surgery, confirm proper ICD function; reprogram the device if necessary.

PATIENT WITH PACEMAKER

HSIUPEI CHEN, MD
WILLIAM A. SHAPIRO, MD

OVERVIEW

Definitions
■ Asynchronous: no sensing circuit to detect intrinsic R waves
■ Synchronous: includes a circuit that detects intrinsic depolarizations & then either activates or inhibits the pacemaker
■ Five-letter generic code for classification
■ Letter 1 = chamber paced (A, atrium; V, ventricle; D, both)
■ Letter 2 = chamber sensed (A, atrium; V, ventricle; D, both; O, none)
■ Letter 3 = response to sensing (T, triggered; I, inhibited; D, both; O, none)
■ Letter 4 = programmable functions (P, programmable for rate and/or output; M, multiprogrammable; C, communicating; R, rate modulation)
■ Letter 5 = antitachyarrhythmic functions (O, none; P, pacing; S, shock; D, both)
■ Possible indications
   ➤ Complete heart block
   ➤ Second-degree AV block
   ➤ MI
   ➤ Sick sinus syndrome
   ➤ Chronic bifascicular or trifascicular block
   ➤ Syncope
   ➤ CHF

PREOP

Issues/Evaluation

- Determine native rhythm & indication for pacemaker.
  - ➤ Old electrophysiologic testing (EPS).
  - ➤ Other cardiac test results.
  - ➤ Most recent pacemaker interrogation report.
- High likelihood of CAD, HTN, DM, peripheral vascular disease.
- Continue all perioperative cardiac meds, including beta blockers & antiarrhythmics.
- Correct any electrolyte abnormality, especially if pt taking digoxin or diuretics.
- Recognize potential sources of electromagnetic interference (EMI) on pacemakers (adapted from Hayes & Strathmore, Levine & Love, Atlee & Bernstein).
  - ➤ EMI source: electrocautery
    - Generator damage: yes
    - Complete inhibition: yes
    - One-beat inhibition: yes
    - Asynchronous pacing: yes
    - Rate increase: yes
  - ➤ EMI source: external defibrillation
    - Generator damage: yes
    - Complete inhibition: no
    - One-beat inhibition: no
    - Asynchronous pacing: yes
    - Rate increase: yes
  - ➤ EMI source: MRI scanner
    - Generator damage: possible
    - Complete inhibition: no
    - One-beat inhibition: yes
    - Asynchronous pacing: yes
    - Rate increase: yes
  - ➤ EMI source: lithotripsy (ESWL)
    - Generator damage: yes
    - Complete inhibition: yes
    - One-beat inhibition: yes
    - Asynchronous pacing: yes
    - Rate increase: yes
  - ➤ EMI source: RF ablation
    - Generator damage: yes
    - Complete inhibition: yes

- One-beat inhibition: no
- Asynchronous pacing: no
- Rate increase: yes
➤ EMI source: electroconvulsive therapy (ECT)
  - Generator damage: no
  - Complete inhibition: yes
  - One-beat inhibition: yes
  - Asynchronous pacing: yes
  - Rate increase: yes
➤ EMI source: transcutaneous electrical nerve stimulation (TENS)
  - Generator damage: no
  - Complete inhibition: yes
  - One-beat inhibition: no
  - Asynchronous pacing: yes
  - Rate increase: yes
➤ EMI source: radiation therapy
  - Generator damage: yes
  - Complete inhibition: no
  - One-beat inhibition: no
  - Asynchronous pacing: no
  - Rate increase: yes
➤ EMI source: diagnostic radiation
  - Generator damage: no
  - Complete inhibition: no
  - One-beat inhibition: no
  - Asynchronous pacing: no
  - Rate increase: yes

What To Do
- Identify the pacer make & model number, date of insertion, indication for implantation.
  ➤ Ask pt for device ID card.
    - Check medical record.
    - Call cardiologist/device manager/pacemaker clinic.
    - Call device representatives (numbers below) to see if they know pt.
    - Obtain CXR of the pulse generator; may reveal the unique radiopaque company code.
- Contact numbers
  ➤ Biotronik® 1-800-547–9001
  ➤ Guidant® 1-800-227–3422

➤ Medtronic ® 1-800-328–2518

➤ Saint Jude Medical ® 1-800-777–2237

■ Check pacer function, battery status, programmed setting, intrinsic rhythm, magnet response (consult the hospital's pacer clinic/service).

■ Reprogram to an asynchronous mode (with adaptive-rate pacing feature off) if EMI likely to cause inhibition & if pt does not have an adequate intrinsic rhythm.

■ Surgery that poses little risk to pulse generator or leads may not require pacer reprogramming (eg, lower extremity surgery, eye cases, or when bipolar cautery is used).

In an Emergency

■ If unable to reprogram the pacer & possible EMI-related malfunction unavoidable, place magnet directly over pulse generator to pace asynchronously.

■ If unable to determine pacer mode, have magnet available for cautery.

INTRAOP

Management

■ Place grounding pad as far as possible from the pacer & in a way that a line drawn between the grounding pad & the cautery does not cross the pacer. Use the lowest possible energies & shortest duration of electrocautery.

■ In case of pacemaker failure, use ACLS protocols including transcutaneous pacing.

➤ Place pads on opposite sides of the heart to allow defibrillation & pacing.

■ Isoproterenol may be infused at a rate of 1–3 mcg/min to increase the ventricular rate.

■ When the magnet is removed, the pacer should revert to the previously programmed mode.

■ Defibrillation will allow current tracking down a pacemaker lead & may make the heart unresponsive to pacemaker stimulation for a period of time.

POSTOP

■ Immediately after surgery, confirm proper pacer function.

■ Reprogram pacer if necessary.

PEDIATRICS

PATRICK ROSS, MD

OVERVIEW
- This chapter presents an overview of important issues in pediatric anesthesia.
- Remember that children are not just small adults!

PREOP

Issues/Evaluation

Airway/Breathing
- Infants & neonates are obligate nasal breathers.
- The cricoid cartilage is the narrowest point in the airway in children <5 y. In adults the narrowest portion is the glottis.
- Recognize the impact of airway edema in children.
  - ➤ Small decreases in airway size in infants dramatically increase the resistance.
  - ➤ Resistance is inversely proportional to radius to the 4th power (Poiseuille's law).
  - ➤ The smaller the child the greater the impact from airway edema.
- Uncuffed ETT is usually selected for children <10 y to decrease the risk of postintubation croup. Subglottic region at cricoid level is narrowest part of the airway.
- Cuffed ETT may be used in pediatric pts, but cuff inflation should be adjusted to desired leak. Choose size 0.5 smaller than recommended for uncuffed ETT.
- As a general guide choose ETT size based upon pt age. Also prepare ETT one size above & below. ETT size is based on tracheal diameter at the cricoid ring rather than the glottic opening. Age vs. uncuffed ETT size:
  - ➤ Preterm neonate: 2.5 – 3.0
  - ➤ Full-term neonate: 3.0 – 3.5
  - ➤ 3 mo to 1 y: 4.0
  - ➤ 2 y: 4.5
  - ➤ 4 y: 5.0
  - ➤ 6 y: 5.5
  - ➤ 8 y: 6.0
  - ➤ 10 y: 6.5

➤ Alternate formula: ETT size $= 4 + $ age$/4$. Can also choose ETT w/ similar diameter to child's 5th finger.

■ Important: Assess leak around ETT after placement.
  ➤ There should be a leak at 10–25 cm water pressure to decrease pressure on tracheal mucosa. Change ETT size accordingly if leak is inappropriately high or low.
  ➤ Infants & children have very compliant chest walls & when subject to high ventilatory pressure are prone to barotraumas.

■ Intubation may be facilitated by placing a towel under the shoulders to move the head into a sniffing position. Infants & children have a large head & prominent occiput relative to their body.

■ Straight laryngoscope blades are more useful than curved in creating a good view w/ laryngoscopy.
  ➤ The cephalad position of the larynx makes the angle between the base of the tongue & glottic opening more acute.
  ➤ Epiglottis can be long & flexible in small children. Straight blade is better for lifting the epiglottis.

■ Can use laryngeal mask airway (LMA) in infants & children but they are much more prone to obstruction with twisting or small movements. Choose LMA size based on pt weight:
  ➤ #1 LMA <5 kg
  ➤ #1.5 LMA 5–10 kg
  ➤ #2 LMA 6.5–25 kg
  ➤ #2.5 LMA 20–30 kg
  ➤ #3 LMA 25 kg to small adult

■ Important: Anticipate short time to desaturation w/ apnea.
  ➤ Infants have a high metabolic rate & increased oxygen consumption.
  ➤ They are more prone to alveolar collapse & have lower FRC than adults.

■ Apnea & bradycardia following anesthesia not uncommon in infants <60 wks post-conceptual age. They should be monitored overnight following procedures.

Cardiovascular

■ Important: Bradycardia is a grave warning sign of hypoxemia, hypercarbia, metabolic acidosis, hypotension, or other insults. Cardiac arrest may follow bradycardia if the underlying condition is not corrected.

■ Stroke volume is relatively fixed in infants & children as the ventricles are relatively noncompliant; therefore, cardiac output is increased by increasing heart rate.

- Baseline heart rate & BP vary with age. As a rough guide:
  - Preterm neonate: HR 120–180, SBP 45–60, DBP 30
  - Term neonate: HR 100–180, SBP 55–70, DBP 40
  - 1 y: HR 100–140, SBP 70–100, DBP 60
  - 3 y: HR 85–115, SBP 75–110, DBP 70
  - 5 y: HR 80–100, SBP 80–120, DBP 70
- Remove all air bubbles from IV lines since there is a high incidence of patent foramen ovale, which increases the risk of coronary or cardiac embolism.

Fluids/GI

- Consider replacement fluid, maintenance, & intraop fluid when estimating fluid requirements.
  - Tailor replacement fluid to the clinical situation. Factors include:
    - Length of NPO status
    - Whether pt has had preoperative fluid restriction (eg, for a PDA in a premature infant)
  - Maintenance fluid is based upon weight:
    - 1–10 kg = 4 cc/kg/h
    - 10–20 kg = 40 cc/h + 2 cc/kg/h
    - >20 kg = 60 cc/h + 1 cc/kg/h
  - Intraop fluid replacement
    - Minor fluid loss such as eye, dental, or endoscopic procedures: 0–10 mL/kg/h
    - Mild to moderate fluid loss such as hernia or cleft lip/palate: 10–20 mL/kg/h
    - Large fluid loss procedures such as intra-abdominal, spine, or craniofacial: 20–30 mL/kg/h
- Consider placement of an intraosseous needle when IV access is extremely difficult to obtain.
- NPO guidelines for children undergoing elective surgery. Consider longer fasting time if pt has delayed gastric emptying.
  - A clear liquid is anything you can read the newspaper through, such as water or apple juice.
  - Normal children <3 y
    - Hold milk, formula, or solids for 6 h prior to surgery.
    - Hold breast milk for 4 h.
    - Hold clear liquids for 2 h.
  - Normal children >3 y
    - Hold milk or solids for 8 h prior to surgery.
    - Hold clear liquids for 2 h.

➤ For all children: if surgery is delayed, consider IV fluids to prevent dehydration.

■ Mean weight for children of different ages:
  ➤ Term newborn: 3.2 kg
  ➤ 6 mo: 7.8 kg
  ➤ 1 y: 10.2 kg
  ➤ 2 y: 12.5 kg
  ➤ 3 y: 15 kg
  ➤ 5 y: 19 kg
  ➤ 7 y: 23 kg
  ➤ 10 y: 32 kg

Hematology

■ Infants are born w/ a high hemoglobin that falls in the first few months & reaches its normal physiologic nadir at age 3 mo.
■ Normal range of Hgb:
  ➤ Term newborn: 13.5–19.5
  ➤ 1 mo: 10.7–16.1
  ➤ 2 mo: 9.4–13.0
  ➤ 6 mo to 6 y: 11.5–13.5
  ➤ 6–12 y: 11.5–15.5
■ Transfusion threshold must be individualized when dealing w/ intraop blood loss.
  ➤ Consider PRBC transfusion for >30–40% blood volume loss.
  ➤ Factors include age of child, associated medical problems, starting Hct, & further anticipated blood loss.

ID

■ URIs (see also "Coexisting Disease: URI")
  ➤ It is quite common for small children to have a cold or URI every month during the winter.
  ➤ The decision whether to anesthetize these children must be done on a case-by-case basis.
  ➤ A recent viral illness puts the child at increased risk of periop wheezing, hypoxemia, atelectasis, laryngospasm.
  ➤ However, in rescheduling the surgery, the child may return again w/ another infection.
  ➤ Factors to consider:
    • Urgency of surgery
    • Health of child
    • Coexisting illnesses
    • Impact of waiting on the family

Thermoregulation
- Children have a larger surface area per kg body weight than adults; this contributes to heat loss in cold ORs.
- Monitor temp closely.
- Measures to maintain temp:
  - ➤ Increase room temp.
  - ➤ Warm IV fluids.
  - ➤ Humidify inspired gases.
  - ➤ Use a warming blanket or warming lights.

Family
- Pay very close attention to the family's role in the anesthetic.
  - ➤ They will not be happy if their issues are not addressed. Subsequently, the child may not be happy & you will not be happy.
  - ➤ If they have reasonable suggestions of what worked w/ a prior anesthetic consider them or explain why it may not be appropriate for this surgery.

INTRAOP

Induction of Anesthesia
- Infants <6–8 mo old may be taken to the OR w/o sedation to proceed w/ an inhalation induction.
- Children 6 mo & older may benefit from an oral premed, inhalation induction w/ the parents present, or both. If there is no induction room close to the OR then strongly consider premed.
  - ➤ Oral midazolam syrup given in dose range of 0.25–0.5 mg/kg is a typical premed. Onset is usually 20 min but may vary w/ each child. Monitor child closely after premed.
- Children can be induced in their parent's arms.
  - ➤ Warn parents that the child will become limp like a rag doll during induction.
  - ➤ Child may also show excitatory symptoms of "stage 2" anesthesia.
  - ➤ This is a time of great fear for many parents. Clearly outlining the likely sequence of changes in their child's behavior will help most parents cope.
- To improve the child's cooperation, consider applying scent to the mask w/ food flavoring & letting the child play w/ it before starting.
- In a cooperative child:
  - ➤ Hold mask close to but not touching the face.
  - ➤ Start oxygen & nitrous oxide, & after a few moments sevoflurane or halothane.
  - ➤ Increase inhaled agent gradually.

➤ When the child loses muscle tone, support the airway & escort the parents out of the room.
- If the child becomes uncooperative during induction:
  ➤ Hold the mask on the face.
  ➤ Increase the inspired gas flow as well the inhaled agent (eg, 4–5% halothane or 7–8% sevoflurane).
  ➤ When the child loses muscle tone, support the airway & escort the parents out of the room.
- For children who are extremely uncooperative or developmentally delayed:
  ➤ Consider induction of anesthesia w/ ketamine 4–10 mg/kg IM. Onset will occur in 3–5 min. Can add atropine 0.02 mg/kg IM to reduce the increased salivation seen w/ ketamine.
  ➤ Prepare to support the airway & provide supplemental oxygen.
  ➤ Start IV as soon as possible.
  ➤ Increase depth of anesthesia w/ an inhaled agent if necessary.
- Children > 10–12 y old may consider IV induction if given the choice & a clear explanation of IV vs inhaled induction. Consider local anesthesia for IV, or EMLA if time permits.

Muscle Relaxants
- Consider avoiding succinylcholine for routine elective surgery in children.
  ➤ In children, succinylcholine may be more likely to produce cardiac dysrhythmias, hyperkalemia, myoglobinemia, malignant hyperthermia.
  ➤ Many children can be intubated w/o muscle relaxants by deepening their level of anesthesia.
  ➤ Succinylcholine 2–4 mg/kg IM still useful for emergent control of the airway in a child w/ no IV access. Can mix w/ atropine 0.02 mg/kg IM to decrease risk of bradycardia.
- Rocuronium can be used in children in dose range of 0.9–1.2 mg/kg IV for emergency or routine intubation if necessary.

Maintenance of Anesthesia
- MAC is higher in infants than in neonates or adults.

Emergence From Anesthesia
- Watch carefully for laryngospasm on emergence.
  ➤ Children are more prone to laryngospasm during emergence than adults.
  ➤ Suction the airway immediately before & after extubation.

➤ Treat laryngospasm initially w/ positive pressure & jaw thrust. but prepare airway equipment & medications if this is ineffective.

POSTOP
■ Can place child in lateral position for transport & recovery so that oral secretions can drain away from the vocal cords & prevent laryngospasm.
■ Transport to PACU w/ supplemental oxygen & monitor breathing pattern closely.
■ Consider bringing parents to PACU as early as possible to relieve anxiety for both parents & child.
■ Order appropriate pain meds & monitor closely for side effects such as respiratory depression.

PERICARDITIS

JAMES BRANDES, MD

OVERVIEW
■ Pericarditis can be classified as acute, subacute or chronic based on duration.
➤ Acute pericarditis: <6 wks
➤ Subacute: 6 wks to 6 mo
➤ Chronic: >6 mo
■ Infectious etiology of pericarditis
➤ In the U.S., viral pericarditis is common, typically after a URI prodrome.
➤ Other infectious causes include bacterial, fungal & tuberculous infections.
• Worldwide, TB is the most common cause of pericarditis.
■ Noninfectious etiologies
➤ Uremia
➤ Myxedema
➤ Autoimmune disease (SLE, rheumatoid)
• Drug-induced (eg, procainamide)
• Post-MI Dressler's syndrome
• Post-cardiac surgery
➤ Chest radiation
➤ Neoplastic disease
• Primary tumor
• Metastatic disease

■ Chronic constrictive pericarditis is a long-term sequela of acute pericarditis (or chronic pericardial effusion) w/ significant morbidity & mortality.

PREOP

Issues/Evaluation

■ Acute pericarditis typically presents w/
  ➤ Chest pain worse w/ inspiration
  ➤ ECG changes
    • Widespread ST segment elevation, sometimes w/ upward concave shape
  ➤ Pericardial friction rub on auscultation
  ➤ Other potential findings: tachycardia, pulsus paradoxus, enlarged cardiac silhouette on CXR from pericardial effusion
■ Most important characteristics of pericardial effusion
  ➤ Normal amount of pericardial fluid is ~25 cc.
  ➤ The volume of effusion is not as crucial as the pressure exerted by the fluid in the pericardial space.
    • If fluid has accumulated over a long period of time, the pericardium will stretch & the effects will typically be subclinical to mild.
    • However, the acute accumulation of even 100 cc of fluid can cause cardiac tamponade.
  ➤ Pulsus paradoxus will usually be present in the setting of significant pericardial effusion.
■ Features of chronic constrictive pericarditis
  ➤ May see calcifications on CXR
  ➤ May hear precordial knock on auscultation
  ➤ Cardiac output is HR- & preload-dependent secondary to impaired diastolic filling of all four chambers.
  ➤ On a CVP tracing, a prominent Y-descent is present secondary to impaired late diastolic filling.
  ➤ Equilibration of diastolic pressures & wedge pressure will be seen w/ a PA catheter.
  ➤ May see Kussmaul's sign in severe cases (increase in CVP w/ inspiration)
  ➤ May see secondary hepatic congestion & ascites

What To Do

■ Postpone elective surgery in pts w/ newly diagnosed pericarditis until workup has been completed.

- Evaluation is directed toward determining the presence of an effusion & signs of cardiac tamponade or myocardial depression.
  - If no effusion present & no component of myocarditis, there are usually no major anesthetic consequences, except for the difficulty of evaluating for ischemic changes by ECG.
  - Important: pt w/ cardiac tamponade can rapidly develop significant hemodynamic instability & may require urgent pericardiocentesis or pericardial window.
- Look for clinical signs of low cardiac output/right or left heart failure.
  - Hypotension
  - Elevated JVD
  - Laterally displaced cardiac impulse
  - Peripheral edema
  - Pulmonary rales
  - Hepatomegaly
  - Ascites
- Obtain cardiac echo to evaluate for effusion, signs of tamponade, or myocardial dysfunction.
  - If a large effusion is present, pericardiocentesis may be performed preop.
  - If the cause is unknown, look for infectious cause, check renal function & thyroid panel & evaluate for stigmata of collagen vascular disease.
- Important: ensure adequate volume status prior to induction, as anesthetics & positive-pressure ventilation can unmask or worsen cardiac tamponade physiology, leading to severe hypotension or cardiovascular collapse. (See also Critical Event chapter "Cardiac Tamponade.")

INTRAOP

- Monitors/line placement
  - Arterial line useful to watch for sudden BP changes.
  - CVP or PA catheter may be useful for severe constrictive disease.
  - TEE may also be useful for severe disease.
- Maintain filling pressure & cardiac output, especially w/ induction of anesthesia.
  - Avoid bradycardia.
  - Aggressively treat hypovolemia.
  - Anticipate hypotension from induction drugs & positive-pressure ventilation.

➤ Coughing at emergence may increase intrathoracic pressure & reduce venous return.
■ Watch for arrhythmias.
■ Pt may develop airway edema from venous congestion.

POSTOP
■ Monitor closely for arrhythmias & signs of low cardiac output.
■ Other monitoring depends on the underlying disease & nature of surgical procedure.
■ If surgical procedure included drainage of pericardial fluid, then cardiac physiology may have improved.

PERIOPERATIVE MYOCARDIAL INFARCTION

ART WALLACE, PHD, MD

OVERVIEW
■ Definitions
  ➤ Myocardial infarction (MI) during periop period. Highest frequency within 72 hours postop.
  ➤ Q-wave MI: transmural infarction w/ new Q waves on ECG.
  ➤ Non-Q-wave MI (NQWMI): non-transmural infarction w/ myocardial enzyme release but no Q wave on ECG (usually has T wave or ST changes).
  ➤ Rule-in for MI in noncardiac surgery: troponin I greater than threshold for hospital w/ or w/o ECG changes.
  ➤ Rule-in for MI in cardiac surgery: troponin I > 10 times threshold for hospital w/ or w/o ECG changes.
  ➤ Coronary artery disease (CAD) is coronary atherosclerosis.
■ Acute mortality from perioperative MI can be substantial (>20%), w/ extremely poor 2-year survival (20%).
■ Usual Rx.
  ➤ Avoid myocardial ischemia: A single 1-minute episode increases risk of MI 10-fold. Periop myocardial ischemia occurs in 40% of pts at risk:
    • Known CAD (prior MI, angina).
    • Known peripheral vascular disease.
    • Two risk factors for CAD (hypertension, age >=65, diabetes, cigarettes, cholesterol >=240).
  ➤ Start beta blockers. All pts w/ CAD, prior MI, angina, peripheral vascular disease, or two risk factors for CAD (hypertension,

age >=65, diabetes, cigarettes, cholesterol >=240) must be on periop anti-ischemia therapy (beta blockers) unless absolutely contraindicated.
> If absolute contraindication for beta blockade, consider alpha-2 agonist therapy w/ clonidine (0.2 mg PO night before surgery, #2-TTS patch for 4 days placed night before surgery).
■ Most common events leading to ischemia
> Preop anxiety: pts should be beta blocked preop.
> Tachycardia from reversal of neuromuscular blockade.
> Atrial fibrillation from postop mobilization of fluid.
> All of these events can be reduced with beta blocker therapy.

PREOP

Issues/Evaluation
■ Evaluate the risk of CAD: known, unknown, at risk for CAD.
■ Evaluate the stability of known CAD.
> Change in anginal pattern
> Congestive failure
■ If CAD is stable
> Pt should be placed on beta blockade (preop atenolol or metoprolol).
> High-risk pt should be on beta blocker for at least 7 days.
> Low-risk pt: give beta blocker ASAP
■ If CAD is unstable: pt should be risk stratified for possible PTCA, CABG or additional medical therapy.

What To Do
■ If acute MI occurs despite anti-ischemia therapy
> Stabilize BP, HR.
> If systolic BP >100 mmHg: nitroglycerine infusion (25–400 mcg/min).
> If systolic BP <100 mmHg: phenylephrine infusion.
> HR should be 50–75 bpm. Maintain w/ esmolol infusion.
> If hemorrhage is not an issue, administer aspirin 325 mg PO.
> Admit to ICU; rule out w/ serial troponin I measurements & ECG.

INTRAOP
■ Rarely occurs intraop in noncardiac surgery w/ appropriate anti-ischemia therapy & good hemodynamic control
■ In cardiac surgery usually presents as new ischemia

➤ Prebypass: anticoagulate w/ heparin, maintain BP & HR, cannulate for bypass, revascularize ASAP
➤ Postbypass: test grafts for patency, consider placement of additional graft, maintain BP & HR, administer nitroglycerin if possible

Management
■ Decrease risk of ischemia & infarction by using periop beta blockade.
■ Control BP & HR.
  ➤ Low systolic pressure: Neo-Synephrine infusion.
  ➤ Normotension or hypertension: nitroglycerine infusion.
  ➤ Tachycardia (HR >80): esmolol infusion.
■ Consider aspirin.
■ Admit to ICU; rule out w/ troponin & ECG, cardiology consult.

POSTOP
■ Consult cardiologist.
  ➤ He/she will administer medical therapy including beta blockers, aspirin, angiotensin-converting enzyme (ACE) inhibitors.
  ➤ Cardiologist will consider risk stratification w/ thallium scintigraphy, echocardiography & coronary catheterization for possible PTCA or CABG.

PERIPHERAL VASCULAR DISEASE (PVD)

MARK ROLLINS, MD

OVERVIEW
■ Definition: atherosclerotic disease affecting blood vessels & perfusion in the extremities
  ➤ Often results in tissue ischemia & associated morbidity
■ Risk factors for PVD include
  ➤ Age >40 yrs
  ➤ Smoking
  ➤ Diabetes mellitus
  ➤ Hyperlipidemia
  ➤ HTN
■ Severity of PVD correlates w/ risk of death from
  ➤ MI
  ➤ Ischemic stroke
  ➤ Other vascular causes
■ Medical therapy may include

- Exercise training program
- Smoking cessation
- Lipid-lowering therapy
- Pentoxifylline therapy
- Antiplatelet therapy
■ Surgical intervention may include
  - Balloon angioplasty and/or stenting
  - Endarterectomy
  - Endovascular grafts
  - Patch angioplasty
  - Vascular bypass surgery w/ autologous vein or synthetic grafts
  - Amputation

PREOP

Issues/Evaluation

■ PVD may result in claudication, rest pain, nonhealing wounds & ulcers, acute thrombosis, cellulitis, osteomyelitis, gangrene.
  - Most pts have reduced functional capacity & lifestyle limitations.
■ Associated medical conditions are common & may include
  - CAD
  - Cerebral vascular disease
  - Diabetes mellitus
  - Smoking
  - HTN
  - COPD
  - Coagulopathies
  - Renal insufficiency
■ Severity of PVD can be noninvasively assessed w/ pulse palpation, ankle brachial index, duplex examination.
  - Angiograms may be done for more detailed evaluation & surgical planning.

What To Do

■ Thorough evaluation for coexisting diseases listed above, w/ particular attention to presence of
  - CAD, including recent MI
  - Cerebral vascular disease
  - Hypercoagulable states
■ Optimize cardiac status prior to surgery.
  - Consider whether further cardiac workup is indicated.
  - Consider periop beta blocker therapy to decrease risk of cardiac complications.

- ➤ Correct anemia in pts w/ CAD.
- ➤ Control HTN prior to surgery & continue antihypertensive regimen in periop period.
- ■ Consider regional anesthesia when appropriate for possible reduction in postop hypercoagulation & adrenergic stress.
  - ➤ Check for coag status & anticoagulant meds that may increase risk of regional block.

INTRAOP
- ■ Monitor for myocardial ischemia, arrhythmias.
- ■ Use of invasive monitoring will depend on coexisting disease & stress of proposed surgery.
  - ➤ Consider invasive monitoring for severe CAD, CHF or labile BP.
- ■ For pts w/ CAD, maintain tight control of HR & hemodynamics throughout case, w/ particular attention to intubation & induction.
- ■ Prevent hypothermia, anemia.
- ■ Monitor extremities for adequacy of perfusion & signs of ischemia.

POSTOP
- ■ Consider ICU monitoring depending on severity of coexisting disease, stress of surgery, intraop course.
  - ➤ Close monitoring may permit detection of myocardial ischemia, CHF, arrhythmias, peripheral ischemia.

PHEOCHROMOCYTOMA

MARC SCHROEDER, MD
JULIN TANG, MD, MS

OVERVIEW
- ■ Definition: epinephrine- & norepinephrine-secreting tumor
  - ➤ 90% made of chromaffin-containing ectodermal cells of the adrenal medulla
  - ➤ 90% benign
  - ➤ 90% unilateral
- ■ Incidence
  - ➤ 0.03–0.04% in general population at autopsy
  - ➤ 0.1% in pts w/ sustained HTN
- ■ Pathophysiology: alpha-1 stimulation results in increased PVR, increased BP. Alpha & beta stimulation lead to
  - ➤ Intravascular volume depletion
  - ➤ Renal failure

➤ Hemorrhage
➤ Tachycardia
➤ Myocardial ischemia
➤ Ventricular hypertrophy/ectopy
➤ Cardiomyopathy
➤ CHF
➤ Glucose intolerance
■ Surgical excision is curative.
➤ Surgery may be performed as open or laparoscopic procedure.
➤ See also Procedure chapter "Pheochromocytoma Resection."
■ Pt w/ known pheochromocytoma should not undergo elective surgery other than resection of the tumor.
➤ If pt requires urgent surgery prior to tumor resection, follow precautions discussed below.

PREOP

Issues/Evaluation
■ Common presenting symptoms
➤ Excessive sweating
➤ Headache
➤ Hypertension
➤ Orthostatic hypotension
➤ Psychosis
■ Diagnosis
➤ Urinary excretion of vanillylmandelic acid (product of catecholamine metabolism) & unconjugated norepinephrine
➤ Increased blood levels of norepinephrine/epinephrine (not in all cases)
➤ MRI
➤ I-123 MIBG
➤ CT or ultrasound can be used to localize tumor.
■ Pheochromocytoma crisis: catecholamine excess w/ hypertensive crisis resulting in hemorrhage/infarct of vital organs
➤ Look for clinical symptoms like fever, tachycardia & changes in mental status.
■ Mortality rate 0–3% even w/ appropriate preparation for tumor resection. Highest for undiscovered cases undergoing unrelated surgery.
■ Evaluate for multiple organ system involvement.
➤ CV: HTN, dysrhythmias, A-fib, sinus tachycardia, mitral valve prolapse, CHF, myocarditis. Decreased exercise tolerance, SOB,

palpitations. Previous hypertensive or arrhythmic response to induction of anesthesia or to abdominal exam.

➤ GI: weight loss, diarrhea, dehydration. Abdominal palpation of tumor can trigger crisis.

➤ Heme: mild polycythemia, thrombocytopenia (decreased intravascular volume)

➤ GU: renal stones from dehydration

➤ CNS: headache, tremor, anxiety, decreased pain threshold, fatigue

➤ Metabolism: glucose intolerance (alpha-adrenergic-induced gluconeogenesis, decreased insulin secretion)

What To Do

■ Goal is to avoid crisis by preop adrenergic blockade. Prehydrate & increase alpha blockade over 10 days up to 2 mo.

➤ Use oral phenoxybenzamine (a long-acting alpha-antagonist) or prazosin for preop alpha blockade. It decreases SVR, increases intravascular volume, corrects glucose intolerance.

➤ If not emergent, try to delay surgery if blockade is not present prior to surgery. If emergent operation, use alpha & beta blockers & nitroprusside. Admit pt to ICU until postop pain issues are resolved.

➤ Adequate blockade if BP normalized/stabilized (no reading >165/90 for 48 h), reduction of sweating, no ST changes on EKG, resolution of glucose intolerance. Adequate blockade takes an average of at least 10–14 days.

➤ Do not administer beta blockade prior to alpha blockade because epinephrine & norepinephrine will produce unopposed alpha stimulation & result in hypertension crisis. The hypertrophied myocardium may not be able to handle the increased workload w/o the beta-1 stimulation.

INTRAOP

■ Monitors: arterial line prior to induction (avoid pain), consider CVP, TEE or PA catheter, monitor temp & glucose level.

■ No difference in outcome w/ GA vs regional anesthesia.

■ Consider epidural for pain relief w/ open procedure.

Management

■ Up to half of undiagnosed pheochromocytoma pts who die in hospital do so during induction of GA, during stress in periop period, or during labor and delivery.

- Prehydrate aggressively if pt can tolerate it.
- Use nitroprusside infusion to treat hypertension during induction. Anticipate exaggerated stress response.
- Anticipate hypotension after surgeon ligates venous drainage of tumor.
  - Have dopamine infusion ready before ligation of adrenal vein.
- Phentolamine IV is often used for intraop alpha blockade (disadvantage: slow onset/long duration, tachyphylaxis).
- Avoid agents or conditions that release catecholamines or block reuptake (eg, ketamine, desflurane).
  - Fasciculations of the abdominal musculature due to succinyl-choline may cause release of catecholamines from abdominal tumor.
  - Vagolytic drugs (anticholinergics, pancuronium) will worsen the sympathetic imbalance.
  - Histamine can cause catecholamine release by the tumor (tubocurare, atracurium, MS, meperidine).
  - Use beta blockers to treat tachycardia & ventricular dysrhythmias.
  - Avoid halothane as it sensitizes the heart to ventricular irritability due to catecholamines.
  - Droperidol (alpha antagonist) may cause paradoxical hypertensive crisis.

POSTOP
- Pts have a tendency to go into CHF (if source of endogenous catechols has been removed) if overhydrated to push urine output.
- For POD 1–3, 50% of all pts remain hypertensive. Aggressive pain mgt w/ epidural, PCA, IV narcotics is indicated.
- Pts may experience postop psychiatric problems.

PNEUMONIA

ANNEMARIE THOMPSON, MD

OVERVIEW
- Definition: lower respiratory tract infection characterized by a new infiltrate on CXR not attributable to pulmonary edema (cardiogenic or neurogenic). Usually associated w/ fever/hypothermia, cough, dyspnea, impaired gas exchange

- Causes decrease in lung compliance due to extravascular fluid/debris in the interstitium and/or the alveoli
- Bacterial pneumonia: antibiotics are the mainstay of therapy
- Viral pneumonia: usually supportive care only
- Aspiration pneumonia: supportive care only

PREOP

Issues/Evaluation
- Elective surgeries should be postponed until pneumonia resolves.
- Consider pneumonia if the following history/physical exam findings are present:
  - Fever
  - Cough
  - Decreased breath sounds on auscultation
  - Egophony
  - Dullness to percussion of chest over lung fields
  - Decreased oxygen saturation
  - Underlying pulmonary disease

What To Do
- CXR
- Consider ABGs to establish baseline oxygenation.
- Discuss findings/plan w/ primary caregiver.

INTRAOP

Management
- Postpone elective surgery.
- If urgent/semiurgent surgery, consider
  - $FiO_2 = 1$ to maximize oxygen content in normal alveoli
  - Routine monitors, plus arterial line for blood gas monitoring
- Pt may require aggressive pulmonary toilet through large endotracheal tube to clear secretions.
- Continue antibiotic therapy if bacterial etiology of pneumonia is suspected.

POSTOP
- Pts w/ pre-existing pneumonia may require postop mechanical ventilation, particularly if undergoing upper abdominal/thoracic surgery, since these surgeries decrease functional residual capacity postop.
- Extubation should be performed when pt is awake w/ intact airway reflexes.

PORPHYRIA

WYNDA W. CHUNG, MD

OVERVIEW
- Definition
  - Inherited or acquired enzymatic defects of heme biosynthesis.
  - These defects lead to accumulation of porphyrins, which are molecular precursors of heme.
- There are various forms of porphyria, depending on the specific enzyme defect & the metabolic intermediate that accumulates.
  - ALA (aminolevulinic acid) synthetase is the rate-limiting enzyme in heme biosynthesis. In porphyria, enzymes subsequent to this step are deficient, leading to an increased activity of ALA synthetase via feedback. This leads to overproduction of heme precursors & accumulation of the precursors before the deficient step.
- Manifestations include
  - Neuropsychiatric: severe abdominal pain, muscle weakness, nausea/vomiting, postural hypotension, HTN
    - Pts can develop a motor & sensory neuropathy related to demyelination.
  - Cutaneous
  - Mixed forms
- Acute attacks are associated w/ the following types, all of which have autosomal dominant inheritance:
  - Acute intermittent porphyria
    - The most common of the acute porphyrias
  - Hereditary coproporphyria
  - Variegate porphyria
- Usual Rx: avoidance of exacerbating factors. Treatment of acute crisis is described below.

PREOP

Issues/Evaluation
- Clinical features of acute attack include the following. Pts are most commonly women in their 30s. Frequency & severity of attacks vary widely.
  - Severe abdominal pain
  - Tachycardia, HTN

- Neurologic manifestations
  - Mental status changes (including confusion, agitation, hallucinations)
  - Cranial nerve palsies
  - Peripheral neuropathy
  - Autonomic dysfunction
- Vomiting, constipation
- Dark-colored urine (varying from red to purple
- Electrolyte imbalances (low Na^+, K^+, Mg^{+2} levels)
  - Hyponatremia may cause seizures.
- Symptoms may be exacerbated by various factors:
  - Drugs (including certain anesthetic agents)
  - Fasting/dehydration
  - Infection
  - Psychological stress
  - Hormonal variation: menstruation; pregnancy may exacerbate or provoke attack
  - Alcohol & substance abuse
- 1% mortality of an acute attack
- Diagnosis of acute attack
  - Laboratory diagnosis is important, as symptoms may not be due to acute porphyria. Typical findings include
    - Increased urinary porphobilinogen
    - Increased aminolevulinic acid

What To Do

- Determine frequency & nature of acute porphyria attacks. Pts w/ active symptoms & frequent attacks are at increased risk of drug-induced acute attack.
- Avoid drugs that are likely to precipitate attacks (see below for drugs commonly encountered in the periop period).
  - For drugs not listed below, consider consultation w/ a more comprehensive list of so-called "safe" & "unsafe" drugs. However, some drugs on these lists appear in both categories.
  - Consider risk & benefit of any drug administered, as there may be lack of evidence of the safety of a particular drug.

INTRAOP

- GA
  - Avoid administration of the following drugs, because they may precipitate a crisis:
    - Thiopental & other barbiturates

- Etomidate
- Ketamine
- Phenytoin
- Diazepam & other benzodiazepines
- Sulfonamide antibiotics
- Sulfonylureas
- Ergot derivatives
- Carbamazepine
- Valproic acid
- Meprobamate
- Pentazocine

➤ Drugs considered safe for anesthesia include
- Propofol
- Volatile anesthetics (particularly nitrous oxide)
- Narcotics (except pentazocine)
- Nondepolarizing & depolarizing muscle relaxants
- Anticholinesterases
- Anticholinergics
- Acetaminophen

■ Signs of an acute crisis during anesthesia
➤ Autonomic instability: HTN & tachycardia are common features of an acute attack.
➤ Generalized convulsions: treatment of seizures is difficult because all commonly used antiseizure drugs are porphyrogenic.
➤ Dark-colored urine.

■ Treatment of an acute crisis
➤ Maintain hemodynamic stability.
➤ Propranolol may improve tachycardia & HTN from sympathetic stimulation.
➤ For generalized convulsions: treat hyponatremia, if present. Gabapentin may be effective for seizure control & is not considered porphyrogenic.
➤ Maintain airway patency & respiratory support, as necessary.
➤ Hydration & correction of electrolyte disturbances
➤ Administer IV dextrose (may decrease serum sodium; use caution in pts w/ hyponatremia).
➤ Treatment w/ heme products suppresses endogenous heme synthesis & decreases excretion of porphyrin compounds.
- Heme arginate: give early in attack; dose is 3 mg/kg/day IV x 4 days. Give in a central vein over 15 min.
- Hematin

■ Regional anesthesia

➤ Limited experience w/ anesthesia in pts w/ porphyria. Some practitioners avoid regional anesthesia because of the following factors:

- Neuropathy from an acute porphyria crisis may be rapid & differentiation between regional anesthesia effects & neuropathy may be obscured.
- Hypovolemia & labile autonomic response increase the risk of hemodynamic instability during sympathectomy from spinal or epidural anesthesia.

➤ Despite these concerns, regional anesthesia has been successfully used in pts w/ porphyria.

POSTOP

■ The rate of recovery from an acute attack depends on the degree of neuronal damage; may be rapid (1–2 days) w/ prompt supportive therapy.

■ Recovery from severe motor neuropathy may continue for months or years.

■ Prompt identification & avoidance of inciting factors can hasten recovery from a crisis & prevent future events.

POTASSIUM DISORDERS

JASON WIDRICH, MD

OVERVIEW

■ Definition: plasma potassium concentration outside normal range (3–5.5 mEq/L)

■ Usual Rx
➤ Diagnosis & treatment of underlying condition
➤ Supplementation or removal of potassium to ameliorate symptoms in the acute setting

PREOP

Issues/Evaluation

■ Hypokalemia [K+] <3.5 mEq/L
➤ Manifestations
- ECG changes: T-wave flattening, prominent U waves, PR prolongation, atrial & ventricular arrhythmias
- Other cardiac effects: myocardial dysfunction; exacerbation of digoxin toxicity with K+ between 3–4 mEq/L

- Neuromuscular: muscle weakness, prolonged neuromuscular blockade, rhabdomyolysis, ileus
- Renal: polyuria, increased bicarbonate reabsorption
- Endocrine: decreased insulin & aldosterone secretion

➤ Etiology
- ECF to ICF shift: acute alkalosis, insulin tx, beta adrenergic activity, hypokalemic periodic paralysis
- Renal loss: mineralocorticoid excess, hyperaldosteronism, hypomagnesemia, diuretics, vomiting, NG suction, amphotericin
- GI loss: vomiting, diarrhea, GI fistula

■ Hyperkalemia serum [K+] >5.5

➤ Manifestations
- Cardiac: peaked T waves, QRS widening, ventricular arrhythmias, wide complex "sine wave," cardiac arrest
- Neuromuscular: muscle weakness

➤ Causes
- Pseudohyperkalemia: hemolysis, leukocytosis or thrombocytosis
- ICF to ECF shift: acidosis, rhabdomyolysis, severe exertion, succinylcholine, tissue catabolism
- Decreased renal excretion: renal failure, hypoaldosteronism (including drug rx with ACE inhibitor, spironolactone, NSAIDs)
- Increased intake: oral or IV

What To Do

■ For mild, asymptomatic hypokalemia (K >2.5), not necessary to postpone elective surgery

■ For symptomatic or severe hypokalemia, consider postponing elective surgery & starting potassium replacement.

➤ For patients taking digoxin, K^+ >4 mEq/L should be the goal prior to surgery.

■ For hyperkalemia, determine cause & initiate treatment prior to surgery.

➤ Verify response to therapy prior to induction of anesthesia.

➤ Hyperkalemia, if untreated, can lead to life-threatening arrhythmias & cardiac arrest.

➤ See also Critical Event chapter "Hyperkalemia."

INTRAOP

■ Do not administer succinylcholine to a pt w/ known hyperkalemia.

➤ Some conditions are associated w/ exaggerated & life-threatening K^+ elevation w/ succinylcholine:
  - Pts w/ burn injury (>48 h), massive trauma, myopathies, prolonged immobilization, paraplegia, denervation of skeletal muscle

■ Suspicion of hyperkalemia or hypokalemia may begin in the intraop period w/ recognition of cardiac arrhythmias or ECG changes.
  ➤ Obtain stat serum potassium level.
  ➤ Determine etiology of the potassium disorder based on pt history, presentation or intraop course.

■ Consider other lab studies to evaluate full electrolyte & acid-base status.
  ➤ ABGs (acid-base changes causing intracellular shifts)
  ➤ Serum electrolytes & anion gap
  ➤ Magnesium
  ➤ Calcium
  ➤ Creatine kinase (CK) (large elevation suggests rhabdomyolysis)
  ➤ Glucose (insulin deficiency or DKA)
  ➤ Creatinine (renal failure)

Management

■ Hyperkalemia (see also Critical Event chapter "Hyperkalemia")
  ➤ Stabilize cardiac membranes:
    - IV calcium gluconate (10 mL of a 10% solution) or calcium chloride (1 g)
    - May repeat in 5 min if no change in ECG
  ➤ Facilitate intracellular shift of potassium:
    - 10 units regular insulin IV.
    - 25–50 g glucose IV.
    - Treat acidosis: hyperventilation, sodium. bicarbonate 50–100 mEq IV, treat underlying metabolic acidosis.
    - Consider inhaled beta agonist (eg, albuterol).
  ➤ Remove potassium from body.
    - Facilitate urine output: administer IV fluid & diuretics (eg, furosemide 10–20 mg).
    - Consider urgent hemodialysis. Will need to call nephrologist & place hemodialysis catheter.
  ➤ Avoid potassium-containing IV solutions.

■ Hypokalemia (see also Critical Event chapter "Hypokalemia")
  ➤ Use continuous ECG monitoring during IV K^+ replacement.
  ➤ KCl IV infusion rate: 0.2–0.5 mEq/kg/h

- 10–20 mEq/h KCl can be given by peripheral IV.
- Higher rates should be given via central access (max replacement should be <240 mEq/24 h).

➤ Use glucose-free IV solutions.

➤ Follow serum potassium level during replacement.

➤ If potassium is slow to increase, look for hypomagnesemia.

- May need to increase magnesium level before potassium will rise appropriately.

POSTOP

■ Follow electrolytes at an appropriate interval (may range from q30min to q24h).

➤ Interval for follow-up will depend on acuity, symptoms, method of correction & concomitant problems that could further complicate potassium balance (eg, acute renal failure, cardiac arrhythmias, DKA).

PREGNANCY

EMILY REINYS, MD

OVERVIEW

■ Surgery is performed during pregnancy in approximately 0.3–2.2% of all parturients.

■ Appendicitis, acute cholecystitis, adnexal masses are the most common nonobstetric conditions requiring surgery during pregnancy.

PREOP

Issues/Evaluation

■ Women of childbearing age should be screened regarding the possibility of pregnancy prior to elective surgery; testing should occur if diagnosis is in doubt.

■ Greatest concerns: prevention of preterm labor, maternal safety, avoidance of teratogens, avoidance of fetal hypoxemia

■ Significant alterations in maternal physiology occur during pregnancy.

➤ Respiratory: increased O_2 consumption, increased alveolar ventilation, decreased FRC, increased airway edema & vascularity.

➤ Cardiovascular: increased intravascular volume, increased cardiac output, dilutional anemia, aortocaval compression.

➤ GI: decreased tone of lower esophageal sphincter.

➤ CNS: decreased MAC requirements for inhalational anesthetics, increased sensitivity to local anesthetics.

What To Do

- Elective surgery should be delayed until 6 wks after delivery.
- Consider delaying necessary surgery until the second or third trimester.
- Emergent surgery during first trimester can be performed w/ general or regional anesthesia. The available data about anesthetic agent teratogenesis do not allow conclusions that any commonly used agent should be avoided during the period of organogenesis.
- Case reports indicate that laparoscopic procedures may be performed safely during all trimesters of pregnancy.
- Aspiration prophylaxis w/ preop antacid should be administered to all women past the first trimester.
- Administration of benzodiazepine to the anxious pt is considered safe at any gestational age (although chronic use during pregnancy is not).
- Ensure adequate preload before performing neuraxial blocks.

INTRAOP

- Prepare for potential difficult intubation due to increased airway edema.
- Avoidance of maternal hypotension/hypoxia is essential to maintain uterine perfusion.
- Teratogenic/adverse effects of anesthetics are inconclusive; data from animal studies conflict with clinical data & species differences are well recognized.
- Large clinical studies of women undergoing surgical procedures during pregnancy suggest no association of anesthetic administration (of any agent, including nitrous oxide) w/ congenital anomalies. However, statistical power does not allow absolute conclusions.
- Nitrous oxide may vasoconstrict uterine vasculature & decrease uterine blood flow if not combined w/ another inhalational agent; there is no evidence that it is deleterious to the developing fetus owing to methionine synthetase inactivation. Very prolonged exposure is not recommended
- Ketamine used in doses >2 mg/kg in first trimester may cause uterine hypertonus.
- Inhalational agents, opioids, most IV & local anesthetics have a good safety profile during pregnancy.

Management

- General anesthesia: left uterine displacement, rapid sequence induction, keep inhalational agents <2.0 MAC, slow reversal of neuromuscular blocking agents (increase in acetylcholine may induce uterine contractions)
- Avoid nitrous oxide w/o concurrent use of another inhalational agent.
- For laparoscopic surgery, keep maternal end-tidal CO_2 30–35 mmHg to prevent fetal acidosis.
- Maternal monitoring: BP cuff, pulse oximeter, end-tidal CO_2 monitor, temp, EKG, arterial line for long or complex cases; blood glucose may be checked in longer cases or pts w/ gestational diabetes; apply compression stockings to avoid lower extremity stasis.
- Fetal monitoring: intermittent or continuous fetal monitoring is recommended after 20–24 wks to check for HR decelerations; consider involvement of a perinatologist/obstetrician to optimize periop mgt.
- Regional anesthesia: decrease dose of neuraxial local anesthetic by 1/3 from that of nonpregnant pt; treat hypotension aggressively w/ ephedrine (phenylephrine is an acceptable second choice).

POSTOP

- Tocolytic therapy in combination w/ continuous monitoring of uterine activity during postop period may help prevent preterm delivery; this is particularly important if surgery was intra-abdominal.

PRIMARY PULMONARY HYPERTENSION

JOSEPH COTTEN, MD, PHD

OVERVIEW

- Definition
  - ➤ Pulmonary hypertension: mean pulmonary artery pressure >25 mmHg at rest or >30 mmHg w/ exercise
  - ➤ Primary pulmonary hypertension: pulmonary hypertension in the absence of a secondary cause
  - ➤ Secondary pulmonary hypertension causes include
    - Pulmonary venous hypertension (wedge pressure >12 mmHg); also called postcapillary pulmonary hypertension
    - Pulmonary hypertension in the first year of life
    - Congenital respiratory disease (lung, thorax, diaphragm)
    - Congenital or acquired cardiac disease (myocardial, valvular)

- Pulmonary artery or pulmonary valve stenosis
- Chronic pulmonary thromboembolism
- Sickle cell anemia
- IV drug abuse
- Obstructive lung disease
- Interstitial lung disease
- Arterial hypoxemia & hypercarbia
- Collagen vascular disease
- Extrinsic compression

■ Pulmonary vascular disease similar to primary pulmonary hypertension can occur w/ HIV, portal hypertension, inhaled cocaine use & appetite suppressant drug use (fenfluramine, dexfenfluramine).

■ Disease is characterized by progressive obliteration of the pulmonary vasculature (especially precapillary arteries). Causes of mortality include right heart failure & sudden death. Pathogenesis includes
  ➤ Endothelial dysfunction (vasoconstriction & impaired vasodilation)
  ➤ Vascular wall remodeling: proliferation of endothelial & smooth muscle cells
  ➤ *In situ* thrombosis

■ Prognosis
  ➤ Mortality highest in pts w/ low CO (<2.5 L/min)
  ➤ Capacity for pulmonary vasodilation also predicts survival

■ Treatment
  ➤ Conventional medical therapy includes
    - Anticoagulants
    - Oral vasodilators (especially calcium channel blockers)
    - Diuretics
    - Cardiac glycosides
    - Supplemental oxygen
  ➤ Continuous IV epoprostenol (prostacyclin, Flolan) shown to improve hemodynamics, exercise capacity, short-term survival
  ➤ Inhaled iloprost (a stable analog of prostacyclin w/ a longer duration of vasodilation) shown to improve symptoms & NYHA class
  ➤ For selected pts w/ severe pulmonary hypertension, balloon atrial septostomy may increase cardiac output, at the expense of hypoxemia.

■ Therapy under investigation includes
  ➤ Oral endothelin receptor antagonist bosentan

- ➤ Other prostacyclin analogs: IV iloprost, SC troprostinil, PO beraprost
- ➤ Inhaled nitric oxide, oral L-arginine
- ■ Surgical therapy includes lung transplantation

PREOP

Issues/Evaluation
- ■ History
  - ➤ Dyspnea, fatigability are early signs.
  - ➤ Angina & syncope w/ exertion are signs of severely limited CO.
  - ➤ 10% report Raynaud's phenomenon, usually women.
- ■ ABGs
  - ➤ Hypoxemia may be present.
- ■ Echocardiogram
  - ➤ Used to evaluate right ventricular function, estimate PA pressure, rule out congenital, myocardial, valvular disease.
- ■ Right heart catheterization
  - ➤ Measures PA pressure, cardiac output, pulmonary capillary wedge pressure
  - ➤ Extreme right ventricular dilatation can compromise left ventricular filling & elevate diastolic pressures.
- ■ ECG
  - ➤ Right axis deviation w/ signs of right ventricular hypertrophy & right atrial enlargement may be observed.

What To Do
- ■ Since these pts are usually followed as outpts by a cardiologist, consider cardiology consultation to define previous & optimal therapy.
- ■ For severe disease in a pt undergoing stressful surgery, consider preadmission to ICU for optimization of pharmacologic therapy. This may include
  - ➤ Placement of PA catheter to assess progress in treating pulmonary hypertension
  - ➤ IV vasodilators
  - ➤ 100% oxygen
  - ➤ Inhaled nitric oxide
  - ➤ IV dobutamine or milrinone to improve right ventricle function

INTRAOP
- ■ Take measures to avoid increases in pulmonary vascular resistance:

➣ Avoid hypoxia, hypercarbia, acidosis, high intrathoracic airway pressure.
➣ Use 100% oxygen (alveolar oxygen tension may be more potent vasodilator than arterial oxygen tension).
➣ Maintain normothermia.
➣ Provide adequate depth of anesthesia.
■ Frequently monitor blood gas & acid-base status.
■ Considerations for nitric oxide or prostacyclin vasodilator therapy (if used)
➣ Nitric oxide can cause methemoglobinemia (treat w/ methylene blue).
➣ Prostacyclin can induce platelet dysfunction.

Management
■ Monitors depend on severity of disease & stress of proposed surgery. May include
➣ Arterial line
➣ PA catheter
➣ TEE
■ Administer suitable pulmonary vasodilator identified preop.
■ Prepare inotropic drugs & consider prophylactic administration to prevent right ventricle dysfunction & failure.
■ Epidural & general anesthesia (alone or in combination) have been used successfully in pts w/ severe pulmonary hypertension.
■ During induction of GA
➣ Ask pt to voluntarily hyperventilate during preoxygenation.
➣ Initiate positive-pressure ventilation cautiously.
➣ Anticipate that stress from intubation will increase pulmonary artery pressure.
■ During maintenance of GA
➣ Avoid factors that increase PVR (discussed above).
➣ Hyperventilate to induce respiratory alkalosis (recognize that end-tidal carbon dioxide may be inaccurate due to abnormal pulmonary blood flow).
➣ Administer bicarbonate based on base deficit to maintain alkalosis.
■ For severely symptomatic pts w/ RV failure, consider potential need for cardiopulmonary bypass. Discuss w/ cardiac surgeon & perfusionist & prepare necessary equipment prior to induction.
➣ Cardiopulmonary bypass equipment
➣ Heparin 300 U/kg

➤ Consider cannulation of femoral vessels under local anesthesia prior to induction.

POSTOP

■ Depending on severity of disease, intraop course & stress of surgery, consider postop ICU care for closer monitoring & further pharmacologic therapy of pulmonary hypertension or right heart failure.

➤ Consider need for postop mechanical ventilation.

PROLONGED QT SYNDROMES

ART WALLACE, PHD, MD

OVERVIEW

■ Definition: Disorder of cardiac repolarization characterized by prolonged QT interval on ECG. QT interval >=450 ms. Can lead to syncope or death due to rapid, polymorphic VT (torsades de pointes).

■ Congenital
  ➤ Rare
  ➤ In conjunction with T-U wave abnormalities
  ➤ Symptoms precipitated by adrenergic stress, exercise, or fright
  ➤ Romano-Ward, Jervell & Lange-Nielsen, SIDS

■ Acquired
  ➤ Complication of drugs that prolong QT (listed below)
  ➤ Can result in syncope, death, torsades (VT)
  ➤ Exacerbated by:
    • QT-prolonging drugs
    • Electrolyte disturbances (see below)
    • Bradycardia

■ No associated cardiac structural abnormality

■ May be an abnormal sodium or potassium channel in congenital long QT

■ Risk factors for sudden cardiac death in congenital long QT
  ➤ History of torsades
  ➤ Family history of sudden cardiac death
  ➤ Excessive QT prolongation or T wave alternans on ECG
  ➤ Deafness: indicating Jervell & Lange-Nielsen syndrome

■ Risk factors for developing long QT syndrome
  ➤ Baseline QT prolongation
  ➤ Congenital long QT syndrome

- ➤ Female gender
- ➤ Hypokalemia
- ➤ Hypomagnesemia
- ➤ Bradycardia
- ➤ Increased dispersion of QT interval
- ➤ Diuretic use
- ➤ Recent cardioversion for atrial fibrillation
- ➤ Congestive heart failure
- ➤ Cardiac hypertrophy
- ➤ Rapid IV drug infusion or high concentration of drugs
- ■ Usual Rx
- ■ Removal of offending agent (drug) – More common in women (2:1)
  - ➤ Droperidol
  - ➤ Quinidine
  - ➤ Sotalol
  - ➤ Ibutilide
  - ➤ Amiodarone
  - ➤ Nonsedating antihistamines
  - ➤ Tricyclic antidepressants
  - ➤ Phenothiazines
  - ➤ Antibiotics
  - ➤ Antifungals
  - ➤ Cisapride
  - ➤ Inhibition of terfenadine or cisapride metabolism by erythromycin & ketoconazole through P450 enzyme CYP3A4

PREOP

Issues/Evaluation
- ■ Identify prolonged QT.
- ■ Identify possible etiologies.
- ■ Eliminate offending drug(s) in pts w/ acquired long QT
- ■ Mainstay of therapy in pts w/ congenital long QT: beta blockers

What To Do
- ■ Congenital
  - ➤ Beta blockers
  - ➤ Cervicothoracic sympathectomy
  - ➤ Cardiac pacing
  - ➤ Implantable cardioverter-defibrillator
- ■ Acquired

➤ Eliminate causative drug or condition
➤ Magnesium sulfate for nonsustained ventricular tachycardia or torsades even with a normal magnesium
➤ Administration of potassium to maintain serum K^+ >4.5 mEq/L
➤ Increase heart rate — pacing, isoproterenol

INTRAOP
■ Eliminate offending medication if possible prior to case.
■ Monitor w/ arterial line & standard monitors.
■ Magnesium for torsadesa.

POSTOP
■ ECG telemetry is appropriate in the postop care of these pts.

PULMONARY EDEMA

LINDA LIU, MD

OVERVIEW
■ Definition: Increased pulmonary capillary pressure that results in leakage of intravascular fluid into the interstitium of the lungs
■ Usual Rx
➤ Diuresis w/ Lasix (10–20 mg IV; if no response within 30 min, administer progressively larger doses) to decrease pulmonary capillary pressure
➤ Inotrope support (dobutamine, dopamine) to increase cardiac output
➤ Morphine sulfate (1–4 mg IV q10–15min) to decrease venous return
➤ Sublingual or IV nitroglycerin to decrease venous return & relieve ischemia
➤ Some pts can benefit from afterload reduction, but this has to be performed w/ caution since low blood pressures can worsen end-organ ischemia.

PREOP

Issues/Evaluation
■ Physical exam findings: rales on lung exam, S3, elevated jugular venous pressure, lower extremity edema, hepatojugular reflux

- Low cardiac output due to ischemia cardiac disease: need evaluation for CAD (EKG, echo, stress test)
- Hypoxia from pulmonary edema: check room air sat or arterial blood gas, CXR
- Electrolyte abnormalities from poor renal function, diuresis & poor peripheral perfusion: check recent electrolytes

What To Do
- If case is not emergent, it should be cancelled since pts are at high risk for postop morbidity & mortality.
- Pts should be medically optimized w/ diuresis, afterload reduction, inotropic support.

INTRAOP
- Arterial line to monitor A-a gradient.
- Consider invasive monitoring (CVP or PA) to help assess fluid balance & intraop fluid shifts.
- TEE can help assess LV function & wall motion abnormalities.
- PEEP can help improve poor A-a gradient.
- May need to give Lasix to decrease capillary pressures or start inotropes to increase cardiac output.

Management
- Cancel elective case to medically optimize pt.
- Otherwise:
  - Treat supportively.
  - Anticipate worsening cardiac function under anesthesia.
  - Consider etomidate for induction if BP is marginal to start.

POSTOP
- Pt will need attention to fluid status postop.
- Leave pt intubated if hemodynamically unstable or PaO_2 is low.

PULMONARY EMBOLISM (PE)

PERRY LEE, MD

OVERVIEW
- Definition: PE is due to the entry of foreign material (eg, clot, air, fat, neoplastic cells, talc, septic emboli, amniotic fluid) into the pulmonary circulation, specifically the pulmonary arteries. Thrombus

is the most common cause; therefore, this chapter will focus on pulmonary thromboembolism.

■ Obstruction of the pulmonary arteries can
  ➤ Increase dead space
  ➤ Result in hypoxia
  ➤ Increase pulmonary vascular resistance
  ➤ Produce reflex bronchoconstriction
  ➤ Cause RV dysfunction & cardiac arrhythmias

■ Usual Rx: anticoagulation, possibly IVC filter placement

■ There are several scenarios in which pts w/ PE may present to the OR.
  ➤ Pts may present to the OR w/ acute PE for placement of vena caval filters to prevent further embolic events, or less often for pulmonary embolectomy.
  ➤ Other pts having unrelated surgery may present with a history of a PE event or have chronic recurrent PE.

PREOP

Issues/Evaluation

■ Prevention of further embolic events is of paramount importance in all pts w/ PE.
  ➤ This often involves systemic anticoagulation w/ Coumadin, unfractionated heparin, or low-molecular-weight heparin (LMWH).
  ➤ In pt w/ an acute embolic event and/or known sources for embolic events (DVTs), continuation of systemic anticoagulation may be necessary until the placement of a vena caval filter or embolectomy.
  ➤ In pts w/ recent or remote embolic events, no data currently exist as to the risk of further embolic events w/ the cessation of anticoagulation; however, in pts w/ a history of an embolic event >1 yr, the risk of further events is probably small.

■ If diagnosis of PE is in doubt, consider further diagnostic measures to confirm the diagnosis & evaluate for pulmonary hypertension & right ventricular failure.
  ➤ Such studies may include spiral CT scans, echocardiography, pulmonary angiography, ventilation/perfusion scans.
  ➤ ABGs may reveal hypoxemia, hypercarbia.

■ Evaluation for further sources of emboli (DVT) should be performed, such as ultrasound or impedance plethysmography.

What To Do

■ Important: if pt is on anticoagulants or if postop DVT prophylaxis includes LMWH, risk of epidural hematoma w/ central neuraxial block is increased. Discuss risk/benefit ratio w/ pt & surgeon. Consider following guidelines in Critical Events chapter "Spinal & Epidural Complications."

➣ If pt is on anticoagulants, determine previous history of thrombosis & assess risk of DVT/PE if anticoagulants are stopped. May need to consult hematology to define this risk, especially for thrombotic disorders.

➣ Important: decide, in conjunction w/ surgeon & hematologist, whether to stop anticoagulant, & when to stop.

➣ Obtain PT if pt on warfarin, PTT if pt on unfractionated heparin. PTT not useful in assessing anticoagulation w/ LMWH.

■ To prevent DVT, consider intermittent pneumatic compression device & elastic stockings. Place at start of case or preop.

INTRAOP

■ Regional anesthetic techniques, where appropriate, may decrease the incidence of DVTs & PE when compared to general anesthetic techniques. For instance, vena caval filters can be placed percutaneously under local anesthesia.

■ Pts w/ PE often display enhanced sensitivity to the circulatory effects of most anesthetic agents & may poorly tolerate hypovolemia or further cardiac insults.

■ Monitoring central venous pressures & invasive BP monitoring may be useful in maintaining adequate venous filling & coronary perfusion pressures.

■ Pts presenting for pulmonary embolectomy are critically ill, often requiring the administration of multiple inotropic & vasoactive agents, during induction & prior to the initiation of cardiopulmonary bypass.

➣ Increased pulmonary vascular resistance & right ventricular failure often persist immediately postop, requiring continued support & positive-pressure ventilation.

Management

■ Avoid factors that will increase pulmonary vascular resistance, such as hypothermia, hypercarbia, hypoxia, acidosis, lung hyperinflation.

■ Watch for signs of worsening or additional PE during surgery. Signs may include

➤ Impaired oxygenation
➤ Decreased end-tidal CO_2
➤ Increased end-tidal CO_2 to PCO_2 gradient
➤ Unexplained hypotension
➤ TEE may be useful intraop diagnostic test

POSTOP
■ Take steps to prevent further embolic events, including appropriate DVT prophylaxis.
  ➤ For high-risk pts, options include
    • LMWH
    • Warfarin
    • Heparin plus intermittent pneumatic compression devices & elastic stockings
  ➤ Other options
    • Low-dose unfractionated heparin or LMWH alone
    • Intermittent pneumatic compression devices or elastic stockings
    • Early ambulation
■ Maintain appropriate vigilance for DVT or worsening PE.

PULMONARY VALVE STENOSIS

RICHARD PAULSEN, MD

OVERVIEW
■ Definition: narrowing of the pulmonary valve causing reduced & turbulent systolic blood flow
  ➤ Most cases are congenital & rarely due to rheumatic disease
■ Usual Rx: balloon dilation, valvulotomy, or replacement, depending on severity

PREOP
Issues/Evaluation
■ Pts are usually asymptomatic & do not require intervention.
■ Signs/symptoms include tachypnea, syncope, angina, hepatomegaly.
■ Pressure gradient >15 mmHg is diagnostic.
■ Pressure gradient >100 mmHg indicates severe disease.
■ RV hypertrophy & subendocardial ischemia common in severe cases

- Prominent A-wave
- Tricuspid regurgitation & atrial fibrillation common

What To Do
- CXR
- ECG
- Echo
- Antibiotics for endocarditis prophylaxis

INTRAOP
- Hemodynamic goals
  - Maintain high preload.
  - Maintain normal sinus rhythm.
  - Avoid bradycardia.
  - Minimize negative inotropes.
  - Maintain SVR.
  - Decrease pulmonary vascular resistance.

Management
- Light premedication, avoiding hypoventilation.
- Standard ASA monitors.
- Other monitors (arterial line, CVP, PA line, TEE) depend on pt disease & stress of proposed surgery.
- With GA or regional, avoid decreasing SVR.

POSTOP
- ECG
- Maintain adequate analgesia

RESPIRATORY ACID-BASE DISORDERS

DAVID SHIMABUKURO, MDCM

OVERVIEW
- Definition
  - Respiratory acidosis: increased pCO_2 from decreased alveolar ventilation
    - Compensation involves renal hydrogen ion excretion, which takes 3–5 days for maximum response.
  - Respiratory alkalosis: decreased pCO_2 caused by hyperventilation
    - Renal compensation occurs through bicarbonate loss in urine, w/ decreased plasma bicarbonate

- Acute disorder
  - 0.08 change in pH for every 10-mmHg change in $PaCO_2$
  - 2-mEq change in serum bicarbonate for every 10-mmHg change in $PaCO_2$
- Chronic disorder
  - 5-mEq change in serum bicarbonate for every 10-mmHg change in $PaCO_2$
- Primary disorder causes pH to shift in that direction.
  - pH <7.35 w/ respiratory acidosis.
  - pH >7.45 w/ respiratory alkalosis.
  - Pt may have a mixed respiratory & metabolic acid-base disorder.
  - As a general rule, the body never overcompensates for any acid-base disorder.
  - Calculate expected metabolic response to the respiratory disorder & consider additional primary metabolic disorder.
- Usual Rx: treat underlying cause of respiratory disorder.

PREOP

Issues/Evaluation
- Determine the cause (primary).
- Common causes of acute respiratory acidosis
  - Drug therapy: opiates, sedative-hypnotics, IV & inhaled anesthetics, muscle relaxants
  - Muscle weakness (related to drug therapy or pt neuromuscular disease)
  - Upper airway obstruction
  - Acute pulmonary process (eg, pulmonary edema, bronchospasm, pneumonia, pneumothorax, hemothorax)
  - Acute exacerbation of chronic lung disease (eg, asthma, COPD)
  - Acute CNS process (eg, stroke, intracranial hemorrhage)
  - Pt on mechanical ventilation
    - Iatrogenic hypoventilation
    - Intentional hypoventilation (permissive hypercapnia)
- Causes of chronic respiratory acidosis
  - Obesity-hypoventilation syndrome
  - Neuromuscular disease (eg, myasthenia gravis, polio, amyotrophic lateral sclerosis, multiple sclerosis, Guillain-Barré syndrome)

➤ Chronic lung disease (COPD, chronic bronchitis, emphysema)
➤ For pt w/ minimal primary medical care, periop presentation of respiratory acidosis may represent a chronic process

■ Signs/symptoms of respiratory acidosis
➤ Overall, symptoms much more common w/ acute respiratory acidosis
➤ Neurologic: headache, blurred vision, restlessness, anxiety, delirium, somnolence
➤ Cardiac: arrhythmias, hypotension

■ Other manifestations of acidosis
➤ Impaired uptake of oxygen by Hgb (right shift of oxyhemoglobin dissociation curve)
➤ Multiple effects on drug handling, including decreased protein binding of anesthetic drugs (eg, thiopental)
➤ Decreased efficacy of local anesthetics due to decreased ionization
➤ Prolonged action of some nondepolarizing neuromuscular blockers (vecuronium, pancuronium, atracurium)

■ Common causes of respiratory alkalosis
➤ Central respiratory stimulation: pain, anxiety, head trauma, brain tumor, stroke, pregnancy
➤ Peripheral respiratory stimulation: hypoxemia, pulmonary emboli, CHF, pneumonia, interstitial lung disease, asthma
➤ Multiple or other mechanisms: liver failure, sepsis, mechanical ventilation
➤ Pt on mechanical ventilation
  • Iatrogenic hyperventilation
  • Intentional hyperventilation (eg, pt w/ elevated ICP)

■ Signs/symptoms of respiratory alkalosis
➤ Important physiologic effect: decreased cerebral blood flow, CNS vasoconstriction
➤ CNS symptoms: irritability, light-headedness, paresthesias, carpopedal spasm, circumoral numbness
➤ Cardiac symptoms: arrhythmias
➤ Other: decreased potassium, decreased ionized calcium, left shift of oxyhemoglobin dissociation curve

■ Consider postponing surgery when
➤ Instrumentation of the trachea is not prudent (eg, severe asthma exacerbation)
➤ Ventilation/oxygenation will not be adequate with OR ventilators (high PIPs & PEEP)

➤ Pt will not tolerate transport to the OR or will not tolerate anesthesia

What To Do
■ If possible, correct the cause before surgery
■ Inform pt of possible postop intubation

INTRAOP
■ Consider arterial line placement.
  ➤ Depending on exact cause of respiratory disorder, frequent blood gases may be necessary, especially towards the end of the case, when extubation is being considered.
■ With acidosis, hyperventilate pt prior to induction; during induction, $PaCO_2$ may rise from initial hypoventilation w/ a further drop in pH.
■ For pt w/ severe pulmonary disease requiring mechanical ventilation, consider whether pt requires ICU ventilator.
  ➤ Most ICU ventilators do not allow delivery of inhaled anesthetics, so may have to use IV anesthetics only.
■ W/ mechanical ventilation & muscle relaxation, can usually normalize pCO_2, but the underlying cause of the respiratory disorder may still be present postop.

POSTOP
■ Arrange ICU care if pt remains intubated.
■ If extubated, pt may require PACU or ICU care overnight to closely monitor respiratory status.
■ Frequent ABGs may be necessary to follow $PaCO_2$ & pH until a steady state is reached.
  ➤ If oxygenation is not an issue, then venous blood gases (VBG) can be used
  ➤ Normal VBG: pH = 7.36; $PaCO_2 = 45$
■ Continue to evaluate & treat the underlying cause of the respiratory disorder.

RESTRICTIVE CARDIOMYOPATHY

MICHAEL J. YANAKAKIS, MD

OVERVIEW
■ Definition: restrictive cardiomyopathy is a pathologic state of impaired diastolic filling that can lead to compromised cardiac output in the setting of increased filling pressures

- Usual Rx: No definitive therapy exists, but ensuring adequate preload & increasing diastolic filling time w/ beta blockade or calcium channel blockade can be beneficial

PREOP

Issues/Evaluation

- Restrictive cardiomyopathy results from a wide variety of pathologic conditions, including
  - ➤ Amyloidosis
  - ➤ Glycogen storage diseases
  - ➤ Hemochromatosis
  - ➤ Sarcoidosis
  - ➤ Fabry's disease
  - ➤ Endomyocardial fibrosis
- Often extremely difficult to distinguish from constrictive pericarditis, even when PA catheter & echo data are available
- Similar to constrictive pericarditis, right & left ventricular pressures may be identical.
  - ➤ However, in restrictive cardiomyopathy, as filling pressures increase, left ventricular pressure will exceed right ventricular pressures.
  - ➤ Therefore, preload augmentation can be helpful in distinguishing restrictive cardiomyopathy from constrictive pericarditis.

What To Do

- There is no definitive therapy for restrictive cardiomyopathy, but ensuring that pt has adequate preload w/o inducing a state of congestive heart failure is the challenge that faces anesthesiologists.
- Preload should be monitored w/ a central venous catheter or PA catheter to follow CVP & PCWP, respectively.
- Anticipate higher filling pressures to ensure adequate cardiac output, but be vigilant about the development of pulmonary edema.
- Rate control w/ beta blockade or calcium channel blockade may be beneficial in that they will increase diastolic filling time.

INTRAOP

- The decreased ventricular compliance mandates increased ventricular filling pressures. This can be facilitated by the use of CVP or PCWP monitoring.

- Ventricular volume cannot be accurately assessed by left ventricular end-diastolic pressures. Therefore, aim for higher filling pressures while monitoring closely for evidence of congestive heart failure.
- Intraop TEE can be helpful for assessing ventricular filling.
- Consider placement of arterial catheter prior to induction of general anesthesia for close BP monitoring.
- Consider use of an induction agent such as etomidate, given the potential for significantly decreased cardiac output.

Management
- Achieve & maintain adequate preload.
- Consider using continuous arterial pressure monitoring, especially prior to induction of general anesthesia.
- Consider monitoring CVP and/or PCWP.
- Consider intraop TEE.
- Control HR w/ beta or calcium channel blockade.
- Be aware of the development of congestive heart failure.

POSTOP
- In postop setting, pay close attention to hemodynamics.
- Continue to achieve adequate HR control (relative bradycardia), using beta & calcium channel blockade when appropriate.
- Monitor closely for signs of congestive heart failure.
- Consider monitoring pt w/ telemetry, given the proclivity for cardiac arrhythmias in the setting of infiltrative cardiomyopathy.

RESTRICTIVE LUNG DISEASE

SUE CARLISLE, PHD, MD

OVERVIEW
- Definition: decrease in total lung capacity resulting from
  - Decrease in elasticity of the lung (eg, interstitial lung disease)
  - Chest wall deformity (eg, kyphoscoliosis)
  - Neuromuscular disease (eg, myasthenia gravis)
  - Extrinsic compression (eg, obesity)
- May be acute (eg, pulmonary edema, acute lung injury) or chronic (eg, diseases that cause pulmonary fibrosis)
- Reduced vital capacity (VC) is found in restrictive lung disease but must be in the presence of a normal FEV1/VC% to be diagnostic

■ Usual Rx: depends on the etiology of restrictive lung disease for a given pt

PREOP

Issues/Evaluation

■ Issues include determination of pts at risk for postop pulmonary complications, including the need for prolonged mechanical ventilation, infections, death.

■ History should elicit risk factors such as
  ➢ Smoking
  ➢ Coexisting diseases
  ➢ Poor exercise tolerance
  ➢ Occupational exposures
  ➢ Drug exposures

■ Symptoms to be concerned about include dyspnea, cough.

■ Signs include cyanosis, chest deformity, tachypnea.

■ Site of surgery is an important risk factor: thoracic & upper abdominal procedures carry a much higher risk of postop complications.

What To Do

■ Preop evaluation of pt w/ a positive history & physical might include
  ➢ Spirometry
  ➢ Pulse oximetry for evaluation of oxygenation
  ➢ ABGs to rule out hypercapnia
  ➢ CXR to look for interstitial changes
  ➢ CT for interstitial, pleural or mediastinal changes
  ➢ Formal PFT may be needed in the case of mixed disease or to quantify the degree of compromise if lung reduction or other high-risk surgery is contemplated. For lung resection, postop complications such as inability to wean from mechanical ventilation are associated w/
    • VC <50% predicted
    • FEV1 <2 L or 50% predicted
    • Hypoxia
    • Hypercapnea
    • Reduced DLCO

INTRAOP

■ Lung volumes must be maintained w/o excessive pressures.

■ A combination of lower tidal volumes (ie, 6 mL/kg) & PEEP should prevent barotrauma & atelectasis.

Management

- Use of neuraxial or selective nerve blocks is associated w/ decreased postop pulmonary complications as compared to general anesthesia.
- Complete reversal of neuromuscular blockade is essential if general anesthesia is used.
- Maintenance of normal calcium, magnesium & potassium levels is important.
- Maintain normal intravascular volume.
- May need an arterial line.
- May need central pressure monitoring, either w/ central line or TEE.

POSTOP

- Adequate pain control w/o respiratory depression is best achieved w/ epidural anesthesia if possible.
- Lung expansion maneuvers such as incentive spirometry or deep breathing & coughing exercises are important.
- Noninvasive ventilation (ie, bilevel positive-pressure ventilation) can be used immediately postop to maintain lung volumes & decrease the work of breathing during recovery.
- Invasive ventilation w/ low TV & PEEP may be necessary in the immediate postop period in high-risk pts or procedures.

RHEUMATOID ARTHRITIS (RA)

KALEB JENSON, MD

OVERVIEW

- Definition: chronic autoimmune disease producing arthritic changes in joints as well as affecting multiple organ systems
- Usual Rx
  - NSAIDs
  - Other disease-modifying antirheumatic drugs: methotrexate, tumor necrosis factor blockers, hydroxychloroquine, sulfasalazine, gold
  - Steroids if the above therapies are inadequate

PREOP

Issues/Evaluation

- Pt may have difficult laryngoscopy/intubation secondary to decreased neck extension, TMJ mobility.

➤ Atlanto-occipital subluxation may result in cervical cord injury.
- Other potential organ system manifestations
  ➤ Cardiac dysfunction such as pericarditis or cardiac tamponade, myocarditis may be present.
  ➤ Pulmonary dysfunction (restrictive lung disease, pulmonary fibrosis) increases risk for complications.
  ➤ Renal insufficiency
  ➤ Decreased exercise tolerance

What To Do
- Check range of motion of neck & TMJ.
  ➤ Consider whether pt may need awake intubation.
- Thorough cardiopulmonary exam; ECG, echo, CXR, PFTs as indicated
- Thorough exam of range of motion of joints so that joints will be properly positioned in the OR

INTRAOP
- Maintain low threshold for awake fiberoptic intubation if pt has decreased neck extension, TMJ, or CNS symptoms.
- If pt has laryngeal arthritis, consider a smaller-than-usual ETT size.
- Careful positioning
- Pt may be more prone to developing hypotension if myocardial function is impaired.

Management
- For pt on chronic glucocorticoid therapy, consider stress-dose steroids.

POSTOP
- Increased risk for laryngeal edema & postop respiratory failure.

SCLERODERMA

DWAIN SKINNER, MD

OVERVIEW
- Definition: Scleroderma (systemic sclerosis) is a chronic, collagen vascular disease that affects the skin, joints & visceral organs.

- Microvascular changes & tissue fibrosis w/ abnormal deposition of collagen are prominent.
- Derangements in humoral & cellular immunity are implicated in the pathogenesis of this autoimmune disease.

PREOP

Issues/Evaluation

- Consequences of microvascular changes include
  - ➤ Dermatologic
    - Skin may be thickened & swollen or, as the disease progresses, atrophic, w/ loss of hair & sweat glands.
  - ➤ Extremities
    - Raynaud's phenomenon occurs in 95% of pts.
  - ➤ Musculoskeletal
    - Joint mobility may become severely restricted.
    - Because of possible TMJ involvement, mouth opening may be affected.
  - ➤ GU
    - Renal involvement is common; destruction of renal blood vessels leads to hypertension, anemia, chronic proteinuria, progressive renal failure.
  - ➤ Pulmonary
    - Gas exchange is affected due to interstitial fibrosis & thickening of alveolar septa.
    - That, together w/ sclerosis of the chest wall, may result in a severe restrictive disease pattern.
    - >30% of scleroderma pts have some degree of pulmonary hypertension w/ possibility of developing cor pulmonale.
  - ➤ Cardiac
    - Myocardial fibrosis occurs in 60% of pts, resulting in
    - Vascular compromise, evidenced by abnormal perfusion scans; however, only approx 20% have decreased resting EF.
    - Conduction defects: fibrosis of cardiac conduction system may cause atrioventricular conduction & supraventricular dysrhythmias.
    - Pericardial effusion is also common.
  - ➤ GI
    - Esophagus is involved in most pts, leading to gastroesophageal reflux & aspiration.
    - There is often decreased small intestinal motility.

What To Do

- Detailed airway exam focusing on TMJ & cervical range of motion. Consider fiberoptic or nasal intubation (the latter may result in hemorrhage due to mucosal fragility) if required.
- Assess range of motion of extremities to guide need for greater care in padding intraop.
- Obtain baseline creatinine & renal function tests.
- Assess preop pulmonary function. Preop ABG, PFTs, CXR may be required.
- EKG & possibly echocardiography to assess effect on cardiac conduction & function.
- Promotility agents & antacids may be required to decrease aspiration risks & sequelae.
- Due to skin manifestations (thickness & edema), venous access may be difficult.
- Arterial access may be a challenge due to arterial sclerosis.

INTRAOP

- Airway may be affected by disease & more difficult to manage.
- Pulmonary manifestations of disease may lead to hypoxemia.
- Cardiovascular function may be affected.
- Extremity positioning due to disease may affect joint range of motion & muscle function.

Management

- Awake and/or fiberoptic intubation if difficult airway suspected
- Rapid sequence intubation for gastroesophageal reflux disease
- Pulmonary status may necessitate high FiO_2 & arterial acid-base measurements as well as judicious fluid therapy, as pts often have renal impairment & leaky vasculature.
- Cardiac involvement may require invasive monitoring (eg, arterial line, CVP & PA monitoring and/or TEE)
- Venous and/or arterial cutdowns may be necessary for vascular access.
- Due to high incidence of Raynaud's, pulse oximetry may be difficult, necessitating intermittent ABG measurements.

POSTOP

- Monitor pulmonary status & oxygenation w/ continuous pulse oximetry (if possible) and/or intermittent ABGs.

SICKLE CELL ANEMIA

JASON LICHTENSTEIN, MD

OVERVIEW
- Definition: hereditary hemolytic anemia resulting from abnormally formed hemoglobin (Hb S), resulting in the sickling & destruction of red blood cells
- The polymerization & precipitation of hemoglobin & consequently the sickling of red blood cells is aggravated by the following conditions:
  - Arterial hypoxemia
  - Acidosis
  - Intravascular dehydration
  - Circulatory stasis
  - Hyperthermia
  - Hypothermia
- Prevalence
  - Disease (0.2% African-Americans)
  - Trait (8% African-Americans)
- Usual Rx: oxygen, hydration w/ IV fluid, pain control, sometimes exchange transfusions

PREOP

Issues/Evaluation
- Pts can be in acute crisis.
  - Vaso-occlusive: causes pain, can result in infarction of organs & thrombosis.
  - Aplastic: red cell production in marrow is either exhausted or prevented, resulting in marked anemia.
  - Splenic sequestration: usually in children <6 y, resulting in sudden entrapment of blood in the spleen, causing significant hypotension.
- Pts predisposed to anemia
- Pts predisposed to infection
- Pts may have pulmonary complications such as
  - Acute chest syndrome: a vaso-occlusive crisis resulting in fever, chest pain, dyspnea, tachypnea, cough. This may lead to acute pulmonary HTN & death.

➤ Sickle cell lung disease: generalized pulmonary fibrosis & hypoxemia leading to cor pulmonale
- Pts are predisposed to cholelithiasis, peptic ulcer disease, ischemic colitis, leg ulcers, priapism, neurologic deficits, nephrotic syndrome, inability to concentrate urine.

What To Do

- Optimize medical condition by treating acute crisis prior to surgery.
- Supplemental oxygen to optimize systemic oxygenation & reduce sickling.
- Optimize circulatory flow & hydration status w/ IVF.
- Check Hgb/Hct & consider exchange transfusions to decrease blood viscosity & increase oxygen carrying capacity (goal: Hct 35–40% w/ 40–50% normal hemoglobin).
- Check BUN/Cr to screen for dehydration & renal abnormalities secondary to infarction.
- Control all infections; many of these pts have infarcted their spleens & are particularly susceptible to encapsulated organisms.
- Manage pain in pts w/ vaso-occlusive crisis.
- Avoid preop meds that result in decreased respiration.
- Regional techniques are often advisable, although most evidence is still inconclusive.

INTRAOP

- Maintain FiO_2, even during regional anesthesia.
- Maintain adequate hydration status.
  ➤ CVP monitor may be useful in certain instances (eg, surgery w/ large fluid shifts).
- Keep pt normotensive to maintain perfusion & circulatory flow.
- Avoid hypothermia/hyperthermia.
- Avoid acidosis.
- Tourniquets & vascular clamps may produce ischemia & promote sickling.
- Cardiopulmonary bypass is particularly dangerous in these pts.

Management

- Goal is to avoid sickling.
- Use regional technique if possible.
- Provide supplemental oxygen & IV fluids.
- Use warming blanket to prevent vasoconstriction; must avoid hyperthermia also, as it promotes sickling.
- Use pressors to support BP if necessary.

POSTOP

- Similar goals as intraop mgt: maintain oxygenation & perfusion, manage pain, prevent hypothermia.
- Close monitoring in postop period; special attention to pulmonary complications, as acute chest syndrome in the postop period is a significant cause of morbidity & mortality.
  - ➤ Good pulmonary toilet is important.
  - ➤ Early ambulation
- Pain mgt in these pts can be quite difficult as many are narcotic-tolerant & respiratory depression should be avoided.

SINUS BRADYCARDIA

ART WALLACE, PHD, MD

OVERVIEW

- Definition: Cardiac rhythm w/ sinus node as the pacemaker but rate slower than normal
  - ➤ 40–60 bpm. If on beta blockers, <50 bpm.
  - ➤ Regular rhythm
  - ➤ 1:1 relationship between P & QRS waves
- Etiology
  - ➤ Hypoxia
  - ➤ Acute inferior MI
  - ➤ Vagal stimulation
    - Ophthalmic traction
    - Uterine traction
    - Sneezing
    - Coughing
    - Micturition
    - Vomiting
    - Defecation
  - ➤ Carotid sinus hypersensitivity
  - ➤ Neurocardiac syncope
  - ➤ Intracranial hypertension
  - ➤ Hypothyroidism
  - ➤ Electrolyte disturbance
  - ➤ High sympathetic blockade from spinal or epidural anesthesia
  - ➤ Athletes
  - ➤ Drug effects

- Beta blockers
- High-potency narcotics
- Calcium channel blockers
- Antiarrhythmics
- Antihypertensives
- Cardiac glycosides
- Lithium
- Cimetidine
➤ Sick sinus syndrome
➤ Intrinsic causes
  - Idiopathic degeneration
  - Chronic ischemia
  - Infiltrative disease
  - Inflammatory disease
  - Musculoskeletal disease
  - Connective tissue disorders
  - Surgical trauma
  - Familial diseases
■ Usual Rx: Identify etiology.
  ➤ Correct hypoxia if etiology.
  ➤ Heart rate <35 bpm poorly tolerated & should be evaluated on basis of effect on cardiac output.
  ➤ Treatment is needed if hypotension, ventricular arrhythmia, or low cardiac output is present.
  ➤ Anticholinergics or sympathomimetics
    - Glycopyrrolate 0.2–1.0 mg IV
    - Atropine 0.4–2 mg IV
    - Ephedrine 5–25 mg IV
    - Isoproterenol 2–10 mcg/min IV
  ➤ Pacing

PREOP

Issues/Evaluation
■ Identify etiology.
■ Correct if possible.

What To Do
■ If associated w/ symptoms, identify etiology & correct.
■ Chronic: If no symptoms are present & etiology is benign, observe.
■ Acute: If new onset, identify etiology & correct.

INTRAOP
- If new onset, identify etiology.
- Correct if symptomatic.
- Sudden bradycardia can represent vagal stimulation that may lead to asystole. Identification & mgt are essential.
- Bradycardia from hypoxia is an absolute medical emergency that should be treated by correction of the etiology of the hypoxia.
- Significantly more injury can occur to pts w/ CAD by administration of atropine w/ resulting tachycardia & subsequent myocardial ischemia than commonly occurs in the hemodynamically stable pt w/ sinus bradycardia of benign origin.

POSTOP
- If etiology of bradycardia was benign (eg, narcotics, beta blockers), observe.
- If etiology was hypoxia or acute MI, appropriate ICU follow-up is required.
- Vagal episodes are transient. Obtain 12-lead ECG to rule out other etiologies.
- If etiology is unknown, further workup may be required.

SINUS TACHYCARDIA

ART WALLACE, PHD, MD

OVERVIEW
- Definition: cardiac rhythm w/ sinus node as pacemaker, but rate is faster than normal
  - 100–170 bpm
  - Regular rhythm
  - 1:1 relationship between P & QRS waves. Normal P wave morphology. P waves can be lost in QRS or T if rate is high
  - QRS morphology is narrow unless aberrancy is present
- Differential diagnosis
  - Atrial fibrillation
  - Atrial flutter
  - Frequent PACs
  - Paroxysmal supraventricular tachycardia (PSVT)
- Usual Rx: Volume repletion & beta blockade

PREOP

Issues/Evaluation

- Tachycardia in pts w/ or at risk for coronary artery disease can lead to myocardial ischemia & associated morbidity & mortality.
- PSVT can be treated w/ vagal maneuvers, adenosine, calcium channel blockers, beta blockers.
- PACs have little significance unless very frequent. May lead to more serious supraventricular arrhythmias or be a sign of digitalis toxicity.
- Atrial fibrillation/flutter can be managed w/ calcium channel blockers, beta blockers, digoxin, procainamide, quinidine, anticoagulation, cardioversion.

What To Do

- Identify etiology; there are 3:
  - ➢ Physiologic sinus tachycardia: numerous causes, including:
    - Volume depletion
    - Pain
    - Fever
    - Anticholinergic medications
    - Hyperadrenergic states
    - Hyperthyroidism
    - Exercise
    - Anemia
  - ➢ Inappropriate sinus tachycardia
  - ➢ Sinus tachycardia, from sinus node re-entry
- Perioperative beta blockade should be administered to all pts w/ coronary artery disease, peripheral vascular disease, or two risk factors for coronary artery disease (hypertension, smoking, cholesterol >240 mg/dL, age >65, or diabetes).

INTRAOP

- All pts w/ or at risk for coronary artery disease should be on perioperative beta blockade.
- Identify etiology & correct.
- Volume
- Beta blockers
- Analgesics

POSTOP

- All pts w/ or at risk for coronary artery disease should be on perioperative beta blockade.

SODIUM DISORDERS

JASON WIDRICH, MD

OVERVIEW
- Definitions
  - Hypernatremia: increase in plasma sodium concentration >145 mEq/L
  - Hyponatremia: decrease in plasma sodium concentration <135 mEq/L
- Sodium concentration does not necessarily correlate w/ extracellular volume status.
- Usual Rx
  - Depends on underlying cause

PREOP

Issues/Evaluation
- Hyponatremia
  - Manifestations reflect hypo-osmolality of brain & formation of cerebral edema. Symptoms depend on magnitude & rate of onset of hyponatremia.
    - Nausea, headache, lethargy, apathy, confusion, stupor, coma, seizures
  - Etiology
    - Circulating volume depletion: GI losses, renal losses, edematous states (heart failure, liver cirrhosis, nephrotic syndrome), skin losses (sweating, burns)
    - Renal failure
    - Hypotonic IV fluid administration
    - Thiazide diuretics
    - Syndrome of inappropriate antidiuretic hormone secretion (SIADH)
    - Adrenal insufficiency
    - Hypothyroidism
    - Pseudohyponatremia related to mannitol, hyperglycemia, TURP irrigation, severe hyperlipidemia, severe hyperproteinemia
- Hypernatremia
  - Usually occurs in adults w/ altered mental status, or infants

➤ Hypernatremia in hospitalized pt usually results from inappropriate fluid therapy in pt w/ increased water losses.

➤ Thirst & water drinking are important factors preventing hypernatremia.

➤ Manifestations primarily involve CNS findings.

  • Altered mental status, lethargy, weakness, irritability, thirst, nausea/vomiting, muscle twitching, hyperreflexia, seizures

➤ Etiology involves sodium retention or water loss in excess of sodium.

  • Sodium retention: ingestion of sodium, IV administration of hypertonic saline or sodium bicarbonate
  • Insensible water loss: fever, exercise, burns
  • Renal water loss: central diabetes insipidus, nephrogenic diabetes insipidus, osmotic diuresis (eg, glucose, urea, mannitol)
  • GI water loss: osmotic diarrhea
  • Hypothalamic disorders: primary hypodipsia, reset osmostat
  • Intracellular water loss: seizures, extreme exercise, rhabdomyolysis

What To Do

■ Obtain electrolytes, BUN, creatinine in pt suspected of electrolyte disorder or w/ medical condition predisposing to electrolyte disorders.

■ Once sodium disorder diagnosed by lab values, determine etiology for disorder.

  ➤ History & physical, including determination of volume status
  ➤ Additional lab studies as required

■ Acute, severe, symptomatic sodium disorders should be corrected before surgery.

  ➤ Postpone elective surgery in these pts.
  ➤ Pt may require hospitalization for treatment.

■ Decision to proceed with surgery in pts w/ asymptomatic sodium disorders depends on etiology & duration of disorder, magnitude of abnormality, coexisting disease & stress of proposed surgery.

  ➤ Consider whether surgical procedure is likely to result in fluid & electrolyte abnormalities:
    • Prolonged surgery
    • Surgery w/ large fluid shifts (eg, extensive intra-abdominal surgery)

- Surgery w/ high blood loss potential (trauma, burns, major abdominal surgery, aortic vascular surgery, liver transplantation)
- Surgery associated w/ sodium abnormalities (neurosurgery, trauma, TURP, hysteroscopy)

■ Cautions
  ➤ Severe hyponatremia can result in cerebral edema, seizures, increased ICP.
  ➤ Rapid correction of hyponatremia to normal or hypernatremic level can lead to central pontine myelinolysis or osmotic demyelination. Other factors are also important, such as presence of hypoxia, alcoholism, burns, hypokalemia.
  ➤ Rapid correction of hypernatremia can lead to cerebral edema.

■ Management depends on disorder, underlying cause, presence of symptoms. Volume status is crucial to determining treatment. General considerations include
  ➤ Hypovolemic hyponatremia
    - Administration of normal saline until volume status restored
  ➤ Hypervolemic hyponatremia
    - More challenging to treat because underlying disease is typically chronic (eg, liver cirrhosis, CHF, nephrotic syndrome)
    - Loop diuretics commonly used in addition to sodium & fluid restriction
  ➤ Euvolemic hyponatremia
    - Acute, symptomatic pt (hyponatremia developing in <48 h): consider ICU admission; hypertonic saline w/ possible use of loop diuretic (eg, furosemide) may be necessary. Typical goals: 2 mEq/L per hour sodium increase until symptoms improve.
    - Chronic symptomatic pt: consider ICU admission; hypertonic saline or normal saline w/ loop diuretic (eg, furosemide) may be necessary. Typical goals: slow increase until symptoms improve, or until sodium increases by 25 or reaches 130 mEq/L.
    - Asymptomatic pt: usually does not require aggressive therapy
  ➤ Hypovolemic hypernatremia
    - Normal saline until euvolemic, then hypotonic IV fluid (eg, D5W, 0.45% NS) based on water deficit
  ➤ Hypervolemic hypernatremia
    - Least common form of hypernatremia
    - Diuretics plus D5W
    - Dialysis for renal failure pt

➤ Euvolemic hypernatremia
  • IV D5W or enteral water based on total body water deficit

INTRAOP
■ If pt w/ sodium disorder requires surgery, consider general treatment approach required. Treatment of underlying causes is always important.
■ Check electrolytes & glucose regularly during procedures associated w/ fluid & electrolyte changes.

POSTOP
■ Assess neurologic status promptly.
■ Continue mgt previously stated.
■ Underlying condition that caused the sodium disorder may need to be readdressed.

SPINAL CORD TRANSECTION

TESSA COLLINS, MD

OVERVIEW
■ Definition: transection of spinal cord. There are 3 phases:
  ➤ Immediate phase
    • Duration: minutes
    • Explosive autonomic discharge is characteristic & results in severe hypertension & arrhythmias.
  ➤ Spinal shock
    • Duration: a few days up to 6–8 wks
    • Results from sudden loss of sympathetic discharge & descending spinal inhibition; this leads to unopposed vagal discharge, bradycardia, hypotension, flaccid paralysis & loss of reflexes
  ➤ Reflex phase
    • Gradual return of sympathetic efferent discharge, muscle tone & reflexes
■ Usual Rx
  ➤ Supportive care, including treatment of BP
  ➤ High-dose methylprednisolone may improve neurologic outcome when administered within 8 h of acute spinal cord injury.
    • Dose regimen is 30 mg/kg IV bolus followed by 5.4 mg/kg/h for 23 h.

PREOP

Issues/Evaluation

- Acute considerations are the ABCs.
  - Airway
    - Mask ventilate; if there is a risk of c-spine injury, ventilate w/o neck hyperextension.
    - Intubate if indicated, w/o neck hyperextension if there is a possibility of c-spine injury.
    - Consider fiberoptic intubation so that neck need not be hyperextended if a c-spine injury is suspected.
  - Breathing: 100% FiO_2
  - Circulation: aggressive fluid resuscitation for hypotension w/ spinal shock; more than one peripheral line should be inserted; pressors should be given as needed. An arterial line is essential for close BP monitoring.
- Chronic phase: main issue is avoidance of autonomic hyperreflexia in lesions above T7. This is characterized by
  - Commonly: hypertension, headache, sweating, flushing or pallor, reflex bradycardia.
  - Less commonly: pupillary changes, Horner's syndrome, nausea, anxiety, penile erection.
  - Triggers: most common are bladder/bowel distention, uterine contractions, acute abdominal pathology.
- Other considerations
  - Respiratory insufficiency due to weakness
  - Muscle: Ach receptor proliferation; avoid succinylcholine; muscle spasms common
  - Impaired thermoregulation
  - Skin ulcers: manipulation could trigger spasm or autonomic hyperreflexia
  - Blood: anemia is common, high risk of DVT
  - GU: bladder distention/urinary retention, renal insufficiency
  - GI: delayed gastric emptying

What To Do

- Preop labs: CBC, electrolytes, BUN, Cr
- PFTs & CXR may be indicated depending on symptoms.

INTRAOP

- Acute transection
  - Minimal anesthetic requirement owing to hypotension.

➤ Hypothermia may be present.
➤ Mechanical ventilation will almost certainly be required.
➤ Steroids may be indicated.
➤ Tracheal suctioning or intubation may cause severe bradycardia or asystole.
■ Chronic transection
➤ Autonomic hyperreflexia syndrome as described above may be seen; it can usually be prevented intraop by adequate anesthesia.

Management
■ Standard monitors
➤ For major surgery in compromised pt, monitoring is as indicated by the pt's condition & the procedure to be performed.
■ Induction
➤ Use nondepolarizing muscle relaxant in pts w/ a chronic transection.
■ Positioning
➤ If acute transection, be careful not to cause more spinal cord damage.
➤ W/ chronic transection, pts may be more vulnerable to poor positioning because of contractures or pressure sores.
■ Fluids: avoid hypovolemia
■ Avoid hypothermia.
■ For BP/HR control
➤ Chronic transection: use a direct-acting vasoactive agent; an exaggerated response to direct-acting sympathomimetic agents is seen due to increased numbers of receptors, so use smaller doses initially
➤ Acute transection: may have severe hypotension requiring significant pressor support
➤ Appropriate agents include phenylephrine (for vasoconstriction), nitroprusside (for vasodilation), or isoproterenol (raise HR), esmolol (lower HR); isoproterenol/esmolol for HR.
■ Autonomic hyperreflexia (see also Critical Event chapter "Autonomic Hyperreflexia")
➤ Spinal anesthesia is very effective in preventing autonomic hyperreflexia; GA or epidural may also be used.
➤ If pt develops autonomic hyperreflexia, first step is to remove the stimulus that elicited the hypertension; this alone may be all that is required to return BP to baseline. While determining

cause, increase depth of anesthesia. Vasodilators (eg, labetalol, nitroprusside) may also be used.

POSTOP

- Careful attention to temp & respiratory function in pts w/ acute cord transection
- Be alert to the development of autonomic hyperreflexia in pts w/ chronic spinal cord transection.

STABLE ANGINA

SAMIR DZANKIC, MD
JACQUELINE M. LEUNG, MD

OVERVIEW

- Definition: clinical syndrome due to myocardial ischemia. Occurs when myocardial oxygen supply does not match myocardial oxygen demand.
- Usual Rx
  - Nitrates, beta-adrenergic antagonists, calcium channel blockers: improve myocardial oxygen supply/demand balance through increasing supply by dilating the coronary vasculature and/or decreasing demand by reducing cardiac work
  - Antiplatelet & antithrombotic agents (aspirin, dipyridamole, ticlopidine)

PREOP

Issues/Evaluation

- Assess disease severity, stability (initial history, physical exam, ECG) & prior treatment.
- Assess functional capacity & comorbid conditions.
- Stratify surgery-specific cardiac risk.
  - High-risk procedures: major emergency surgery, aortic & other major vascular surgery, peripheral vascular surgery, prolonged intraperitoneal & intrathoracic procedures (>3 h) w/ large fluid shifts and/or blood loss.
  - Intermediate-risk procedures: carotid endarterectomy, head & neck surgery, intraperitoneal & intrathoracic procedures, orthopedic procedures, prostate surgery.
  - Low-risk procedures: endoscopic & superficial procedures, cataract surgery, breast surgery.

- Based on clinical history, surgery-specific risk, functional capacity & results of previous studies, further testing may be indicated.
  - ➤ Functional capacity poor in subjects undergoing intermediate-to high-risk procedures; consider pharmacologic stress testing, such as dipyridamole-thallium scintigraphy or dobutamine stress echocardiography. If test results positive, consider coronary angiography.
  - ➤ Functional capacity moderate to excellent in subjects undergoing high-risk procedures, consider exercise treadmill test & follow w/ coronary angiography if indicated. For intermediate- to low-risk procedures, further testing may not be necessary.

What To Do
- Optimize antianginal and/or antihypertensive therapy before surgery (improve supply/demand balance).
- Consider beta-adrenergic blockers if there is no contraindication.
- Continue antianginal therapy up to the time of surgery & also postop.
- In pts w/ unstable angina, postpone procedure, start aggressive medical treatment, consider coronary angiography. Based on results, may proceed w/ PTCA or CABG surgery before noncardiac surgery.
- If emergency surgery, proceed w/ procedure, consider prophylactic anti-ischemic therapy & rigorous control of hemodynamics.

INTRAOP
- Rigorous hemodynamic control to minimize the occurrence of hypertension & tachycardia (increase oxygen demand) or hypotension (decrease oxygen supply). Avoid anemia, hypoxia, volume overload.
- If severe CAD or left ventricular dysfunction is present or high-risk surgery, may need invasive monitoring (arterial line, central line, pulmonary artery catheter).
- Monitor for myocardial ischemia (simultaneous leads V5 & II, possible multiple lead ST segment analysis if available).
- Consider intraop TEE for monitoring global & regional left ventricular function, particularly for pts w/ uninterpretable ECG such as left bundle branch block or ventricular pacemaker, or in a high-risk surgical setting in which rapid changes in loading conditions may occur.

Management
- Preop sedation to avoid anxiety-induced tachycardia & hypertension

- The anesthetic goal is to perform a smooth induction to minimize hypertension, hypotension, tachycardia. Etomidate may be a suitable induction agent in certain high-risk pts.
- Prevent hypertension & tachycardia at the time of intubation or extubation using lidocaine, beta blockade (esmolol, labetalol, metoprolol) or calcium channel blockers, or narcotics.
- Anesthetic depth should be adequate prior to tracheal intubation.
- Adequate analgesia should be established prior to tracheal extubation.
- Any volatile anesthetic is acceptable for maintenance.
- If signs of myocardial ischemia (ST depression/elevation), consider Rx.
  - ➤ Increase supply: correct hypotension, hypoxemia (increasing FiO_2, addition of PEEP if mechanically ventilated), anemia.
  - ➤ Decrease demand: deepen level of anesthesia, vasodilators, calcium channel blockers, beta-adrenergic blockers.
  - ➤ Consider diuresis (furosemide) for fluid overload.
  - ➤ IV nitroglycerin or nicardipine to relieve suspected coronary spasm.

POSTOP
- Continue to monitor hemodynamics & ECG ST-segment changes.
- Continue or consider instituting beta blockade.
- If suspect periop infarction, order 12-lead ECG & cardiac enzymes (CK-MB or troponin I).
- Effective pain mgt to prevent hemodynamic changes.
- Supplemental oxygen.

STATUS POST LUNG TRANSPLANT

BETTY LEE-HOANG, MD

OVERVIEW
- Definition: pt status post single- or double-lung transplant
- For information on the lung transplant procedure, see Procedures chapter "Lung Transplant."

PREOP

Issues/Evaluation
- Determine indication, type (single vs double) & date of transplant.

➤ Look for right ventricular dysfunction, which may have occurred prior to transplant.

➤ Pt may still have residual or recurrent pulmonary disease in the transplanted and/or residual lung, so appropriate mgt for the disease should still be taken.

■ Determine status of graft function (eg, episodes of acute or chronic rejection).

■ These pts will always be on chronic immunosuppressant therapy to prevent organ rejection.

➤ Pts on chronic steroids may require additional stress-dose steroids.

➤ Immunosuppressant drugs may have systemic effects (eg, cyclosporine).

INTRAOP

■ Transplantation disrupts neural innervation, lymphatic drainage & bronchial circulation of the transplanted lung.

■ The cough reflex is abolished below the carina, so pt may be at higher risk of aspiration & may be unable to clear secretions well.

■ Bronchial hyperreactivity may be present.

■ The loss of lymphatic drainage increases extravascular lung water & may predispose the lungs to pulmonary edema. Because of this, fluid replacement should be kept to a minimum.

■ The bronchial suture line may always be at risk of ischemic breakdown due to the loss of bronchial circulation.

POSTOP

■ Pts will need respiratory therapy for pulmonary toilet, especially after undergoing tracheal intubation.

■ Continue immunosuppression.

➤ Post-transplant pts are always at risk for organ rejection.

➤ They may require lung biopsies to rule this out if they experience a change in their pulmonary status.

STROKE

SUNDEEP MALIK, MD

OVERVIEW

■ Definition: acute neurologic change related to impairment of cerebral circulation that lasts >6 h

- 85% of strokes are ischemic; remainder are hemorrhagic.
  - Ischemic stroke most commonly due to thrombus or embolism
  - Risk factors include HTN, smoking, diabetes mellitus.
- Over half of pts who survive a stroke are able to live independently; up to 80% regain ability to walk.
- Usual Rx
  - Acute mgt includes early evaluation, supportive care, possible use of IV thrombolysis or intra-arterial MCA thrombolysis, antithrombotic drug, antiplatelet drug.
  - Rehab phase helps to improve functional status. Potential problems addressed include DVT prevention, dysphagia, incontinence, focal weakness, aphasia, skin injury, tendency for mechanical falls, depression.
  - Long-term goals include prevention of second stroke.

PREOP

Issues/Evaluation

- Evaluation & mgt of acute stroke will not be discussed in detail. Immediate complications of acute stroke that may involve the anesthesia provider (eg, for tracheal intubation & mechanical ventilation) include
  - Airway obstruction
  - Hypoventilation
  - Aspiration pneumonia
  - Coma
  - Seizures
  - Cerebral edema, increased ICP
- Management of HTN immediately after acute stroke is controversial. Antihypertensive therapy to reduce BP may lead to decrease in cerebral blood flow. Decision to treat HTN should be based on clinical status, baseline BP, decision regarding thrombolytic therapy. Most recommend treatment for very severe HTN (SBP >220, mean BP >130, DBP >120).
  - Long-term HTN treatment will reduce risk of stroke.
- Acute ischemic stroke commonly occurs in pts w/ cardiovascular disease, including
  - CAD, including acute MI
  - HTN
  - CHF
  - Arrhythmias, especially atrial fibrillation

■ Hypotension during anesthesia can contribute to morbidity in stroke pts undergoing surgery.

What To Do
■ For pt presenting for surgery w/ history of acute stroke
  ➤ Determine time since acute stroke occurred.
  ➤ Postpone elective surgery in pt w/ acute stroke within 4 wks.
    • Changes in CNS physiology may persist for >4 wks, including loss of carbon dioxide responsiveness, altered cerebral autoregulation, altered blood-brain barrier integrity.
  ➤ Determine symptoms of acute stroke, extent of neurologic deficit, presence of residual deficit.
    • Residual motor weakness is important to detect, since denervation from upper motor neuron lesion predisposes to exaggerated hyperkalemia w/ succinylcholine.
    • Document all preop neuro deficits in case postop neuro deficit occurs.
  ➤ Determine previous workup for cause of stroke, w/ special attention to cardiovascular causes:
    • Arrhythmia (eg, atrial fibrillation)
    • CHF
    • Intracardiac thrombus
    • Carotid or vertebral-basilar vascular disease
    • Valvular disease (eg, mitral stenosis, aortic stenosis, vegetation from endocarditis)
    • Aortic atheroma
  ➤ Determine if pt has fixed stenosis of artery to brain (eg, carotid, vertebral or intracranial stenosis).
    • If there is a fixed stenosis, consider discussion w/ neurologist regarding optimal BP during surgery. These pts are at increased risk of cerebral ischemia from relative hypotension.
  ➤ Pursue further workup of coexisting diseases as necessary.
  ➤ Determine presence of anticoagulation therapy.
    • Consider whether (and when) to discontinue prior to surgery.
    • May affect decision regarding regional blockade.

INTRAOP
■ Tightness of intraop BP control will depend on cause of stroke, residual cerebrovascular disease, time since stroke.
  ➤ Tight BP control is of highest importance in pt w/ residual cerebrovascular disease, especially fixed stenosis of cerebral arterial

blood supply. Reduction in BP may lead to reduction in cerebral blood flow & risk of cerebral ischemia.

➤ Consider placement of arterial line for monitoring.
➤ In pts at highest risk, maintain BP within 20% of baseline.
■ Important concerns regarding neuromuscular blockade.
➤ In presence of residual muscle weakness, do not use succinylcholine beginning 1 week after acute stroke.
➤ Duration of exaggerated hyperkalemia risk in these pts is unclear.
➤ Nondepolarizing muscle relaxants do not have risk of hyperkalemia.
➤ Monitor neuromuscular blockade on a nonparalyzed extremity.
   • Extremity w/ weakness may not display appropriate evidence of neuromuscular blockade.
■ Monitor hematocrit & transfuse appropriately.

POSTOP
■ Issues include
➤ Evaluation of neurologic status & comparison to preop state to detect new deficits
➤ Restarting anticoagulation
➤ BP control
➤ Maintenance of hematocrit

SUBSTANCE ABUSE (INCLUDING COCAINE ABUSE)

DON TAYLOR, MD, PHD

OVERVIEW
■ Considerations largely determined by
➤ Class of substance
   • Stimulants such as methamphetamines & cocaine have similar physiologic effects.
➤ Route of intake
   • Injection drug users may have specific problems based on route of administration (eg, infectious risks such as HIV & hepatitis C from needle sharing, difficult IV access, endocarditis, pulmonary HTN).
■ In general, acute intoxication leads to decreased anesthetic requirements.

➤ Stimulants are the major exception; the sympathetic stimulation caused by cocaine & amphetamines may increase anesthetic requirements.

■ Chronic substance use generally increases anesthetic requirements or has no effect.

➤ Stimulants are the exception; withdrawal may decrease anesthetic needs.

■ Physical dependence is most likely with agents acting at GABA receptors (ETOH, barbiturates, benzodiazepines) & opioids.

➤ These are also the only agents for which specific antagonists are available (eg, naloxone, flumazenil).

• Use caution when administering these antagonists; titrate to effect.

• Agonist drug may outlast antagonist effects, requiring redosing.

• Naloxone may precipitate acute pulmonary edema.

• Flumazenil lowers seizure threshold, even in pts lacking history of seizure disorder.

PREOP

Issues/Evaluation

■ Concomitant abuse common; elicit drug history (timing, amount, frequency, route, length of addiction)

■ Consider postponing elective surgery in presence of acute intoxication or withdrawal.

■ Opiate abusers have increased analgesic requirements; titrate to effect.

■ Consider drug testing.

Organ System Effects of Drugs of Abuse

■ CV effects

➤ Cocaine/stimulants

• Hypertension

• Tachycardia

• Increased risks of MI (risk reported to be increased by a factor of 24 in otherwise healthy patients in first hour following use). Cocaine-induced MI may be difficult to identify as ECG specificity is decreased & serum CK levels are an unreliable indicator (elevated in 1/2 of users w/o MI, presumably secondary to rhabdomyolysis).

- Arrhythmia: acutely increased incidence of arrhythmia secondary to circulating catecholamines may make halothane relatively contraindicated.
- Sudden death
- Cocaine may alter LV function & generation & conduction of impulses by a variety of mechanisms: sympathomimetic qualities increase ventricular irritability; lowers fibrillation threshold; prolongs QRS & QT intervals (similar to class I antiarrhythmic); increases intracellular calcium; decreases vagal activity.
  - ➤ Opiates
    - Bradycardia
    - Hypotension
- ■ Respiratory effects
  - ➤ Cannabis: respiratory effects of 3–4 cannabis cigarettes per day roughly equivalent to 1 pack per day tobacco
  - ➤ Cocaine: bronchospasm, pulmonary edema, pulmonary hemorrhage, "crack lung" (diffuse alveolar infiltrates on CXR)
  - ➤ Opiates: ventilatory depression (primarily rate), apneic threshold & hypoxic drive altered. Chest wall rigidity may occur. Synergistic effects on respiratory drive w/ benzodiazepines, barbiturates.
- ■ Neurologic effects
  - ➤ Cocaine/stimulant use can produce headaches, seizures, hyperthermia, intracranial hemorrhage.
  - ➤ Barbiturates/benzodiazepines: withdrawal decreases seizure threshold
- ■ Heme effects
  - ➤ Cocaine use can lead to thrombocytopenia.
- ■ Renal
  - ➤ Cocaine may produce rhabdomyolysis.
- ■ Metabolic
  - ➤ Barbiturates may induce hepatic enzymes.
- ■ Pregnancy
  - ➤ Cocaine/stimulants can lead to premature labor, precipitate delivery.

INTRAOP
- ■ Stabilize hemodynamics prior to induction.
- ■ Ketamine relatively contraindicated due to sympathomimetic effects.
- ■ Use direct rather than indirect pressors for treatment of hypotension.

■ Cocaine-induced coronary artery vasoconstriction is reversed by phentolamine (alpha antagonist), exacerbated by propranolol and labetalol (controversial): esmolol may be better choice due to beta-1 selectivity. Consider NTG & calcium channel blockers (verapamil) as agents of choice for cocaine-induced chest pain; also, aspirin & benzodiazepines may be of benefit.

POSTOP
■ Withdrawal from substance may occur.
■ Pain mgt may be an issue.
■ Relapse may be a consideration in pts wishing to remain abstinent.

SUPRAVENTRICULAR TACHYCARDIA

ART WALLACE, PHD, MD

OVERVIEW
■ Definition: Tachycardia originating in or that uses the atrium or atrioventricular junction & that requires participation of the bundle of His for propagation of the tachycardia circuit
■ AV node-dependent junctional tachycardias
➤ Atrioventricular node re-entrant tachycardia (AVNRT)
➤ Atrioventricular re-entrant tachycardia (AVRT)
➤ Junctional ectopic tachycardia
■ AV node-independent atrial tachycardias
➤ Sinus tachycardia
• Physiologic
• Inappropriate
• Sinus node re-entry
➤ Atrial tachycardia
• Unifocal
• Multifocal
➤ Atrial flutter
➤ Atrial fibrillation
■ Pathophysiology of SVT
➤ Baseline rhythm disorder
➤ Sinus node-based arrhythmias are response to physiologic stress:
• Fever
• Exercise
• Thyrotoxicosis
• Caffeine

- Aminophylline
- Alcohol

PREOP

Issues/Evaluation
- Prognosis of SVT linked to prognosis of structural heart disease.
- Prognosis of SVT is benign in absence of structural heart disease.
- Radiofrequency ablation eliminates problem.

What To Do
- Identify arrhythmia.
- Assess severity & frequency of symptoms.
- If pt is anticoagulated (afib/aflutter), check PT/PTT & decide on strategy for management of anticoagulation. If decision is made to stop anticoagulation, assess PT/PTT prior to surgery.
- Review history of prior pharmacologic therapy & level of success; use what worked well before.
- If pt is on beta blockade, continue.
- If pt has CAD, PVD, or risk factors for CAD (HTN, smoking, age >65, diabetes, cholesterol >240), start perioperative beta blockade.

INTRAOP
- Monitor.
- Maintain antiarrhythmic therapy if present.
- In cases w/ hemodynamically significant SVT or structural heart disease, A-lines are helpful.

Management
- Usual Rx: acute treatment of regular tachycardia
  - Stable BP >90/60 mm Hg w/ narrow QRS & regular RR
    - Vagal maneuvers (Valsalva, carotid massage, ice water)
    - Adenosine 6–12 mg IV
    - Verapamil, diltiazem
    - Propafenone, sotalol
    - Procainamide
    - Amiodarone
    - Atrial pacing
    - Synchronous cardioversion
- Stable blood pressure w/ wide complex QRS
  - Vagal maneuvers
  - Adenosine 6–12 mg IV

- ➤ Procainamide
- ➤ Atrial pacing
- ➤ Synchronous cardioversion
- ➤ CONTRAINDICATION TO DIGOXIN OR VERAPAMIL
- ■ Unstable BP <90/60 mm Hg
  - ➤ Synchronous cardioversion
- ■ Acute pharmacologic therapy of SVT
  - ➤ Adenosine 6–2 mg IV bolus
  - ➤ Verapamil 0.07 mg/kg IV over 2 min
  - ➤ Diltiazem 0.25–0.35 mg IV over 2 min
  - ➤ Digoxin 8 mcg/kg over 10 min, give 50% daily dose then wait 4–12 hours for subsequent doses, check ECG
  - ➤ Propranolol 1–3 mg IV (1 mg/min)
  - ➤ Quinidine 0.25 mg/kg IV at 10 mg/min
  - ➤ Procainamide 10–15 mg/kg IV not to exceed 20 mg/min, followed by 1–4 mg/min
  - ➤ Disopyramide 1–2 mg/kg IV at 10 mg/min
  - ➤ Flecainide 100 mg po BID up to 400 mg/day
  - ➤ Sotalol 80 mg PO BID up to 320 mg/day
  - ➤ Amiodarone 150 mg over 10 min, then 1 mg/min for 6 hours, then 0.5 mg/min

POSTOP

- ■ Base mgt on course of operation.
- ■ In pts w/ structural heart disease, additional postop monitoring in an ICU or step-down unit may be appropriate.

SYSTEMIC LUPUS ERYTHEMATOSUS

JAMES BRANDES, MD

OVERVIEW

- ■ Autoimmune disease, most often w/ onset in young to middle-aged women
- ■ Immune complex deposition occurs throughout the body, inciting the inflammatory response, which results in tissue destruction & remodeling that impairs end-organ function
- ■ Broad clinical spectrum of manifestations that may affect every organ system of the body

PREOP

Issues/Evaluation
- Cardiac involvement includes
  - Pericarditis
  - Myocarditis
  - Endocarditis
  - Heart block
- Serositis may present as abdominal or chest pain.
- Pleuritic involvement may cause restrictive pattern on PFTs.
- Lupus anticoagulant is common (this term is a misnomer, as this makes people more prone to thrombosis).
- Renal insufficiency is common; many of these pts require dialysis & may present for renal transplants.
- Pulmonary hypertension may also be present.
- Nervous system involvement: neuropathy, altered mental status may be present
- Chronic anemia, thrombocytopenia, and/or neutropenia may occur.
- Pt may be on steroids and/or potent immune-suppressing medications.
- Airway involvement may occur in the form of TMJ disease or involvement of arytenoids.
- Exacerbation w/ pregnancy is common; fetal demise is more common in these pts.

What To Do
- Careful history & physical to asses all major organ systems for involvement
- Antibiotic prophylaxis for cardiac valvular disease
- Administer stress-dose steroids IV for pts on chronic steroid therapy.
- Careful fluid replacement & medication selection in renal failure
- Evaluate coag & hematologic status prior to regional.

INTRAOP
- Monitoring related to specific organ system pathology (eg, consider PA line if pulmonary HTN or CHF is present & surgery is stressful)
- Beware of arrhythmias from cardiac conduction system involvement.
- Drugs that may exacerbate disease include hydralazine, procainamide, phenytoin, penicillin.
- Avoid renally excreted drugs if renal insufficiency is present.
- Careful positioning of involved joints/extremities

POSTOP

- Continued steroid dosing may be necessary if pt is steroid-dependent.
- Symptoms may be exacerbated in the postop period.

THE ELDERLY PATIENT

JASON WIDRICH, MD

OVERVIEW

- Definition
  - ➤ Can be arbitrarily defined as pt >65 years old
  - ➤ Physiologic age more important than biologic age
- Elderly pts frequently have multiple coexisting diseases

PREOP

Issues/Evaluation

- Understand the typical physiologic changes that occur with aging, although not all changes may be present in a particular pt. Cardiovascular & respiratory changes, as well as changes in drug metabolism, have the biggest impact on anesthesia care.
- Cardiovascular
  - ➤ Fibrosis of conduction system
  - ➤ Increased vagal tone, decreased sensitivity of adrenergic receptors
  - ➤ Diminished cardiac reserve can cause BP drop w/ anesthetic induction.
  - ➤ Decreasing maximal HR w/ age
  - ➤ Decreased baroreceptor reflex
- Respiratory
  - ➤ Closing capacity begins to exceed functional residual capacity.
  - ➤ PaO_2 falls with age: $PaO_2 = 102$ (age/3)
  - ➤ Increased chest wall rigidity
  - ➤ Decreased cough, muscle strength, peak flow
  - ➤ Blunting of response to hypoxia & hypercapnia
- Renal
  - ➤ Decreased GFR, renal blood flow, tubular function
  - ➤ Impaired ability to concentrate or dilute urine
  - ➤ Sodium & potassium balance may be affected.

- BUN increases 0.2/year
- Creatinine remains unchanged (muscle mass changes)
- GI
  - Hepatic blood flow, liver function, biotransformation decrease
  - GI motility often altered
- CNS
  - Cerebral blood flow & brain volume decrease
  - Higher likelihood of cognitive impairment preop
- Musculoskeletal
  - Arthritic joints, decreased bone density
- Dermatologic
  - Skin more friable & likely to bruise
- Airway
  - Laryngeal, pharyngeal, airway reflexes are decreased. With GA, consider delaying tracheal extubation until pt is awake
  - Fewer cilia in bronchial tree, decreasing secretion mobilization
  - There may be limitations to mouth opening & neck extension due to arthritis or disease
  - Teeth may be loose from decay. Dentures are often present & must be removed prior to intubation

What To Do
- Look for common coexisting diseases that occur in this population, including
  - HTN
  - Renal dysfunction
  - Coronary artery disease
  - COPD
  - Diabetes mellitus
- Workup depends on pt & proposed surgery
- Medication history is particularly important because of the common occurrence of polypharmacy & the potential for adverse drug interactions

INTRAOP
- Drug effects
  - Drugs that are renally or hepatically cleared will have prolonged effects.
  - Lower albumin levels may require lower doses of barbiturates, opioids, benzodiazepines.

➤ Barbiturate doses are altered by slow redistribution from central compartment.

➤ MAC is decreased w/ inhaled anesthetics.

■ Regional anesthesia issues

➤ Lower vertebral body height, reduced epidural space & increased spread will require lower doses.

• Decrease local anesthetic dose in spinals.

• Decrease volume of local anesthetic dose in epidurals.

➤ Usually not necessary to decrease LA dose in peripheral blocks

■ Production of body heat decreases, reducing ability to maintain core temp in cold environments like OR.

Management

■ May choose to avoid or decrease benzodiazepine dose to decrease cognitive dysfunction

■ Pay close attention to positioning secondary to arthritis and "stiff joints." Risks of neurologic & dermatologic (tape/Bovie pads/pinching) injury is much higher in the elderly.

■ No proven difference between regional vs general in producing postop delirium

■ Assess volume status; expect lability of BP & HR at anesthetic induction/emergence & in PACU.

■ Pts w/ comorbid conditions (cardiac/respiratory/renal/hepatic) should be treated according to recommendations for their specific conditions.

■ Use forced air warming or other therapy as necessary to avoid hypothermia & maintain core temp.

POSTOP

■ Use any measures to assist in reorientation to prevent postop delirium (window view, presence of family).

■ Aggressive pulmonary rehabilitation may be necessary to prevent postop respiratory dysfunction or pneumonia.

TRICUSPID VALVE REGURGITATION

RICHARD PAULSEN, MD

OVERVIEW

■ Definition: incompetent tricuspid valve causing systolic reverse blood flow.

➤ Etiologies include IVDA endocarditis, trauma, RV failure, Ebstein's anomaly.
■ Usual Rx: valvular plication, annuloplasty or replacement, depending on severity.

PREOP

Issues/Evaluation
■ Usually associated w/ other valve disease (mitral stenosis)
■ Isolated disease well tolerated
■ Blowing murmur best heard at left fifth intercostal space
■ Most symptoms related to increased RV afterload
■ A-fib common
■ Giant V-wave seen on CVP or jugular venous pulsations

What To Do
■ CXR
■ EKG
■ Echo
■ Antibiotics for endocarditis prophylaxis

INTRAOP
■ Hemodynamic goals
➤ Maintain high preload.
➤ Maintain elevated HR.
➤ Maintain NSR if possible.
➤ Minimize negative inotropes.
➤ Maintain SVR.
➤ Avoid increasing pulmonary vascular resistance.
■ Alter mgt accordingly if mixed valvular lesion present.

Management
■ Standard ASA monitors.
■ Other monitors (arterial line, CVP, PA line, TEE) depend on pt disease & stress of proposed surgery.
➤ May be difficult to pass PA line.
■ With GA or regional, avoid decreasing SVR.

POSTOP
■ ECG.
■ Maintain adequate analgesia.

TRICUSPID VALVE STENOSIS

RICHARD PAULSEN, MD

OVERVIEW

- Definition: narrowing of the tricuspid valve causing reduced & turbulent diastolic blood flow.
  - ➤ Etiologies include rheumatic valvulitis, SLE, endomyocardial fibroelastosis, carcinoid syndrome.
- Usual Rx: commissurotomy or valve replacement, depending on severity.

PREOP

Issues/Evaluation

- Long asymptomatic period until valve area <1.5 cm^2
- Pressure gradient of >3 mmHg is significant
- Harsh diastolic murmur, best heard at left fifth intercostal space
- Signs of right heart failure (hepatic dysfunction, ascites, edema)
- Giant A-waves seen on CVP or jugular venous pulsations
- Associated w/ mitral stenosis

What To Do

- CXR
- EKG
- Echo
- Antibiotics for endocarditis prophylaxis
- LFTs, PT if suspicious of hepatic dysfunction

INTRAOP

- Hemodynamic goals.
  - ➤ Maintain high preload.
  - ➤ Avoid tachycardia.
  - ➤ Minimize negative inotropes.
  - ➤ Avoid decrease in SVR.

Management

- Preop reduction in hepatic congestion (diuretics, salt restriction, digitalis).
- Anxiolytic premed.
- Standard ASA monitors.

- Other monitors (arterial line, CVP, PA line, TEE) depend on pt disease & stress of proposed surgery.
  - ➤ May be difficult to pass PA line.
- With GA or regional, avoid decreasing SVR.

POSTOP
- ECG.
- Follow hepatic function.
- Maintain adequate analgesia.

UNSTABLE ANGINA

SAMIR DZANKIC, MD
JACQUELINE M. LEUNG, MD

OVERVIEW
- Definition: clinical syndrome due to myocardial ischemia that is characterized by
  - ➤ Accelerating angina (ie, change from chronic stable angina to angina that is more frequent, severe, prolonged, or precipitated by less exertion than previously)
  - ➤ Resting angina (occurrence of angina when pt is sedentary or awakening from sleep)
  - ➤ New-onset angina
- Usual Rx: requires admission to coronary care unit (CCU) & treatment w/ heparin, nitrates, beta-adrenergic blocking agents, calcium channel blockers or intra-aortic balloon pump in refractory cases

PREOP

Issues/Evaluation
- Type of procedure (emergency or elective)
- Disease severity & stability (initial history, physical exam, ECG), current treatment, functional capacity, comorbid conditions, existing diagnostic studies
- Rule out acute MI (order 12-lead ECG, cardiac enzymes).

What To Do
- For elective surgery
  - ➤ Surgery should be delayed & pt medically stabilized (transfer to CCU & start aggressive IV therapy).

➤ Order pharmacologic stress testing such as dipyridamole-thallium scintigraphy or dobutamine stress echocardiography if not already available.

➤ Consider angiography based on the results of noninvasive studies.

➤ Plan subsequent care based on diagnostic findings (medical mgt only or CABG vs PTCA).

■ For emergency surgery, aggressive medical therapy w/ IV nitroglycerin, beta-adrenergic blockers or calcium channel blockers should be started, as well as optimization of all comorbid conditions.

INTRAOP

■ Rigorous hemodynamic control to minimize the occurrence of hypertension & tachycardia (increase oxygen demand) or hypotension (decrease oxygen supply). Also avoid anemia, hypoxia, fluid overload.

■ Invasive monitoring (arterial line, PA catheter) likely required.

■ Monitor for myocardial ischemia (simultaneous leads V5 & II; possible multiple lead ST-segment analysis if available).

■ Consider intraop TEE for monitoring global & regional left ventricular function, particularly for pts w/ uninterpretable ECG such as left bundle branch block or ventricular pacemaker, or in a high-risk surgical setting in which rapid loading conditions changes may occur.

■ Continue all previous IV therapy up to the time of surgery.

Management

■ Preop sedation to avoid anxiety-induced tachycardia & hypertension.

■ The anesthetic goal is to perform a smooth induction to minimize hypertension, hypotension & tachycardia, or worsening of the ischemic state. Etomidate, narcotics are suitable induction agents.

■ Preop anti-ischemic therapy such as nitroglycerin should be continued intraop; however, dosing may need to be adjusted in the settings of general anesthetic.

■ Prevent hypertension & tachycardia at the time of intubation or extubation using lidocaine, beta blockade (esmolol, labetalol or metoprolol) or calcium channel blockers, or narcotics.

■ Anesthetic depth should be adequate prior to tracheal intubation.

■ Establish adequate analgesia prior to tracheal extubation.

■ Treat myocardial ischemia (ST depression/elevation) aggressively.

➤ Increase supply: correct hypotension, hypoxemia (increasing FiO_2, addition of PEEP if mechanically ventilated), anemia. Use caution when using vasoconstrictor in the setting of myocardial ischemia: myocardial ischemia may be worsened w/ the increase in wall stress.

➤ Decrease demand: deepen level of anesthesia, vasodilators, calcium channel blockers, beta-adrenergic blockers.

POSTOP
■ Transfer to CCU for further medical care.
■ Continue IV anti-ischemic treatment.
■ Continue to monitor hemodynamics & ECG ST-segment changes.
■ Periop MI should be ruled out w/ serial 12-lead ECG & cardiac enzymes (CK-MB, troponin).
■ Effective pain mgt to prevent hemodynamic changes.
■ Supplemental oxygen or continue tracheal intubation w/ sedation until stable.

UPPER RESPIRATORY TRACT INFECTION (URI)

ATSUKO BABA, MD

OVERVIEW
■ Definition: A usually viral infection of the upper respiratory tract causing cough, rhinitis, fever, malaise, myalgias, increased airway reactivity.
■ Usual Rx: A prophylactic annual vaccine can be helpful. Amantadine, an antiviral medication, may shorten the illness but does not shorten the duration of airway reactivity. If the URI is a bacterial infection, antibiotics can be helpful.

PREOP
Issues/Evaluation
■ Active or recent URI can increase postop pulmonary complications when the trachea is intubated.
■ Pts w/ active or recent URIs have bilateral myringotomy/tympanostomy & tonsillectomy/adenoidectomy performed more frequently.
■ There is no increased risk of pulmonary complications in short procedures that do not require intubation of the trachea (eg, BM & T).
■ W/ tracheal intubation there is increased incidence of bronchospasm, laryngospasm, intraop/postop oxygen desaturation.

- Symptoms indicating lower respiratory involvement/more serious illness are fever, purulent drainage, productive cough, decreased activity.
- Airway hyperreactivity does not return to baseline for 2–7 wks after pt is asymptomatic. Most pediatric pts have multiple URIs per year, making it impractical to wait for this period.
- Periop pulmonary complications are most significant in pts <1 y of age & less significant in pts >5 y of age, presumably secondary to airway size.

What To Do

- Elective surgery should be postponed in a pt w/ URI symptoms <1 y old.
- Elective surgery should be postponed in pts w/ URI symptoms indicating lower respiratory tract involvement or more serious illness, w/ a consultation w/ the primary pediatrician if symptoms do not improve.
- The period of delay should be at least 2 wks.
- Pts w/ URIs should be treated as if they have reactive airway disease.

INTRAOP

- For short procedures, mask/LMA general anesthesia if possible will decrease pulmonary complications.
- Be prepared for bronchospasm, laryngospasm, or oxygen desaturation, esp w/ endotracheal intubation.

POSTOP

- Be especially cautious of pulmonary complications during transport from OR to recovery room.
- Since postop oxygen desaturation can be expected, prolonged supplemental oxygen & pulse oximetry monitoring should be available.

VENTRICULAR FIBRILLATION (VF)

ART WALLACE, PHD, MD

OVERVIEW

- Definition: Chaotic cardiac rhythm characterized by presence of multiple simultaneous circulating waveforms in varying states of depolarization & repolarization.
- Usual Rx: Defibrillation as soon as possible.

- Check responsiveness.
- Activate emergency response system.
- Call for a defibrillator.
- A: Airway: Open the airway.
- B: Breathing: Provide positive-pressure ventilation.
- C: Circulation: Give chest compressions.
- D: Defibrillation (200 J, 200–300 J, 360 J)
- E: Epinephrine 1 mg IV bolus, repeat every 3–5 min
- Vasopressin 40 U IV, single dose IV
- Defibrillation 360 J
- Amiodarone 300 mg IV bolus, 150 mg IV bolus in 3–5 min, then 1 mg/min for 6 h, then 0.5 mg/min. Max cumulative dose: 2.2 g/24 h.
- Lidocaine 100 mg IV (1.0–1.5 mg/kg IV) followed by 0.5–0.75 mg/kg IV bolus. Max dose: 3 mg/kg.
- Magnesium 1–2 g IV push
- Procainamide 20 mg/min IV. Max dose: 17 mg/kg, 100 mg IV bolus q5min is acceptable.
- Consider sodium bicarbonate.
- Defibrillate.

PREOP

Issues/Evaluation
- Implies presence of structural heart disease or prior disaster.
  - Coronary artery disease: monomorphic VT or VF implies prior MI.
  - Dilated cardiomyopathy: common.
  - Mitral valve prolapse.
  - Hypertrophic cardiomyopathy.

What To Do
- Identify primary etiology of VF.
- All pts w/ CAD, prior MI, angina, peripheral vascular disease, or two risk factors for CAD (hypertension, age >=65, diabetes, cigarettes, cholesterol >=240) must be on perioperative anti-ischemia therapy (beta blockers) unless absolutely contraindicated.
- Pts w/ history of VF frequently have more severe CAD w/ ischemia or dilated cardiomyopathy. Preoperative beta blockade should be begun at least 7 d prior to surgery & continued for at least 30 d postop.

■ If pt has implanted defibrillator, will need to be shut off for surgery w/ electrocautery.

INTRAOP
■ Standard monitoring + arterial line
■ Shut off implanted defibrillators.

Management
■ For acute episode of VF, manage as above.
■ Identify etiology of VF & correct if possible.
   ➤ Hypoxia.
   ➤ Acidosis.
   ➤ Ischemia.
   ➤ Electrolyte abnormalities.
   ➤ Mechanical or electrical stimulation of myocardium.
      • Touching.
      • Lithotripsy.
      • Microshock.

POSTOP
■ Turn implanted defibrillator back on.
■ Base mgt on course of operation & severity of disease. In pts w/ structural heart disease & a history of VF, additional postop monitoring in an ICU or step-down unit is appropriate.
■ For acute episodes of VF, postop telemetry is required. Pts should be admitted to monitored bed & ruled out for MI. This should include serial enzymes (troponin) & ECG.
■ If evidence of acute myocardial ischemia or infarction is present, consider mgt w/ antiplatelet drugs, beta blockade, nitrates, & possible emergent clot lysis w/ streptokinase, TPA, or angioplasty.

VENTRICULAR TACHYCARDIA (VT)

ART WALLACE, PHD, MD

OVERVIEW
■ Definition: A rapid rhythm originating in ventricular tissue caused by re-entry, triggered activity, or enhanced automaticity. VT is classified as:
   ➤ Monomorphic: scarred myocardium w/ structural heart disease.

- Polymorphic: abnormalities in repolarization.
- Sustained/nonsustained.

■ Usual Rx
  - Unstable
    - Check responsiveness.
    - Activate emergency response system.
    - Call for defibrillator.
    - Airway: open the airway.
    - Breathing: provide positive-pressure ventilations.
    - Circulation: give chest compressions.
    - Defibrillation: 200 J, 200–300 J, 360 J
    - Epinephrine 1 mg IV push, repeat q3–5min. Or vasopressin 40 U IV, single dose.
    - Amiodarone 300 mg IV bolus, 150 mg IV bolus in 3–5 min. Max cumulative dose: 2.2 g/24 h.
    - Lidocaine 100 mg IV bolus (0.5–0.75 mg/kg IV).
    - Magnesium 25–50 mg/kg over 10–20 min, 2 g max IV.
    - Procainamide.
    - Consider sodium bicarbonate.
  - Stable: medical therapy.
    - Monomorphic VT: Can use cardioversion if any problems.

■ Normal ejection fraction.
  - Amiodarone 150 mg over 10 min, then 1 mg/min for 6 h, then 0.5 mg/min.
  - Lidocaine 100 mg IV (0.5–0.75 mg/kg IV) bolus.
  - Procainamide 10–15 mg/kg IV not to exceed 20 mg/min, followed by 1–4 mg/min.
  - Sotalol 1.0–1.5 mg/kg, then 10 mg/min.

■ Poor ejection fraction.
  - Amiodarone 150 mg IV over 10 min.
  - Lidocaine 100 mg IV (0.5–0.75 mg/kg IV) bolus.
    - Polymorphic VT: Can use cardioversion if any problems.

■ Normal baseline QT interval.
  - Treat ischemia.
  - Correct electrolytes.
  - Any one of the following:
    - Beta blockers.
    - Lidocaine.
    - Amiodarone.
    - Procainamide.
    - Sotalol.

- Prolonged baseline QT suggests torsades de pointes.
  - ➤ Correct abnormal electrolytes.
  - ➤ Any one of the following:
    - Magnesium 1–2 g IV over 5 min, 0.5–1.0 g/h IV
    - Overdrive pacing
    - Isoproterenol
    - Phenytoin
    - Lidocaine
  - ➤ Chronic: implantable defibrillator

PREOP

Issues/Evaluation
- Implies presence of heart disease
  - ➤ Coronary artery disease: monomorphic VT implies prior MI
  - ➤ Dilated cardiomyopathy: common
  - ➤ Mitral valve prolapse
  - ➤ Hypertrophic cardiomyopathy

What To Do
- Identify primary etiology of VT.
- All pts w/ CAD, prior MI, angina, peripheral vascular disease, or two risk factors for CAD (hypertension, age >=65, diabetes, cigarettes, cholesterol >=240) must be on perioperative anti-ischemia therapy (beta blockers) unless absolutely contraindicated.
- Pts w/ history of VT frequently have more severe CAD w/ ischemia or dilated cardiomyopathy. Preop beta blockade should be begun at least 7 d prior to surgery & continued for at least 30 d postop.
- If pt has implanted defibrillator, will need to be shut off for surgery employing electrocautery.

INTRAOP
- Standard monitoring + arterial line
- Shut off implanted defibrillators.

Management
- For acute episode of VT, manage as above.
- Identify etiology of VT & correct if possible.
  - ➤ Hypoxia.
  - ➤ Acidosis.
  - ➤ Ischemia.
  - ➤ Electrolyte abnormalities.
  - ➤ Mechanical or electrical stimulation of myocardium.

- Touching.
- Lithotripsy.
- Microshock.

POSTOP

- Turn implanted defibrillator back on.
- Base mgt on course of operation & severity of disease. In pts w/ structural heart disease & a history of VT, additional postop monitoring in an ICU or step-down unit is appropriate.
- For acute episodes of VT, postop telemetry is required. Pts should be admitted to monitored bed & ruled out for MI. This should include serial enzymes (troponin) & ECG.
- If evidence of acute myocardial ischemia or infarction is present, consider mgt w/ antiplatelet drugs, beta blockade, nitrates, & possible emergent clot lysis w/ streptokinase, TPA, or angioplasty.

WOLFF-PARKINSON-WHITE/PRE-EXCITATION SYNDROMES

ART WALLACE, PHD, MD

OVERVIEW

- Definition: Activation of part of the ventricle by an anomalous connection before it is depolarized by the normal atrioventricular (AV) conduction system
  - 98% AV: connection in four locations: midseptal, anteroseptal, para-Hisian, posteroseptal
  - 2% atriofascicular: duplication of normal conducting system. AV node-like remnant is connected to the right bundle branch or to the distal right ventricle.
  - 30–50% asymptomatic
  - Can be associated w/ sudden death
- Diagnosis: Delta waves w/ short PR interval
- Usual Rx
  - Catheter ablation (primary & most appropriate therapy)
  - Beta blockers
    - Atenolol
    - Sotalol
    - Esmolol
  - Propafenone
  - Flecainide

PREOP

Issues/Evaluation
- Rapid atrial tachycardias can be conducted 1:1 to ventricle w/ hemo-dynamic collapse.
- Atrial fibrillation or flutter can lead to sudden death.
- Catheter ablation of aberrant pathway is most appropriate therapy.

What To Do
- Identify arrhythmia.
- Assess frequency & severity of symptoms.
- Consider catheter ablation for anyone w/ Wolff-Parkinson-White plus:
  - Ventricular fibrillation
  - Rapid atrial fibrillation
  - Recurrent SVT
- Not recommended for completely asymptomatic pre-excitation

INTRAOP
- Monitor.
- Consider arterial line.

Management
- Avoid atrial fibrillation or flutter.
- Avoid calcium channel blockers.
- Avoid digoxin.

POSTOP
- Base mgt on course of operation. In pts w/ symptomatic SVT, additional postop monitoring in an ICU or step-down unit may be appropriate.

PART TWO

Procedures

ABDOMINAL AORTIC ANEURYSM (AAA) REPAIR

CHRISTOPHER G. HATCH, MD

PREOP

Preop Considerations

- Aortic disease is indicative of other vascular disease listed below. AAA surgery has high risk of periop myocardial ischemia. Strongly consider perioperative beta blockade in these pts.
  - Coronary artery disease. Manifestations include:
    - MI
    - Stable or unstable angina
    - LV dysfunction/CHF
    - Atrial fibrillation
    - Arrhythmias; cardiac pacemakers not uncommon in this population
  - Peripheral vascular disease
  - Carotid artery disease: always listen for carotid bruits & ask about TIA/CVA symptoms
- Other common comorbidities
  - COPD
  - HTN
  - DM
    - Because AAA surgery is a major stressor, consider perioperative insulin infusion for type 1 DM.
  - Renal dysfunction
    - Often exacerbated by periop angiograms/IV contrast
    - Can give acetylcysteine (Mucomyst) 600 mg PO BID × 2 days for renal protection from IV contrast injury
- Drug therapy issues
  - Pts should take all their cardiac medications up to & including day of surgery.
  - Continuation of ACE inhibitors is controversial; they have been assoc w/ severe hypotension during GA.
  - Diuretics may be held on the morning of surgery.
  - Many pts are diabetics on insulin.
    - Pts coming from home can check their glucose at home & bring their insulin with them.

- For brittle diabetics or pts already in the hospital, IV glucose & insulin may be instituted prior to surgery.
- See also Coexisting Disease chapter "Diabetes Mellitus."
➢ Pts are often taking anticoagulation or antiplatelet agents.
- Coumadin: generally discontinued 7 days prior to procedure; bridge therapy w/ LMWH may be necessary depending on indication for Coumadin (eg, DVT, heart valve)
- ASA: discontinue 7 days prior to surgery
- Plavix: discontinue 7 days prior to surgery
- Ticlid: discontinue 7 days prior to surgery
■ Geriatric population undergoing this procedure is at risk of postop delirium
➢ See also Coexisting Disease chapter "The Elderly Patient."
■ Reduce risk of cardiac complications.
➢ Periop beta blockade has been shown to greatly decrease the risk of MI.
➢ Consider involving cardiology service to follow patients in the periop period.

Physical Findings
■ Pts commonly have coexisting diseases mentioned above. Findings may be present in multiple organ systems, including
➢ Neck
- Carotid bruits
- Increased jugular venous pressure
➢ Pulmonary
- Wheezes
- Rales
- Rhonchi
- Distant breath sounds
- Barrel chest
➢ Cardiovascular
- Check for regular vs irregular rhythm
- Presence of S3 or S4
- Murmurs
- Displaced apical impulse
➢ Abdomen
- Bruits
- Pulsatile masses
- Obesity

> Extremities
> - Diminished or absent lower extremity pulses
> - Nonhealing ulcers
> - Distal embolic phenomena

Workup

- Ask about functional status/exercise tolerance as guide to severity of cardiovascular & pulmonary disease.
- Cardiac complications account for most (50–65%) of the periop morbidity & mortality associated w/ AAA surgery. Special care should be given to cardiac evaluation of these pts.
  > Incidence of periop MI: 4–5%.
  > ECG.
    - Obtain an old ECG for comparison when diagnosing postop ECG changes.
  > Based on history & physical findings, special studies such as echocardiography (TTE or TEE), stress tests (ie, dobutamine or thallium) or coronary angiography may be indicated.
  > Persantine thallium test/dobutamine echo: consider using these tests for cardiac risk stratification in pts w/
    - New or changing anginal pattern
    - New ECG changes
    - Recent CHF/MI
    - Multiple cardiac risk factors in setting of poor functional status
  > Periop beta blockade has been shown to reduce risk of cardiac complications.
- Carotid ultrasound is indicated if bruits are present, especially if there is a history of stroke or TIA.
- PFTs or ABGs are usually not indicated.
  > However, in pts w/ moderate to severe pulmonary disease & upper abdominal incisions, PFTs may help guide preop medical therapy for optimal pulmonary status & estimate risk.
  > Functional status is also predictive of pulmonary complications.
- Smoking cessation is a crucial step in minimizing pulmonary complications.
  > 6–8 weeks of smoking abstinence is optimal.
- Labs
  > CBC
  > BUN, creatinine
  > PT/PTT

- ➤ Electrolytes for pts on diuretics, ACE inhibitors, or history of renal insufficiency or failure
- ■ Surgeon typically orders CT scan w/ contrast or MRA to evaluate the extent of the aortic disease (position [infra- or suprarenal], diameter, involvement of the mesenteric vessels).

Choice of Anesthesia
- ■ GA preferred for open AAA repair.
- ■ Epidural may be used for postop analgesia or as an adjunct to GA.
  - ➤ Weigh the potential benefits of epidural against the risk of epidural hematoma in the pt on periop anticoagulants.

INTRAOP
Monitors/Line Placement
- ■ Because of rapid hemodynamic changes & the potential for hypotension & myocardial ischemia, standard monitors plus the following are required:
  - ➤ ECG w/ ST segment analysis
  - ➤ Arterial line
  - ➤ Central venous line
- ■ Additional monitors may include TEE and/or PA catheter to evaluate myocardial function & cardiac output & to calculate systemic vascular resistance.
- ■ Two large-bore peripheral IVs (or central introducer sheath) needed for possible rapid fluid & blood administration

Intraop Concerns
- ■ Maintenance of hemodynamic stability
  - ➤ Close titration of IV & inhalation agents w/ emphasis on hemodynamic stability, not speed of onset
  - ➤ Thiopental, propofol, etomidate, fentanyl or other synthetic narcotics, and benzodiazepines have all been used successfully to this effect.
  - ➤ Esmolol & nitroglycerin may be useful for additional hemodynamic mgt of hypertension or tachycardia.
  - ➤ Esmolol or opioids may be necessary to blunt the pt's response to tracheal intubation.
  - ➤ Maintaining HR & MAP within 20% of baseline is generally appropriate; agents should be readily available to achieve that goal.
- ■ Muscle relaxation is necessary for surgical exposure.

- Obtain baseline ABG & ACT.
- Keep blood products in the OR in case of significant hemorrhage.
- Avoid hypothermia by warming IV fluids & using forced air warming.
- Preservation of renal function is an important concern, though there is controversy as to the utility of these therapies.
  - Renal perfusion may be enhanced by using a dopamine infusion ($\sim$2 ug/kg/min) throughout the case.
  - Mannitol may be given (12.5–25 g) prior to cross-clamp application.
  - After the cross-clamp is released, some advocate using furosemide to improve urinary output.
- Prior to cross-clamping of the aorta, give heparin IV to achieve an ACT >300 (normal 110–140 sec).
- Cross-clamping of the aorta results in significant cardiac stress.
  - Acute left ventricular strain produces a major cardiovascular stress; magnitude is related to clamp position.
    - MAP may increase only 2% w/ infrarenal clamping & 5% w/ suprarenal, but may increase up to 54% w/ supraceliac placement.
  - Preload & afterload may increase. Ejection fraction may decrease. This may lead to myocardial ischemia in pts w/ significant CAD.
- Mgt of hemodynamic changes w/ aortic cross-clamp
  - NTG, beta blockers and/or sodium nitroprusside may be used to prevent the hypertensive response.
  - Increasing anesthetic depth can also be helpful prior to cross-clamping.
  - Anticipation of the increase in SVR is important; in general, any of the agents mentioned above can be used to reduce MAP 10–20% prior to clamping. Clearly, this is most applicable w/ a supraceliac clamp.
  - Some vascular surgeons clamp the iliac arteries first to prevent distal embolization due to the aortic clamp.
- Other changes w/ aortic cross-clamp
  - Ischemia/hypoperfusion of the kidneys, abdominal viscera, spinal cord
  - Accumulation of acid metabolites in tissues & vasculature below the level of the clamp
- After cross-clamping, the aneurysm is opened, thrombotic material is removed & the anterior & lateral walls are removed, leaving the posterior wall intact. Bleeding vessels are ligated, the graft is sewn

in place, the cross-clamp is removed & the iliac arteries are anastomosed.

■ Anticipation of clamp removal is important.
  ➤ Prior to clamp removal, increase preload.
    • Some clinicians advocate increasing the PCWP (if PAC used) by 3–4 mmHg above baseline to offset the anticipated hypotension assoc w/ unclamping.
  ➤ Discontinue agents such as NTG, nitroprusside & esmolol & decrease anesthetic depth as necessary.
  ➤ Agents such as calcium, phenylephrine, ephedrine & epinephrine may be necessary due to decreases in SVR & CO. Raising BP 20–30% above baseline with such agents prior to clamp release is often necessary to avoid significant hypotension.
  ➤ Duration & location of the aortic clamp determine the degree of hypotension observed.
  ➤ A supraceliac clamp can result in significant bowel & liver ischemia; decrease in SVR & CO after release of such a clamp can be significant.

■ Upon unclamping, acidic metabolites from the ischemic tissues below the clamp are washed back into the circulation.
  ➤ Make prophylactic ventilatory adjustments to accommodate this increased acid load.
  ➤ Profound acidosis may require buffer therapy (bicarbonate or THAM) to adjust the pH until the acidosis resolves.
  ➤ Frequent ABGs are necessary to monitor this acidosis & guide appropriate therapy.

■ After unclamping, reverse the heparin effect w/ protamine. Discuss timing of reversal w/ surgeon.

■ As bleeding may present or worsen after unclamping, monitoring of blood loss & serial hematocrits are necessary to aid in fluid mgt & blood product transfusion.

■ If epidural is being used for postop analgesia, consider whether to dose epidural intraop.
  ➤ Epidural usually dosed after the aortic cross-clamp is released, hemostasis is adequate & BP is stable. One regimen is 1/8% bupivacaine with 3–5 mcg/mL fentanyl at 8–12 cc/hr after a divided-dose bolus of 8–10 cc.

■ At end of case, decide whether tracheal extubation should be considered, depending on intraop course & coexisting disease.

■ Pts benefit from postop care in an ICU or monitored setting, given the high risk of cardiac complications.

POSTOP

Pain

- Moderate to severe
- Pts usually require epidural or PCA.
  - ➤ While continuous epidural infusions can be used for pain control, they are often avoided in these pts due to intraop or preop coagulopathy & concerns regarding epidural hematoma.
- IV opioids may also be given via PCA or intermittent IV bolus, depending on the pt's mental status & postop course.
- Pain control is essential in the postop mgt of these pts, as increased pain & anxiety result in catecholamine release, resulting in increased myocardial oxygen demand & ischemia.
  - ➤ In addition, recovery of pulmonary function is improved w/ adequate pain control.

Complications

- The major complication is myocardial ischemia. It occurs more frequently postop than in the preop or intraop periods.
  - ➤ Postop period is marked by increased myocardial oxygen demand, increased catecholamine levels, hypoxia, hypercoagulability, large fluid shifts.
  - ➤ Watch for myocardial ischemia, CHF, pulmonary edema.
  - ➤ See also Critical Events chapter "Myocardial Ischemia."
- Surgical complications include lumbar muscle rhabdomyolysis, anastomotic bleeding, coagulopathy, renal dysfunction/failure, visceral ischemia & infarction, lower extremity ischemia/emboli, spinal cord ischemia/injury.
- The incidence of spinal cord injury is reported to be 0.15% in unruptured AAA repair. The artery of Adamkiewicz arises from above L3 in most people; therefore, clamping at or above this level increases the risk of spinal cord injury.

SURGICAL PROCEDURE

Indications

- A ruptured AAA is an indication for an emergent repair; unfortunately up to 60% of these pts die prior to reaching the hospital.
- Elective surgery is recommended for pts w/ an asymptomatic aneurysm >5 cm in diameter.
- Severe coexisting disease may be a contraindication to surgery; endovascular surgery may be an alternative for these pts.

Procedure
- Generally, a midline incision is made from the xiphoid to the pubic symphysis to expose the aneurysm & iliac arteries & isolate the renal arteries & ureters.
- A cross-clamp is placed proximal to the aneurysm, which is then opened. Thrombotic material is removed & the anterior & lateral walls are removed, leaving the posterior wall intact.
- Bleeding vessels are ligated, the graft is sewn in place, the cross-clamp is removed & the iliac arteries are anastomosed.

Surgical Concerns
- Aneurysm rupture prior to cross-clamp placement
- Aneurysmal involvement of renal or mesenteric arteries
- Duration of cross-clamping & consequent ischemia
- Renal ischemia & consequent dysfunction
- Spinal cord ischemia

Typical EBL
- Extremely variable, from <500 cc to >1 blood volume
  - ➢ Type & cross-match always indicated; cell saver can be useful if available
  - ➢ Pts w/ ruptured AAA are more likely to have large blood loss, coagulopathy & thrombocytopenia.

ACUTE AORTIC DISSECTION REPAIR

RICHARD PAULSEN, MD

PREOP

Preop Considerations
- Two classifications of aortic dissection
  - ➢ DeBakey
    - Type I: origin of dissection in ascending aorta; extends distal to aortic arch
    - Type II: origin of dissection in ascending aorta; extent confined to aortic arch
    - Type III: origin of dissection in descending aorta
  - ➢ Stanford
    - Type A: all dissections involving ascending aorta
    - Type B: all dissections distal to left subclavian artery (sparing ascending aorta)

- Usual Rx
  - Surgical therapy of type A dissection
  - Medical therapy of most type B dissections
- Dissection is considered acute when diagnosis made within 14 days of symptom onset
- Symptoms
  - 90% of pts have abrupt, severe chest pain, often w/ migration of pain to back.
  - Complications of dissection can result in additional symptoms (see below).
    - Fatal rupture of the ascending aorta or aortic arch
    - Altered mental status
    - Renal insufficiency
    - Visceral ischemia
    - Myocardial ischemia
- Complications of aortic dissection include the following. Two-day mortality is at least 50%.
  - Acute aortic insufficiency (AI)
  - Pericardial effusion & tamponade (w/ ascending aorta involvement)
  - Acute congestive heart failure
  - Hemothorax
  - Aortic branch occlusion
    - Arms or legs (20% incidence)
    - idney (15%)
    - Brain (5%)
    - Heart (10%); can cause acute myocardial ischemia
    - Bowel or spinal cord (3%)
- Causes or factors predisposing to aortic dissection
  - Trauma
  - Infection
  - Marfan syndrome
  - Iatrogenic (eg, cardiac surgery, vascular catheters)
  - Atherosclerosis
  - HTN
  - Some congenital lesions (eg, aortic coarctation, bicuspid aortic valve, aortic arch hypoplasia)
  - Pregnancy
  - Age >60
- Common coexisting diseases in this population
  - Coronary artery disease

➤ HTN
➤ COPD
➤ Peripheral vascular disease
➤ DM
➤ Chronic renal insufficiency
■ If dissection suspected, control BP using vasodilators (NTP, NTG) & beta blockers (eg, esmolol, metoprolol).
➤ Goal: SBP 105–115, HR 60–80.
➤ For hypotension, do not administer agents that increase contractility (eg, ephedrine). Instead, consider alpha-agonist agent such as phenylephrine.

Physical Findings
■ Depend on extent of dissection & branch occlusion
■ General
➤ Anxiety, diaphoresis
■ Cardiovascular
➤ Shock
➤ CHF
➤ Hypotension (from hemorrhage)
➤ HTN (related to pain or anxiety)
➤ New murmur from AI
➤ Asymmetric pulses
■ CNS
➤ Hemiparesis or hemiplegia
➤ Document neuro exam findings in case a new deficit develops postop
■ Other
➤ Hoarseness (from recurrent laryngeal nerve compression), dyspnea, stridor (from tracheal compression)
➤ Abdominal pain (bowel ischemia)
➤ Oliguria

Workup
■ Lab studies
➤ CBC, electrolytes, BUN, creatinine, PT, PTT, fibrinogen, LFTs, ABGs
■ ECG: check for LVH, ischemia/infarction; low QRS voltage is suggestive of tamponade
■ CXR: check for widened mediastinum, tracheal compression, or pleural effusion (from hemothorax)

- Specific diagnostic imaging
  - ➤ Echocardiography
    - Evaluate heart & valve function, location of aortic tear, presence of flap, pericardial effusion/tamponade, wall motion abnormalities from coronary occlusion
    - TEE can be used if pt cannot tolerate transport to radiology for other type of imaging study. Not as useful in detecting more distal dissections.
  - ➤ MRI or CT scan
    - Location & extent of dissection
  - ➤ Aortography
    - Location of tear, involvement of other arteries
- Blood products
  - ➤ Type & cross-match 4 units PRBC
  - ➤ Consider FFP or platelets as indicated

Choice of Anesthesia
- GA required
- Thoracic epidural is an option if pt stable & no contraindications; however, would avoid in pts likely to undergo heparinization & cardiopulmonary bypass
- Cautious use of premed to control pain/anxiety
- Depending on risk of aspiration, consider Bicitra, H2 antagonist, metoclopramide

INTRAOP

Monitors/Line Placement
- Standard monitors.
- Foley catheter.
- Arterial line: place prior to transporting pt.
  - ➤ Artery cannulated depends on type of surgery, location of injury.
  - ➤ For type A dissection, consider bilateral radial arterial lines.
  - ➤ Ideally, place arterial lines pre- and postdissection to assess proximal & distal perfusion.
- Central line
  - ➤ Consider large-bore introducer sheath to facilitate rapid transfusion.
- PA line
  - ➤ May be useful in assessment of cardiac output & volume status.
- TEE can be useful in evaluating
  - ➤ Aortic pathology.

➤ Global & regional LV function.
➤ Integrity of valve function.
➤ Intracardiac air.
■ Consider benefits of neurologic monitoring (eg, EEG, SSEP).
■ Two large peripheral IVs or peripheral rapid infusion catheter.
■ For type A dissection, avoid placing lines in left arm & left IJ if possible.
■ Place invasive monitors prior to induction if possible.

Intraop Concerns
■ Prior to induction
➤ Place arterial line for close BP monitoring.
➤ Control HTN & reduce contractility w/ combination of vasodilators & beta blockers.
➤ Consider potential for undiagnosed pericardial effusion, which can predispose to tamponade. (See also Critical Event chapter "Cardiac Tamponade.")
■ Concerns during induction
➤ Control hemodynamics closely, especially during laryngoscopy.
➤ Can use combination of anesthetic agents (eg, narcotics, etomidate, midazolam) & vasoactive agents (eg, beta blockers, nitroprusside, nitroglycerin) to control BP & HR & minimize chance of HTN & tachycardia.
➤ Maintain cricoid pressure in pts at risk of aspiration.
■ Can maintain anesthesia w/ a variety of agents (eg, narcotics, inhaled agent, benzodiazepines)
■ If surgical approach is thoracotomy (eg, type B dissection), double-lumen ETT (DLT) may be required.
➤ In general left-sided DLT is preferred.
➤ Consider right-sided DLT if left mainstem bronchus is compressed.
■ For type A dissection (involving the aortic arch)
➤ Can have massive hemorrhage when pericardium is opened.
➤ Tamponade may improve w/ drainage of pericardial blood.
➤ Cardiopulmonary bypass will be required (possibly via femoral artery).
➤ Hypothermic circulatory arrest may be used.
➤ Possible procedures include aortic valve replacement, reimplantation of coronary arteries or great vessels.
■ For type B dissection (descending lesions)
➤ Aortic cross-clamping may result in liver, bowel, renal ischemia.

- ➤ Left atrial to aortic shunt may be used to improve blood flow distal to aortic cross-clamp.
- ➤ Pt at risk for paraplegia from decreased spinal cord perfusion (anterior spinal artery syndrome).
  - Some surgeons employ a closed lumbar CSF drain & remove CSF to maintain pressure 10 mmHg.
- ■ Potential for end-organ ischemia from aortic cross-clamp
  - ➤ Spinal cord: discussed above
  - ➤ Bowel
  - ➤ Liver
  - ➤ Renal
- ■ For descending aortic dissection repair w/o bypass, concerns regarding aortic cross-clamping & unclamping are similar to AAA repair. See Procedures chapter "Abdominal Aortic Aneurysm Repair."
- ■ After repair, keep mean BP 60–80 & HR <100 to reduce risk of repeat dissection.

Intraop Therapies
- ■ Protection from renal ischemia: consider using mannitol, furosemide, dopamine or fenoldepam during aortic cross-clamp.
- ■ Consider hemostatic agent such as aprotinin or aminocaproic acid to reduce bleeding, especially for bypass & circulatory arrest.
- ■ Heparin to maintain ACT >400 for bypass case
- ■ Mgt of circulatory arrest
  - ➤ Cool to 15–18 degrees C.
  - ➤ Consider steroids & mannitol (controversial).
  - ➤ Administer thiopental (decrease cerebral metabolic rate) & consider EEG monitoring (controversial).
  - ➤ Prevent hyperglycemia & acidosis.
  - ➤ Maintain neuromuscular blockade (prevents shivering).
- ■ At end of surgery, change to single-lumen ETT if DLT used. Facilitates postop mechanical ventilation in ICU.
- ■ Reverse neuromuscular blockade in ICU to allow immediate evaluation of spinal cord function.

POSTOP

Pain
- ■ Moderate to severe
- ■ IV narcotics via PCA when awake
- ■ Consider epidural for thoracotomy incision if no contraindication

Complications
- MI
- Hemorrhage
- Dysrhythmias
- Coagulopathy
- Renal failure
- Bowel ischemia
- Paraplegia
- Infection
- Intracoronary air
- Death

SURGICAL PROCEDURE

Indications
- Type A dissection.
- Type B dissection not amenable to medical treatment.

Procedure
- Type A dissection
  - Median sternotomy.
  - Identify lesion location.
  - Cardiopulmonary bypass, potentially via femoral route
  - Graft placement.
  - Possible use of circulatory arrest for distal anastomosis.
  - Other procedures as needed: reimplantation of great vessels or coronary arteries, CABG.
  - Wean from bypass.
  - Reverse heparin.
  - Establish hemostasis.
  - Close chest.
- Type B dissection
  - Left thoracotomy w/ left lung deflated.
  - Identify lesion.
  - Consider need for cardiopulmonary bypass.
  - Consider need for left atrial to aortic shunt.
  - Aortic cross-clamp.
  - Graft placement.
  - Unclamp aorta.
  - Wean from bypass.
  - Reverse heparin.
  - Establish hemostasis.
  - Close chest.

Surgical Concerns

- Minimizing aortic cross-clamp time (ideally <30 min) to decrease incidence of spinal cord ischemia.
- Graft patency.
- Organ ischemia.
- Emboli.
- Removing intracardiac air.
- Hemostasis.

Typical EBL

- Blood loss not usually recorded for cardiopulmonary bypass cases.
- Transfusion requirements can be significant (>1 blood volume), especially for type A dissection.

ADULT HEART TRANSPLANTATION

RICHARD PAULSEN, MD

PREOP

Preop Considerations

- Pt typically has end-stage cardiac failure (NYHA class III or IV) w/ poor long-term prognosis.
  - ➤ See also Coexisting Disease chapter "Congestive Heart Failure."
- Typical clinical features include the following:
  - ➤ Because of low cardiac output (CO), pts often "bridged" to transplant w/
    - Inotrope therapy (eg, dobutamine, milrinone).
    - LV assist devices.
    - Intra-aortic balloon pump.
  - ➤ Pts often have pulmonary hypertension, neuroendocrine abnormalities, hepatic dysfunction.
  - ➤ Because of thromboembolism risk, pts often on anticoagulants & may need FFP prior to surgery.
  - ➤ Pt may have had previous cardiac surgery (increases risk of hemorrhage).
  - ➤ Arrhythmias are a common cause of pretransplant death.
- Immunosuppression med may be started immediately preop.
- Note condition of donor heart & preharvest inotropic support.

Physical Findings

- Vital signs & hemodynamics: note current status & recent trends.

■ Evaluate findings of CHF.

Workup
■ CBC, electrolytes, BUN, creatinine, PT, PTT, fibrinogen.
■ Type & cross-match for PRBCs; consider need for additional blood products (eg, FFP, platelets, cryoprecipitate).
■ ECG.
■ CXR.
■ Review results of most recent cardiac evaluation.
  ➤ Right & left heart catheterizations: note PA pressure, note PVR response to vasodilators
  ➤ Echo: ejection fraction typically 10–20%

Choice of Anesthesia
■ GA
  ➤ Do not induce GA until donor heart has been evaluated & cleared for use.
  ➤ Decide whether to place invasive monitors prior to induction.
  ➤ Anticipate slower-than-usual IV induction secondary to low CO.
  ➤ Anticipate hemodynamic effect of induction drugs & provide inotrope or vasopressor support as necessary.
    • Options for induction drugs include etomidate, w/ narcotic or benzodiazepine.
  ➤ Maintain anesthesia w/ inhaled agent or narcotic-based technique w/ benzodiazepine for amnesia.
■ Be prepared to initiate inotropic support before, during or after induction.

INTRAOP

Monitors/Line Placement
■ Standard monitors
■ Arterial line
■ Central line
  ➤ Consider use of left IJ, since cardiologist will use right IJ for future endomyocardial biopsies
■ TEE
■ PA catheter
  ➤ Will need to withdraw prior to removal of native heart
■ One or two large-bore peripheral IVs
  ➤ Consider 7 or 8.5 F rapid infusion catheter for pt w/ previous cardiac surgery.
■ Important: place monitors using strict aseptic technique

Intraop Concerns

- Standard preparation for cardiopulmonary bypass (CPB), including heparin to maintain ACT >400 sec
- Postbypass, must understand physiologic differences of transplanted heart
- Cardiac physiology changes
  - ➢ Since both sympathetic & parasympathetic innervation is lost in the transplanted heart, many of the reflex arcs are lost (eg, vagal maneuvers are ineffective)
  - ➢ Light anesthesia, hypoxia, hypotension & hypovolemia usually do not promote tachycardia
  - ➢ CO is dependent on preload since the reflex tachycardia found w/ hypotension & hypovolemia is severely blunted.
- Important drug pharmacology issues posttransplant
  - ➢ Certain agents will not produce their expected hemodynamic response because of the altered cardiac physiology (especially denervation)
  - ➢ Agents having usual effects include isoproterenol, epinephrine, dopamine, dobutamine, beta blockers.
  - ➢ The usual changes in HR associated w/ atropine, glycopyrrolate, edrophonium, neostigmine, pancuronium, succinylcholine & phenylephrine will not be seen
  - ➢ Cyclosporine may exacerbate renal dysfunction
- Target posttransplant HR is 90–120
- Postop RV failure can occur immediately from severe pulmonary hypertension

Intraop Therapies

- Consider hemostatic agent to reduce blood loss (eg, aprotinin, aminocaproic acid or tranexamic acid)
- Issues w/ weaning & terminating CPB
  - ➢ Same degree of preharvest inotropic support may be needed for donor heart
  - ➢ Isoproterenol (10–150 mcg/min) useful for inotropic support, pulmonary vasodilation & maintenance of adequate HR ("chemical pacemaker")
  - ➢ For additional inotropic support, consider dopamine and/or epinephrine
  - ➢ TEE is useful for evaluation & mgt of
    - Preload
    - Global & regional LV function

- Residual Intracardiac air
- Left atrial suture line
➤ Consider agents to manage pulmonary HTN:
- Inhaled nitric oxide
- Epoprostenol (Flolan)
- Nitroprusside
- Nitroglycerin
➤ Consider need for temporary pacemaker to achieve adequate HR
■ Discuss postbypass immunosuppression therapy w/ surgeon
➤ May include methylprednisolone 500 mg
■ Maintain full monitoring upon transport to ICU & ensure that all inotropes & vasopressors are continued

POSTOP

Pain
■ Moderate
■ IV sedatives to tolerate mechanical ventilation
■ IV narcotics for analgesia
■ Consider need for PCA after extubation

Complications
■ Immediate complications
➤ RV failure
➤ Hemorrhage
- May require emergency surgery if bleeding is severe, or if tamponade develops
- See also Procedures chapter "Cardiac Surgery Re-Exploration."
➤ Oliguria
➤ Intracoronary air causing ischemia
➤ Hyperacute rejection
■ Later complications
➤ Drug side effects: cyclosporin, corticosteroids, azathioprine
➤ Early acute rejection (10–21 days)
➤ Infection

SURGICAL PROCEDURE

Indications
■ End-stage cardiac failure w/ poor prognosis

Procedure
■ Donor heart examined
■ Median sternotomy

- Open pericardium preserving phrenic nerve
- Cannulate aorta & vena cava (bicaval cannulation)
- CPB initiated
- Cross-clamps applied
- Aorta & PA transected, followed by incision through the atria
  - Cuff of native tissue w/ pulmonary veins remains & may cause dual P waves on ECG
- Recipient heart removed
- Donor heart attached via the atria; then the PA & aorta are anastomosed
- Intracardiac air removed
- Aorta unclamped & pt rewarmed
- NSR established
- CPB discontinued
- Pacing wires placed
- Heparin reversed, hemostasis confirmed, chest closed

Surgical Concerns
- Donor heart function
- Removal of Intracardiac air
- Hemostasis & hemorrhage
- RV function postbypass

Typical EBL
- Not usually measured for CPB case
- Blood loss & transfusion requirement may be significantly higher for repeat sternotomy

---

AMPUTATION, LOWER EXTREMITY

JASON WIDRICH, MD

PREOP

Preop Considerations
- Pts for lower extremity amputations typically have many coexisting diseases. Because of this, preop considerations may include
  - Respiratory: COPD
  - Cardiovascular: HTN, CAD, PVD (30% of pts)

- Preop beta blockers should be started in pts w/ coronary artery disease
➤ Metabolic: diabetes (70% of pts)
➤ Neurologic: sequelae of vascular disease: neuropathies, CVA, TIA
➤ Renal: renal insufficiency may be present secondary to vascular disease
➤ Hematologic: pts may be anemic or hypovolemic preop due to chronic disease
➤ ID – pt may have chronic infection/osteomyelitis. May also present as critically ill pt w/ sepsis related to lower extremity gangrene.
■ Aspirin or anticoagulants may need to be stopped preop.

Physical Findings
■ May include
➤ Cardiac: distant heart sounds, elevated jugular venous pressure, S3, S4
➤ Respiratory: rales
➤ Extremities: infection, ulcers, neuropathy; extremities may be cold, pulseless, or painful

Workup
■ Will depend on coexisting disease.
■ In general, check electrolytes, blood glucose, BUN, Cr, PT, PTT, CBC.
■ ECG.
■ CXR.
➤ Consider for pts w/ significant pulmonary disease or recent CHF.

Choice of Anesthesia
■ General or regional anesthesia may be used; however, regional procedures may reduce the incidence of phantom limb pain, particularly if continued postop.
■ Lumbar epidural or spinal anesthetic should cover to T12 level.
■ If considering regional block, assess ability to lie flat w/o respiratory distress.

INTRAOP

Monitors/Line Placement
■ Standard monitors
■ At least one IV of 18 g or larger

- Foley catheter
- Other monitors as indicated by pt condition

Intraop Concerns
- Careful positioning & padding are needed to prevent ischemic pressure ulcers.
- Tourniquet may be used to reduce blood loss.
  - ➤ Deflation can lead to embolization of thrombus that may have formed in the leg & possible PE.
- Blood loss not usually excessive, but transfusion may be necessary, especially in anemic pts.
- Operative time will depend on type of surgery. In critically ill pt w/ sepsis, surgeon may perform "guillotine" amputation with surgical time <30 min.

Intraop Therapies
- Glucose mgt in diabetic pts

POSTOP

Pain
- Moderate
- Pain can be managed acutely w/ IV narcotics, PCA or spinal narcotics.
- However, pts are at risk of developing phantom limb pain; continuous regional anesthesia or analgesia postop may reduce the probability of this occurrence.

Complications
- Anemia or hemorrhage
- Phantom limb pain
- Deep venous thrombosis
- Myocardial infarction
- CVA
- Wound infection
- Depression

SURGICAL PROCEDURE

Indications
- Peripheral vascular disease, diabetes, gangrene, trauma, tumor.

Procedure
- Above-the-knee amputation
  - ➤ Starts at distal third of femur.

➤ A stump is often made from suturing the anterior and posterior muscle groups together.

➤ Multiple debridements may be necessary in an infected or dirty wound before a stump can be made.

■ Below-the-knee amputation

➤ May be performed at different levels on the lower leg due to the health of the underlying tissue that will be used to form the flap.

➤ After the muscular & neurovascular tissues are ligated, the bones may be cut.

➤ The posterior tissues are more likely to form the bulk of the flap.

➤ A drain is often left & a compression dressing is placed.

➤ Before closing the wound, a determination will need to be made if it is contaminated & in need of debridements before stump closure.

Surgical Concerns

■ Bleeding, wound infection, wound breakdown.

Typical EBL

■ 200–250 mL

ANORECTAL SURGERY

JASON WIDRICH, MD

PREOP

Preop Considerations

■ Performed for a variety of conditions: hemorrhoids, prolapse, fecal incontinence, fistulas, condyloma

■ Pt may require bowel prep prior to surgery, which may alter electrolyte balance.

■ Pt may have severe pain that limits ability to sit. Positioning for start of procedure may require significant analgesic premed.

Physical Findings

■ None typical

Workup

■ Consider electrolytes if bowel prep performed.

■ Other tests as needed based on history & physical.

Choice of Anesthesia
- Premed for pain may be needed prior to positioning.
- Procedure may be performed w/ general anesthesia, spinal or epidural anesthesia or MAC.
  - ➤ Surgeon may supplement the anesthetic w/ local block of the pudendal nerves.

INTRAOP

Monitors/Line Placement
- Standard monitors.
- One peripheral IV usually adequate.

Intraop Concerns
- Positioning issues
  - ➤ Lithotomy position can cause peroneal nerve damage.
  - ➤ Prone jack-knife position may create difficulty w/ ventilation.
    - Airway mgt may be difficult if pt in prone position develops respiratory depression or apnea.
- Highest levels of stimulation include
  - ➤ Injection of local anesthetic.
  - ➤ Instrumentation of sphincter.
  - ➤ Anoscope insertion & probing of anal fissures.

Intraop Therapies
- For pt undergoing anorectal surgery under MAC in the prone position.
  - ➤ Carefully titrate analgesic agents to avoid respiratory depression, given potential difficulties w/ airway mgt while prone.
  - ➤ Ketamine may provide analgesia w/ reduced risk of respiratory depression compared to opioids. May supplement w/ midazolam or propofol to prevent dysphoric reaction.

POSTOP

Pain
- Mild to moderate, depending on procedure
- In PACU, IV narcotics may be necessary
- PO analgesics required if pt discharged home on day of surgery
- Consider PCA or neuraxial opioid if pt has severe pain & will be admitted to the hospital overnight
- Sitz baths & stool softeners often prescribed to prevent pain or breakdown of surgical repair

Complications
- Urinary retention
- Nerve damage from positioning or compression

SURGICAL PROCEDURE

Indications
- Rectal prolapse, fecal incontinence, hemorrhoids, condyloma, various other indications.

Procedure
- Depends on reason for surgery
  - For hemorrhoids, an anoscope is inserted & hemorrhoids are either ligated via rubber band or resected surgically.
  - Anal fissures/fistulas are explored & drained & either closed or resected.
  - Fecal incontinence is treated by removing weak or fibrotic tissue in a longitudinal section from the anus. The remaining tissues are sutured together to recreate an intact sphincter mechanism.
  - Care must be taken to identify & avoid the internal hemorrhoidal nerves.

Surgical Concerns
- Prevention of infection
- Constipation
- Stricture
- Urinary incontinence

Typical EBL
- Minimal (<100 mL)

ANTERIOR CERVICAL DISKECTOMY

EDWIN CHENG, MD

PREOP

Preop Considerations
- Usual diagnosis is herniation or degeneration of cervical disk causing spinal nerve root compression.

- Symptoms include neck pain, often radiating down one arm. Pt may progressively develop weakness & atrophy of arm muscle groups.
- For pain control, pt may be taking aspirin, NSAIDs, or opioid-containing analgesic.

Physical Findings

- Limited neck flexion, extension or rotation. Determine the extent of neck movement pt can tolerate w/o eliciting pain or other neurologic symptoms.
- Airway exam.
- Document preop sensory & motor deficits.
- Stop any antiplatelet agents at least 1 week prior to surgery.

Workup

- CBC.
- Pt usually has had MRI of spine.
- Other tests as indicated by coexisting disease.

Choice of Anesthesia

- General endotracheal anesthesia.

INTRAOP

Monitors/Line Placement

- Standard monitoring
- Consider arterial line if NIBP monitoring unreliable due to body habitus or positioning.
- Specialized neuromonitoring may be used.
  - ➤ If monitoring somatosensory evoked potentials (SSEP), use <0.5 MAC volatile anesthetic, no nitrous oxide.
    - Supplement the anesthetic w/ propofol, narcotics & muscle relaxation.

Intraop Concerns

- Potential difficult airway mgt
  - ➤ For pts w/ neck instability or limited neck extension, consider awake fiberoptic intubation.
  - ➤ Secure ETT well, since access to the airway is hindered by drapes & incision site.
- Pt position is supine w/ shoulder roll & neck extension.

- Autologous bone grafts may be removed from iliac crest, requiring additional analgesia.
- After retraction of carotid artery, surgeon may request palpation of temporal artery pulse to ensure adequate perfusion.
- On emergence from GA, leave ETT in place until pt is awake & has satisfactory respiratory pattern.
- Prior to extubation, evaluate for upper airway edema.
  - Examine neck & trachea.
  - Consider performing a leak test by deflating the ETT cuff & allowing pt to breathe around the ETT.

Intraop Therapies
- To minimize coughing on emergence, consider IV or tracheal lidocaine, or IV narcotics.

POSTOP

Pain
- Minimal to moderate in immediate postop period
- IV narcotic administration provides satisfactory analgesia.

Complications
- Airway obstruction
  - See also Critical Event chapter "Airway Obstruction."
  - Differential diagnosis includes neck hematoma, soft tissue swelling, airway edema, superior laryngeal nerve damage.
  - Notify surgeon & OR staff immediately.
  - Neck hematoma treated by opening the wound & removing blood & clot prior to attempting tracheal intubation.
  - Tracheal intubation & surgical airway may be difficult due to tracheal deviation & soft tissue swelling.
- Pneumothorax
  - See also Critical Event chapter "Pneumothorax."
  - May occur due to entrainment of air through the surgical wound; may manifest as dyspnea & respiratory insufficiency.
  - Simple pneumothorax may evolve into hemodynamically significant tension pneumothorax.
  - Check CXR if pt is hemodynamically stable.
  - If pt is unstable, insert 20g needle anteriorly at second intercostal space on the side of the pneumothorax.
- Other causes of postop respiratory distress include phrenic nerve dysfunction related to surgery.

SURGICAL PROCEDURE

Indications
- Cervical radiculopathy, myelopathy, instability, disk disease

Procedure
- Anterolateral neck incision
- Dissection between carotid sheath & esophagus
- Curettage & removal of disk & other bony elements causing root or cord compression
- Fusion of neck may be performed using bone graft (autologous or bone bank) & additional hardware may be placed to ensure neck stability

Surgical Concerns
- Massive bleeding due to carotid or jugular injury
- Neurologic injury to peripheral nerves, spinal nerves, spinal cord
- Esophageal perforation

Typical EBL
- W/o fusion, 50–200 cc
- W/ fusion, 200–500 cc

AORTIC VALVE REPLACEMENT

LUNDY CAMPBELL, MD

PREOP

Preop Considerations
- Pts undergoing aortic valve replacement usually have aortic stenosis (AS), aortic insufficiency, or both.
- Aortic stenosis creates a fixed obstruction to outflow. These pts are extremely sensitive to increases in heart rate & decreases in afterload & preload.
- Pts w/ critical AS have angina, CHF, or syncope related to the valve lesion. Such pts have a poor survival rate w/o aortic valve replacement.
- Respiratory compromise may occur secondary to LV failure & pleural effusion.
- Both AS & aortic insufficiency (AI) lesions may predispose pt to CHF, hepatic congestion, syncope & renal failure.
- See also Coexisting Disease chapters "Aortic Stenosis," "Aortic Insufficiency."

Physical Findings

- AS: Systolic ejection murmur at second right interspace w/ radiation to great vessels. Second heart sound may be decreased. Decreased carotid upstroke on palpation.
- AI: Pandiastolic murmur over left sternum to lower left sternal border. Pulse pressure may be wide.

Workup

- ECG.
- Echocardiogram to evaluate valve lesions & ventricular function.
- Coronary angiography: pt may need this to rule out coexisting coronary disease. If significant stenosis found, pt may also require CABG surgery.
- CBC.
- Liver function tests.
- PT, PTT, electrolytes, BUN, Cr.

Choice of Anesthesia

- GA w/ cardiopulmonary bypass.
  - ➤ Many techniques acceptable, as long as careful attention is paid to maintenance of blood pressure & SVR & avoidance of tachycardia. This is especially important during induction.
- Consider use of intrathecal narcotic for postop analgesia.

INTRAOP

Monitors/Line Placement

- Standard ASA monitors
- Foley catheter
- Arterial line
- Central line w/ CVP monitoring
- TEE
- Pulmonary artery catheter may be useful. Will depend on pt's LV function as well as local practice of surgeon & anesthesia provider

Intraop Concerns

- Induction of anesthesia
  - ➤ Pts w/ AS require maintenance of afterload & preload & a stable, moderately slow heart rate to maintain an adequate cardiac output.
    - Most anesthetic agents will decrease SVR.
    - Pt w/ critical AS has relatively fixed stroke volume & will not have appropriate compensation.

- Tachycardia will increase myocardial oxygen demand & reduce LV filling period.
- Combination of hypotension & tachycardia can produce severe myocardial ischemia.

➤ Pts w/ AI require adequate filling pressures, fast heart rate & low SVR to maintain adequate cardiac output.

■ Ensure baseline ACT is drawn ASAP.
■ Maintenance of anesthesia includes attention to
  ➤ Adequate muscle relaxation.
  ➤ Adequate level of anesthesia, which may include:
    - Narcotic
    - Volatile agent
    - Benzodiazepines to ensure adequate amnesia
■ Consider administration of hemostatic agent to decrease blood loss. This is controversial & will vary by surgeon & practice setting.
■ Ensure heparin is given prior to starting cardiopulmonary bypass & ACT is >400.
■ During bypass: Ensure perfusionist maintains adequate MAP & amnestic agent (volatile agent or benzodiazepine).
■ Weaning from bypass
  ➤ AS pts may require high filling pressures due to the hypertrophied noncompliant ventricle.
  ➤ AS/AI pts may require inotropic support.
  ➤ Monitor closely for signs of ischemia.
  ➤ Temporary pacing or mechanical support may be required.
    - Pts are at risk of heart block.
    - Atrial "kick" is important to maintaining cardiac output after valve replacement.
■ Hemostatic issues
  ➤ Ensure heparin completely reversed w/ protamine.
  ➤ Treat any remaining coagulopathy aggressively. Platelets that have circulated through the pump are usually dysfunctional, so platelets & any prebypass blood removed should be given back to pt.
■ Emergence: Transport intubated pt w/ full monitors & any inotropic agents to ICU.

Intraop Therapies
■ To maintain adequate SVR/MAP in pts w/ AS prior to valve repair: phenylephrine.
■ Hemostatic agents: aminocaproic acid, aprotinin.

- Post-bypass inotropic agents may include dopamine, epinephrine, dobutamine, amrinone, milrinone.

POSTOP

Pain
- Moderate
- Parenteral opioids or intrathecal narcotics usually required.
- Intubated pt may receive propofol or benzodiazepines for sedation.

Complications
- Hemorrhage: may require reoperation if severe or persistent.
- Tamponade: may require emergent bedside drainage.
- Cardiac failure: may require left ventricular assist devices or intra-aortic balloon pumps to assist a failing left ventricle.
- Arrhythmias relatively common, especially atrial fibrillation. Some pts receive prophylactic antiarrhythmics (eg, amiodarone).
- Heart block: temporary pacer wires usually placed at time of surgery.
- Ischemia/myocardial infarction: avoid ventricular overload, consider perioperative beta blockade if possible.

SURGICAL PROCEDURE

Indications
- Typical indications include critical or symptomatic AS, severe AI, or evidence of worsening CHF w/ end-organ involvement.

Procedure
- Involves median sternotomy, cannula placement, cardioplegia w/ cooling, cardiopulmonary bypass, sewing in of prosthetic valve, weaning from bypass, removal of cannula, closure

Surgical Concerns
- Risk of air embolization requires adequate venting of heart & changing patient position during refilling of heart.
- Perivalvular leaks may occur after valve is placed. TEE helps monitor this.
- Weaning from bypass is a critical time. Pt may require placement of intra-aortic balloon pump or return to bypass.

Typical EBL
- Not usually estimated for cardiopulmonary bypass cases.

APPENDECTOMY

JONATHAN CHOW, MD

PREOP

Preop Considerations
- Pt may have hypovolemia from fever, vomiting, anorexia.
- Pt may have delayed gastric emptying.
- If appendix has ruptured, pt may develop abdominal sepsis, especially if diagnosis is delayed.

Workup
- CBC, physical exam
  - Surgeon may obtain an ultrasound and/or CT scan as part of evaluation.

Choice of Anesthesia
- General anesthesia is customary, although epidural & spinal anesthesia can be used.
  - If general anesthesia is used, a rapid sequence intubation is indicated.

INTRAOP

Monitors/Line Placement
- Standard monitors unless pt status indicates more invasive monitoring.

Intraop Concerns
- Full stomach precautions: rapid sequence IV induction.
  - Consider placement of NG or OG tube to decompress stomach & remove oral contrast if used in radiographic studies, or if prolonged ileus likely.
  - Pt will probably need preop hydration because hypovolemia is often present.

POSTOP

Pain
- Moderate; consider PCA

Complications
- Sepsis
- Paralytic ileus

SURGICAL PROCEDURE

Indications
■ Appendicitis

Procedure
■ Pt is supine. Appendix is removed via a small right lower quadrant incision.
■ Can also be performed via laparoscopic approach. For anesthetic considerations, see Procedures chapter "Laparoscopic General Surgery."

Typical EBL
■ <75 mL

BLALOCK TAUSSIG SHUNT (BTS)

KIM SKIDMORE, MD

PREOP

Preop Considerations
■ Modern modified BTS consists of a Gore-Tex tube graft connecting the right subclavian artery to the pulmonary artery.
■ BTS is useful for congenital heart disease w/ poor pulmonary blood flow. Common diseases requiring BTS:
  ➢ Tetralogy of Fallot
  ➢ Pulmonary atresia
  ➢ Pulmonic stenosis
■ Diseases for which BTS may be part of surgical staging or palliation
  ➢ Hypoplastic left heart, Norwood stage I
■ Procedure is usually performed <6 months of age.

Workup
■ CXR
■ EKG
■ Echo
■ Cardiac cath if indicated

Choice of Anesthesia
■ Premed
  ➢ If >12 months of age, consider midazolam 0.5–1 mg/kg PO, not to exceed 20 mg.

➤ If pt refuses oral premed, consider ketamine 4 mg/kg IM or morphine 0.2 mg/kg IM.
■ General endotracheal anesthesia is induced by either inhaled or IV route.

INTRAOP

Monitors/Line Placement
■ Two peripheral IVs usually adequate.
■ Arterial line.
➤ Avoid right radial arterial line because of clamps & shunts involved in BTS procedure.
■ ACT to manage heparin dosing.
■ TEE not always done because site of surgery cannot be seen.
➤ TEE may be useful for confirming diagnosis, monitoring ventricular function, or monitoring for intracardiac air.

Intraop Concerns
■ To optimize PVR, must maintain key metabolic parameters. For pts w/ profound hypoxemia, monitor arterial blood gas approx every 20–30 min.
➤ pH: Diagnose & treat acidosis.
➤ Hct: If pt has hypoxemia & shunting, transfuse to keep Hct > 40.
➤ $PaCO_2$ & PaO_2: Maintain w/in normal limits to optimize pulmonary vascular resistance.
■ Maintain FiO_2 at 0.21 to simulate normal life & to allow the correct choice of shunt size.
■ For redo operation, anticipate higher blood loss.
■ On transport to ICU, continue ventilation via ETT on room air.

POSTOP

Pain
■ Moderate
■ Pts usually remain intubated immediately postop & receive IV opiates
■ Complications
■ Potential clotting of shunt, w/ hypoxemia
■ Sometimes prophylactically treated w/ rectal aspirin & IV heparin to keep ACT >200

SURGICAL PROCEDURE

Indications
■ BTS may be useful for congenital heart disease w/ reduced pulmonary blood flow.

Procedure
- BTS is creation of an aortic to pulmonary window; first performed in 1945 for tetralogy of Fallot.
- Modern modified BTS consists of one end of a Gore-Tex tube graft connecting to the side of the right subclavian artery w/ the other end connecting to the pulmonary artery.
  - ➤ Size of shunt in infants typically 2.5, 3.0, 3.5, or 4.0 mm ID.
- Performed via median sternotomy or right thoracotomy, depending on pt stability & potential need for cardiopulmonary bypass.
- For most BTS, perfusionists are on standby.

Surgical Concerns
- Shunt can thrombose & cause hypoxemia.
- Shunt size could be too large & cause systemic hypoperfusion, acidosis, hypotension.

Typical EBL
- Usually not excessive, but blood transfusion usually required.

BOWEL RESECTION

JAMES MITCHELL, MBBS

PREOP

Preop Considerations
- Two major pt groups
  - ➤ Young pts w/ inflammatory bowel disease (IBD)
  - ➤ Older pts for cancer resections
- Pts w/ IBD are typically
  - ➤ Slim
  - ➤ Otherwise well
  - ➤ May be on long-term corticosteroids & opioids
- Cancer pts may have
  - ➤ Anemia
  - ➤ Hypercoagulability
  - ➤ Hepatic dysfunction from metastases
  - ➤ Electrolyte disturbance from secretory adenocarcinomas
- Other pts may include critically ill pt (usually elderly) w/ bowel ischemia and/or perforation
- Bowel prep may cause dehydration, electrolyte disturbance

Physical Findings
- Signs of bowel obstruction if present

Workup
- Preop investigations as indicated: hematology, electrolytes, liver function, coags
- Investigation of usual comorbidities in elderly pts
- Cross-match blood

Choice of Anesthesia
- General anesthesia
  - ➤ Rapid sequence induction indicated in pts w/ GI obstruction
- Additional epidural anesthesia & postop analgesia supported by literature: less opioid use, faster wakeup, earlier return of bowel function, diminished inflammatory response, protection against DVT, better respiratory function
  - ➤ Contraindicated in pts w/ sepsis or coagulopathy
  - ➤ Consider testing for coagulopathy prior to placing epidural catheter

INTRAOP

Monitors/Line Placement
- Bowel resection has potential for substantial bleeding & third-space loss of fluids. This dictates choice of monitors & lines.
- Large IVs, arterial line, central line are often indicated, depending on the extent of resection & anticipated surgical difficulty.
- Otherwise standard monitors appropriate.
- Surgeon will commonly request nasogastric tube.

Intraop Concerns
- Positioning, particularly if in lithotomy position for perineal approach
- Fluid shifts
- Heat loss
- Usual concerns w/ stress of surgery in older pts

Intraop Therapies
- Fluid mgt guided by CVP, urine output, observed blood loss, duration of surgery. Fluid balance often positive several liters on paper.
- Active warming of upper body (& legs if possible).

POSTOP

Pain
- Moderate to severe
- Typical mgt options include PCA, epidural.

➤ Epidural dilute local anesthetic plus fentanyl by infusion usually provides good analgesia.

Complications
- Anastomotic leak may require reoperation. This may also cause sepsis.
- Respiratory, cardiac, or renal complications are more common in the elderly.
  - ➤ Pts usually benefit from postop respiratory care (eg, incentive spirometry).

SURGICAL PROCEDURE

Indications
- Bowel cancer
- IBD refractory to medical mgt
- Nonmalignant disease causing obstruction
- Ischemic or nonviable bowel

Procedure
- Laparotomy w/ resection of affected bowel & its mesentery.
- If anal canal or rectum is to be resected, perineal approach is often required as well.
- Primary anastomosis commonly performed. Two- or three-stage procedures w/ temporary or permanent stomas are sometimes required.

Surgical Concerns
- Dissection in pelvis for low anterior resections may be difficult.

Typical EBL
- Highly variable

BREAST RECONSTRUCTION

JASON WIDRICH, MD

PREOP

Preop Considerations
- Often performed in conjunction w/ or after a mastectomy
- See also Procedures chapter "Mastectomy."
- Pt w/ metastatic breast cancer may have multiple manifestations.
  - ➤ Respiratory: lung mets or effects of previous radiation therapy to the chest, including pleural effusion or obstructive pneumonia

➤ Cardiovascular: cardiotoxicity from previous chemotherapy (eg, doxorubicin)
➤ Neurologic: mental status change from brain mets, major depression after mastectomy, weakness from spinal cord metastasis
➤ Hematologic: anemia secondary to chronic disease or drug toxicity
➤ Musculoskeletal: bone mets may be present

Physical Findings
■ May have palpable breast mass or nipple discharge, if premastectomy

Workup
■ CBC
■ Consider type & screen
■ Further workup determined by coexisting diseases
■ Pt may have workup for metastatic disease prior to procedure

Choice of Anesthesia
■ GA required for breast reconstruction
➤ Extent of muscle or tissue dissection required for reconstruction will influence the choice of adjunctive regional anesthesia (eg, thoracic epidural or intercostal blocks).
■ If TRAM or abdominal flap breast reconstruction is planned, a thoracic epidural may be useful for postop pain control.

INTRAOP

Monitors/Line Placement
■ Standard monitors
■ One or two peripheral IVs
■ Foley catheter
■ ECG pads need to be positioned away from surgical field

Intraop Concerns
■ Arms are usually "out" (abducted). They must be positioned & padded carefully because the surgeon may want to evaluate the appearance of the reconstruction w/ pt in sitting position.
■ Do not place monitors or IVs on the side on which the mastectomy was performed.
■ Because of the proximity of the airway to the surgical field, consider whether an ETT rather than an LMA should be used to secure the airway.
■ Normally low blood loss, but transfusions may be necessary in anemic pt or if loss is larger than usual.

Intraop Therapies

- Surgeons may request that pt is placed in seated position at various times during the case to assess cosmetic appearance of reconstruction.
  - ➤ A safety belt at the hip level & placement of the foot of the bed in a slightly upward position will prevent sliding of pt.
  - ➤ In addition, the arms may be secured to arm boards extended laterally to prevent pt from sliding when placed in the seated position.
  - ➤ This will likely require extensions of the ventilator circuit.
- At the conclusion of surgery, a compressive dressing may be placed around the entire chest/torso. This is done with the least difficulty w/ pt in the seated position.
- Third-space fluid loss: usually 4–6 mL/kg/h
- Prophylactic antiemetics should be administered.

POSTOP

Pain

- Moderate
- IV narcotics or PCA
- Epidural, if used, should cover to T4–6 area for postop pain control

Complications

- Nausea/vomiting
- Pneumothorax
- Pt may have a compressive dressing around the chest & torso that may limit ability to perform deep breathing
- Impaired cough related to use of an abdominal flap

SURGICAL PROCEDURE

Indications

- Status post mastectomy

Procedure

- Reconstruction is accomplished with a prosthetic implant or a rotational flap.
- Reconstruction can be performed at the same time as a radical mastectomy or at a later period after resection.

Surgical Concerns

- Lymphedema, nerve damage, wound infection, hematoma, ischemia or necrosis of flap, imperfection of cosmetic repair.

Typical EBL

- 150–500 mL

BRONCHOSCOPY

ALISON G. CAMERON, MD

PREOP

Preop Considerations

- For visualization of bronchi & upper airway for diagnostic or therapeutic interventions.
- Pts can vary from healthy to those w/ severe airway obstruction.
- Tobacco use is frequent in this pt population, w/ associated COPD, pulmonary infiltrates.
- Many pts also have cardiovascular disease.
- If lung cancer, may have Eaton-Lambert (myasthenic) syndrome, which can result in increased sensitivity to nondepolarizing neuromuscular blockers.

Physical Findings

- Findings depend on pt disease. Possible findings include
  - ➤ Dyspnea, which may be positional (eg, w/ a large tumor impinging on the airway)
  - ➤ Wheezing
  - ➤ Stridor
  - ➤ Hemoptysis

Workup

- Dental assessment
- Careful airway assessment
- Depending on symptoms & comorbid conditions
  - ➤ CBC, platelets
  - ➤ ABG
  - ➤ PFTs
  - ➤ ECG
  - ➤ CXR

Choice of Anesthesia

- Antisialogogue (glycopyrrolate 0.2 mg IV)
- Avoid heavy premeds that may impair respiratory status postop.
- Three types of scopes can be used: flexible fiberoptic, rigid-ventilating, rigid-Venturi (Sanders injector) type.
- Flexible fiberoptic scope
  - ➤ MAC w/ sedation can be used w/ flexible fiberoptic scope, if pt is not likely to develop respiratory distress postop.

- ➤ Topical anesthesia can also be used w/o involvement of anesthesia provider.
- ➤ Flexible scope allows use of regular ETT (8.0 or larger; if smaller size is used, should use pediatric scope) & ventilation of both lungs during the procedure. High flows must be used, however, due to the large leak around the scope.
- ■ Rigid bronchoscopy
  - ➤ General anesthesia is required for rigid scope & requires better pt relaxation due to higher risk of tracheal tear or pneumothorax.
  - ➤ This is often done in concert w/ mediastinoscopy or thoracotomy.
  - ➤ Ventilator circuit will attach to side port of rigid scope if jet ventilation is not used.
- ■ Sanders injector-Venturi ventilation w/ a rigid scope
  - ➤ Depending on circuit available, use either oxygen flush valve or hand trigger to ventilate.
  - ➤ Oxygen at 3–5 PSI is delivered via 16g or 18g needle inside & parallel to the length of the rigid scope, or attached to side arm of scope.
  - ➤ Keep inspiratory time to 1–2 sec.
  - ➤ Watch chest rise to assess for adequate amount of ventilation.
  - ➤ Ensure chest deflates prior to initiating next inspiration.
  - ➤ The burst of oxygen entrains room air into the pt's airway.

Airway nerve blocks prior to induction may help keep hemodynamics stable, since BP swings are likely due to periods of little stimulation interspersed w/ those of significant stimulation.

INTRAOP

Monitors/Line Placement
- ■ Standard ASA monitors
- ■ One peripheral IV
- ■ Arterial line usually not necessary
- ■ Tooth guards, eye protection

Intraop Concerns
- ■ Shoulder roll often placed to improve head position.
- ■ Pt is supine w/ neck extended at upper cervical level & head elevated, so be careful w/ the cervical spine, particularly if there is a question of cervical spine stability or C-spine symptoms.
- ■ Inadequate ventilation
  - ➤ Prolonged jet ventilation (>1 hour) may be required if an airway tumor is treated w/ laser.

- Dysrhythmias possible secondary to elevated PCO_2 due to inadequate ventilation (CO_2 will rise at rate of 3 mm Hg/min during apneic oxygenation).
- Tracheobronchial injury
- Debris aspiration
- $ETCO_2$ reading will not be accurate if ventilating via rigid scope side port due to dilution of entrained air.

Intraop Therapies

- Complete muscle relaxation for rigid scope (either succinylcholine infusion or short-acting nondepolarizing muscle relaxant)
  - ➣ Monitor train of four closely w/ nerve stimulator.
- IV anesthesia is useful for cases w/ interruption of ventilation.
- Hyperventilate w/ rigid scope to prepare for times of apnea.
- Frequent suctioning may be necessary, but this may decrease the FIO_2 & therefore drop the PaO_2.
- Prepare for rapid recovery as procedure may end abruptly.
- If rigid scope used, intubate pt w/ ETT at end of procedure & wait to extubate pt until fully awake.

POSTOP

Pain

- Minimal to mild
- Acetaminophen, NSAID, or parenteral opioids usually adequate
- Avoid allowing pt to eat or drink for several hours postop until airway block resolved (if used).

Complications

- Airway edema (may necessitate administration of steroids)
- Airway obstruction
- Tracheal tear
- Barotrauma
- Dental damage
- Aspiration
- Pneumothorax
- Pneumomediastinum
- Hemothorax
- Airway fire (if laser used)

SURGICAL PROCEDURE

Indications

- Multiple. Partial list includes
  - ➣ Cough, wheeze, atelectasis

➤ Preop evaluation
➤ Unresolved pneumonia
➤ Carcinoma of lung (primary or metastatic)
➤ Benign tumor
➤ Hemoptysis
➤ Obstruction
➤ Lung abscess
➤ Removal of foreign bodies (spontaneous ventilation is best for this to not move object further into airway)
➤ Diagnostic/therapeutic visualization/biopsies of tumors
➤ Tracheoesophageal fistula

Procedure
■ Surgeon stands at head of bed. Depending on type of scope, anesthesia provider will vary intubation/airway plan.
■ W/ flexible scope, scope is passed through large ETT (8.0 or larger preferred) w/ special adapter that attaches to top of ETT that can be closed when scope is pulled out to prevent w/air leak.
■ W/ rigid bronchoscopy, scope is inserted via right side of mouth until epiglottis is visualized, & then advanced into the upper airway. If foreign body is to be removed, forceps will be passed through the scope. Biopsies may be taken. Ventilation is performed via rigid-Venturi jet or special adaptor (Racine).
■ Laser bronchoscopy may also be performed via rigid scope.

Surgical Concerns
■ Inadequate muscle relaxation resulting in inability to adequately open mouth for scope placement
■ C-spine instability limiting neck extension
■ Aspiration

Typical EBL
■ Minimal

CABG WITH CARDIOPULMONARY BYPASS (CPB)

ERIC BROUCH, MD
MARTIN J. LONDON, MD

PREOP

Preop Considerations
■ Premedication

➤ Order all antianginals & antihypertensives to be given prior to surgery.
➤ Provide adequate anxiolysis & analgesia using premeds to minimize ischemia on arrival to OR.
  • Outpts: consider oral diazepam 5–10 mg PO w/ IV midazolam (1–2 mg) and/or low-dose fentanyl.
  • Inpts: consider IM morphine 0.1–0.15 mg/kg w/ lorazepam 1–2 mg IM on call to OR.
➤ Order supplemental oxygen w/ premedication. Avoid oversedation in the elderly.
■ For unstable angina pt on IV heparin, discuss d/c orders w/ surgeon.
  ➤ Can usually stop heparin 4 h preop in pts w/o chest pain or left main disease.
■ Prophylactic antibiotics: cefazolin 1 g or vancomycin 1 g most common

Physical Findings
■ Airway exam & ID of difficult airway crucial to avoid hypoxemia, hypercarbia, catecholamine release, which may cause ischemia.
  ➤ Consider awake fiberoptic intubation in high-risk pt, using esmolol, remifentanil, or other short-acting agents to control hemodynamics.
■ Evaluate pt's daily range of BP & HR & maintain intraop values w/in 20% to minimize cardiac, cerebral, or renal ischemia.
■ Evaluate for CHF.
■ Evaluate for occlusive carotid disease.

Workup
■ Evaluation includes
  ➤ Cardiac catheterization
  ➤ Echocardiogram
  ➤ CXR
  ➤ Carotid duplex ultrasound
  ➤ Pulmonary function tests
■ Need to ascertain
  ➤ Number of diseased vessels
  ➤ Presence of significant left main disease
  ➤ Status of collateral circulation
  ➤ Ejection fraction
■ Look for
  ➤ Concurrent valvular disease, particularly ischemic mitral regurgitation (may require annuloplasty).

> Aortic stenosis (because of propensity for subendocardial ischemia).
> Aortic insufficiency (because anterograde cardioplegia via the aortic root may distend the ventricle).

Choice of Anesthesia

- GA w/ controlled ventilation is required.
  > Use any combination of opioid (eg, fentanyl, sufentanil, remifentanil), volatile agent (eg, isoflurane, sevoflurane, desflurane) & IV adjuvant (midazolam, propofol) as long as hemodynamics are carefully managed.
  > Typical regimen: fentanyl (10–20 mcg/kg), midazolam (0.05–0.10 mg/kg) and/or propofol infusion w/ volatile agent supplementation.
  > Avoid nitrous, given risk of hypoxemia & potential hazards of coronary or cerebral air embolus.
- Most centers practice "fast tracking": pt is extubated as soon after surgery as he/she meets criteria (responsive, intact neuro status, stable hemodynamics & cardiac rhythm, normothermic, minimal bleeding).
- Avoid tachycardia, which is the key factor precipitating pre-CPB ischemia.
- Regional used in some pts, esp thoracotomy incision.
  > A single-shot spinal (morphine 0.01 mg/kg) is most common, although thoracic epidurals are also used.
  > Place epidural the night before surgery because of bleeding concerns w/ anticoagulation for CPB.

INTRAOP

Monitors/Line Placement

- Place 14g or 16g IV radial arterial line prior to induction.
- Central access, usually via right internal jugular vein, is needed for all pts for pressure monitoring & IV heparin.
- PA catheter use depends on surgeon & center.
  > Availability & expertise w/ TEE, comorbidities & postop recovery facilities guide CVP vs PA catheter use.
  > Consider preinduction PA catheter in pts w/ poor ejection fraction and/or associated valvular disease.
- TEE can be helpful for evaluation of regional wall motion, global contractility, valvular lesions & aortic arch atheromatous disease.
  > Ensure the pt is well anesthetized prior to probe insertion.

➤ Decompress the stomach w/ an OG tube before & after TEE use.
- Activated clotting time measurement is required to manage heparin dosing & reversal.
- Measure core temp (bladder or rectal) & surrogate of cerebral temp (nasopharyngeal) to manage cooling & rewarming from CPB.
  ➤ Avoid increasing core to cerebral temp gradient (this is associated w/ jugular venous desaturation).

Intraop Concerns
- Perfusionist & cardiac surgeon should be available prior to induction.
  ➤ CPB machine should be primed in case rapid institution of CPB is required.
- During induction, avoid hemodynamic instability & maintain MAP & HR w/in 20% of baseline.
- Anesthetics
  ➤ Avoid thiopental in pts w/ impaired LV function.
  ➤ Use low-dose opioids, volatile anesthesia, and/or short-acting beta blockers (eg, esmolol) to blunt response to laryngoscopy & intubation.
  ➤ Consider early nondepolarizing muscle relaxant to offset muscle rigidity from opioids,& maintain throughout case.
    • Alternate strategy: "light" or no relaxation to monitor for light anesthesia
- After induction obtain baseline ACT & ABG, cardiac output if a PA catheter is being used & TEE basic exam.
- Antifibrinolytics are commonly used (epsilon-aminocaproic acid, tranexamic acid), esp in pts undergoing repeat sternotomy (see Procedure chapter "Redo CABG") or those who refuse blood products.
  ➤ Most common regimens: single IV bolus of aminocaproic acid 5 g administered w/ heparin & after protamine, or by constant infusion prior to sternotomy
- Consider prebypass phlebotomy in pt w/ adequate Hct to prevent platelet degranulation during CPB.
  ➤ Sequester blood gradually during IMA harvesting via the central line, or have perfusionist drain via venous cannula just prior to CPB.
- Saphenous vein & radial artery harvest may begin prior to sternotomy.
- Sternotomy is highly stimulating & requires adequate anesthesia to avoid hemodynamic changes.
  ➤ Important: deflate the lungs immediately prior to sternotomy.

- After sternotomy, the left IMA is usually harvested, the pericardium is opened & the heart & aortic arch are exposed.
- Prior to aortic cannulation
  - Heparin (300–400 U/kg) is administered.
  - An ACT of 450–500 sec is required prior to initiation of CPB.
  - Heparin resistance, usually due to prolonged preop heparin use w/ depletion of antithrombin III substrate, can occur.
    - Treat heparin resistance w/ 1 unit FFP or recombinant anti-thrombin III if available.
- Cannulation
  - Surgeon places aortic cannula first.
    - Perfusionist can use this to transfuse from the CPB machine prior to bypass if the pt is hypovolemic and hypotensive. (BP improvement is greater w/ infusion into the arterial resistance side of the circulation compared to the venous capacitance side.)
    - Keep systolic blood pressure <110 mmHg during cannulation to decrease chance of aortic dissection.
  - A venous cannula is placed into the IVC via the RA appendage.
  - A cannula is often placed in the coronary sinus through the RA for retrograde cardioplegia.
  - LV vent may be placed via the right superior pulm. vein to prevent LV distention during CPB.
- Prior to CPB, withdraw PA catheter 3–5 cm to avoid wedging. Can use TEE to visualize tip of PA catheter.
- After testing the venous & arterial cannulas, CPB is started.
  - Stop ventilation when full flow confirmed by perfusionist.
- Myocardial preservation during CPB
  - Exclude heart from circulation (aortic cross-clamping).
  - Arrest heart w/ high-potassium cardioplegia.
  - Induce regional hypothermia w/ cold cardioplegia.
  - Other strategies can be used.
- During CPB, assess adequacy of tissue perfusion by
  - Online arterial & venous oxygen saturation monitoring
  - Serial ABG/Hct determinations
  - Arterial blood pressure monitoring
    - Maintain MAP >50 mmHg (65 mmHg or greater in pt w/ CVD or renal insufficiency).
  - Urine output
- Monitor ACT & give additional heparin as needed.
- Keep HCT >20–22% w/ PRBCs.

- Considerations prior to weaning from bypass.
  - Rewarm.
  - Establish stable rhythm & rate.
  - Prepare for pacing.
  - Re-establish ventilation.
  - Optimize lab values (esp pH, hematocrit, potassium & calcium).
  - Plan for maintaining adequate cardiac output & systolic blood pressure.
    - Pre-CPB LV function & cross-clamp time are major determinants of need for inotropic support post-CPB.
    - Use PA catheter-derived CO & SVR & TEE LV function to guide therapy.
- Wean CPB gradually by occluding venous return to the pump, increasing preload, allow ventricle to eject & override the arterial flow. Then reduce pump flow & stop CPB.
- Then give 1-cc test dose of protamine & observe for hypotension, anaphylaxis, or PA hypertension.
  - Give standard protamine dose of 1–1.3 mg per 100 units of heparin over at least 5 min.
  - Confirm ACT returns to baseline & give additional protamine if needed.
  - Watch for rise in ACT if heparin-rich blood from the CPB circuit is reinfused.
- Notify surgeon when protamine is started.
  - Surgeon will d/c venous cannula & perfusionist will drain residual blood for reinfusion.
  - Can give blood to pt in 100-cc increments, guided by PA diastolic pressure and/or LV end-diastolic area on TEE transgastric short-axis view.
  - Use reverse Trendelenburg position to facilitate volume administration.
- Optimize fluid/blood therapy prior to ICU transfer.
  - Monitor invasive BP, HR, ECG & O_2 saturation during transport.
  - Bring meds to treat BP, HR, ischemia & arrhythmias.

Intraop Therapies

- Keep bolus vasopressors (phenylephrine, ephedrine & epinephrine) ready to treat hypotension due to vasodilation, hypovolemia, or impaired contractility.
  - Surgical manipulation of the heart causes hypotension but is transient.

➤ Closely watch the surgical field & communicate w/ surgeon about BP, HR changes.
■ Pacing
  ➤ Dual-channel pacemaker must be immediately available.
  ➤ Ischemia & impaired AV conduction due to potassium cardioplegia commonly cause AV block & bradycardia.
  ➤ Maintain HR at 80–90 bpm for several hours after CPB to avoid LV/RV distention.
■ Weaning from bypass
  ➤ Calcium chloride (1 g incrementally) commonly used
  ➤ May need infusion of catecholamines (dopamine, epinephrine, dobutamine) or phosphodiesterase inhibitors (amrinone, milrinone), esp if pt has impaired LV function.
  ➤ Use intra-aortic balloon counterpulsation when inotropic support alone is inadequate (systemic hypotension, cardiac index $<2.0\,L/min/m^2$, high filling pressures) to augment diastolic coronary perfusion & forward flow.
    • Aortic insufficiency is a relative contraindication to IABP.
    • Can use TEE to check position of IABP (must be placed below the level of the left subclavian & carotid vessels).

POSTOP

Pain
■ "Fast tracking" & early extubation should not preclude adequate pain control. Options:
  ➤ IV short-acting opioids (eg, low-dose IV morphine)
  ➤ IV NSAID (eg, ketorolac)
    • Avoid NSAIDs in pt w/ renal insufficiency.
■ CABG w/ IMA dissection is more painful than CABG w/ saphenous vein harvest alone.

Complications
■ HTN is a common problem, often unresponsive to sedation or narcotics.
  ➤ May need nitroprusside or nitroglycerin infusions or careful use of beta blockers (esmolol, metoprolol).
■ Bleeding is most common cause of return to OR. Manifestations:
  ➤ Continued output from chest tubes.
  ➤ Hypotension.
  ➤ Need for fluid & blood products.

➤ Cardiac tamponade may occur if excessive blood accumulates in mediastinum.

■ Coagulopathy is common.
➤ Usually from impaired platelet function. Platelet count usually drops by 50%.
➤ Coagulation factor dilution occurs but is rarely severe enough to cause bleeding.
➤ Hypothermia after CPB enhances bleeding Treat w/ forced air rewarming in the ICU.

■ Atrial fibrillation
➤ Occurs in 20–40% of pts, most commonly on POD 2–3.
➤ Can be associated w/ hypotension.
➤ A more serious complication is CVA due to thrombus & embolization.
➤ Useful therapy: diltiazem, amiodarone, procainamide, beta blockers and/or digoxin. Synchronized cardioversion may be required.

■ Low cardiac output syndrome
➤ Most common in pt w/ poor preop LV function and/or pt w/ inadequate myocardial preservation on CPB, or technically poor revascularization (eg, small distal targets, excessive calcification, intramyocardial vessels).
➤ IABP usually required for LV failure.
➤ RV failure is less common & more difficult to treat; may require insertion of a PA balloon (technically difficult).
➤ If CO remains low despite IABP, consider placement of ventricular assist device.

■ Stroke/neuropsychological changes
➤ Overt CVA may occur in 1–3% of pts but is most common in the elderly, diabetics, females, pt w/ prior CVA, pt w/ aortic arch atheroma and/or concurrent carotid disease.
➤ Subtle degrees of dysfunction & cognitive disturbances are common.

SURGICAL PROCEDURE

Indications
■ Typical indications include multivessel CAD or significant left main CAD.

Procedure
■ Involves sternotomy, dissection of grafts (saphenous veins, left or right internal mammary artery, radial artery or other arteries) w/

anastomoses to vessels distal to obstructing lesions after initiation of CPB & ischemic arrest.

Surgical Concerns
- Adequate conduits for performing multiple anastomoses.
- Adequate surgical exposure for cannulating the heart & aorta.
- Performing distal anastomoses on a nonbeating, well-protected heart is the primary reason for performing CABG on bypass. Long-term graft patency may be optimized using this approach. Other approaches: off-pump CABG.

Typical EBL
- Very variable & surgeon-specific.
- Exact EBL is difficult to quantitate & rarely done.
- 2–4 units of blood loss common.
- RBC transfusion threshold widely variable based on surgeon, center, & pt factors.

CARDIAC SURGERY RE-EXPLORATION

ART WALLACE, PHD, MD

PREOP

Preop Considerations
- Is the case an emergency take-back or a redo case? For redo see "Coronary Artery Bypass Graft Redo" chapter.
- For emergency cardiac re-exploration, move quickly to the OR to avoid cardiac arrest from tamponade. Obtain the following information:
  - ➤ Hemodynamic condition: Is it tamponade or stable? Even if stable, it may decompensate to tamponade rapidly.
  - ➤ Hct, platelet count, PT/PTT, use of antifibrinolytics. Most cardiac surgery re-explorations are for surgical bleeding that has led to medical bleeding. One can debate the primary problem, but both the surgical & the medical sources of bleeding must be treated.
  - ➤ Blood products: How many units of RBC, PLT, FFP are available? Is cross-matching difficult?
  - ➤ Availability of OR
  - ➤ IV access?
  - ➤ Monitoring: Is it adequate? Is it still working? Arterial line, ECG, pulse ox are essential.
  - ➤ Is pt still intubated?

Physical Findings
- Blood pressure, cardiac output, PAD, chest tube drainage rate

Workup
- Dictated by urgency of case.
- H&P: Read the last note & update. Check labs, CXR.
- Review intraop events (new wall motion abnormalities, what was the surgery, how easily was pt weaned from bypass? Was it off pump?)
- Know the lines (arterial line, IVs, endotracheal tube, PA catheter).
- Know what infusions the pt is on.
- Know when the next dose of prophylactic antibiotics is due.

Choice of Anesthesia
- If pt is intubated & sedated, must continue that regimen (eg, continue propofol infusion, fentanyl-midazolam).
- Add sufficient agent to guarantee amnesia (eg, midazolam, inhaled agent).
- Nondepolarizing muscle relaxants helpful.

INTRAOP

Monitors/Line Placement
- Most lines will already be in place from previous case. Arterial line, ECG, & big IV are essential.

Intraop Concerns
- Controlling hemodynamics despite surgical manipulation of the heart.
- Correcting coagulopathy.

Intraop Therapies
- Redose the prophylactic antibiotics.
- Send labs: ABG, electrolytes, Ca, Mg, HCT, PLT, PT/PTT, fibrinogen.
- Transfuse platelets, FFP, RBC, cryoprecipitate (rarely needed) as appropriate.

POSTOP
- Postop pain not a major issue.
- Continue sedation until oxygenation, ventilation, level of consciousness, hemodynamics, coagulopathy allow extubation.
- Complications
- Mediastinitis.
- ARDS.

- Pneumonia.
- Transfusion reactions/sequelae.

SURGICAL PROCEDURE

Indications
- Uncontrolled excessive hemorrhage despite normal coag status.
- Hemodynamic instability suggesting tamponade.

Procedure
- Open the sternotomy.
- Clear the clot.
- Check all operative sites: distal anastomosis, proximal anastomosis, cannulation & vent sites, internal mammary artery graft site, sternal wire sites.

Surgical Concerns
- Hemorrhage.
- Hemodynamic instability/arrest from tamponade.

Typical EBL
- Highly variable.

CARDIOVERSION

LUNDY CAMPBELL, MD
WILLIAM A. SHAPIRO, MD

PREOP

Preop Considerations
- Ventricular rate control.
- Duration of AF.
- Overall left ventricular function.
- Anticoagulation.
- Pt size.
- NPO status.

Physical Findings
- Evaluate HR, BP.
- Evaluate for evidence of rhythm intolerance such as altered mental status, syncope, pulmonary edema.
- If pt has altered mental status, pulmonary edema, or significant hypotension, immediate cardioversion is indicated.

■ Ventricular rate control can be achieved w/ IV beta-blocking or calcium channel-blocking agents if blood pressure is within normal limits.

Workup
■ Evaluate for cause of AF; obtain electrolytes, BUN, Cr; check acid/base status.
■ Correct any abnormality predefibrillation if possible.
■ Evaluate for cardiac causes such as acute MI & noncardiac causes such as thyroid disease.

Choice of Anesthesia
■ Ultra-short-acting IV agent preferred.
  ➤ Propofol.
  ➤ Barbiturate.
  ➤ Benzodiazepine.

INTRAOP

Monitors/Line Placement
■ Working IV.
■ Oxygen, airway equipment, suction available.
■ Standard ASA monitors.
■ Defibrillator type: Monophasic or biphasic waveform defibrillation.

Sequence
■ Preoxygenation via mask w/ a good seal.
■ IV sedation, typically w/ propofol 1.0–2.0 mg/kg.
■ Synchronized cardioversion after loss of consciousness.
■ Airway mgt as required before & after cardioversion.

Concerns: Urgent or emergent cardioversion may require endotracheal intubation for airway protection.
■ Use anterior-posterior pad placement whenever possible.
■ Start cardioversion w/ 100 joules or more.
■ If pt is large, use machine w/ biphasic defibrillation, if available.
■ Cardioversion may produce ventricular fibrillation. If so, turn off synchronization & defibrillate.

POSTOP

Pain
■ Generally none; sometimes chest pain if multiple defibrillations

Complications
- Airway: Observe in PACU/ICU until recovery from IV sedation
- Arrhythmia monitoring: Keep defibrillator equipment at pt bedside

SURGICAL PROCEDURE
N/A

CAROTID ENDARTERECTOMY

MANUEL PARDO, JR., MD
JAMES M. SONNER, MD
DHANESH GUPTA, MD
DANIEL M. SWANGARD, MD

PREOP

Preop Considerations
- Pt symptoms include TIAs.
- Pt may already have neuro deficit.
- Common coexisting diseases: HTN, CAD, COPD, DM.
- Pt may be receiving aspirin, other antiplatelet drugs or heparin (pts w/ crescendo TIA sx).

Physical Findings
- Possible carotid bruit.
- Examine pt carefully & document pre-existing neuro deficits.
- Document baseline BP in both arms.

Workup
- High likelihood of coexisting CAD. Pt may need eval for ischemic heart disease.

Choice of Anesthesia
- GA. Possible advantages: Control of airway, ability to control minute ventilation & CO_2 tension. Technique should be designed to facilitate prompt wakeup so that neuro status can be evaluated immediately postop.
- Regional anesthesia. Requires motivated pt & surgeon. Can use deep or superficial cervical plexus block, although superficial block w/ 15 cc 0.5% bupivacaine usually adequate. Possible advantages: Ability to detect an intraop neuro deficit from cerebral ischemia during carotid clamping. Because of the deficit, pt may become confused & move, making surgical conditions difficult. Subsequent sedation or induction of GA may be difficult because of limited access to airway.

INTRAOP

Monitors/Line Placement
- Arterial line is usually placed for close BP monitoring.
- ACT machine to manage heparin dosing.

Intraop Concerns
- During induction & maintenance of GA, closely monitor BP to minimize risk of hypoperfusion & cerebral ischemia. Maintain BP within 20% of baseline.
- Possible monitors for cerebral ischemia: stump pressure, SSEP, EEG, transcranial Doppler.
- Stump pressure is measured by surgeon. A catheter is placed in the carotid artery & connected to a pressure transducer. The carotid is clamped proximal to the catheter. The measured pressure reflects the collateral cerebral blood flow. Mean pressure <50 mm Hg suggests inadequate collateral flow & need for carotid shunt placement.
- On carotid clamping, EEG or SSEP may show ischemic changes such as decreased amplitude. If this occurs, surgeon may decide to place carotid shunt.
- Some surgeons request thiopental to reduce the cerebral metabolic rate during carotid clamping.
- Because of delicate nature of the surgery, pt movement must be minimized. Deeper levels of anesthesia may lead to hypotension. Muscle relaxants may be useful in minimizing movement.
- Essential: Cardiac ischemia monitoring w/ a 5-lead EKG.
- On emergence from GA, pt may develop hypertension, resulting in bleeding from the suture line & wound hematoma.
- Minimize coughing on emergence to decrease chance for wound hematoma formation. Consider IV lidocaine, tracheal lidocaine, narcotic admin, or deep extubation.

Intraop Therapies
- Vasopressors may be needed to maintain adequate cerebral perfusion: phenylephrine infusion or boluses.
- Rx for hypertension on emergence: May include nitroglycerin infusion, nitroprusside infusion, esmolol, metoprolol, or labetalol.

POSTOP

Pain
- Typically minimal

Complications

- Airway obstruction
  - In addition to usual causes of postop airway obstruction, neck hematoma from carotid bleeding poses a unique, life-threatening risk. Also consider recurrent laryngeal nerve injury, esp w/ history of contralateral carotid or other neck surgery.
  - Neck hematoma may be superficial or deep to platysma muscle.
    - Superficial hematoma can cause more impressive swelling.
    - Deeper hematomas more dangerous, as they are more likely to cause airway compression & deviation.
  - Tracheal intubation may be difficult & may require hematoma evacuation at bedside.
  - Surgical airway may be difficult due to neck swelling & tracheal deviation.
  - Exploratory surgery is usually required to repair bleeding blood vessel.
- Mgt of airway obstruction
  - Notify surgeon & OR staff promptly because hematoma can enlarge rapidly.
  - Prepare equipment for difficult airway mgt prior to intubation attempts. Consider tracheal intubation before development of stridor.
  - If pt has airway obstruction or respiratory symptoms that could be related to neck hematoma, remove neck sutures at pt's bedside to decompress the hematoma. This may improve mask ventilation & ease of direct laryngoscopy.
  - Ask surgeon to prepare equipment for tracheotomy or cricothyrotomy in case of failed intubation.
- Stroke
  - Usually from emboli; can also result from global cerebral hypoperfusion.
  - Mgt may include carotid ultrasound or head CT scan.
  - If pt is comatose, consider tracheal intubation for airway protection.
- Myocardial ischemia
  - May present on emergence or in first few days after surgery.
  - Depending on severity, mgt may involve pt transfer to monitored setting, nitroglycerin, beta blockers, cardiac echo, or cardiac cath.
- Recurrent laryngeal nerve injury
  - May be related to cervical plexus blockade (if used) or to surgery itself.

> Unilateral nerve injury usually causes hoarseness but rarely causes stridor & airway obstruction.
> Diagnose by fiberoptic or indirect laryngoscopy.
> In absence of airway obstruction, no specific therapy needed initially.

SURGICAL PROCEDURE

Indications
■ Typical indications: asymptomatic high-grade carotid stenosis & symptomatic carotid stenosis

Procedure
■ Involves dissection of the carotid artery, application of a cross-clamp, arteriotomy, removal of obstructive plaque, patch placement, skin closure

Surgical Concerns
■ Cerebral perfusion may be inadequate with carotid cross-clamping. May consider placement of a shunt. Other concerns include embolic stroke from embolization of plaque
■ Typical indications for shunt
> Recent neuro deficit
> Stump pressure <50 mm Hg
> SSEP or EEG changes of ischemia w/ carotid clamping

Typical EBL
■ 100–300 mL

CATARACT WITH OR WITHOUT IOL

RENÉE J. ROBERTS, MD
ERIC HUANG, MD

PREOP

Preop Considerations
■ Coexisting diseases are those seen in the elderly population, such as
> HTN
> CAD
> COPD
> DM
> Osteoarthritis

■ Assess for ability to lie still and flat: elicit history of
  ➤ Claustrophobia
  ➤ Back pain
  ➤ Cough
  ➤ Orthopnea
  ➤ Reflux
  ➤ Tremor

Physical Findings
■ Decreased visual acuity
■ Findings of associated or comorbid diseases

Workup
■ Routine labs or EKG not necessary unless clinically indicated from history & physical findings

Choice of Anesthesia
■ GA used uncommonly, in select pts only
  ➤ Pts w/ severe claustrophobia, back pain, or coughing may benefit from GA due to inability to remain still.
  ➤ Succinylcholine transiently increases intraocular pressure, but use not contraindicated.
  ➤ Adequate depth of anesthesia, preferably w/ muscle relaxation, is essential to prevent a sight-threatening injury if the pt coughs or moves during surgery.
■ MAC w/ local anesthesia is the most common approach. The pt receives sedation for comfort at the time a block (eg, facial nerve & retrobulbar block) is performed.
  ➤ Requires cooperative pt
  ➤ Less hemodynamic changes than GA.
  ➤ Risk of CO_2 rebreathing due to drapes.
  ➤ Retrobulbar block has more reliable anesthesia & akinesia than peribulbar block but is more invasive, w/ higher complication risk.
  ➤ Topical anesthesia w/o retrobulbar or peribulbar block is increasingly common but requires an even more cooperative pt.

INTRAOP

Monitors/Line Placement
■ Standard monitors
■ Due to drapes over face, fresh air flow under the drapes must be provided to minimize rebreathing.

■ Concurrent use of electrocautery & supplemental oxygen beneath drapes creates fire hazard.

Intraop Concerns
■ For MAC, typically agents required only for placement of local block (alfentanyl 250–1,000 mcg, propofol 30–60 mg, fentanyl 25–100 mcg)
  ➤ After block is placed, oversedation must be avoided because it will interfere with pt cooperation & pt may move during surgery.
■ Phenylephrine is a direct alpha agonist used for pupillary dilation & ocular vasoconstriction. Topical 10% solution has greater potential for hypertension than 2.5% solution.
■ Use muscle relaxants during GA to prevent movement.
■ After GA, aim to minimize coughing & vomiting.
  ➤ Consider deep extubation or lidocaine 1 mg/kg at emergence.
  ➤ For vomiting, consider orogastric decompression & antiemetic agent.
■ Look for serious complication of retrobulbar block.
  ➤ Subarachnoid block (SAB) may occur w/ local anesthetic dissection along perineural sheath of optic nerve, resulting in brain stem anesthesia w/ apnea or loss of consciousness. Treatment is supportive.

Intraop Therapies
■ Oculocardiac reflex: Ocular traction may cause bradycardia due to a trigeminal-vagal reflex; other dysrhythmias may be seen as well.
  ➤ The treatment is to stop surgical stimulation until an acceptable rhythm returns.
  ➤ Atropine or glycopyrrolate can be given for refractory bradycardia or to prevent recurrence of bradycardia w/ surgery.

POSTOP

Pain
■ Minimal
■ Diplopia & nausea & vomiting are typically more common & disturbing than pain
■ Complications
■ Corneal edema, eye infection & rarely retinal detachment or wound dehiscence

SURGICAL PROCEDURE

Indications
- Cataracts

Procedure
- Via small anterior capsular incision, the lens is removed. Ultrasonic phacoemulsion is often used to break up lens for removal by suction.
- A new lens is inserted. The incision is closed.
- Surgical Concerns
- Akinesis of eye essential. Coughing or pt movement while the globe is open could cause permanent ocular damage.

Typical EBL
- Insignificant

CEREBRAL ANEURYSM RESECTION

RENÉE J. ROBERTS, MD
DHANESH K. GUPTA, MD

PREOP

Preop Considerations
- Mortality from unruptured aneurysms is <5%, ruptured aneurysms is 20%.
- Leading causes of morbidity & mortality are rebleeding & vasospasm.
  - Risk of recurrent subarachnoid hemorrhage (SAH) is highest in first 48 hr after rupture (at least 4% risk, but may be as high as 10–20%). SAH has a 25% mortality.
  - Subsequent risk of recurrent SAH is 1–2% per day for first 2 wks.

Physical Findings
- Pts w/ unruptured aneurysm typically have no symptoms of findings, unless the aneurysm causes mass effect.
  - Mass effect more commonly occurs w/ large aneurysm.
  - Symptoms of mass effect depend on aneurysm location & can include:
    - Headache
    - Third nerve palsy
    - Visual field defects
    - Brain stem dysfunction
    - Seizures

- If pt has SAH, findings may include:
  - Headache
  - Nuchal rigidity
  - Cranial nerve palsy (especially CN III & CN VI)
  - Hypertension
  - ECG changes
  - Increased ICP (decreased level of consciousness)
  - Motor or sensory changes
- SAH classified by clinical findings (Hunt-Hess grade)
  - Grade I: Asymptomatic, or minimal headache, slight nuchal rigidity
  - Grade II: Moderate to severe headache, nuchal rigidity, no neuro deficit other than cranial nerve palsy
  - Grade III: Drowsiness, confusion, or mild focal deficit
  - Grade IV: Stupor, moderate to severe hemiparesis, early decerebrate rigidity
  - Grade V: Deep coma, decerebrate rigidity, moribund appearance
- Head CT grading of SAH (Fisher grade) correlates w/ severity of vasospasm
  - Grade I: No subarachnoid blood
  - Grade 2: Diffuse vertical layers <1 mm
  - Grade 3: Localized clot and/or vertical layer >1 mm
  - Grade 4: Intracerebral or intraventricular clot w/ diffuse or no subarachnoid blood

Workup
- Document baseline BP & any neuro deficits
- Angiogram to document location of aneurysm
  - Hypovolemia may result from contrast-induced diuresis
- Approximately 1/3 of pts have ECG changes consistent w/ myocardial ischemia (ST segment depression or symmetric T-wave inversions)
  - No relationship between any ECG abnormality & cardiac mortality or morbidity has been found
- Cardiac workup for pt w/ SAH
  - Proceed to surgery w/o further workup after ECG & CPK-MB if:
    - No increase in CPK-MB
    - No ischemic changes on ECG
    - No clinical pulmonary edema
    - No hypotension
  - Obtain echocardiogram prior to surgery if any of the following:

- Increase in CPK-MB ($>2\%$)
- ST depression or symmetric T-wave inversion
- Clinical hypotension
- Clinical pulmonary edema
➤ Echo findings
  - Wall motion abnormalities (WMA) in coronary artery distribution: Consider cardiac catheterization for possible treatment of coexisting coronary artery disease
  - WMA NOT in coronary artery distribution: Consider invasive hemodynamic monitoring (CVP vs PA catheter vs TEE), esp if EF $<30\%$, clinical persistent hypotension, or mod-severe pulmonary edema
  - No WMA: Proceed w/ surgery

Choice of Anesthesia
■ GETA

INTRAOP

Monitors/Line Placement
■ Arterial line
  ➤ Place prior to induction or prior to laryngoscopy if labile BP to allow tighter control.
■ 2 large PIVs w/ blood tubing.
■ Consider need for CVP monitor, PA line, or TEE as determined by cardiac status.
■ Consider SSEP or EEG to monitor cerebral ischemia & titrate cerebroprotective agents.

Intraop Concerns
■ Aneurysm rupture
  ➤ Periods of greatest risk: induction, pin placement for Mayfield head holder, & vessel dissection.
■ Cerebral ischemia
  ➤ Cerebral ischemia can occur from brain retraction.
  ➤ Consider use of special neuromonitoring technique: eg, monitor for ischemia during temporary or permanent clipping using EEG (if not using burst suppression) or SSEP.

Intraop Therapies
■ Aneurysm rupture
  ➤ Maintain normal BP.

- Avoid large increases in MAP that will increase aneurysm transmural pressure & possibly cause rupture.
- Avoid large decreases in MAP that may cause ischemia due to inadequate CPP.

➤ Useful to prepare short-acting dilute vasodilator (eg, nitroprusside) & vasoconstrictor (phenylephrine) to treat extremes of blood pressure.

➤ If rupture occurs
- Aggressively treat hypovolemia.
- Communicate w/ surgeon regarding decreasing CBF to allow "bloodless field."

■ Cerebral ischemia
➤ Mild hypothermia (34–35 degrees C) to decrease $CMRO_2$.
➤ Barbiturates/propofol titrated to EEG burst suppression (dec $CMRO_2$).

POSTOP

Pain
■ Mild to moderate: pt typically receives intermittent IV morphine & does not require PCA.

Complications
■ Ischemic injury of brain supplied by aneurysmal vessel (or perforators near base of aneurysm), or from intraop retraction
■ Vasospasm (25% incidence).
➤ Usually presents 4 days to 2 wks after SAH.
➤ Symptoms can include altered mental status, focal neuro finding.
➤ Some centers monitor for this in the ICU w/ transcranial Doppler.
➤ Rx w/ nimodipine, hypervolemia, hypertension, hemodilution, papaverine, or angioplasty.

SURGICAL PROCEDURE

Indications
■ Any intracranial aneurysm, especially if pt has already had evidence of hemorrhage

Procedure
■ Craniotomy to identify vessels & nonimportant perforators
■ Possible use of temporary clip after PRN burst suppression to control inflow of blood & to soften aneurysm
■ Permanent clip of neck of aneurysm

Surgical Concerns
- Cerebral ischemia from clipping, low CPP, or retraction
- Rupture: most likely during induction, clipping, or dissecting neck of aneurysm

Typical EBL
- 300–800 mL w/o rupture

CESAREAN-HYSTERECTOMY

JOHN P. LEE, MD
SAM HUGHES, MD
MARK ROSEN, MD

PREOP

Preop Considerations
- Anesthetic implications of physiologic changes of pregnancy
  - ➤ Need for left uterine displacement
  - ➤ Presence of decreased FRC
  - ➤ Requirement for full stomach precautions: administer nonparticulate antacid (eg, bicarbonate) preop; metoclopramide and/or ranitidine optional
- Procedure can be elective, or an intraop emergency (eg, uterine atony or accreta)
- Pt may suffer considerable blood loss, particularly if nonelective procedure.
- Volume load (10–20 mL/kg crystalloid), particularly before regional anesthesia & in fasted pts
- Consider awake fiberoptic intubation for difficult airway (elective procedure)

Physical Findings
- Possible difficult airway from weight gain of pregnancy & capillary engorgement
- Expect systolic murmur
- BP: Intraop BP may remain essentially normal w/ hemorrhage; tachycardia typical first sign; cardiovascular collapse can appear suddenly

Workup
- CBC, coags, blood type & cross-match
- Work up any preexisting pregnancy-related complications

■ Confirm fetal heart rate & reason for cesarean hysterectomy to help select anesthetic choice & timing

Choice of Anesthesia
■ GA. Potential advantages:
  ➤ Airway remains protected during potential episodes of hypotension
  ➤ Discomfort, nausea, vomiting & restlessness avoided during prolonged procedure involving intraperitoneal manipulation & traction
  ➤ Reliable abdominal muscle relaxation can be achieved for optimal surgical field
■ GA
  ➤ Before birth
    • Rapid sequence induction (thiopental 4–5 mg/kg—succinylcholine 1.5 mg/kg)
    • 50% nitrous oxide in oxygen &
    • 0.5 MAC volatile agent until birth
  ➤ After birth
    • 70% nitrous oxide
    • 0.25 MAC volatile agent &
    • Opioids (150–250 mcg fentanyl)
    • May add benzodiazepine
    • Neuromuscular blockade helpful
    • Awake extubation
■ Epidural anesthesia has been used w/ high degree of success. However, there may be an increased need to induce GA compared w/ cesarean alone
■ Lumbar epidural anesthesia, T4-S4
  ➤ 20 mL (after test dose & administered in divided doses) of: 2% lidocaine w/ epinephrine 1:200,000 (2 mL of 8.4% bicarbonate optional to speed onset)
  ➤ 50–100 mcg fentanyl may improve intraop block
■ Continuous spinal anesthesia is another option

INTRAOP

Monitors/Line Placement
■ Large-bore venous access required (eg, two 16g catheters)
■ Arterial line & CVP should be considered; provision to place one intraop should be available
■ Availability of rapid transfusion blood warmer (eg, Level 1)

- Blood availability must be ensured.
- Intraop Concerns
- Same for nonemergent C-section
- Hemorrhage, DIC, hypotension, dilution coagulopathy; blood products may be needed
- If regional anesthesia used & there is significant blood loss, airway can be compromised, and/or attention to nausea, vomiting, discomfort may distract from aggressive blood/fluid replacement
- Intraop Therapies
- Blood, factors, & fluid replacement
- Rx w/ vasopressors may be needed for short duration. Ephedrine, phenylephrine, & dopamine should be readily available

POSTOP

Pain

- Epidural morphine (4–5 mg) for postop pain control
- Consider ketorolac (15–30 mg IV/IM) for synergism
- Narcotics via PCA
- Continuous epidural infusion of dilute local anesthetic; rarely indicated
- Consider removing epidural catheters only after resolution of DIC, if it occurs
- If GA used, consider postop regional block for analgesia if appropriate
- Complications
- Rebleeding
- Respiratory complications from massive transfusion
- DIC

SURGICAL PROCEDURE

Indications

- Uterine rupture, atony, or placenta accreta, increta or percreta
- Postpartum hemorrhage unresponsive to conservative measures (oxytocin, methylergonovine, 15-methylprostaglandin F2-alpha [Hemabate], hypogastric, uterine, ovarian, or internal iliac artery ligation, or embolization)

Procedure

- Cesarean delivery followed by hysterectomy

Surgical Concerns

- Enlarged, engorged uterus

- Difficult exposure
- Blood loss (massive hemorrhage possible)
- Trauma to ureters

Typical EBL
- 3,500 mL (range extends to massive hemorrhage)

CIRCUMCISION

ATSUKO BABA, MD

PREOP

Preop Considerations
- Most commonly done in infancy
- Routine circumcisions are controversial, but some studies show that there is an increased incidence of urinary tract infections in uncircumcised boys
- Less common in adults, but may be done for medical reasons (eg, phimosis, paraphimosis) or for personal or religious reasons

Physical Findings
- Possible phimosis

Workup
- No additional workup is necessary if pt is otherwise healthy

Choice of Anesthesia
- Children
  - ➤ GA w/ a mask, LMA, or ETT w/ or w/o a caudal block for postop analgesia
  - ➤ An inhalational induction w/ or w/o premed of oral midazolam or IM ketamine
- Adults
  - ➤ Usually done as local procedure, w/ surgeon performing penile nerve block w/ possible ring block

INTRAOP

Monitors/Line Placement
- Standard monitoring
- IV line started after GA induction

Intraop Concerns
- No special concerns

Intraop Therapies
- A caudal injection of 0.25% bupivacaine (1 cc/kg) prior to incision provides effective postop analgesia.

POSTOP

Pain
- Intraop caudal w/ bupivacaine
- Intraop ring block around the penis or penile block (usually performed by the surgeon if a caudal is contraindicated)

Complications
- Bleeding/infection

SURGICAL PROCEDURE

Indications
- Phimosis
  - Phimosis is often used as a vague term to indicate inability to retract foreskin, although this can be a normal finding.
  - True phimosis, also called preputial stenosis, refers to scarring of the prepuce.

Procedure
- Excision of the preputial skin of the penis for full exposure of the glans of the penis
  - Either freehand excision or devices (eg, Gomco or Mogen) can be used.
  - Techniques include dorsal slit technique & sleeve technique.

Surgical Concerns
- Postop bleeding/infection

Typical EBL
- Minimal

CLEFT LIP REPAIR

GERALD DUBOWITZ, MB CHB

PREOP

Preop Considerations
- Pt may be any age, but typically is a child >10–12 wks old.
- Cleft lip may be assoc w/ other, undiagnosed anomalies.

Physical Findings

- Pt may have a bilateral or unilateral cleft lip, which may be assoc w/ a cleft palate.
- May be other midline embryonic defects (eg, congenital heart disease)
- Pt may have a syndrome assoc w/ a difficult airway (eg, Pierre-Robin).

Workup

- Standard history & physical, emphasis on identifying coexisting defects (eg, cleft palate, cardiac defects).

Choice of Anesthesia

- Local/regional
  - ➤ Can be done by local infiltration w/ or w/o infraorbital nerve block in older pts.
- GA
  - ➤ Favored by many practitioners, particularly in younger pts.
  - ➤ RAE ETT favored by many surgeons. Procedure can also be done w/ an LMA.
  - ➤ GA may be supplemented w/ regional block. (infraorbital nerve) or infiltration of LA.

INTRAOP

Monitors/Line Placement

- Standard monitoring.
- One peripheral IV.

Intraop Concerns

- Pharyngeal pack must be removed prior to extubation.
- Blood may pass into the pharynx or stomach.

POSTOP

Pain

- Minimal to mild.
- Pain rarely a problem if local anesthesia is used intraop or adequate analgesia given intraop.
- Local infiltration w/ ropivacaine reported to last longer than lidocaine or bupivacaine for postop pain control & therefore may be the local anesthetic of choice.
- Mild analgesics (eg, acetaminophen) usually effective.
- Avoid eating "sharp" foods in the immediate postop period (eg, potato chips).

- A solution of aluminum-magnesium hydroxide & diphenhydramine (Maalox & Benadryl) can often help if the child is very fussy; helps coat the mouth, easing transition to oral intake.

Complications
- Early: Bleeding is usually self-limiting but in more extensive repairs may require return to OR.
- Late: Rare (<1%) wound breakdown at the suture line, usually due to trauma (eg, bumping into caregiver's shoulder) or infection. Fistula formation is possible if suture line breaks down.

SURGICAL PROCEDURE

Indications
- Congenital cleft lip

Procedure
- Involves apposition of lip defect, often employing small rotational flaps rather than simple apposition of the two sides

Surgical Concerns
- The size of the defect may make it a bigger procedure, w/ consequent increases in pain.
- Bilateral clefts lips are generally done at the same time.

Typical EBL
- Minimal

CLEFT PALATE REPAIR

GERALD DUBOWITZ, MB CHB

PREOP

Preop Considerations
- Typically performed in children aged 10–12 mo.
- Consider long-lasting preop pain relief (eg, q24h Cox-2 inhibitor).

Physical Findings
- Cleft may be partial or complete depending on the length & depth of the defect.
- Often but not always assoc w/ cleft lip.
- Cleft lip tends to be repaired in earlier childhood & palate repairs later, preferably before phonation & speech development.

■ May be assoc w/ other midline embryonic defects (eg, congenital heart disease).

Workup
■ Standard history & physical.

Choice of Anesthesia
■ GA
➢ Inhaled or IV anesthesia may be used.
➢ Oral RAE ETT.
■ Administration of local anesthetic by surgeon is good for minimizing anesthetic & for postop pain relief.
■ Can also consider supplemental nerve blockade (eg, infraorbital block, though this block will not provide adequate anesthesia on its own).

INTRAOP

Monitors/Line Placement
■ Standard monitoring

Intraop Concerns
■ May include the possibility of blood passing into the pharynx or stomach. This is rarely significant since most surgeons infiltrate the field w/ epinephrine.
■ Ropivacaine has been reported to last much longer than lidocaine or bupivacaine postop & hence may be the local anesthetic of choice.

POSTOP

Pain
■ Mild to moderate
■ Can be a significant problem
➢ Can be minimized if local anesthetic is used intraop and/or adequate preop analgesia given
■ Moderate analgesics are usually effective (eg, NSAIDs, acetaminophen w/ opiate). Avoid eating "sharp" foods in the immediate postop period (eg, potato chips).
■ A solution of aluminum-magnesium hydroxide & diphenhydramine (Maalox & Benadryl) can often help if the child is very fussy; it helps coat the mouth, easing transition to oral intake.

Complications
■ Early

➤ Bleeding is usually self-limited but in more extensive repairs may require return to OR.

■ Late
  ➤ Rare (<1%) wound breakdown at the suture line. Usually due to trauma (eg, bumping against caregiver's shoulder) or infection.
  ➤ Fistula formation is possible if suture line breaks down.
  ➤ Bleeding may also occur up to 2–3 weeks postop.

SURGICAL PROCEDURE

Indications
■ Congenital cleft palate

Procedure
■ Correction of central palatal defect
■ Achieved by releasing lateral palate, apposing the central portion & leaving the lateral palate to heal by secondary intention

Surgical Concerns
■ The bigger the defect, the greater the potential blood loss & postop pain
■ Cleft lips may be done at the same time or as a separate procedure

Typical EBL
■ Minimal

CORNEAL TRANSPLANT (PENETRATING KERATOPLASTY)

JASON WIDRICH, MD

PREOP

Preop Considerations
■ Done for a variety of indications. Disease may be limited to eye.
  ➤ In the U.S., approx 40,000 corneal transplants performed each year.

Physical Findings
■ None typical.

Workup
■ Based on coexisting disease.
■ Stop aspirin or anticoagulant drugs.

Choice of Anesthesia
- GA or MAC w/ regional block
  - During transplant pt will have an open globe. Most surgeons will request GA for the procedure.
  - Regional anesthetic may be unsuitable for pt who is uncooperative, has a chronic cough, or cannot lie flat.

INTRAOP

Monitors/Line Placement
- Standard monitors
  - One peripheral IV.

Intraop Concerns
- Minimize pt movement during surgery, especially during placement of donor cornea.
- Oculocardiac reflex can result from tension on ocular structures, causing bradycardia & other arrhythmias.
- If liquid vitreous substitutes are needed to replace a vitreous leak, avoid nitrous oxide during the procedure & for the next 4–6 wks. N_2O can cause IOP increases.

Intraop Therapies
- Oculocardiac reflex is treated by halting the stimulus, increasing depth of anesthesia & administering IV glycopyrrolate or atropine if bradycardia persists.
- Consider prophylactic antiemetics.

POSTOP

Pain
- Minimal
- PO analgesics

Complications
- Nausea/vomiting
- Corneal abrasion

SURGICAL PROCEDURE

Indications
- Corneal dystrophy
- Keratoconus
- Aphakic bullous keratopathy
- Keratitis

Procedure
- A central portion of the recipient's cornea is removed w/ a trephine.
- Donor cornea is sutured in place.

Surgical Concerns
- Open globe, extrusion of lens
- Wound dehiscence
- Visual outcome
- Infection
- Graft rejection, failure
- IOP control, postkeratoplasty glaucoma

Typical EBL
- Minimal

CRANIOTOMY FOR TUMOR

ROBERT M. DONATIELLO, MD

PREOP

Preop Considerations
- Consider characteristics of the pt's neuro illness & general medical conditions that may affect anesthesia care.
- Neuro history
  - ➤ Symptoms & duration; includes
    - Seizure activity (type, frequency, duration, related characteristics)
    - ICP characteristics (headache, nausea, vomiting, mentation issues, visual problems)
    - Focal signs (specific characteristics depend on lesion location)
    - Neurocirculatory status (TIAs, stroke history)
    - Peripheral nervous system (strength, sensation, autonomic changes)
  - ➤ Interventions to date; includes
    - Chemotherapy (more often instituted w/ metastatic disease; ascertain which drugs & seek side effects)
    - Steroid therapy (eg, dexamethasone)
    - Radiation (local radiation more of an issue w/ metastatic disease)
    - Surgery/anesthesia (review any past operative & anesthetic records)

➤ Neurobehavioral evaluation: allows determination of neuro baseline to compare w/ postop. Often performed as part of neuro consult. Should include
- Memory
- Attention span
- Spatial perception
- Higher cognition

■ Medical history: pertinent issues for craniotomy include
➤ Renal disease: must investigate because mannitol or furosemide commonly used intraop for diuresis
➤ Hematologic: coagulopathy increases surgical bleeding & anemia decreases oxygen content

■ Medications
➤ It is especially important to note these types of medications:
- Cardiovascular
- Antiseizure (pts often taking Dilantin or Tegretol)
- Pain (NSAIDs & aspirin especially)
- Steroids

Physical Findings
■ Perform & document neuro exam, w/ particular attention to
➤ Level of consciousness
➤ Motor or sensory deficit (eg, hemiparesis)
➤ Cranial nerve palsies

■ Evaluate evidence of increased ICP: pt may exhibit visual changes, papilledema, or changes in mental status

■ Evaluate evidence of mass effect: may be noted peripherally ("sided" weakness, sensory changes) or centrally (cranial nerve defects)

■ Assess airway & potential difficulties w/ intubation. Unforeseen problems may lead to disastrous changes in ICP

Workup
■ CBC, coag studies
■ Electrolyte status: fluid shifts induced by osmotic agents may alter the pt's electrolyte status considerably, contributing to postop obtundation
■ Head CT or MRI
➤ Note size & location of tumor.

➤ Look for evidence of elevated ICP, cerebral edema, mass effect, midline shift, herniation.

Choice of Anesthesia

■ GA used for most cases. Allows control of airway & a stable operative field for the surgeon. ICP can be modified by hyper- or hypoventilation.

➤ Important: choose an anesthetic regimen that promotes rapid wake-up & minimal respiratory depression. Neuro status will be evaluated immediately postop, & slow awakening may lead to emergent head CT.

➤ A typical anesthetic could consist of:
  • Midazolam premed
  • Minimal narcotic premed (could lead to respiratory depression & hypercarbia prior to induction)
  • Induction w/ propofol or thiopental
  • <0.5 MAC inhalation agent
  • Nitrous oxide 60–70%
  • Continuous infusion of fentanyl at 1–5 mcg/kg/h
  • Paralysis w/ a nondepolarizing muscle relaxant
  • Total IV anesthesia (TIVA) may be useful approach, especially when neuromonitoring is used (see below)

■ MAC: for "awake" craniotomies
  ➤ Allows pt's mental status to be continually monitored
  ➤ Allows cortical or speech mapping
  ➤ More eloquent cortical areas may be spared by this technique
  ➤ Pt discomfort & potential movement & airway difficulties may raise the difficulty level

INTRAOP

Monitors/Line Placement

■ Arterial line allows close management of BP & CPP.
  ➤ In awake craniotomies, use adequate local anesthetic when placing the arterial line.
■ Two peripheral IVs usually adequate.
■ Central line rarely needed.
■ Neuromonitoring may be provided to assess functional integrity of awake or asleep pts. Certain modifications necessary to the anesthetic are discussed below.

Intraop Concerns

- Mgt of ICP is the primary concern during craniotomy for tumor resection.
  - Elevated ICP may be present preop, may develop during surgery, or may occur postop.
- Other major concerns include
  - Maintaining CPP > 70 mmHg to minimize cerebral ischemia from retraction.
  - Providing good surgical conditions ("relaxed brain") to facilitate exposure.
- At induction, ensure minimal change in ICP.
  - Provide adequate preoxygenation & encourage hyperventilation.
  - Use IV propofol or thiopental. Both decrease cerebral blood flow & can decrease ICP.
  - To minimize coughing w/ tracheal intubation, provide adequate depth of anesthesia & muscle relaxation.
    - Consider lidocaine, 1–2 mg/kg IV 90 sec prior to laryngoscopy.
  - Further therapy discussed in "Intraop Therapy" section below.
- A lumbar drain may be placed by the surgeon or anesthesiologist.
  - Pay particular attention to it intraop, making sure it does not drain unexpectedly.
  - Surgeon may request withdrawal of CSF to reduce intracranial volume.
- For neuromonitoring, consider the following anesthetic recommendations:
  - Motor mapping asleep
    - No muscle relaxant during mapping.
    - Use 70% N_2O & <0.5 MAC inhaled agent.
    - Keep pt temp >36 degrees C.
  - Speech mapping awake
    - Goal is to have awake, cooperative pt during mapping.
    - Narcotic infusion OK.
    - Propofol OK.
  - SSEP & motor evoked potential (MEP) studies
    - Avoid nitrous oxide.
    - Avoid inhaled agents.
    - Propofol + narcotic OK.
    - Muscle relaxant OK for SSEP.
    - Do not use muscle relaxant for MEP.

- If SSEPs diminish, may be a sign of cerebral hypoperfusion. Discuss w/ surgeon & neurophysiologist whether to increase mean BP by 10–20%.
■ For awake craniotomy
  ➢ Sedative or analgesic infusions will be highest during most painful parts: placement of pins for head holder & opening of skull.
  ➢ Otherwise, pt should be easily responsive & comfortable until mapping is completed. Then, anesthetic level can be increased.
  ➢ Airway & respiratory concerns
    - Be exceptionally vigilant of the airway: intubation is extremely difficult in a pt whose head is pinned.
    - Titrate sedatives & analgesics carefully to minimize airway obstruction.
    - Use a nasal airway early in pts w/ signs of obstruction.
    - Prepare an LMA as alternate form of airway mgt.
    - Ensure a reliable end-tidal CO_2 tracing w/ the nasal cannula, but remember that pCO_2 will be higher than $ETCO_2$.
  ➢ Create access to oberve the pt.
    - Move surgical drapes aside.
    - Clear the areas likely to be affected by intraop seizure.
    - Modulate the depth of anesthesia as needed.
■ When working in the posterior fossa, brain stem manipulations may cause profound cardiovascular changes; if such changes occur, alert the surgeon & treat appropriately for persistent changes.
■ When waking pt from a craniotomy, maintain same concerns regarding ICP & hemodynamics.
  ➢ Consider IV lidocaine to prevent coughing on emergence.
  ➢ Consider IV labetalol to minimize hypertension & tachycardia on emergence.
■ Avoid volume overload, as this might worsen cerebral edema in the injured brain.
■ For a sitting craniotomy, see Procedure chapter "Craniotomy in the Seated Position."

Intraop Therapies

■ At start of case, surgeon may request mannitol 0.25–1 g/kg IV. Also, surgeon will likely request prophylactic antibiotics & dexamethasone 4–10 mg IV.

- Atropine may be necessary for severe bradycardia w/ posterior fossa manipulation, but use could cause undesirable tachycardia.
- For increased ICP
  - Facilitate cerebral venous drainage.
    - Keep head & neck position neutral.
    - Consider elevation of head of bed.
    - Minimize elevations in intrathoracic pressure: use adequate neuromuscular blockade or opiates to prevent coughing or breathing.
  - Discontinue inhaled agent & N_2O to reduce effects of cerebral vasodilation on ICP.
  - To avoid cerebral vasodilation from inhalation agent, administer IV propofol & oxygen.
  - Mild hyperventilation to $PaCO_2$ 30–35 mmHg.
  - Diuresis w/ mannitol or furosemide if necessary.

POSTOP

Pain

- Typically mild to moderate. Pts usually have adequate analgesia w/ intraop fentanyl & postop intermittent IV morphine. PCA not usually needed.

Complications

- Mental status changes
  - All craniotomy pts should be observed at a level equivalent to ICU monitoring for at least 8 h postop.
  - Oversedation or residual effects of anesthetics are potential causes of postop altered mental status.
  - May also be due to elevated ICP, cerebral edema secondary to surgical trauma, or electrolyte imbalance secondary to fluid shifts.
  - Consider treatment of specific causes.
    - Mannitol for suspected cerebral edema or elevated ICP.
    - Naloxone for undesired opiate effect.
  - Head CT may be useful in selected pts to look for structural abnormalities (eg, cerebral edema, hemorrhage, hematoma, tension pneumocephalus).
  - Notify surgeon of significant mental status changes, as pt may require reintubation, urgent head CT, even re-exploration.

- Postop airway swelling & obstruction
  - May be an issue in sitting or prone posterior fossa craniotomies, as facial or lingual edema may compromise airway patency
  - If pt has obvious facial or lingual swelling
    - Do not extubate immediately.
    - Observe pt in PACU or ICU with head of bed elevated.
    - Consider cuff leak test, fiberoptic exam of airway, or direct laryngoscopy to assess airway swelling & likelihood of airway obstruction postextubation.
- Seizures: may require additional phenytoin loading, possible reintubation.

SURGICAL PROCEDURE

Indications
- Tumor
  - Different types & classifications, including
    - Supratentorial vs infratentorial
    - Intra-axial (astrocytoma, oligodendroglioma, glioblastoma) vs extra-axial (meningioma, acoustic neuroma)

Procedure
- Varies based on location of tumor. Common pt positions include supine (craniopharyngiomas, subfrontal), lateral (temporal, parietal), prone (occipital, cerebellar), sitting (posterior fossa, pineal).
- Pt's head often placed in Mayfield pins or a head holder.
- Skull is removed over access point by bur holes & bone saw.
- Dura is opened & tumor is exposed w/ the use of image-guided navigation system (eg, StealthStation) when necessary.
- Neuromonitoring tests may be used to discern functional tissue from tumor.
- Tumor is resected, dura is closed, bone (vascularized or free) or plating is placed, skin is closed.

Surgical Concerns
- ICP & cerebral edema may affect localization of tumor. Osmotic diuretics may be instituted to facilitate visualization.
- Neuro exam performed immediately postop, so pt must be alert quickly after procedure.

Typical EBL
- 100–500 mL

CRANIOTOMY IN THE SEATED POSITION

PHILIP BICKLER, MD

PREOP

Preop Considerations
- This procedure carries risks beyond those of a typical craniotomy because of the seated position. The pt's cardiovascular status deserves particular attention because of the following:
  - Venous air embolus (VAE) is a common occurrence in the seated position & pts w/ a patent foramen ovale are at risk for arterial air embolism.
    - Can lead to significant cardiac & neurologic morbidity, or death
  - Venous return is compromised in the seated position. Even young healthy pts will have decreased venous return & decreased cardiac output in the seated position during GA.
  - Those w/ poor cardiac function, atrial fibrillation, or right heart failure may not tolerate the position w/o dangerous declines in CPP.

Workup
- In addition to the routine preop testing request, a cardiac echo study to look for a patent foramen ovale.
- Pts w/ posterior fossa tumors may have dysphagia, abnormal airway reflexes, or altered respiratory & cardiovascular control.
- Hydrocephalus may be present.

Choice of Anesthesia
- GA w/ ETT to control CO_2 & possible postop ventilation.
- No particular anesthetic is superior for craniotomies. Bear in mind the following goals:
  - Maintain adequate cerebral perfusion. Consider pt's underlying disease & possible altered autoregulation of blood flow.
  - The anesthetic should be as compatible as possible w/ any neuromonitoring procedures.
  - Plan emergence to allow timely postop assessment of neuro function.
  - Ensure an appropriate depth of anesthesia to obviate movement or recall.
  - A typical anesthetic could consist of:
    - Low-dose inhalational agent

- Nitrous oxide 60% (if VAE occurs, change to 100% O_2)
- Continuous infusion of fentanyl at 1–5 mcg/kg/h
- Maintain paralysis w/ nondepolarizing muscle relaxant.

INTRAOP

Monitors/Line Placement

■ Two large peripheral IVs, one before induction
■ Arterial line
  ➤ Place the arterial pressure transducer at the level of the circle of Willis to reflect CPP.
  ➤ If transducer placed at right atrial level, calculate distance to brain to properly assess CPP.
■ Central line
  ➤ Measure CVP w/ an air aspiration catheter (eg, a Bunnegin-Albin type catheter) placed in the right atrium under ECG monitoring (observing change in p-wave morphology in ECG signal from catheter tip).
  ➤ Use the catheter to aspirate air in the event of a VAE.
  ➤ A subclavian or brachial catheter is preferred over internal jugular because of minimal manipulation of head & neck.
■ A precordial Doppler probe is positioned in the right second intercostal space near the sternum to aid in early detection of air embolization.
  ➤ Be sure that venous air embolism can be detected: rapidly inject 5 cc of saline agitated w/ a bubble of air into an IV line: the Doppler should detect the microbubbles.
■ An esophageal stethoscope should also be placed as an auxiliary means to detect a large air embolism (a machinery murmur may be heard).
■ Respiratory gas analysis: anesthetic agent, CO_2 & nitrogen
■ Neuromonitoring: EEG, SSEPs, or other modalities to monitor cerebral function.
■ Be sure the pt is wearing antiembolism hose (aids in preventing venous pooling & dependent edema) & sequential compression devices on both legs.
■ A forced air warming/cooling blanket should be in place as well.

Intraop Concerns

■ When surgery is in the posterior fossa, brain stem manipulations may cause profound cardiovascular changes. If such changes occur,

alert the surgeon & treat appropriately if suspension of stimulation doesn't extinguish the response.
- Review how to move OR table to resuscitation position.
- High risk for VAE (see also "Venous Air Embolism" chapter)
  - From the time of incision onward VAE can occur. Reduce risk by keeping CVP slightly elevated.
  - Essentials of mgt
    - 100% O_2
    - Flood surgical field w/ saline.
    - Aspirate right atrial catheter (can help confirm dx).
    - Ask surgeon to compress jugular veins to reduce air entry.
    - Circulatory support/fluid resuscitation.
- Maintain adequate CPP.
- In most cases moderate hyperventilation ($PaCO_2$ 30–35 mmHg) is desirable.
- Mannitol, 0.5–1.0 g/kg, may be requested by surgeons to relax the brain.
- Maintain paralysis during surgery.
- Consider mild hypothermia to achieve cerebral protection.
  - Consider effect of hypothermia on neuromonitoring method.

Intraop Therapies
- Vasopressors may be needed to maintain adequate CPP: phenylephrine boluses or infusion.

POSTOP

Pain
- Typically minimal.

Complications
- Neuro
  - Delayed awakening.
  - New neuro deficits, stroke.
  - Intracranial hemorrhage, edema potential causes.
  - Respiratory failure secondary to brain stem edema or surgical trauma.
- Management of neuro changes
  - Notify surgeon.
  - Depending on clinical presentation, pt may require:
    - Tracheal intubation for airway protection or respiratory failure.
    - Emergent head CT.
    - Emergency re-exploration.

- Postop hypothermia due to inability to rewarm pt.
- Postop hypertension common in posterior fossa surgery.
- Myocardial ischemia may present immediately or days later.

SURGICAL PROCEDURE

Indications
- Tumors & other lesions (eg, AVMs, aneurysms) of the midline posterior fossa or deep midline supratentorial region not accessible w/ pt in prone, lateral, or other positions.

Procedure
- Craniectomy, retraction of cerebellum, other structures as required. Procedures may take many hours.

Surgical Concerns
- Adequate exposure; influenced by $PaCO_2$. May need mannitol to reduce brain volume to achieve surgical access.

Typical EBL
- 300–500 cc; may be much greater w/ neurovascular procedures.

CRANIOTOMY/TRAUMA

TESSA COLLINS, MD
MIMI C. LEE, MD, PHD

PREOP

Preop Considerations
- Pts often have associated injuries, including:
  - Intraabdominal
  - Orthopedic
  - Spinal cord
  - Other organ trauma
- Ventilation & oxygenation may be inadequate
- Tracheal intubation may be indicated if:
  - Hypoxemic
  - Hypercapnic
  - Gag reflex absent
  - Glasgow Coma Scale score <=8
- ICP may be elevated

- Systemic hypotension (SBP <80) correlates w/ poor outcome
- Skull fractures often occur in assoc w/
  - Underlying contusions
  - Epidural hematomas, which may expand in size over time
  - Subdural hematomas, which may expand in size over time
- Severe head injuries can be assoc w/
  - DIC
  - ARDS

Physical Findings
- Hypotension
- Hypoxemia & hypercapnia
- Periodic increases in arterial blood pressure w/ reflex bradycardia (Cushing's response), assoc w/ abrupt increases in ICP
- Altered level of consciousness and/or focal neuro deficits
- Basilar skull fracture, suggested by:
  - CSF rhinorrhea/otorrhea
  - Hemotympanum
  - Ecchymosis of periorbital tissue (raccoon eyes)
  - Ecchymosis of periaural tissue (Battle's sign)

Workup
- Radiologic studies
  - C-spine x-ray
  - Abdominal & chest x-ray
  - Pelvis x-ray
  - Head CT w/o contrast w/ bone & brain windows when pt is stable
- Blood work
  - CBC w/ platelet count
  - Coag studies
  - Electrolytes, BUN, creatinine
  - ABG
  - Type & cross
  - Drug & alcohol screen

Choice of Anesthesia
- GA
- Intubate the trachea using
  - RSI (see under Preop) or
  - "Modified" RSI in more stable pts. May give, prior to laryngoscopy:

- Lidocaine (1.5 mg/kg) and/or
- Fentanyl (1–4 mcg/kg)

- Insert a large-bore orogastric tube.
- Choice of anesthetics.
  - IV anesthetics
    - **Barbiturates** (thiopental, pentobarbital) decrease CBF, CBV & ICP.
    - **Etomidate** has similar neuro effects but may be preferred because of decreased chance for systemic hypotension.
    - **Propofol** can result in severe hypotension. Prior intravascular volume resuscitation is critical.
    - **Benzodiazepines** may be used for sedation.
  - Inhalational anesthetics
    - Halothane increases ICP & CBF.
    - Isoflurane decreases $CMRO_2$.
    - Sevoflurane is similar to isoflurane.
    - Desflurane increases ICP at high doses.
    - Nitrous oxide can cause cerebral vasodilation & thus elevated ICP. It should be avoided in pts w/ pneumocephaly or pneumothorax.
- Local anesthetics may decrease the required depth of anesthesia.
- Opioids can minimize breathing & coughing, which could otherwise lead to elevated intrathoracic pressure & interfere w/ cerebral venous drainage.
- Muscle relaxants facilitate adequate ventilation & reduce coughing.
- Avoid ketamine, which raises ICP.

INTRAOP

Monitors/Line Placement
- Standard monitors plus intra-arterial BP monitor, ideally placed prior to induction.
- 2 large-bore peripheral IV catheters.
  - Consider femoral vein or subclavian vein introducer sheath.
  - Consider right subclavian instead of jugular vein, because less head manipulation is necessary & carotid puncture not a risk.
- CVP monitoring may be necessary to evaluate volume status.
- ICP monitor may be placed by neurosurgeons.

Intraop Concerns
- Maintain CPP 70–110 mmHg.

- Avoid systemic hypotension (<=80 mmHg).
- Avoid increasing CVP or ICP.
- Maintain mild hypothermia.
- Avoid hypoxemia & hypercarbia.
- Treat anemia, coagulopathy & DIC.
- Volume resuscitate w/ isotonic, glucose-free solution, colloid, blood & blood products as indicated. Do not fluid overload.
- Avoid hyperglycemia (keep glucose <180 mg/dL).

Intraop Therapies
- Elevated ICP
  - Hyperventilate to $PaCO_2$ of 25–30 mmHg.
  - Increase depth of anesthesia (barbiturates or propofol particularly useful; avoid high levels of volatile anesthetics, which can cause cerebral vasodilation).
  - Diurese: Osmotic agents (mannitol 0.25–1 mg/kg IV bolus over 10–20 min) or loop diuretics (furosemide).
  - Drain CSF through ventricular drainage catheter placed by neurosurgeons.
  - Maintain temp at 33–35 degrees C.
- Hypotension
  - Use pressors or inotropes as necessary.
- Avoid vasodilators for HTN before dura is opened.
- Treat DIC as needed w/ FFP, platelets & cryoprecipitate.
- Use PEEP as required for ARDS or neurogenic pulmonary edema, but wait until dura is opened.

POSTOP

Pain
- Minimal. However, sedation may be required if pt is left intubated postop.

Complications
- Primary intrinsic brain damage
- Secondary brain insult
- DIC
- ARDS
- Aspiration pneumonitis and/or pneumonia
- Neurogenic pulmonary edema w/ decreased cardiac output
- Diabetes insipidus

- Brain herniation
- Death

SURGICAL PROCEDURE

Indications
- Open, depressed skull fractures.
- Subdural or epidural hematomas.
- Intraparenchymal hemorrhages or contusions resulting in significant mass effect or midline shift.

Procedure
- Bur hole(s) placement
  - Often relieves pressure immediately; used as an initial effort to lower ICP until bone flap can be removed & dura opened, if necessary.
- Craniotomy
  - Open skull fractures are elevated & dura evaluated, debrided & repaired if necessary. Antibiosis is imperative perioperatively.
  - Trauma flap for epidurals (EDH) & subdurals (SDH): large, temporo-fronto-parietal craniotomies are performed on the side of injury to thoroughly examine & identify bleeding vessels.
    - In SDH, bridging dural veins are often the source of bleeding.
    - In EDH, meningeal arteries are often torn.
- Craniectomy is sometimes performed & bone flaps replaced if & only when massive cerebral edema subsides.

Surgical Concerns
- Beware of overaggressive reduction of CBF & ICP, which may lead to further SDH due to sudden shrinking of parenchyma, leading to breakage of bridging dural veins.
- Beware of possible brain herniation w/ dural opening.
- Beware of venous air emboli.
- Beware of subtle subdural hematomas, epidural hematomas & focal contusions that may blossom over time.
  - A hematoma not requiring therapy initially may worsen & require emergent decompression.

Typical EBL
- Highly variable; may be significant if pt develops DIC.
- Be prepared to transfuse large quantities of blood and/or blood products rapidly.

CYSTECTOMY

JASON WIDRICH, MD

PREOP

Preop Considerations
- Type of cystectomy depends on diagnosis.
  - Partial: can be done for bladder diverticula, fistulas (colovesical, vesicovaginal), cystitis, localized endometriosis.
  - Radical: generally for bladder cancer.
    - In men, usually involves prostatectomy, possible urethrectomy
    - In women, procedure may include pelvic exenteration. (See also Procedures chapter "Pelvic Exenteration.")
    - Radical cystectomy requires urinary diversion or neobladder construction.

Physical Findings
- None typical

Workup
- CBC, electrolytes, BUN, creatinine, PT, PTT.
- Workup for metastatic disease.

Choice of Anesthesia
- Spinal, epidural or general anesthesia.
- Consider GA or GA & epidural for larger resections or prolonged surgery.

INTRAOP

Monitors/Line Placement
- At least one large-bore peripheral IV.
- Standard monitors.
- Consider arterial line or central line depending on coexisting disease & size of resection.
- Foley catheter will be used at beginning of procedure but may be removed during surgery (except for partial cystectomy).

Intraop Concerns
- Hemorrhage.
- Potential for lengthy surgery related to urinary diversion or neobladder construction.
  - Increased risk of hypothermia, third-space fluid losses.

■ Will be difficult to evaluate urine output when bladder is removed.

POSTOP

Pain
■ Moderate
■ PCA or epidural adequate

Complications
■ Ileus
■ Infection
■ Anastomotic leak
■ Acute renal failure

SURGICAL PROCEDURE

Indications
■ Bladder cancer
■ Nonmalignant disease
  ➤ Bladder diverticula
  ➤ Hemangiomas
  ➤ Cystitis
  ➤ Fistulas (colovesical, vesicovaginal)
  ➤ Localized endometriosis

Procedure
■ Midline lower abdominal incision.
■ A simple cystectomy involves removal of the bladder only & is reserved for nonmalignant disease.
■ A partial cystectomy is done for pts w/ nonmalignant disease or localized tumors.
■ Radical cystectomy involves removal of the bladder & the lower ureters & may require pelvic lymph node dissection or resection of the urethra.
  ➤ In men, it includes the prostate & the seminal vesicles.
  ➤ In women, the uterus, ovaries & vaginal wall may be involved in the resection (pelvic exenteration).
■ A segment of bowel may be taken from terminal ileum to fashion a urinary diversion through the abdominal wall.
■ For a bladder substitution, a section of vascular bowel may be used to fashion a pouch that can then be connected to the ureters & the urethra to re-establish the flow of urine.

Surgical Concerns
- Bladder drainage
- Hemorrhage
- Infection
- Ileus
- Hematuria
- Fistula formation

Typical EBL
- Minimal for partial resections to >1,500 mL for radical cystectomy.

DILATATION AND CURETTAGE/EVACUATION (D&C, D&E)

DWAIN SKINNER, MD

PREOP

Preop Considerations
- Determine reason for performing procedure:
  - ➤ Diagnosis or treatment of abnormal uterine bleeding due to hormonal changes, polyps, dysplasia, complications due to IUDs, miscarriages.
- Determine gestational age of fetus if pt is pregnant.
- Maternal changes w/ pregnancy to be considered include cardiovascular, pulmonary, GI, renal, neurologic sensitivity to anesthetics.
  - ➤ See also Coexisting Disease chapter "Pregnancy."
- If pt has suffered intrauterine fetal demise, a coagulopathy (DIC) may be present.
- If there is a postpartum retained placenta, prior blood loss from delivery needs to be considered.
- Evaluate for anemia or hypovolemia.

Physical findings (in pregnant pts)
- Uterine size, gestational age.
- Impact of abdominal girth on respiratory & GI systems.
- Effects of fetal size on maternal physiology.

Workup
- CBC, blood products, coagulation studies may be required.
- Choice of Anesthesia
- Conscious sedation or MAC.
  - ➤ Paracervical block w/ or w/o sedation.

➤ Neuraxial block (eg, spinal).
➤ Consider GA if pt is undergoing therapeutic abortion of fetus beyond second trimester as increased risk for aspiration w/ sedation due to mechanical & hormonal effects on GI system.
  • Consider antacid administration & rapid sequence induction of GA in these pts.

INTRAOP
■ Standard ASA monitors
■ Additional vascular access if excessive blood loss considered possible
■ Availability of blood products if coagulopathy present

POSTOP

Pain
■ Usually mild & controlled w/ PO analgesics

Complications
■ Bleeding
■ Infection
■ Coagulopathy

SURGICAL PROCEDURE

Indications
■ Abnormal uterine bleeding (diagnostic or therapeutic)
■ Therapeutic abortions
■ Retained placenta postpartum

Procedure
■ Procedure is preceded by the insertion of laminaria tents on the day prior to, or cervical dilators on the day of, surgery to gradually dilate cervix.
■ Through dilated cervix, curet or gentle suction is used to scrape & loosen lining of uterus.
■ Hysteroscope sometimes used for visualization

Surgical Concerns
■ Excessive blood loss if coagulopathy present

Typical EBL
■ Minimal to >100 cc

ELECTROCONVULSIVE THERAPY (ECT)

WYNDA W. CHUNG, MD

PREOP

Preop Considerations

- Pts w/ the following conditions may require special considerations:
  - Pts w/ intracranial lesions require invasive monitoring (ie, arterial line), w/ tight hemodynamic control.
  - Pregnant pts should be intubated, w/ close fetal monitoring & left uterine displacement.
  - Pts w/ gastroesophageal reflux disease may require aspiration prophylaxis & rapid sequence induction/intubation.
  - Pts w/ severe cardiac dysfunction may require invasive monitoring.
  - Those w/ pacemakers may safely undergo treatment, but a magnet should be readily available if there is a need to convert to a fixed mode.
- Psychiatric drug interactions
  - Tricyclic antidepressants (including amitriptyline, nortriptyline, imipramine, doxepin).
    - Inhibit reuptake of norepinephrine & serotonin.
    - As a result, the response to indirect-acting sympathomimetics (eg, ephedrine) may be attenuated.
    - There may be an exaggerated pressor response to direct-acting sympathomimetics, as well as anticholinergics.
    - ECG changes (eg, widened QRS complex, prolonged PR interval, T wave abnormalities) are common in these pts.
  - MAO inhibitors (including phenelzine, isocarboxazid)
    - Inhibition of MAO leads to an increase in intracellular epinephrine, norepinephrine, dopamine & serotonin levels. This has the potential to adversely affect hemodynamic instability.
    - Meperidine & ephedrine should be avoided because of potential drug interactions.
    - Discontinuation of MAO inhibitors before anesthesia is unnecessary.
  - Selective serotonin reuptake inhibitors (including sertraline, fluoxetine, paroxetine).

- No significant anesthetic drug interactions.
- These drugs may increase ECT-induced seizure duration.

Physical Findings
- None typical

Workup
- Careful history & physical exam, w/ evaluation of comorbid conditions

Choice of Anesthesia
- GA is required for only a brief period (1–5 min). Accordingly, only small doses of short-acting agents are used, in conjunction w/ succinylcholine.
- Methohexital is the traditional induction agent for ECT, but thiopental, propofol, or etomidate may be used.
- The seizure itself usually results in a brief period of amnesia, somnolence & often confusion.

INTRAOP

Monitors/Line Placement
- Routine monitoring for GA.
- One peripheral IV.
- Seizure activity is sometimes monitored by an EEG.
  - Seizure activity can also be monitored in an isolated extremity.
    - Tourniquet is inflated around one extremity prior to injection of succinylcholine, thereby preventing entry of muscle relaxant & allowing observation of convulsive motor activity in the extremity.

Intraop Concerns
- Seizure activity is associated w/ an initial parasympathetic discharge, followed by a more sustained sympathetic response.
  - Bradycardia, mild hypotension & increased secretions characterize the initial phase.
  - Marked bradycardia (<30 bpm) & even transient asystole (up to 6 sec) are occasionally seen.
  - The hypertension & tachycardia that follow are typically sustained for several minutes.
- Transient autonomic imbalance can produce:
  - Arrhythmias (atrial or ventricular).

- ➤ PR-interval prolongation.
- ➤ Increased QT interval.
- ➤ T wave abnormalities on the ECG.
- ■ An increase in cerebral blood flow & cerebral metabolic rate leads to an increase in ICP.
- ■ Intragastric & intraocular pressure may also transiently increase.

Intraop Therapies
- ■ Following adequate preoxygenation, administer IV induction agent.
  - ➤ Methohexital 0.5–1 mg/kg is most commonly employed.
    - • In very small doses, methohexital may actually enhance seizure activity.
  - ➤ Propofol 1–1.5 mg/kg may be used, but higher dosing may result in reduced seizure duration.
  - ➤ Minimize or avoid benzodiazepines, since they raise seizure threshold & decrease duration.
  - ➤ Ketamine increases seizure duration but also increases incidence of delayed awakening, nausea & ataxia.
  - ➤ Etomidate may also prolong recovery.
  - ➤ Short-acting opioids such as alfentanil alone do not produce amnesia.
    - • However, alfentanil (10–25 mcg/kg) can be a useful adjunct when small doses of Brevital are required in pts w/ high seizure threshold.
  - ➤ Increases in seizure threshold are often observed w/ each subsequent ECT.
- ■ Administer muscle relaxant.
  - ➤ Muscle paralysis is required from the time of electrical stimulation until the end of the seizure to prevent injury from tonic-clonic contracture (eg, long bone fracture).
  - ➤ A short-acting agent, such as succinylcholine (0.25–0.5 mg/kg), is most often used.
- ■ Place bite block or tongue protector.
- ■ Psychiatrist will administer a unilateral or bilateral electrical stimulus to induce seizure.
- ■ Continue controlled mask ventilation w/ 100% oxygen until spontaneous ventilation resumes.
- ■ Hyperventilation can increase seizure duration by up to 20%.
- ■ Mgt of common cardiovascular events
  - ➤ Treat pronounced parasympathetic effects w/ atropine.

➤ Alpha & beta-adrenergic blockade & nitroglycerin have been successful in controlling sympathetic manifestations:
  • Labetalol 10–20 mg IV.
  • Esmolol 40–80 mg IV.
  • However, high doses of beta-adrenergic blockade (esmolol 200 mg) may be assoc w/ decreased seizure duration.
➤ As noted above, pts w/ pacemakers may safely undergo treatment, but a magnet should be readily available if there is a need to convert to a fixed output mode.

POSTOP
■ Following the procedure, pt needs to be monitored in PACU.
■ Pt may subsequently be discharged to home or transferred to the hospital ward.

Pain
■ Minimal, although myalgias are possible.

Complications
■ Most common: headaches, myalgias.
■ Postictal confusion is common; anterograde & retrograde memory loss do occur.
  ➤ Most pts recover from memory loss in 1–3 weeks following treatment.
■ Cardiac events (comprised mainly of malignant arrhythmias & myocardial infarctions) account for 67% of all ECT-related mortalities.
■ Pulmonary events (eg, pulmonary edema, emboli, or obstruction) account for most other mortality.
■ Cerebrovascular events have rarely been cited w/ ECT.

SURGICAL PROCEDURE
Indications
■ Depression

Procedure
■ ECT
  ➤ Electrical stimuli are administered until a therapeutic seizure is induced (approx 30–60 sec in duration).
  ➤ A good therapeutic effect is generally not achieved until a total of 400–700 sec of seizure has been induced.

➤ Since only one treatment is given per day, pts are usually scheduled for a series of treatments, usually 2 or 3 per wk.

➤ Progressive memory loss often occurs w/ an increasing number of treatments (esp when electrodes are applied bilaterally).

➤ Of those receiving ECT, 75–85% have a favorable response.

Surgical Concerns
■ Contraindications
  ➤ Absolute contraindications: recent myocardial infarction (usually <3 mo), recent stroke (usually <1 mo), intracranial mass or increased ICP.
  ➤ Relative contraindications: angina, poorly controlled heart failure, significant pulmonary disease, bone fractures, severe osteoporosis, glaucoma, retinal detachment, thrombophlebitis, pregnancy.
■ Lithium is associated w/ post-therapy confusion, delirium.
■ Current mortality rate for ECT is estimated to be one death per 10,000 treatments.

Typical EBL
■ None

EMERGENT CESAREAN SECTION

JOHN P. LEE, MD
SAM HUGHES, MD
MARK ROSEN, MD

PREOP

Preop Considerations
■ An OR should be set up & ready for emergent ("crash") C-section at all times, w/ anesthetic machine, monitors, drugs, & supplies immediately available
■ Anesthetic implications of physiologic changes of pregnancy
  ➤ Need for left uterine displacement
  ➤ Presence of decreased FRC
  ➤ Requirement for full stomach precautions: administer nonparticulate antacid (eg, bicarbonate) preop
■ Rapid consultation w/ obstetrician regarding indication & timing of C-section

Physical Findings
- Possible difficult airway from weight gain of pregnancy & capillary engorgement
- Expect systolic murmur

Workup
- Abbreviated history & PE (perform airway exam at least)

Choice of Anesthesia
- Indication for emergency (hemorrhage, preeclampsia, medical disease, amniotic fluid embolism or other obstetric problem) can help guide anesthetic choice.
- Communication w/ obstetrician essential for balancing maternal risk vs fetal benefit.
- Rapidity of regional vs general anesthesia, risk of maternal airway mgt w/ general anesthesia, & gravity of fetal condition must be considered.
  - GA: Most rapid & reliable, but includes airway mgt risks.
    - Regional anesthesia takes longer than GA.
    - Spinal anesthesia preferred regional technique if no existing block or functioning epidural catheter is present.
    - If there is a functioning indwelling epidural catheter: Most rapid agent is 3% 2-chloroprocaine (2% lidocaine has an onset of about 8–12 min if there is a functioning labor epidural).

INTRAOP

Monitors/Line Placement
- Pulse oximeter, blood pressure cuff, EKG in that order.
- Continue fetal monitoring (FHR) for as long as possible. Check FHR upon arrival in OR.
- Need large-bore IV.
- Consider induction before all monitors placed & patient prepped & draped (controversial).

Intraop Concerns
- Same as for nonemergent C-section.
  - Failed intubation.
  - Aspiration.
  - Hemorrhage.
  - Hypotension.
  - Seizure from accidental rapid injection of local anesthetic IV.

➤ Rare: air or amniotic fluid embolus.
➤ Uterine exteriorization often causes nausea.

Intraop Therapies
■ Aspiration and/or failed intubation
  ➤ Maintain cricoid pressure.
  ➤ Ventilate by mask or LMA.
  ➤ Proceed w/ general anesthetic.
  ➤ After delivery, re-attempt to secure airway.
■ Inadequate ventilation by mask or LMA
  ➤ Consider cricothyrotomy.
  ➤ Otherwise awaken mother & consider regional anesthetic (continuous spinal).
  ➤ Maternal life should be guarded compared w/ fetal life.
■ Maternal hypotension w/ regional anesthesia is common. Rx is:
  ➤ Left uterine displacement.
  ➤ Fluids.
  ➤ Ephedrine 10–25 mg IV or 10–50 mcg phenylephrine (if ephedrine unsuccessful after 3 doses).
■ Patchy block can be supplemented by additional local anesthetic (epidural), or conscious sedation (IV fentanyl, midazolam, propofol, and/or ketamine, 0.25 mg/kg).
■ Uterine atony & hemorrhage: Observe uterine tone after placenta delivered for indication of possible hemorrhage. Rx is:
  ➤ Uterine massage.
  ➤ Oxytocin administered after placenta delivered: 20–40 IU in 1 L by rapid infusion, not IV push (hypotension, cardiac arrest reported).
  ➤ Methylergonovine (Methergine) 0.2 mg IM or prostaglandin F 2-alpha (Hemabate) 0.25 mg IM if atony unresponsive to oxytocin alone. Doses may be repeated.
  ➤ Consider fluid resuscitation w/ colloid, additional IV access, & call for blood if bleeding persists or profound.

POSTOP

Pain
■ Intrathecal (0.15–0.2 mg) or epidural morphine (4–5 mg) for postop pain control
■ Consider ketorolac (15–30 mg IV/IM) for synergism.
■ Narcotics via PCA
■ Continuous epidural infusion of dilute local anesthetic; rarely indicated

Complications
- Postpartum hemorrhage from uterine atony, genital tract disruption, retained placenta & membranes (may require manual removal of placenta, D&C, reoperation [hysterectomy])

SURGICAL PROCEDURE

Indications
- Fetal "distress" (imprecise term for variable gravity of fetal well-being)
- Maternal hemorrhage (eg, abruption, uterine rupture, placenta previa)
- Breech
- Prolapsed cord

Procedure
- Involves incision through the uterus, delivery of the baby, exteriorization of the uterus, repair of the uterine incision, manual massage of the uterus to promote a contracted uterus
- Persistent bleeding may require cross-clamp of uterine arteries or even hysterectomy

Surgical Concerns
- Fast but safe time from incision to delivery

Typical EBL
- 1,000 mL (more if maternal hemorrhage indication for procedure)
- Hard to estimate due to amniotic fluid

ENDOSCOPIC SINUS SURGERY

JASON WIDRICH, MD

PREOP

Preop Considerations
- Most pts scheduled for endoscopic sinus surgery have recurrent acute sinusitis or chronic sinusitis that has not improved w/ medical therapy.
  - ➤ Medical therapy of sinusitis may include antibiotics, decongestants, topical steroids, antihistamines.
- Increasing use of endoscopic sinus surgery has reduced use of more invasive procedures such as Caldwell-Luc operation.

Physical Findings

- None typical, though may have tenderness over sinuses

Workup

- Prior to endoscopic sinus surgery, pt will have nasal endoscopy to evaluate
  - Middle turbinate
  - Middle meatus & osteomeatal complex
  - Nasal polyps
  - Mucus or purulent discharge
  - Anatomic causes of obstruction
- CT scan typically done to evaluate sinus anatomy & relationship to other vital structures (eg, carotid artery, optic nerve, orbit)

Choice of Anesthesia

- GA or MAC w/ local anesthesia

INTRAOP

Monitors/Line Placement

- Standard monitors
- One peripheral IV

Intraop Concerns

- Positioning: head of bed is usually elevated & turned toward surgeon
- Arrhythmias or hypertension from use of cocaine or epinephrine-containing local anesthetic
- Aspiration of blood

Intraop Therapies

- For GA, suction pharynx thoroughly prior to extubation

POSTOP

Pain

- Mild
- IV or PO narcotics
- Acetaminophen

Complications

- Bruising around eye
- Worsening or persistence of facial pain (sphenopalatine ganglion often implicated)
- Rare but serious complications

➤ Blindness from optic nerve damage

➤ CSF leak causing rhinorrhea

SURGICAL PROCEDURE

Indications

- Recurrent acute sinusitis
- Chronic sinusitis
- Nasal polyps

Procedure

- Nasal mucosa is packed w/ local anesthetic & vasoconstrictor solution.
- Endoscopes used for visualization.
- Goal of surgery is to remove osteomeatal blockage, restore normal sinus ventilation & mucociliary function.
- Tissues can be removed or biopsied w/ a variety of equipment under endoscopic guidance.
- Image-guided navigation system may be used.

Surgical Concerns

- Infection
- Postop bleeding & orbital hematoma
- CSF leak (rare)
- Blindness (rare)

Typical EBL

- 50–300 mL

ENDOSCOPY, GI

DAVID SHIMABUKURO, MDCM

PREOP

Preop Considerations

- Although performed in the GI suite, fluoroscopy room, or ICU, GI endoscopy should be treated like an OR case.
  - ➤ The procedures include upper (EGD, ERCP) and lower (colonoscopy) procedures for evaluation & treatment of GI bleeding, biliary stent placement, or other diagnostic/therapeutic interventions.

Anesthesia providers are usually requested only in difficult cases (eg, failed prior attempt secondary to inadequate sedation, hemodynamically unstable, active bleeding, multiple comorbidities leading to high risk) & pediatric cases.

Physical Findings
- Flow murmur w/ acute anemia from a significant GI bleed may be present.
- Hepatic findings may occur from chronic liver disease & are related to severity. They can range from none to jaundice, ascites, palmar erythema & spider nevi.

Workup
- Dictated by comorbidities.
- In pts w/ liver disease, consider full coagulation panel & platelet count.
- In pts w/ end-stage liver disease or cancer, also consider CXR & 12-lead ECG.

Choice of Anesthesia
- Depends on procedure being performed & reason it is being done. In most cases, MAC is all that is required; otherwise, GA is indicated.
- The procedure can be as short as a few minutes or as long as several hours.
- In pts undergoing an upper endoscopy, if the pt is vomiting or actively bleeding and/or hemodynamically unstable, then the trachea should be intubated.
- Both upper & lower procedures are done w/ pt in the left lateral decubitus position.

INTRAOP
Monitors/Line Placement
- Routine monitors are usually sufficient, but this depends on comorbidities.
- Arterial line
  - Should be used in any hemodynamically unstable pt (and considered in pts who have required multiple blood transfusions to maintain an adequate hemoglobin level).
  - Should also be considered in pts w/ probable bleeding esophageal varices, as they can decompensate very quickly.
- Peripheral IV access

➤ In a pt who is bleeding, two large-bore peripheral IVs (16g or larger) are required.
➤ If peripheral access is difficult, one peripherally placed rapid infusion catheter (eg, 7 Fr), a double-lumen 8 Fr central venous line (CVL), or introducer catheter CVL (any size) can be used instead.

Intraop Concerns
- Universal precautions (especially eye protection) are imperative as there is a high incidence of hepatitis among these patients.
- In patients undergoing an upper endoscopy, the airway is shared.
- The endoscope can be removed immediately should it be necessary for airway mgt.
- In pts w/ end-stage liver disease, benzodiazepines should be avoided, as their metabolism is extremely slow, w/ prolongation of drug effect.
- Epinephrine is sometimes used for sclerotherapy in peptic ulcer disease & can be systemically absorbed; if it is inappropriate for the pt, discuss its use with the endoscopist.
- Bleeding: normal EBL is none to minimal but can be liters if there is an active bleed w/ difficult hemostasis.
- These procedures are normally done outside the OR, where assistance from other anesthesiologists or OR staff is not readily available.

Intraop Therapies
- For bleeding pts, banding, sclerotherapy, and/or cauterization.
- An IV octreotide infusion may be requested.
- For esophageal or biliary strictures, dilation and/or stent placement.
- During diagnostic procedures, polypectomies & biopsies commonly done.

POSTOP
- Typically, pts are extubated at the end of the procedure when they are awake & able to protect their airway.
- These pts are recovered as would any pt receiving GA or MAC (eg, in the PACU or ICU).

Pain
- Usually none

Complications
- Usually limited to aspiration, MI, infection.
- Perforation of the GI tract can always occur.

- Secondary to insufflation of gas, subcutaneous emphysema can also occur.

SURGICAL PROCEDURE

Indications
- Diagnostic and/or therapeutic interventions for GI disorders

Procedure
- Involves placement of an endoscope via the oral cavity or anus
- Normally uncomfortable but not painful

Surgical Concerns
- Gag reflex normally blunted by topical anesthesia and/or IV meds
- During an upper endoscopy, the airway is shared

Typical EBL
- Minimal, but can be liters in a pt w/ an active GI bleed

ENDOVASCULAR AAA REPAIR

DANIEL M. SWANGARD, MD

PREOP

Preop considerations
- ➤ Pts selected for endovascular technique have often been refused open aortic repair.
  - ➤ Hence, moderate or severe coexisting disease(s) may be present.
- Aortic disease is indicative of other vascular disease:
  - ➤ Coronary artery disease
    - MI
    - Stable or unstable angina
    - LV dysfunction/CHF
    - Atrial fibrillation
    - Arrhythmias; cardiac pacemakers are not uncommon in this population
  - ➤ Peripheral vascular disease
  - ➤ Carotid artery disease
- Other common comorbidities include
  - ➤ COPD
  - ➤ HTN

- ➤ Diabetes
- ➤ Renal dysfunction
    - Renal dysfunction is often exacerbated by perioperative angiograms/IV contrast.
    - Can give Mucomyst 600 mg PO BID for renal protection (see NEJM 2000;343:180–4)
- ■ Pts are often taking anticoagulation or antiplatelet agents:
    - ➤ Coumadin
    - ➤ **Heparin**
    - ➤ ASA
    - ➤ Plavix
    - ➤ Ticlid
- ■ Geriatric population undergoing this procedure is at risk of postop delirium.

Physical Findings
- ■ Neck
    - ➤ Carotid bruits
    - ➤ Increased jugular venous pressure
- ■ Pulmonary
    - ➤ Wheezes
    - ➤ Rales
    - ➤ Rhonchi
    - ➤ Distant breath sounds
    - ➤ Barrel chest
- ■ Cardiovascular
    - ➤ Regular vs irregular rhythm
    - ➤ Presence of S3 or S4
    - ➤ Murmurs
    - ➤ Displaced apical impulse
- ■ Abdomen
    - ➤ Bruits
    - ➤ Pulsatile masses
    - ➤ Obesity
- ■ Extremities
    - ➤ Diminished or absent lower extremity pulses
    - ➤ Nonhealing ulcers
    - ➤ Distal embolic phenomena

Workup
- ■ Ask regarding:

➤ Functional status/exercise tolerance as guide to severity of cardiovascular & pulmonary disease

➤ Can pt lie flat for duration of procedure?

■ ECG: Obtain an old ECG to help assess for changes

■ Persantine thallium test/dobutamine echo: Consider using these tests for cardiac risk stratification in pts w/:

➤ New or changing anginal pattern

➤ New ECG changes

➤ Recent CHF/MI

➤ Multiple cardiac risk factors in setting of poor functional status

■ Carotid ultrasound is indicated if bruits are present, esp if there is a history of stroke or TIA.

■ PFTs or ABG usually not indicated; consider plasma HCO_3 level to assess for CO_2 retention.

■ Lab tests

➤ CBC

➤ Cr

➤ PT/PTT

➤ Consider electrolytes for pts on diuretics, ACE inhibitors, or history of renal insufficiency or failure.

■ Start beta blockade.

➤ This reduces cardiac risk in at-risk pts.

■ Consider involving cardiology service to follow pts in periop period.

Choice of Anesthesia

■ Regional technique preferred

➤ Lumbar epidural

• Check if pt is on anticoagulants before attempting epidural; may need to check coags (eg, PTT) to establish whether epidural can be placed safely.

• Epidural placement is NOT contraindicated by usual intraop heparinization.

• T12 level needed

• 8–10 cc of local anesthetic (eg, 2% lidocaine or mepivacaine) often adequate

• If blood is obtained w/ epidural needle or catheter aspiration, attempt catheter placement up or down one level.

➤ Spinal or continuous spinal

• Check if pt is on anticoagulants before attempting spinal; may need to check coags (eg, PTT) to establish whether regional technique can be performed safely.

- Spinal or continuous spinal placement is NOT contraindicated by usual intraop heparinization.
- Length of procedure is determined by center experience (may be >3 h); for lengthy cases, use a continuous spinal: titrate 0.75% bupivacaine to obtain a T12 level (total of ~8–10 mg total first dose is often adequate) w/ redosing q60–90 min using 1/3–1/2 initial dose & close monitoring of level of anesthesia.

■ General anesthesia acceptable

INTRAOP

Monitors/Line Placement

■ Standard monitors

■ Two 14–18g IVs

■ Arterial line: Common for monitoring activated clotting time, other labs, close BP monitoring in population w/ cardiac comorbidities

■ Central line usually not required unless there is a history of significant left ventricular dysfunction or decompensated CHF

■ PA line usually not required

■ TEE may be considered w/ GA as a monitor for ischemia/wall motion abnormality in pts w/ severe CAD/LV dysfunction or symptomatic valvular lesions

Intraop Concerns

■ Regional techniques
  ➤ Anticipate significant decreases in BP due to sympathectomy.
  ➤ Consider gentle fluid bolus (500–1,000 cc) w/ dosing.

■ Stent-graft deployment
  ➤ Deployment is brief.
  ➤ Stents are most often self-expanding.
  ➤ Stent may be further expanded using angiographic balloon; mild increases in SVR w/ balloon inflation do occur.
  ➤ Typical increases in SVR seen w/ open repair are NOT observed.

■ Distal ischemia: Most often brief; changes such as decreased SVR, decreased pH, & increased pCO_2 assoc w/ aortic clamp release in open repairs are not observed.

■ Cardiac ischemia
  ➤ Important to maintain hemodynamic stability
  ➤ Strongly consider beta blockade

■ COPD & its attendant symptoms
  ➤ Secretions
  ➤ Wheezing

- ➤ SOB
- ➤ Coughing in awake pts
- ■ Cerebrovascular Dz
- ■ Maintain BP within 10–15% of baseline values.
- ■ LV diastolic dysfunction
  - ➤ Common due to chronic HTN, LVH
  - ➤ Preload-dependent & sensitive to decreased intravascular volume & decreased sympathetic tone assoc w/ neuraxial anesthesia
- ■ Hemorrhage
  - ➤ May go unrecognized due to retroperitoneal location
  - ➤ Always consider in setting of persistent drops in BP or Hct changes out of proportion to EBL.
- ■ Heparinization
  - ➤ Check baseline activated clotting time (ACT) prior to bolus (normal 100–125 sec).
  - ➤ Desired ACT after dosing usually >2x baseline (ie, 200–250).
  - ➤ Heparin is reversed w/ protamine.
- ■ Diabetes
  - ➤ Follow glucose.
  - ➤ Anticipate insulin resistance due to perioperative stress.
- ■ Diuresis
  - ➤ Can occur due to IV contrast.
  - ➤ Follow U/O.

Intraop Therapies
- ■ Low-dose propofol infusions (10–50 ucg/kg/min) for sedation
- ■ Phenylephrine infusion (10–50 ucg/min) for sympathectomy
  - ➤ Use caution in setting of LV dysfxn.
- ■ Beta blockade (IV metoprolol/esmolol) for cardiac ischemia/risk reduction
  - ➤ Use caution in setting of active COPD or CHF exacerbations.
- ■ Beta agonists & anticholinergics (Atrovent) as needed for COPD
  - ➤ Be aware of resulting tachycardia (B agonists) in setting of CAD.
- ■ Heparin
  - ➤ 100 U/kg IV bolus
  - ➤ Maintenance ~10 U/kg q45–60min
- ■ Protamine
  - ➤ 5–10 mg/1,000 U of initial heparin bolus.
  - ➤ Always use a test dose 5–10 mg.

➤ Observe closely for protamine reactions (more common in pts taking NPH insulin).

POSTOP
Pain
- Usually mild
- Request bupivacaine infiltration to incisions following closure.
- IV opiates first 24 hours followed by oral agents such as Vicodin or Percocet.
- Consider combination therapies: NSAIDs, Tylenol to reduce opiate requirements.
- Remove epidural & intrathecal catheters after documenting normal coag status in PACU.
  - ➤ Intrathecal opiates & postop epidural infusion usually NOT required.

Complications
- Intraop aneurysm rupture
- Conversion to open repair (rare at experienced centers)
- Iliac artery injury, retroperitoneal hemorrhage (rare at experienced centers)
- Cardiac ischemia, MI, CHF, arrhythmias
- HTN
- COPD exacerbation, atelectasis, pneumonia
- Hyperglycemia, ketoacidosis, hyperosmolar state in diabetic pts
- Postop delirium in elderly pts
- Worsening of pre-existing renal dysfunction due to 80–150 cc IV contrast for required intraop angiograms
- Hypovolemia due to hemorrhage; bleeding can be retroperitoneal & go unrecognized
- Graft-related complications: "endoleaks" (see below)
- Postop fever, leukocytosis common; etiology unknown

SURGICAL PROCEDURE
Indications
- Infrarenal abdominal aortic aneurysms
- Suprarenal & thoracic aortic aneurysms (only at experienced centers)
- Procedure goal: Exclusion of aortic aneurysm from circulation using a stent-graft to span proximal & distal extent of aneurysm

- Desired surgical result: Aneurysmal portion of aorta, once excluded from circulation, thromboses & shrinks over time
- Bilateral horizontal infrainguinal incisions
- Dissection, exposure & control of femoral vessels
- Heparinization
- Percutaneous cannulation of femoral vessels w/ 5–6 Fr angiographic sheath; sheath punctures skin, enters vessel under direct vision within operative field
- Angiographic catheters advanced into aorta under fluoroscopic guidance for baseline angiograms
- Seldinger technique employed to exchange angiographic sheaths for 18–24 Fr stent-graft deployment system
- Aortic stent-graft deployed using fluoroscopic guidance
- Stent-graft types: uni-iliac or bifurcated grafts; most devices self-expanding
  - ➤ Uni-iliac stent-graft spans infrarenal aorta (proximal) to one common iliac artery (distal); this necessitates a fem-fem bypass & contralateral iliac artery occlusion to prevent retrograde flow into aneurysm.
- Bifurcated stent-graft spans infrarenal aorta (proximal) to both common iliac arteries (distal); graft can consist of up to 3 components: 1 bifurcated aortic stent-graft, 2 iliac stent-grafts. Deployment is sequential.
- Angiographic confirmation of proper proximal (infrarenal) & distal implantation/positioning
- Reversal of heparin w/ protamine
- Hemostasis & closure
- PACU for recovery; stepdown unit for postop care

Surgical Concerns
- Aortic rupture & conversion to open repair
- Careful deployment of proximal (infrarenal) portion of stent-graft to avoid even partial renal artery occlusion
- Iliac/femoral artery dissection/injury, retroperitoneal hemorrhage
- Type I endoleak: Leak around proximal aortic implantation site into aneurysm
- Type II endoleak: Retrograde flow into aneurysm from IMA
- Type III endoleak: Leak between aortic & iliac components of bifurcated graft into aneurysm

- Flow via endoleak into aneurysm risks aneurysm rupture; often discovered on follow-up CT imaging; most endoleaks repaired by placement of additional stent-grafts
- Graft migration, graft kinking
- Graft infections (rare)

Typical EBL
- ~250 cc

EPILEPSY SURGERY

MIMI C. LEE, MD, PHD
DHANESH K. GUPTA, MD

PREOP

Preop Considerations
- Epilepsy is a chronic condition characterized by recurrent, unprovoked seizures.
- There are many different classes of seizures, including partial (simple or complex) vs generalized.
- There are many underlying causes of seizures, including intrinsic parenchymal pathology (mass lesions, necrosis, maldevelopment), trauma, & other medical conditions (electrolyte abnormalities, chemical toxicities, & psychosis [nonepileptic seizures]).
- Desired outcome of epilepsy surgery is reduction in seizure frequency w/ continued medical therapy.
- Seizure information
  - ➤ Inquire if pt has aura to help determine when seizures occur.
  - ➤ Determine typical seizure events.
  - ➤ This info is useful in case pt has intraop seizure.
- Seizure meds
  - ➤ Meds may be tapered before surgery.
  - ➤ Pts on chronic anticonvulsants may have rapid metabolism of muscle relaxants.

Physical Findings
- None typical

Workup
- MRI brain
- Head CT
- PET, SPECT

- Video-EEG monitoring
  - ➤ Often performed preop to establish clinical correlation of seizure w/ EEG activity.
  - ➤ Scalp or intraop placed subdural electrodes most commonly used. Stereotactically positioned, intracortical depth electrodes may also be used.
- WADA testing (intracarotid Amytal testing)
  - ➤ Used to predict potential outcome of surgical resection.
  - ➤ Identifies dominant hemisphere for language function & evaluates memory function of isolated, noninvolved hemisphere.

Choice of Anesthesia
- Avoid premed that can change seizure threshold.
- Conscious sedation/neuroleptic anesthesia.
  - ➤ Allows for electrocorticography (EcoG) mapping w/o influence of systemic anesthetics.
  - ➤ Allows for localization of speech center in relationship to seizure focus that may minimize chances of aphasia after resection.
  - ➤ Local anesthetic for pinning & for scalp block by surgeon.
  - ➤ Opiate, tranquilizer, and/or propofol may be administered as boluses or continuous infusions. For example:
    - Alfentanil (0.5–2.0 ug/kg/min), remifentanil (0.05–0.25 mcg/kg/min), or fentanyl.
    - Droperidol (1.25–2.5 mg boluses titrated to sedation & loss of spontaneous speech; known risk for torsades).
    - Propofol (25–100 mcg/kg/min) continuous infusion; discontinue at least 20 min prior to electrocorticography.
    - Diphenhydramine (12.5-mg boluses, max 100 mg).
    - All anesthetics should be discontinued appropriately prior to mapping.
- GA
  - ➤ May be preferable, depending on surgeon & pt.
  - ➤ Warn pt preop about possible awareness, given the need to decrease anesthetics during EcoG.
  - ➤ Use agents w/ minimal effect on EcoG. For craniotomy, resection, & closure, consider:
    - Opiate, muscle relaxant, nitrous oxide.
    - Low-concentration inhaled agent.
    - Propofol infusion.
    - Droperidol.

- Important: Discontinue volatile agent/propofol infusion for EcoG.
➤ Anticipate shorter duration of nondepolarizing muscle relaxation if pt on chronic anticonvulsants.

INTRAOP

Monitors/Line Placement

■ Discuss placement of catheters & lines w/ the surgeon, who may have a preference regarding side of epileptic activity to be monitored intraop (eg, no lines on right arm or leg for left-sided cortical lesions).
■ Two well-taped (18g) peripheral IVs, preferably avoiding joints so they are not dislodged by generalized seizure.
■ Routine ECG, pulse oximetry, nasal cannula w/ $ETCO_2$ (for speech mapping cases) & possibly invasive arterial BP monitoring.

Intraop Concerns

■ Seizures
➤ Learn pt's typical seizure pattern & aura.
■ For awake crani
➤ Minimize fluids if bladder not drained by indwelling catheter.
➤ Maximize pt comfort.
  - Establish rapport w/ pt.
  - Discuss positioning preop. Head may or may not be fixed in pins.
  - Ensure that pt understands & can tolerate immobility for duration of awake component of procedure.
➤ Remind pt to speak before attempting to move!
■ For crani under GA
➤ Do not use agents that will interfere w/ seizure threshold until EcoG complete.
  - Avoid benzodiazepines & barbiturates.
➤ Do not use muscle relaxant during mapping procedures.
➤ Etomidate 7-mg boluses may be given to induce seizure focus during EcoG.

Intraop Therapies

■ For awake crani
➤ Discomfort/pain
  - Administer additional local anesthetic, if appropriate.
  - Administer additional opiate or sedative-hypnotic.
  - Coordinate small adjustments in bed & extremity position w/ pt & surgeon.

➤ Airway obstruction
- Attempt to avoid by judicious titration of sedative & opiates.
- Decrease anesthetic level.
- Increase supplemental oxygen, since nasal cannula may be insufficient. Consider 100% face mask, unilateral or bilateral nasal airways (after topical lidocaine), or oral airway placement until anesthetic level has decreased.
- LMA placement or induction & endotracheal intubation may be required.

■ Seizures
➤ Inform surgeon. Application of cold saline directly on exposed cortex is usually sufficient to stop seizure activity.
➤ If continued seizure activity, administer acute anticonvulsive therapy:
- Methohexital 30–50 mg boluses.
- Propofol 10–20 mg boluses.
- Benzodiazepines (lorazepam 0.1 mg/kg IV or diazepam 0.2 mg/kg IV at 5 mg/min every 5 min prn up to 3 doses) & barbiturates (phenobarbital, up to 20 mg/kg IV infused at <100 mg/min) may be used if EcoG is complete.
- Important: Discuss w/ surgeon prior to administration of long-acting epileptic agents.

POSTOP

Pain
■ Minimal, especially after scalp block w/ local anesthetic
■ Commonly manifests as dull, persistent headache, relieved by acetaminophen w/ or w/o low-dose narcotic

Complications
■ Related to craniotomy (hemorrhage, elevated ICP)
■ Awareness
■ Mobility secondary to uncontrolled seizure
■ Inadequate ventilation or airway obstruction due to oversedation, intraop seizure, or subsequent treatment necessitating endotracheal intubation

SURGICAL PROCEDURE

Indications
Severe & medically uncontrollable seizure disorder after >=1 year of satisfactory medical treatment, resulting in disability
■ Pts w/ EEG-proven temporal lobe focus

- Infrequently, pts w/ extratemporal lobe foci, secondary generalized seizures, or unilateral, multifocal epilepsy assoc w/ infantile hemiplegia syndrome

Procedure
- Resection of epileptic focus
  - Lesion resection (lesionectomy)
  - Cortical resection (corticectomy)
  - Temporal lobectomy
    - Amygdalohippocampectomy, more selective resection of temporal lobe
  - Hemispherectomy
- Disconnection techniques
  - Corpus callosectomy
  - Subpial transection

Surgical Concerns
- Whether to use intraop mapping or stimulation to identify seizure foci
- Type of anesthesia: conscious sedation vs. general
- Degree of resection, minimizing functional deficit
- Concerns of craniotomy

Typical EBL
- <100 cc for limited resection, but may be 1–3 L for hemispherectomy

---

ESOPHAGOSCOPY

ALISON G. CAMERON, MD

PREOP

Preop Considerations
- Esophagoscopy is used for visualization of esophagus for diagnostic or therapeutic interventions.
- May be performed as part of "panendoscopy" (eg, laryngoscopy, bronchoscopy, pharyngoscopy, esophagoscopy) in pt w/ head & neck cancer. In this pt group, common coexisting disease includes.
  - Malnutrition, anemia
  - Tobacco use w/ associated COPD
- Esophagoscopy may be part of upper GI endoscopy (eg, for pt w/ GI bleeding).

➤ See Procedure chapter "GI Endoscopy" for further discussion of upper & lower GI endoscopy & use in GI bleeding.

Physical Findings
- Depend on reason for procedure.
- In pt w/ head & neck cancer, consider whether tumor involves upper airway & whether intubation may be difficult.

Workup
- CBC
- ECG
- CXR
    ➤ Check for esophageal dilatation, retained fluids.
    ➤ Evidence of cardiac or pulmonary disease may be more common in this pt population.
- Dental assessment (risk of dental damage w/ scope placement).
- Careful airway assessment, especially in pts w/ head & neck cancer.

Choice of Anesthesia
- Consider antisialogogue (eg, glycopyrrolate 0.2 mg IV).
- GA w/ cuffed ETT is required for rigid esophagoscopy.
- MAC can be used w/ fiberoptic esophagoscopy.

INTRAOP

Monitors/Line Placement
- Standard ASA monitors
- One peripheral IV
- Other monitors as required by other parts of procedure
    ➤ Esophagoscopy may be performed as part of cancer surgery (eg, panendoscopy, radical neck dissection).

Intraop Concerns
- Shoulder roll placed to facilitate neck extension & scope placement.
- Rigid scope may dislodge ETT.
    ➤ Tape securely & observe position closely during surgery.
- Procedure duration may be short, affecting choice of anesthetic agents & muscle relaxants.

Intraop Therapies
- Muscle relaxation may facilitate placement of rigid scope.
- Adequate depth of anesthesia to minimize chance of pt movement & esophageal perforation.

POSTOP

Pain
- Minimal to mild.
- Acetaminophen or IV opioids usually adequate.

Complications
- Perforation or laceration of esophagus.
  - ➤ This can be a catastrophic complication & can result in severe illness, including sepsis, massive hemorrhage, pneumo/ hemomediastinum, mediastinitis, pneumo/ hemothorax, inability to swallow, dehydration, pleural effusion.
  - ➤ Signs include tachycardia, fever, hypotension, upper chest crepitus, mediastinal air on CXR, possible pulmonary insufficiency w/ ensuing cardiac compromise.
  - ➤ Therapy may include surgical repair & drainage.
- Dental damage
- Aspiration

SURGICAL PROCEDURE

Indications
- Removal of foreign bodies.
- Diagnostic/therapeutic visualization/biopsies of tumors.
- Esophageal dilatation for esophageal strictures.
- Tracheoesophageal fistula.

Procedure
- Rigid esophagoscope or flexible gastroscope inserted through mouth to view entire length of esophagus.
- For foreign body removal, forceps will be passed through the scope.
- Biopsies may be taken, as well as ligation/cautery of varices or other bleeding sources.
- For dilatation, balloon or sized dilators may be used.

Surgical Concerns
- Inadequate muscle relaxation resulting in inability to open mouth adequately for scope placement.
- Pt movement, increasing risk of esophageal perforation.
- Cervical spine instability limiting neck extension.
- Aspiration.

Typical EBL
- Minimal, unless indication for procedure is GI bleeding.

EXCISION OF MEDIASTINAL MASS

JAMES HSU, MD

PREOP

Preop Considerations
- See also Coexisting Disease chapter "Patient With Mediastinal Mass."
- Pts can present special challenges because of the possibility of tracheobronchial obstruction & hemodynamic collapse from compression of the heart and/or great vessels.
  - ➤ Tumor obstruction of major airways can occur around the tracheobronchial tree, distal to the ETT.
  - ➤ Also, intubation in a pt w/ an airway distorted from tumor compression may result in complete occlusion of the ETT.
  - ➤ Loss of spontaneous ventilation may cause loss of support of critically narrowed air passages, leading to airway obstruction that may not be overcome w/ positive-pressure ventilation.
- For lymphomas, radiation or chemotherapy generally results in a decrease in tumor size & a reduction in symptoms.
  - ➤ If possible, such treatments should be rendered before GA is used.

Physical Findings
- Seek symptoms & signs in the supine & sitting positions:
  - ➤ Cough.
  - ➤ Dyspnea.
  - ➤ Stridor.
  - ➤ Inspiratory intercostal muscle retraction.
  - ➤ Tachypnea.
  - ➤ Wheezing.
  - ➤ SVC syndrome (distended neck veins, varicosities over chest & upper extremities, increased neck girth).
- Asymptomatic pts can develop airway obstruction during anesthesia, so the absence of symptoms doesn't ensure a patent airway during anesthesia.

Workup
- CT or MRI scan to identify tumor size & location, severity of airway narrowing.
- Echocardiogram.
- Flow-volume loops (obtain in sitting & supine positions).

Choice of Anesthesia
- Anesthetic mgt principles.
    - When possible, perform procedures under local anesthesia, maintaining spontaneous ventilation.
    - If possible, shrink a symptomatic tumor w/ radiation or chemotherapy before undergoing GA.
    - If GA is required, examine the tracheobronchial tree w/ a fiberoptic bronchoscope & consider an awake intubation.
    - Whenever possible, maintain spontaneous ventilation during GA.
- Discuss w/ surgeon whether pt may require cardiopulmonary bypass for the procedure. Ensure that appropriate equipment & personnel are available.

INTRAOP

Monitors/Line Placement
- Standard monitors + arterial line, CVP.
- Consider PA line (for TBT obstruction or compression of PA or heart).
- TEE may be used if pt is under GA.
- Lines
- Consider whether central line should be placed in femoral vein to avoid region of tumor.
- Large-bore IV lines for rapid fluid administration.
- For SVC obstruction, use lower extremity IV lines.

Intraop Concerns
- Tracheobronchial obstruction, loss of airway.
    - Pt may require semi-Fowler's or other position.
    - Maintain spontaneous ventilation when possible.
    - Positive-pressure ventilation may or may not help the airway obstruction.
- Consider armored endotracheal tube: may be less prone to kinking or obstruction.
- Examine airway by fiberoptic bronchoscope preop or immediately after induction.
- Vascular obstruction of great vessels.
    - Consider monitoring w/ TEE.
    - Change pt position to alleviate compression.
- Tumor lysis syndrome if recent chemotherapy.

Maintain close communication w/ surgeons regarding hemodynamic stability w/ intraop manipulation.

Consider whether pt should remain intubated or would benefit from postop ICU care.

POSTOP

Pain

■ Tends to be severe; may be managed by either a thoracic epidural or a PCA. Thoracotomy incision is generally more painful than median sternotomy. A PCA may be preferred if CPB is anticipated.

Complications

■ If surgery not successful in removing tumor, pt is still at risk for previously discussed complications: loss of airway, airway obstruction, inability to ventilate/oxygenate w/ positive-pressure ventilation, hypoxemia, hypercarbia.

SURGICAL PROCEDURE

Indications

■ Adults: majority of tumors involve hilar lymph nodes w/ bronchial carcinoma or lymphoma, but benign conditions such as cystic hygroma, teratoma, thymoma & thyroid tumors can occur.
■ Pediatrics: most masses are benign bronchial cysts, esophageal duplication, or teratomas.
■ W/ tumors involving the tracheobronchial tree & compression of the great vessels, CPB should be immediately available.

Procedure

■ Either a thoracotomy (in the lateral position) or a median sternotomy (in the supine position), depending on tumor involvement of the tracheobronchial tree & great vessels, and/or the chances of requiring CPB

Typical EBL

■ Highly variable depending on involvement of the great vessels & tracheobronchial tree

---

EXTRACORPOREAL SHOCKWAVE LITHOTRIPSY (ESWL)

JASON WIDRICH, MD

PREOP

Preop Considerations

■ ESWL used for treatment of stones in ureter & kidney

- Types of lithotripters
  - Percutaneous
    - Immersion: Pt placed in semi-sitting position, immersed in water to the shoulders. Electrohydraulic shock wave is focused through the fluid toward the stone. Most painful but probably most effective form of ESWL. Less common now than dry coupling methods.
    - Nonimmersion: Electromagnetic or piezoelectric shockwave focused on stone. More comfortable procedure for pt.
  - Laser
    - Involves endoscopy & laser vaporization of stones.
    - Least painful form of lithotripsy.
- Obesity may increase the difficulty of focusing the shockwave blast path.

Workup
- CBC w/platelets, electrolytes, BUN, Cr.
- Urologist may order CXR, KUB, CT scan for stone location.
- Stop aspirin, NSAIDs, & anticoagulant medication. Obtain PT/PTT if history suggests bleeding disorder.
- Pt w/ pacemaker or ICD:
  - Interrogate pacemaker/AICD prior to procedure to prevent triggering or other malfunctions w/ initiation of shockwave.
  - Consider changing pacemaker to fixed output mode (eg, VOO, DOO) to prevent inhibition by shockwave.
  - Consider deactivating defibrillation function of ICD during procedure.

Choice of Anesthesia
- Procedure can be performed under GA, regional anesthesia, or conscious sedation.
- Regional anesthesia should cover to T8 level.
- Pain from ESWL influenced by power of shockwave, size & distribution of shockwave entry point, as well as pt's pain threshold.

INTRAOP
Monitors/Line Placement
- One peripheral IV
- Standard monitors
- Immersion lithotripsy
  - Ensure BP cuff will tolerate immersion.
  - Attach ECG to exposed skin on shoulders or upper chest.

➤ Attach pulse oximeter probe to nose or earlobe.

➤ May need to prepare longer IV tubing, respiratory circuit & monitoring lines.

➤ Measure temp. Maintain immersion fluid at body temp or slightly warmer to prevent hypothermia.

Intraop Concerns

- Cardiac arrhythmias possible, although shockwaves are timed to QRS complex.
- Minimize pt movement, which could affect focus point of shockwave.
- Pacemaker/ICD pt: Keep device away from shockwave blast path.
- Immersion
  - ➤ Anticipate reduced lung volumes: FRC, VC.
  - ➤ Anticipate increased cardiac filling pressures, though may be offset by vasodilation from warm immersion fluid.

Intraop Therapies

- Surgeon may request therapy (atropine, glycopyrrolate) to increase heart rate. Shocks are synchronized w/ the ECG R wave & a rapid heart rate will therefore shorten the procedure.
- Cardiac arrhythmias
  - ➤ Usually disappear when shockwaves are discontinued.
  - ➤ Treat persistent dysrhythmias.

POSTOP

Pain

- PO narcotics are usually sufficient for pain control, & procedure usually done as outpatient.

Complications

- Hematuria, skin abrasion/bruising common.
- Perinephric hematoma: May rarely cause anemia & require blood transfusion.
- Pulmonary contusion rare. For children, consider padding thorax w/ foam.

SURGICAL PROCEDURE

Indications

- Renal or ureteral calculi

Procedure
- Pt placed on OR table. Lithotripter placed on pt's skin. Shockwave focused on stone.
  - Immersion: Pt is placed in metal frame, lowered into immersion bath to shoulders. Shockwaves focused on the stone, guided by fluoroscopy.
- Typically 3,000 shocks administered at one session.

Surgical Concerns
- Stone volume, stone composition, clearance of fragments by functioning renal unit.
- Consideration of alternate procedure (eg, percutaneous nephrolithotomy, ureteroscopy).
- Consider risk in pt w/ abdominal aortic aneurysm, pregnancy, solitary kidney.

Typical EBL
- Minimal to none

EYELID BLEPHAROPLASTY

JASON WIDRICH, MD

PREOP

Preop Considerations
- Surgery for baggy eyelids or "droopy" upper eyelid affecting vision
  - Usually done for cosmetic reasons, although upper eyelid skin can occasionally obstruct peripheral vision
  - May be done as sole procedure or as part of other facial plastic surgery, such as browlift, facelift, or skin resurfacing
- Pt may have ocular or neurologic symptoms
  - Dry eyes, previous infections, visual field abnormality
  - Eyelid droop may be secondary to neuro deficit (eg, Horner's syndrome)

Physical Findings
- Lid droop or excess fatty tissue above or below eye
- Other findings could include
  - Horner's syndrome: ptosis, miosis, anidrosis
  - Cranial nerve deficits
  - Vision or visual field change

Workup

- Surgeon generally evaluates for eye disorders (eg, vision, visual field tests).

Choice of Anesthesia

- For blepharoplasty as the sole procedure, local anesthesia plus conscious sedation is usually adequate.
- Some surgeons feel that local anesthesia may distort anatomy & may request GA.
- GA may be appropriate for pts undergoing multiple cosmetic procedures (eg, facelift, browlift, skin resurfacing).

INTRAOP

Monitors/Line Placement

- Standard monitors
- One peripheral IV

Intraop Concerns

- Pressure from mask ventilation may affect cosmetic repair at emergence.
- Intravascular absorption of epinephrine or local anesthetic.
  - ➤ Not usually a concern if low volumes of local anesthetic used.
- Uncontrolled HTN may cause hematoma or affect surgical repair.
- Oculocardiac reflex may occur, manifest as bradycardia or other arrhythmias.

Intraop Therapies

- For oculocardiac reflex, stop stimulus; glycopyrrolate or atropine for persistent bradycardia.

POSTOP

Pain

- Minimal, especially if local anesthetic used

Complications

- Hematoma
  - ➤ Can occur from coagulopathy or hypertension
  - ➤ Can rarely cause retrobulbar hematoma
    - Symptoms of retrobulbar hematoma include chemosis, mydriasis, proptosis, conjunctival injection
- Blindness
  - ➤ Rare complication

➤ Generally occurs from retrobulbar hematoma w/ optic nerve compression
■ Corneal abrasion
■ Dry eye syndrome (keratoconjunctivitis sicca)

SURGICAL PROCEDURE

Indications
■ Elective for cosmetic effect
■ Lid ptosis that obstructs vision

Procedure
■ Local anesthetic w/ epinephrine is injected into area of incision
■ Skin incision
➤ For the lower eyelid, incisions may be done through transconjunctival approach w/o skin incision
■ Removal of excess skin, fat, muscle
■ Closure

Surgical Concerns
■ Symmetry of eyes
■ Patient satisfaction w/ cosmetic effect
■ Hematoma (subcutaneous or retrobulbar)
■ Blindness (from retrobulbar hematoma & optic nerve compression)
■ Ptosis
■ Entropion
■ Ectropion
■ Infection
■ Facial nerve injury
■ Diplopia

Typical EBL
■ Minimal

FEMORAL-FEMORAL BYPASS, ILIOFEMORAL BYPASS

DANIEL M. SWANGARD, MD

PREOP

Preop Considerations
■ Peripheral vascular disease is associated w/ coronary artery disease (CAD) & cerebrovascular disease

- Obtain history of CAD
  - MI
  - Stable vs unstable angina
  - LV dysfunction or CHF
  - Atrial fibrillation
- Common comorbidities
  - COPD
  - HTN
  - Diabetes mellitus
- Geriatric population at risk of postop delirium
- Renal dysfunction often exacerbated by IV contrast from preop angiogram
- Anticoagulation/antiplatelet agents
  - Pts are often taking Coumadin, ASA, Plavix, Ticlid.
  - Heparin infusions or enoxaparin also possible for acutely ischemic leg

Physical Findings
- Because of common occurrence of coexisting disease, many physical findings are possible
- Vital signs
  - May have elevated BP
  - Increased HR
  - Reduced SpO_2
- Neck
  - Carotid bruits
  - Increased JVP
- Pulmonary
  - Wheezes
  - Rales
  - Rhonchi
  - Distant breath sounds
  - Barrel chest
- CV
  - Note heart rate
  - Regular vs irregular rhythm
  - Presence of S3 or S4
  - Murmurs
  - Displaced apical impulse
- Abdomen
  - Bruits
  - Pulsatile masses

- Extremities
  - Diminished or absent lower extremity pulses
  - Coolness or pallor
  - Nonhealing ulcers
  - Peripheral embolic phenomena

Workup
- Ask about functional status/exercise tolerance as guide to severity of CV & pulmonary disease.
- An old ECG is helpful to assess for changes seen on current ECG.
- Persantine thallium/dobutamine echo: consider these tests for cardiac risk stratification for pts w/ new or changing anginal pattern, new ECG changes, recent CHF/MI, or multiple cardiac risk factors in setting of poor functional status. Inquire about past studies.
- Initiate beta blockade for cardiac risk reduction in appropriate pts.
- Carotid ultrasound indicated if bruits are present, esp if there is a history of CVA/TIA. Inquire about past studies.
- PFTs or ABG usually not indicated; consider HCO_3^- to assess for CO_2 retention.
- Labs: CBC, Cr, PT/PTT; consider electrolytes for pts on diuretics or ACE inhibitors or w/ history of acute renal failure or chronic renal insufficiency.
- Consider involving cardiologist to follow pt perioperatively.

Choice of Anesthesia
- Either general or regional anesthesia can be performed; coexisting morbidities may guide anesthetic choice.
- GA
  - Expect labile BP w/ induction.
  - Give induction agents in divided doses (eg, propofol ~30–50 mg/dose or STP ~50–75 mg/dose) to achieve hypnosis.
  - To prevent HTN w/ laryngoscopy consider fentanyl (1–2 mcg/kg) and/or esmolol (0.5 mg/kg) just prior to laryngoscopy.
  - For hypotension consider small doses of phenylephrine (25–50 mcg), noting that the response to phenylephrine is often exaggerated in this pt population.
  - Gingerly titrate maintenance agents.
  - Phenylephrine is often required for normotension prior to incision.
- Lumbar epidural
  - Check if pt is taking anticoagulants, which contraindicate epidural placement.

➤ Check coagulation parameters when in doubt.

➤ Careful placement of epidural is NOT contraindicated by usual intraop heparinization.

➤ 2% lidocaine or mepivacaine produces good surgical anesthesia. Carefully titrate 5 cc q10min to achieve T8–10 level (10–12 cc is often adequate).

➤ Avoid neuroaxial level >T8 in moderate/severe COPD.

■ Subarachnoid block w/ continuous spinal

➤ Find out if pt is taking anticoagulants, which contraindicate catheter placement.

➤ Check coagulation parameters when in doubt.

➤ Careful placement of spinal catheter is NOT contraindicated by usual intraop heparinization.

➤ For continuous spinal, titrate 0.75% bupivacaine to T8–10 level (~10 mg total initial dose often adequate); redosing q60–90min (1/3–1/2 initial dose); monitor level closely.

➤ Avoid neuroaxial level >T8 in moderate/severe COPD.

INTRAOP

Monitors/Line Placement

■ Standard monitors.

■ Two peripheral 14g–18g IVs.

■ Arterial line.

➤ Common for ACT monitoring & monitoring of other labs as dictated by comorbidities, close BP monitoring in pts in higher cardiac risk group.

■ Central line

➤ Usually not required unless history of significant LV dysfunction or decompensated CHF. Consider for redo procedures, which have increased blood loss.

■ PA line

➤ Usually not required.

■ TEE

➤ May be considered w/ GA as monitor for ischemia/wall motion abnormality in pts w/ severe CAD/LV dysfunction or symptomatic valvular lesions.

Intraop Concerns

■ Regional techniques: anticipate significant decreases in BP due to sympathectomy.

➤ Consider gentle fluid bolus (500–1,000 cc) prophylactically.

- Cardiac ischemia: hemodynamic stability is important to prevent ischemia.
  - Consider beta blockade. Periop ischemia often occurs 24–72 hours postop. If beta blockade indicated & initiated, it must be continued at least 7–10 days postop.
- COPD
  - Exacerbation of COPD may occur due to instrumentation of airway, leading to
    - Increased peak airway pressures
    - Secretions
    - Wheezing
    - Coughing
- BP
  - Because of chronic HTN & peripheral vascular disease, wide fluctuations in BP should be anticipated & minimized w/ induction, incision, blood loss, emergence & due to postop pain.
- Cerebrovascular disease
  - Maintain BP w/in 10–15% of baseline values.
  - LV diastolic dysfunction common due to chronic HTN & left ventricular hypertrophy.
  - Pts are preload-dependent & sensitive to decreased intravascular volume & decrease in sympathetic tone assoc w/ neuraxial techniques.
- Heparinization: check baseline ACT prior to bolus of heparin (normal ACT 100–125 sec).
  - Desired ACT after dosing usually >2x baseline (ie, 200–250).
  - Heparin reversal w/ protamine.
- Diabetes
  - Follow glucose.
  - Anticipate insulin resistance due to periop stress.
  - Consider insulin infusion for IDDM pts; continue until resumption of normal oral intake.
  - See also Coexisting Disease chapter "Diabetes Mellitus."

Intraop Therapies
- Phenylephrine infusion (10–50 mcg/min) PRN for sympathectomy from regional anesthetic
  - Use phenylephrine cautiously in setting of LV dysfunction.
- Beta blockade (IV metoprolol/esmolol) PRN for cardiac ischemia/ risk reduction
  - Use w/ caution in setting of active COPD or CHF exacerbations.

- Inhaled beta agonists & anticholinergics PRN
  - Be aware of resulting tachycardia in setting of CAD w/ beta agonists.
- Heparin
  - 100 U/kg IV bolus.
  - Maintenance ~10 U/kg q45–60min.
- Protamine
  - 5–10 mg/1,000 U of initial heparin bolus.
  - Test dose 5–10 mg always used.
  - Observe closely for protamine reactions (more common in pts taking NPH insulin).

POSTOP

Pain

- Mild to moderate. Options include
  - Infiltration of bupivacaine into the incision if appropriate w/ closure
  - PCA
  - Consider combination therapies: NSAIDs, Tylenol to reduce opiate requirement
  - Intrathecal opiates
    - MSO_4 0.25 mg $\times$ 1
    - Consider dose reduction in elderly or COPD pts.
  - Use oral analgesics or PCA for supplementation.
  - Epidural infusion: ropivacaine or bupivacaine 0.1–0.25% + fentanyl 2–5 mcg/cc at 8–10 cc/h
  - Consider early transition to oral agents to ensure adequate pain control after discharge home
  - Remove epidural & intrathecal catheters after documenting normal coag status

Complications

- Cardiac
  - Ischemia
  - MI
  - CHF
  - Arrhythmias
  - Hypertension
- Pulmonary
  - COPD exacerbation
  - Atelectasis
  - Pneumonia

- Metabolic
  - Hyperglycemia
  - Ketoacidosis
  - Hyperosmolar state in diabetic pts
- Neurologic
  - Postop delirium, particularly in elderly pts
- Renal
  - Worsening of pre-existing renal dysfunction
  - Pts receiving IV contrast for periop angiograms are at particular risk.
  - Mucomyst 600 mg PO BID can be given for renal protection.
- Coagulopathies from heparin, or dilutional coagulopathy.
- Hypovolemia from hemorrhage & inadequate volume replacement.
- Graft-related complications.
  - Hemorrhage
  - Graft thrombosis
  - Infection
- Deep venous thrombosis
- Pulmonary embolism

SURGICAL PROCEDURE

Indications
- Iliac occlusive disease
  - Claudication not responsive to conservative/medical mgt
  - Lower extremity rest pain
  - Nonhealing lower extremity ulcers due to chronic ischemia
  - Acute lower extremity ischemia (cold leg)

Procedure
- Iliofemoral bypass
  - Oblique lower quadrant (kidney transplant) incision
  - Retroperitoneal dissection to expose iliac vessels; infrainguinal incision for femoral artery exposure
  - Graft tunneling
  - Iliac & femoral arteriotomies
  - Endarterectomy PRN
  - Synthetic graft anastomoses
- Fem-fem bypass
  - Bilateral vertical infrainguinal incisions for femoral artery exposure
  - Synthetic graft tunneled subcutaneously across lower abdomen, common femoral arteries clamped

- ➢ Femoral arteriotomies bilaterally
- ➢ Endarterectomies PRN
- ➢ Anastomoses completed
- Infected/redo bypass grafts
  - ➢ Similar sequence as above
  - ➢ However, expect increased blood loss, surgical time
  - ➢ Infected grafts typically excised & replaced w/ autologous superficial femoral or greater saphenous vein, cryopreserved vein, or synthetic graft material

Surgical Concerns
- Proximal & distal control of vessels through good exposure; may necessitate muscle relaxation for iliac exposure
- Ureteral injury
- Iliac vein injury due to posterior proximity to artery
- Sympathetic nerve injury resulting in retrograde ejaculation
- Technically superior anastomoses to prevent bleeding, stenosis, occlusion
- Bleeding, hemostasis
- Distal embolization due to clamping
- Postop complications (see above)

Typical EBL
- 100–250 cc
- Expect larger EBL for redo procedures or operations for infected grafts

---

GASTRECTOMY

JAMES BRANDES, MD

PREOP

Preop Considerations
- Often pts have poor nutritional status, malnutrition.
- May have chronic anemia from bleeding
- May be hypovolemic from poor PO intake, bowel prep
- Considered to have a full stomach because of possible gastric outlet obstruction
- May have electrolyte disturbances from GI losses.
- Rarely, this operation is performed for pts w/ Zollinger-Ellison syndrome (gastrinoma) to remove the affected end organ.

Physical Findings
- Cachexia, clinical signs of hypovolemia.

Workup
- CBC
  - Electrolytes.
  - Orthostatic signs.
  - Evaluation of metastatic disease, CT scan showing tumor location.

Choice of Anesthesia
- GA required. Thoracic epidural may be useful for postop analgesia.
  - Epidural should cover upper midline or subcostal incision.

INTRAOP

Monitors/Line Placement
- Large-bore peripheral access
- Consider arterial line & CVP based on pt overall status & coexisting disease.
- Monitor urine output.
- Warm IV fluids.

Intraop Concerns
- Possibility of bleeding/rapid blood loss.
- Rapid sequence induction to reduce the risk of aspiration.
- Traction on the subcostal area may increase PIP & may impede venous return.
- Avoid nitrous oxide because of bowel distention issues.
- Extubate pt fully awake & fully reversed, or take pt intubated & sedated to ICU.
- Consider typing & cross-matching blood.
  - Prepare to transfuse PRBCs & other blood products as needed.

POSTOP

Pain
- Moderate
- PCA or epidural infusion usually required

Complications
- Hemorrhage
- Atelectasis: prevent w/ incentive spirometry
- Ileus: use of thoracic epidural will decrease this

SURGICAL PROCEDURE

Indications
- Gastric carcinoma, Zollinger-Ellison, uncontrolled hemorrhage Procedure
- Ex-Lap via midline or subcostal incision

Surgical Concerns
- Curative vs palliative operation (gastrojejunostomy)
- Wide en bloc resections including surrounding organs popular in Japan, where gastric disease requiring resection is more prevalent

Typical EBL
- 400–700 cc

GASTRIC BYPASS FOR MORBID OBESITY

MERLIN LARSON, MD
JASON WIDRICH, MD

PREOP

Preop Considerations
- Definition
  - Morbid obesity is often defined as twice the ideal body weight.
  - Alternately, obesity & morbid obesity can be defined in terms of Body Mass Index (BMI), which equals the pt's weight in kilograms divided by the square of the pt's height in meters.
  - Obesity = BMI >25; morbid obesity = BMI >35
- Common comorbid conditions
  - CAD
  - Sleep apnea
  - Hypoventilation syndrome
  - Gastroesophageal reflux disease (GERD)
  - DM
  - HTN
- IV, epidural placement may be difficult.
- Determine if case is open or laparoscopic before anesthetic is started, as this will influence mgt (eg, placement of epidural for pain control).

Physical Findings
- Examine weight distribution: is it primarily abdominal? does it involve the face or airway?

- Conical upper arm shape interferes w/ accurate noninvasive BP
- Careful airway exam is essential since the airway may be difficult to manage in some obese pts.
  - ➤ No clear correlation between BMI & airway difficulty, but consider awake fiberoptic intubation for BMI >50.
  - ➤ Neck circumference >50 cm & Mallampati class >3 may be risk factor for difficult intubation.

Workup
- CBC, lytes, glucose, EKG
- If indicated, ABG, PFT, CXR, or echo (to evaluate pulmonary HTN or right heart strain)

Choice of Anesthesia
- GA necessary for both open & laparoscopic procedures.
- Upper thoracic epidural optional.
  - ➤ Placement may be difficult because of excess subcutaneous tissue.
- 90% oxygen w/ vapor or propofol may improve wound healing & decrease nausea/vomiting compared w/ lower oxygen concentrations or the use of nitrous oxide.
- Some surgeons request avoidance of nitrous oxide, particularly during laparoscopic procedures.
- Some surgeons request 5,000 units SC heparin before incision.

INTRAOP
Monitors/Line Placement
- Noninvasive BP monitoring may be challenging or unreliable; use an arterial line in this case.
- CVP is useful for vascular access but not necessary if a good peripheral IV can be obtained.

Intraop Concerns
- Exposure of intra-abdominal contents requires profound muscle relaxation.
- Before clamping the stomach, pull back NG tube so that the fourth distal mark is at the nose. Surgeon is concerned that NG tube not be incorporated into operative site.
- Changes in pt position during surgery (eg, Trendelenburg) may predispose to atelectasis, V/Q mismatch, hypoxemia.

- For laparoscopic surgery, typical concerns related to initiation & maintenance of pneumoperitoneum. (See also Procedures chapter "Laparoscopic General Surgery.")
- Safety belt should be used & checked, as change in table position could lead to movement on table or a fall.

Intraop Therapies
- Manipulation of NG tube

POSTOP

Pain
- Moderate to severe, less for laparoscopic procedure.
- Epidural beneficial if procedure is open.
- Laparoscopic procedures require less intense analgesics.

Complications
- Postop respiratory failure
  - Ventilatory failure following extubation may occur; pt must be totally awake & breathing adequately before extubation.
  - Careful monitoring of respiratory status is required of all pts, usually in ICU setting.
  - Sleep apnea pts may require mask CPAP, usually benefit from observation in the ICU.
- Increased risk of DVT/PE
  - Consider compression stockings, sequential compression device, or SC heparin.

SURGICAL PROCEDURE

Indications
- Morbid obesity in pts motivated to lose weight

Procedure
- Midline incision for open procedure
- Supine position for open & laparoscopic procedures
- A variety of procedures may be performed. They can be categorized into:
  - Restrictive procedures (eg, vertical banded gastroplasty)
  - Restrictive procedures w/ some malabsorption (eg, Roux-en-Y gastric bypass)
    - Probably most commonly performed procedure

➤ Malabsorptive procedure w/ some restriction (eg, distal Roux-en-Y gastric bypass)

➤ Malabsorptive procedure (eg, jejunoileal bypass)

■ Some procedures are assoc w/ higher long-term complications & have been largely abandoned

Surgical Concerns
■ Exposure of abdominal contents
■ Adequacy of anastomosis

Typical EBL
■ 300 mL

GASTROSCHISIS SURGERY

ATSUKO BABA, MD

PREOP

Preop Considerations
■ External herniation of abdominal viscera through a defect in the anterior abdominal wall lateral to the umbilical cord
■ No hernia sac covering viscera
■ Rarely assoc w/ other congenital anomalies
■ Assoc w/ malrotation & intestinal atresia
■ Incidence of preterm delivery >33%
■ Cover exposed viscera w/ moist dressings & a plastic bowel bag & maintain neutral thermal environment to decrease fluid & heat loss
■ Decompress stomach w/ orogastric tube to decrease risk of regurgitation & pulmonary aspiration
■ Maintain adequate hydration (6–12 cc/kg/h); protein-containing solutions should constitute 25% of replacement fluids to compensate for the protein loss & third-space translocation
■ Mortality 15–23%

Physical Findings
■ External herniation of abdominal viscera through a defect in the anterior abdominal wall lateral to the umbilical cord

Workup
■ Diagnosed in the first trimester of pregnancy w/ fetal ultrasound

- Hypovolemia evidenced by hemoconcentration & metabolic acidosis
- Appropriate workup to rule in/out assoc conditions

Choice of Anesthesia
- General endotracheal anesthesia w/ possible awake intubation after decompression of the stomach

INTRAOP
Monitors/Line Placement
- Two peripheral IVs.
- Arterial line helpful for BP monitoring & ABGs.

Intraop Concerns
- Because of coexisting hypovolemia, titrate anesthetics slowly to avoid hypotension.
- Opioids and/or volatile anesthetics can be used.
- Nitrous oxide may cause intestinal distention, interfering w/ the return of viscera into the abdomen.
- A tight surgical abdominal closure can lead to compression of the inferior vena cava/hypotension, compression of the diaphragm/ decreased pulmonary compliance, & compression of perfusing vessels to abdominal organs.
- Preterm neonates vulnerable to retinopathy of prematurity w/ high oxygen concentrations.
- When primary surgical abdominal closure is not possible, the herniated viscera is temporarily covered with a Dacron-reinforced Silastic silo, w/ the contents being slowly reduced over 1–2 wks.

Intraop Therapies
- Maintain body temp & continue replacement fluids.

POSTOP
Pain
- Moderate to severe.
- Use narcotics judiciously if extubated.

Complications
- Mechanical ventilation postop is usually indicated for 24–48 h w/ monitoring in the NICU.

- May require TPN.
- A tight surgical closure may lead to hemodynamic, pulmonary & abdominal organ dysfunction.
- Infection.

SURGICAL PROCEDURE
Indications
- Abdominal wall defect w/ the goal of safely replacing herniated viscera into the abdomen

Procedure
- Safely replace herniated viscera into the abdominal cavity w/ primary surgical closure or staged repair w/ a Silastic silo & definitive closure in 10–14 days

Surgical Concerns
- Impaired ventilation & venous return will result from overaggressive attempts at closure

Typical EBL
- 5–10 cc/kg

HAND SURGERY

SUNDEEP MALIK, MD

PREOP
Preop Considerations
- A variety of hand & distal forearm surgeries are commonly performed on an outpatient basis.
- For pt w/ rheumatoid arthritis, look for c-spine involvement.
- If hand procedure is related to infection, look for signs of sepsis.

Physical Findings
- Look for bony deformities or contractures that may limit pt positioning.
- If hand is infected, look for lymphatic tract spread up arm, a contraindication to regional.

Workup

■ Based on pt age & coexisting disease.

Choice of Anesthesia

■ GA: Can be used alone or in addition to brachial plexus block
■ Local anesthesia or MAC: Best for soft tissue surgery not requiring large volume of local anesthetic.
  ➤ Some procedures that may be suitable for MAC: Dupuytren's contracture release, trigger finger repair, carpal tunnel repair, DeQuervain's tenosynovitis release, repair of lacerated nerve or tendon.
  ➤ Surgeon may perform digit block or wrist blocks to supplement local anesthesia or MAC.
■ Regional anesthesia: Can block at level of neck, axilla, elbow, wrist, & digits, or Bier block.
  ➤ Bier block: for procedures <45–60 min. Tourniquet pain becomes significant w/ longer procedures.
    • Operative time may vary by surgeon & complexity of surgery.
  ➤ Brachial plexus blocks (axillary, supraclavicular, infraclavicular) tend to be the best to reliably produce surgical anesthesia. They may be useful for longer or more painful procedures that may not be suitable for Bier block or MAC (eg, ORIF distal radius or wrist fracture).
    • Axillary block may be most suitable for most types of hand surgery.
    • Interscalene blocks may spare ulnar distribution. If procedure involves wrist, can perform blockade of lateral & median antebrachial cutaneous nerves.
    • Supraclavicular & infraclavicular blocks have small risk of pneumothorax.
  ➤ Wrist blocks
    • Some surgeons or anesthesia providers perform these to supplement brachial plexus block.
  ➤ Know which nerves innervate the area of surgery
    • Radial nerve: Sensation to lateral dorsum of hand & dorsum of thumb, index, & middle fingers to the distal interphalangeal joint.
    • Median nerve: Sensation to lateral portion of palm including thumb, index, middle, & lateral portion of ring finger.
    • Ulnar nerve: Sensation to dorsum & palmar aspects of medial hand.

INTRAOP

Monitors/Line Placement
- Routine monitors
- Place IVs in opposite extremity

Intraop Concerns
- Proper positioning of extremity
- Tourniquet pain w/ longer operative times
- Nerve blocks: If inadequate block, may need to supplement w/ local or IV agents, or convert to GA

Intraop Therapies
- Analgesics or sedatives to supplement blocks

POSTOP

Pain
- Varies w/ surgery. Bone surgery is more painful than soft tissue surgery
- For outpatient: Oral narcotic, IV or IM ketorolac, regional block
  - ➤ If nerve block used during surgery but pain recurs prior to discharge, consider repeat nerve block w/ long-acting local anesthetic
- For inpatient: PCA, regional block, continuous regional catheter

Complications
- Nerve damage, potentially related to block or to surgery itself

SURGICAL PROCEDURE

Indications
- Vary

Procedure
- Varies

Surgical Concerns
- Relate to specific surgery

Typical EBL
- Minimal, esp if tourniquet used

HEPATIC RESECTION

JAMES BRANDES, MD
MANUEL PARDO, JR., MD
JOHN R. FEINER, MD

PREOP

Preop Considerations
- Liver tumors: include hepatocellular carcinoma (HCC), metastatic cancer, adenomas, hemangiomas, cysts
- Pts w/ HCC commonly have underlying hepatitis B or C.
- Extent of surgery depends on size & location of tumor. Complications & bleeding increase w/ larger resections. Range: wedge resection, left hepatectomy, right hepatectomy, trisegmentectomy.
- Donor hepatectomy also performed for living related transplant. If donation is to child, left or left lateral segmentectomy is performed. For adult, right hepatectomy is most common.

Physical Findings
- Essential: Look for signs of cirrhosis: ascites, peripheral edema, jaundice, spider angiomas, asterixis, caput medusa.
- Evaluate volume status carefully. Pt may have peripheral edema w/ intravascular volume depletion.

Workup
- Most important: Look for evidence of cirrhosis: PT, albumin, AST/ALT.
- PT/PTT: PT may be prolonged from cirrhosis & hepatic synthetic dysfunction; consider IM vitamin K to correct possible vitamin K deficiency.
- AST/ALT: May show elevation c/w chronic hepatitis. If new changes c/w acute hepatitis, consider further workup.
- CBC: Thrombocytopenia common in cirrhotic pt. Pt may have anemia of chronic disease. Cancer pt may have bone marrow suppression from chemotherapy.
- Electrolytes, BUN, creatinine: Cirrhosis & high creatinine may indicate hepatorenal syndrome; electrolytes may be abnormal from diuretics.
- Abdominal CT scan: Look for size & location of tumor & proximity to major vessels, esp IVC.

- T&C for 4–6 units of PRBCs. Order FFP if PT prolonged.
- CXR: May indicate metastatic disease.

Choice of Anesthesia
- GA required. Midthoracic (T7–9) epidural useful for postop pain in noncirrhotic pt. Epidural can be dosed during case; if using local anesthetic watch for vasodilation from sympathectomy.
- Nitrous oxide usually omitted to avoid bowel distention.
- Muscle relaxant usually continued during the case, unless epidural dosed w/ local to provide relaxation.

INTRAOP
Monitors/Line Placement
- Standard monitors + CVP & arterial line. For smaller & more peripheral resections, can omit CVP and/or arterial line.
- Large-bore peripheral IVs
- Place large-bore central access if unable to obtain adequate peripheral IV.
- Foley catheter
- Rarely incision will be thoracoabdominal, & double-lumen ETT may be needed for surgical exposure.

Intraop Concerns
- Massive hemorrhage: Anticipate this, esp during later phases of liver transection. Keep blood in room; reorder promptly. Anticipate FFP & platelet needs as blood loss nears one-half to one blood volume. Consider rapid transfusion device, point-of-care hemoglobin testing. Monitor ABGs/base deficit if blood loss significant.
- Surgeon's approach to bleeding. Surgeon may use Pringle maneuver (reduce hepatic blood inflow by clamping portal vein, hepatic artery, common bile duct at porta hepatis). This causes temporary hepatic ischemia, esp w/ longer clamp times. Venous back-bleeding can still occur. Splanchnic venous pooling behind clamp may cause decreased preload.
- Additional surgical approach. IVC clamp: Surgeon can also clamp suprahepatic & infrahepatic IVC for compete vascular isolation. This causes hypotension from large drop in preload. Mgt: Infuse fluid prior to IVC clamp. Anticipate need for vasopressors. IV access below the diaphragm will be ineffective.
- Fluid mgt: Keep CVP in low or normal range. High CVP may lead to increased venous bleeding during resection.

- Hypotension: Can be severe, esp from bleeding & hypovolemia. Reverse Trendelenburg & epidural local anesthetic can also decrease preload.
- Hypotension, other causes: Temporary IVC compression from surgical manipulation of liver; Rx: IV fluid, & ask surgeon to stop manipulation if possible. Potential: Air embolism from hepatic veins.
- Retractor placement may increase PIP & decrease tidal volumes by pulling up on rib cage.
- Special concerns for cirrhotic pt: Watch for nosebleed or bleeding varices from NG tube placement. Watch urine output closely. If low, consider renal dose dopamine. Concern is risk of causing hepatorenal syndrome. Monitor glucose & electrolytes & PT closely.
- Decision re: extubation & postop ICU vs PACU is based on pt stability, pt coexisting dz, EBL, extent of surgery.

Intraop Therapies
- Forced air warmer to lower body & IV fluid warmer to minimize hypothermia.

POSTOP

Pain
- Moderate to severe. Bilateral subcostal incision more painful than midline incision.
- Epidural infusion w/ local & narcotic.
- PCA if no epidural. Consider intercostal nerve blocks.

Complications
- Hepatic ischemia causing reduced synthetic function, coagulopathy, or DIC. Correct coagulopathy w/ FFP. Don't remove or replace epidural if INR >1.5.
- Liver failure: More common in cirrhotic pt. Surgical team will monitor AST/ALT, PT, & mental status postop.
- Postop hemorrhage: Manifestations include falling HCT, abdominal distention, hypotension, increased drain output.
- Electrolyte imbalance, hypoglycemia.
- Respiratory insufficiency: Factors can include extent of surgery, assoc atelectasis, blood loss, body habitus, pt coexisting disease. Monitor resp status & ABG after extubation, or consider

postop intubation if complicated case. Consider monitoring in ICU setting.

SURGICAL PROCEDURE

Indications
- Liver tumor

Procedure
- Incision: Subcostal, right-sided chevron, or midline.
- Dissect attachments of the liver to the diaphragm & surrounding structures.
- Dissect & ligate arterial & portal blood supplies & biliary drainage. If possible, ligate hepatic vein draining affected lobe. Blood loss typically occurs after this, w/ transection of the liver parenchyma.
- Transection done w/ CUSA (Cavitron ultrasonic suction aspirator), harmonic scalpel, finger fracture, or scalpel. Ligate larger intra-parenchymal vessels & cauterize smaller vessels w/ argon laser or electrocautery.
- If tumor extends into IVC, venovenous bypass may be necessary using venous cannulas in groin & neck. Surgeon should discuss this preop.

Surgical Concerns
- Intraop hemorrhage.

Typical EBL
- Variable depending on extent of resection, location of tumor. Range: 200 cc through 1–2 blood volumes.

HERNIORRHAPHY

EMILY REINYS, MD

PREOP

Preop Considerations
- Most pts are generally healthy
- Procedure usually performed on an outpatient basis

Physical Findings
- Groin pain or lump

- Incarceration leading to strangulation will usually lead to tenderness over the strangulated hernia, sometimes w/ edema & redness of the overlying skin
- Pts w/ strangulated hernias may have abdominal distention & signs of bowel obstruction

Workup
- Consider causes of increased intra-abdominal pressure that could be a precipitating factor in hernia development (eg, chronic cough, constipation)

Choice of Anesthesia
- Local anesthesia w/ sedation, spinal, epidural & general anesthetic are all acceptable techniques. Important considerations are:
  - Pt preference
  - Age
  - Presence of coexisting disease
  - Expected duration of procedure
- Laparoscopic repairs require GA w/ controlled ventilation
- Local w/ sedation
  - Acceptable for simple herniorrhaphy
  - Some discomfort may occur w/ peritoneal manipulation
- Spinal
  - Depending on anticipated duration of surgery, can consider 0.75% bupivacaine, 12–15 mg
- Epidural
  - 1.5–2.0% lidocaine w/ epinephrine 5 mcg/mL, 15–25 mL initial bolus
  - Supplement w/ 5–10 mL as needed
- GA
  - Standard induction
  - Consider LMA use
  - Neuromuscular blockers generally not required
  - In event of strangulation, consider rapid sequence induction w/ cricoid pressure & endotracheal intubation

INTRAOP

Monitors/Line Placement
- Standard monitors.
- One peripheral IV.

Intraop Concerns
- If strangulation has been present for some time, pt may require significant fluid resuscitation.

Intraop Therapies
- When prosthetic mesh is to be used for repair, prophylactic antibiotics may be given at induction.

POSTOP

Pain
- Typically minimal

Complications
- Nausea/vomiting
- Failure to void
- Numbness in the distribution of the ilioinguinal nerve is common postop & sometimes persists

SURGICAL PROCEDURE

Indications
- Defect in the transverse abdominis layer (inguinal hernia) or bulging of tissues over the femoral canal (femoral hernia)

Procedure
- Inguinal hernia
  - Involves opening the external inguinal ring, freeing the spermatic cord & hernial sac off the inguinal canal, dissecting the hernia from the spermatic cord & closing the fascial defect
  - Laparoscopic repair of inguinal hernias has been assoc w/ less postop pain, but greater risk of injury to the bowel or blood vessels
- Femoral hernia
  - Involves exposing the hernial sac as it exits the preperitoneal space through the femoral canal, then suturing the iliopubic tract to Cooper's ligament

Surgical Concerns
- Avoidance of damage to spermatic cord, testicular blood supply & ilioinguinal nerve

Typical EBL
- Usually minimal (25–50 mL)

HYPOSPADIAS REPAIR

KURT DITTMAR, MD

PREOP

Preop Considerations
- Typically pts are healthy.
- Often performed before age 2

Physical Findings
- Varying degrees of defect may be present. The abnormal opening of the urethral meatus can be located anywhere between the glans & the perineum. More proximal lesions may require extensive dissection.
- Associated w/ inguinal hernia, cryptorchidism

Workup
- Standard pediatric preop evaluation, taking into account pt's other medical problems.

Choice of Anesthesia
- GA required
  - ➤ GA + regional block (combined technique) often useful.
    - Typically pt has an inhaled induction using a face mask, then an LMA or ET tube is used to protect the airway.
    - Then a caudal or epidural block is performed.
    - For long cases, a catheter can be left in the epidural space & dosed throughout & at the end of the procedure for postop pain control.

INTRAOP

Monitors/Line Placement
- Standard monitors
- One 22g or 24g IV

Intraop Concerns
- Most of the anesthetic complications pertain to the technique used (total spinal, inadequate control of the airway) & should be treated accordingly.

Intraop Therapies
- In the combined approach, pt typically requires a reduced amount of opioids & inhaled agent.

POSTOP

Pain

- Moderate. Two modalities are usually used to treat postop pain:
- Caudal block, usually one shot.
  - ➤ For complex cases requiring extensive dissection, a catheter may be kept in place.
- Acetaminophen, usually rectal.

Complications

- Disruption of repair through instrumentation of the urethra. Distal repairs may not require urethral catheter.

SURGICAL PROCEDURE

Indications

- Abnormal opening of urethral meatus

Procedure

- Defect is repaired using preputial or meatal skin flaps. If chordee is present, Nesbitt plication or tunica albuginea plication may be necessary.

Surgical Concerns

- Proximal lesions increase the extent of dissection & therefore the difficulty of the case.
- In complex cases bladder or buccal mucosa can be used to repair the urethra.

Typical EBL

- Minimal

ICD PLACEMENT

LYDIA CASSORLA, MD

PREOP

Preop Considerations

- Wide range of general health: athletes to cardiac transplant candidates.
- Determine underlying cardiac function:
  - ➤ Normal: Routine monitoring usually adequate

> Depressed: Deterioration may occur if repeated shocks are necessary for ICD lead placement & testing. Assess monitoring & IV access accordingly. Arterial line may be helpful.

> Severely depressed/CHF: Pt may not tolerate sedation without securing airway. Arterial line helpful to assess recovery from shocks. Proximal venous access such as antecubital & external jugular may speed onset of meds in sicker pts.

■ GERD may influence decision to secure airway.
■ Heart failure pts may be anticoagulated.

Physical Findings
■ Determine if consistent w/ CHF.

Workup
■ Most pts have ischemic heart disease.
■ Pts must lie flat during procedure; assess for orthopnea.

Choice of Anesthesia
■ MAC or GA; local anesthetic often adequate for surgical stimulation.
■ LMA & ET tube used successfully for GA.
■ Muscle relaxation not required.
■ Propofol infusion for MAC or GA permits rapid changes in depth of anesthesia.

Avoid agents w/ antiarrhythmic properties (eg, IV lidocaine) as they may interfere w/ induction of VF, which is necessary for procedure.

INTRAOP

Monitors/Line Placement
■ Place IV in arm opposite vein used by cardiologists for central access.

Intraop Concerns
■ Minimize fluid administration for pts w/ poor ventricular function.
■ Pt will have VF induced & undergo defibrillation, possibly multiple times.
■ Surgery resembles non-ICD pacemaker w/ little stimulation other than pocket for device.
■ Assess ECG ST segments & BP recovery after each shock.
■ Communicate w/ cardiologist regarding recovery from VF; he or she may wish to reinduce arrhythmia as soon as possible for electrophysiologic reasons. Allow adequate time for ST segment & hemodynamic recovery.

- Following arrest, circulating catecholamines often surge due to adrenal release. Peak effect delayed if cardiac output is impaired.
- If refractory hypotension develops, suspect cardiac tamponade due to perforation of cardiac chamber. Assess w/ echocardiography ASAP.

Intraop Therapies
- Be prepared to defibrillate externally if device fails following induction of VF.
- Be prepared for cardiac resuscitation & external pacing.

POSTOP

Pain
- Minimal

Complications
- Deterioration in cardiac performance is possible, esp following multiple shocks in the presence of limited cardiac reserve
- Hematoma in pocket
- Intravascular thrombus formation related to leads
- CHF in pts w/ poor ventricular function

SURGICAL PROCEDURE

Indications
- Indications are in rapid evolution.
- History of cardiac arrest or syncope w/ inducible sustained VT or VF
- Recurrent VT or VF unresponsive to medical mgt & not thought to be due to a recoverable condition (eg, acute MI)
- Inducible sustained VT or VF in high-risk group such as low cardiac output
- Recurrent atrial fibrillation (evolving indication)

Procedure
- Central venous access for placement of intracardiac leads
- Testing of leads for sensing, pacing, & energy required for defibrillation
- Pocket for device
- Newer devices no longer require epicardial access

Surgical Concerns
- Central venous access
- Functional & cosmetic w/ regard to device placement

Typical EBL
- Minimal unless access to central vein is complicated

INFRAINGUINAL BYPASS

DANIEL M. SWANGARD, MD

PREOP

Preop Considerations
- Pts w/ peripheral vascular disease are likely to have CAD & cerebrovascular disease as well.
  - ➤ CAD: Pt may have a history of MI, stable or unstable angina, LV dysfunction/CHF, or atrial fibrillation.
- Cardiac pacemakers are not uncommon in this population.
- Other comorbidities include
  - ➤ HTN
  - ➤ DM
  - ➤ COPD
  - ➤ Renal dysfunction
- The geriatric population on whom these procedures are performed is at risk of postop delirium.
- Anticoagulation/antiplatelet agents are common:
  - ➤ Coumadin
  - ➤ ASA
  - ➤ Plavix
  - ➤ Ticlid
  - ➤ Heparin infusions/enoxaparin for acute ischemic extremity

Physical Findings
- Vital signs: may have elevated BP or HR, low SpO_2
- Neck: may have carotid bruits, increased jugular venous distention
- Pulmonary: wheezes, rales, rhonchi, distant breath sounds, barrel chest may be present
- CV: note rate, regular vs irregular rhythm, S3 or S4, murmurs, displaced apical impulse
- Abdomen: examine for bruits, pulsatile masses
- Extremities: there will be diminished or absent lower extremity pulses, coolness or pallor, nonhealing ulcers, possibly distal embolic phenomena

Workup

■ Ask about functional status/exercise tolerance as guide to severity of CV & pulmonary disease.

■ Obtain a recent as well as an old ECG (to compare to new ECG for changes).

■ PTHAL or dobutamine echo: used for cardiac risk stratification in pts w/ new or changing anginal pattern, new ECG changes, recent CHF/MI or multiple cardiac risk factors in setting of poor functional status

  ➤ Inquire about past studies.

■ Beta blockade will reduce cardiac risk in at-risk pts.

■ Carotid ultrasound should be obtained to evaluate bruits, especially if there is a history of CVA/TIA.

  ➤ Inquire about past studies.

■ PFTs/ABGs are usually not indicated; consider HCO_3 to assess for CO_2 retention.

■ Labs: CBC, Cr, PT/PTT; lytes for pts on diuretics or ACE inhibitors or history of acute renal failure or chronic renal insufficiency.

■ Consider involving cardiology to follow pt perioperatively.

Choice of Anesthesia

■ GA

  ➤ Expect labile BP w/ induction; place arterial line prior to induction for this reason.

  ➤ Gingerly titrate hypnotic agent on induction: for instance, divided doses of propofol (~30–50 mg/dose) or sodium thiopental (~50–75 mg/dose).

  ➤ For hypotension consider small doses of phenylephrine (25–50 mcg); response to phenylephrine is often exaggerated in this pt population.

  ➤ To prevent HTN during airway manipulations, consider fentanyl (1–2 mcg/kg) or esmolol (0.5 mg/kg) just prior to laryngoscopy.

  ➤ Maintenance of anesthesia is often w/ vapor & fentanyl.

  ➤ Neo-Synephrine is often required to maintain normotension prior to incision.

  ➤ Intraop hemodynamic stability is promoted by the use of fentanyl &/or beta blockade.

■ Lumbar epidural

  ➤ Check whether pt is on anticoagulants before placing an epidural.

  ➤ Check PTT if indicated.

➤ Epidural placement is NOT contraindicated by usual intraop heparinization.

➤ 2% lidocaine & mepivacaine are typical agents used via epidural.

➤ 5 cc local anesthetic per dose is titrated q5–10 min to establish block; 8–10 cc total dose is often adequate.

➤ Anesthesia to T12 level is required for surgery.

■ Subarachnoid block (continuous spinal)

➤ Check whether pt is on anticoagulants before performing spinal.

➤ Check PTT if indicated.

➤ Spinal placement is NOT contraindicated by usual intraop heparinization.

➤ For continuous spinal, titrate 0.75% bupivacaine to T12 level (total of ~8–10 mg total initial dose often adequate); redosing q60–90min (1/3–1/2 initial dose); monitor level closely.

■ Coexisting morbidities guide anesthetic choice.

INTRAOP

Monitors/Line Placement

■ Standard monitors

■ One 14g or 16g IV

■ Arterial line

➤ Common for blood pressure & ACT monitoring as well as other labs as indicated by comorbidities

■ Central line

➤ Usually not required unless there is a history of significant LV dysfunction or decompensated CHF

➤ Consider for redo procedures because of increased blood loss

■ PA line

➤ Usually not required

■ TEE

➤ May be considered w/ GA as a monitor for ischemia/wall motion abnormality in pts w/ severe CAD/LV dysfunction or symptomatic valvular lesions

Intraop Concerns

■ Regional techniques: anticipate decreases in BP due to sympathectomy.

➤ A gentle fluid bolus (500–1,000 cc) may help reduce the decrease in BP.

- Cardiac ischemia: hemodynamic stability is important to prevent ischemia.
  - Consider beta blockade.
  - Carefully monitor for ischemia.
- COPD: exacerbation may occur due to airway instrumentation.
  - Symptoms may include increased peak airway pressures, secretions, wheezing, coughing.
  - Avoid neuroaxial block with a level >T8 in pts w/ moderate or severe COPD.
- Blood pressure fluctuations may occur w/ induction, incision, blood loss, emergence & postop pain due to chronic HTN & PVD.
- Cerebrovascular disease: pts are at risk of stroke or TIA
  - Careful BP mgt, within 10–15% of baseline values, is the goal.
  - An awake pt w/ a block permits an excellent assessment of CNS ischemia.
- LV diastolic dysfunction is common due to chronic HTN & LVH.
  - Cardiac output is preload-dependent in these pts (ie, sensitivity to decreased intravascular volume).
- Heparin
  - Check baseline ACT prior to heparin bolus (normal is 100–125 sec).
  - Desired ACT after dosing usually >2x baseline (ie, 200–250).
  - Reversal is w/ protamine at the end of the case.
- DM: follow glucose intraop.
  - Anticipate insulin resistance due to periop stress.

Intraop Therapies
- Phenylephrine infusion (10–50 mcg/min) PRN for hypotension.
  - Use w/ caution in the setting of LV dysfunction.
- Beta blockade (IV metoprolol/esmolol) PRN for cardiac ischemia/ risk reduction.
  - Use w/ caution in setting of active COPD/CHF exacerbations.
- Beta agonists for COPD exacerbation PRN
- Heparin
  - 100 U/kg IV bolus
  - Maintenance ~10 U/kg q45–60 min
- Protamine
  - Reversal dose is 5 mg/1,000 U of initial heparin bolus.
  - Always use a test dose of 5–10 mg, observing closely for protamine reactions.

- Protamine reactions are more common in pts taking NPH insulin.

POSTOP

Pain

- Moderate
- PCA
- Combination therapies can be used, such as NSAIDs or Tylenol to reduce opiate requirement.
- Intrathecal opiates: MSO_4 0.25 mg × 1
  - ➤ Reduce dose in the elderly or in pts w/ COPD.
  - ➤ Oral agents or PCA can be used to supplement intrathecal narcotics.
- Epidural infusion: ropivacaine/bupivacaine 0.1–0.25% + fentanyl 2–5 mcg/cc at 8–10 cc/h
- Discontinue epidural & intrathecal catheters after ensuring normal coag status.

Complications

- Cardiac ischemia, MI, CHF, arrhythmias
- HTN
- COPD exacerbation, atelectasis, pneumonia
- Hyperglycemia, ketoacidosis, hyperosmolar state in diabetic pts
- Postop delirium in elderly pts
- Worsening of pre-existing renal dysfunction, especially in pts receiving IV contrast for periop angiograms
  - ➤ Consider Mucomyst 600 mg PO BID for renal protection.
- Hypovolemia due to hemorrhage &/or inadequate volume replacement
- Graft-related complications: hemorrhage, graft thrombosis, infection
- DVT/PE

SURGICAL PROCEDURE

Indications

- Infrainguinal occlusive disease
- Claudication not responsive to medical mgt
- Rest pain in affected extremity
- Nonhealing leg ulcers due to chronic ischemia
- Acute lower extremity ischemia (cold foot/leg)

- Goal: bypass of occlusive infrainguinal segment(s) w/ shortest graft possible
- Typical procedures: fem-pop bypass, fem-tibial bypass, fem-peroneal bypass

Procedure
- Infrainguinal bypass
  - Ipsilateral or contralateral saphenous vein harvest & preparation if applicable
  - Femoral & distal artery dissection & exposure
  - Tunneling
  - Heparinization
  - Femoral & distal artery clamping
  - Arteriotomies
  - Anastomoses
  - Unclamping & reperfusion
  - Intraop arteriogram PRN
  - Hemostasis/heparin reversal & closure
  - Lower extremity splinting PRN
- Redo &/or infected bypass grafts: similar sequence as above; however, expect
  - Increased blood loss & surgical time
  - If saphenous veins have been previously harvested, then arm veins, cryopreserved vein, or synthetic graft material may be used
  - Harvesting of arm veins may necessitate GA

Surgical Concerns
- Success of infrainguinal bypass procedures is dependent on adequate arterial inflow from aorta/iliac artery
- Proximal & distal control of vessels is achieved through good exposure
- Technically superior anastomoses are required to prevent bleeding, stenosis & occlusion
- Bleeding, hemostasis
- Distal embolization due to clamping
- Vasoconstriction due to hypothermia/hypovolemia postop resulting in poor graft flow & occlusion

Typical EBL
- 100–250 cc
- Expect larger EBL for redo procedures or operations for infected grafts

INTERVENTIONAL NEURORADIOLOGY

MIMI C. LEE, MD, PHD

PREOP

Preop Considerations

- The endovascular approach is used for the diagnosis & treatment of neurovascular diseases of the central & peripheral nervous system.
- Procedures range from diagnostic cerebral angiograms to complex coiling & embolization of cerebral aneurysms, arteriovenous malformations & spinal vascular abnormalities.
- Anesthetic management focuses on
  - ➤ Pt immobility for optimal imaging.
  - ➤ Hemodynamic stability.
  - ➤ Hemodynamic control as required by the specific procedure.
  - ➤ Immediate availability for unexpected problems.

Physical Findings

- Pts who present for neurointerventional procedures are outpts or stable inpts w/ neurovascular disease.
  - ➤ TIA.
  - ➤ Stroke.
  - ➤ Mild intracranial hemorrhage.
  - ➤ Low-grade subarachnoid hemorrhage.
  - ➤ Neuro deficits.
  - ➤ Pts often undergo diagnostic angiograms first to determine whether endovascular intervention is warranted.
- Other pts are critically ill & hospitalized for a serious neurovascular injury.
  - ➤ High-grade subarachnoid hemorrhage.
  - ➤ Severe intracranial hemorrhage.
  - ➤ Major stroke from cerebral ischemia/infarction

Workup

- Perform standard H&P plus a detailed neuro exam to assess preprocedure deficits.
- Evaluate cardiac & pulmonary status; deliberate hyper- or hypotension & hypo/hypercapnia may be necessary for a successful procedure.
- CBC, coagulation studies.

Choice of Anesthesia

- Discuss the procedural goals & anesthetic plan w/ the endovascular surgeon.
- Many diagnostic procedures & some interventional procedures can be performed under conscious sedation or MAC.
  - Pt cooperation is imperative for immobility & high-quality radiologic imaging.
  - Breath holding for improved image quality during angiography may be requested.
- GA may be requested because of control of airway & ventilation, & reduced chance for movement compared to conscious sedation or MAC.
  - While the pt is mechanically ventilated during GA, apnea is often provided to improve image quality during contrast imaging.
  - GA may be needed in case of unexpected emergency or uncooperative pts.

INTRAOP

Monitors/Line Placement

- Standard monitors.
- At least one peripheral IV.
  - Place additional lines or monitors prior to draping.
  - Once procedure commences, access to the pt may be limited due to imaging equipment & sterile drapes.
- Arterial line is recommended for intracranial/spinal cord procedures, especially if deliberate hypertension or hypotension is employed.
- Surgeons will place at least one femoral artery sheath for access.
  - Can request pressure transduction for femoral line
- Central line not necessary for procedure, although may be in place for an ICU pt
  - CVP monitoring may be indicated to facilitate normo- or hypervolemia for treatment of vasospasm after subarachnoid hemorrhage.
- Frequent blood draws may be required for ACT monitoring of heparin therapy. If radial arterial line not used, can request that surgeons draw blood from femoral line.
- EEG, SEP, MEP, TCD or xenon-blood flow studies are sometimes employed for adjunctive monitoring.

Intraop Concerns

- Sudden, unexpected catastrophe may occur, such as vascular injury & subsequent hemorrhage related to
  - The nature of many neurovascular diseases (eg, intracranial aneurysms)
  - Use of microcatheters manipulated from a long distance
- In the worst-case scenario, a cerebral or spinal vessel is ruptured & immediate hemorrhage occurs.
  - Morbidity & mortality high
  - Tamponade eventually occurs in the brain, as the skull is a fixed cavity.
  - Emergency ventriculostomy may be required, necessitating the immediate availability of a neurosurgeon.
  - Less commonly, emergency craniotomy, corticectomy or craniectomy may be required to evacuate space-occupying clot or relieve ICP.
  - Brain herniation & death can occur.

POSTOP

Pain

- Usually isolated to the femoral access site
- Postprocedural headache can be treated w/ PO or IV analgesics

Complications

- Delayed hemorrhage at site of surgery
- Delayed occlusion of artery in CNS
- Complications of femoral arterial access
  - Local hematoma
  - Retroperitoneal hematoma
  - Femoral artery laceration
  - Femoral artery pseudoaneurysm

SURGICAL PROCEDURE

Indications

- Depends on pt disease.

Procedure

- Access
  - Femoral, carotid or brachial artery.
  - May require multiple access sheaths.

- Diagnostic angiography
  - Carotids, vertebrals & selected cerebral arteries.
  - Vein of Galen.
  - Cerebral or spinal vascular malformations.
- Carotid or vertebral artery stenting.
- Angioplasty.
  - For vasospasm or atherosclerotic disease.
- Thrombolysis for acute stroke.
- Balloon occlusion.
  - Temporary prior to planned occlusion (Wada test).
  - For carotid-cavernous fistula.
- Embolization
  - Coiling of aneurysms
  - Intra-arterial chemotherapy.
  - Alcohol injection of facial or superficial vascular malformations

Surgical Concerns
- CNS hemorrhage during intracranial endovascular procedure.
  - Call for help, including neurosurgical consultation.
  - Reverse anticoagulation (protamine 1 mg for every 100 U heparin administered).
  - Secure the airway w/ ETT & hyperventilate w/ 100% FiO_2.
  - Elevate head of bed to 30 degrees (consider CPP).
  - Administer mannitol 0.5–1.0 g/kg by rapid IV infusion.
  - Consider phenytoin, dexamethasone, phenobarbital & thiopental administration.
- Occlusion of intracranial vessel
  - Deliberate hypertension.
  - Titrate according to neuro, angiographic or physiologic improvement.

Typical EBL
- <100 cc
  - Usually limited to femoral access site.
  - Can be greater if hemorrhage occurs in the presence of anticoagulation.
  - Extent of hemorrhage is limited by the fixed cranial vault (intracranial procedure) or closed intradural space (spinal vascular procedure).
  - Influenced by state of concomitant antiplatelet or anticoagulant therapy.

INTRACRANIAL AVM RESECTION

ALEX KAO, MD
DHANESH K. GUPTA, MD

PREOP

Preop Considerations

- Determine if pt has had previous embolization of AVM.
  - ➤ Successful embolization may decrease bleeding during resection.
  - ➤ If recent, contrast-induced diuresis may cause hypovolemia.
- Previous radiosurgery may make resection more complicated because neovascularization & soft tissue fibrosis or parenchymal scarring may occur.
- Look at neuro angiogram results.
  - ➤ Up to 58% incidence of concurrent aneurysm, often of a feeding vessel of the AVM.
  - ➤ Avoid large increases in MAP if an unsecured aneurysm is present.

Physical Findings

Neuro symptoms depend on location & size of AVM.

- Pt may have increased ICP due to hemorrhage.
- Pt may have seizure disorder.
  - ➤ If on anticonvulsants, nondepolarizing muscle relaxants may have shortened duration of action.
- Pt may be on chronic narcotics for headache & therefore have narcotic tolerance.

Workup

- Head CT, MRI, angiogram to document location, size, & angioarchitecture of AVM.
- CBC, coags, lytes, BUN/Cr.
- T&C 4–6 units PRBCs.

Choice of Anesthesia

- GETA
- Limiting volatile anesthetic to <0.5 MAC will minimize cerebral vasodilation & potential for increased ICP.
- For SSEP monitoring, may need to tailor anesthetic drugs.
  - ➤ Limit volatile anesthetics & N_2O.
  - ➤ Consider propofol infusion.
- For motor evoked potential (MEP) monitoring:

> Maintain normothermia.

> Avoid muscle relaxation.

INTRAOP

Monitors/Line Placement

■ Standard monitors

■ Arterial line to assist w/ CPP monitoring

> Keep transducer at level of circle of Willis, or

> Keep transducer at right atrial level & account for height difference to brain

■ CVP line occasionally used for infusion & monitoring of vasopressors

■ Two large-bore IVs for fluid resuscitation

■ SSEP & MEP may be used to monitor for neuro injury during resection

Intraop Concerns

■ Surgical retraction & concern for CNS injury

> Risk will depend on size & location of AVM.

> Maintain CPP at least 70 mmHg.

> Avoid conditions that can lead to increased ICP.

■ Elevated ICP

■ Bleeding

■ Cerebral protection: allow hypothermia to 34–35 degrees C

Intraop Therapies

■ BP control

> Consider mild hypotension (80% of baseline MAP) to reduce bleeding only if CPP can be maintained >70 mmHg

> Consider labetalol therapy on emergence to minimize hypertension

■ ICP control

> Mild hyperventilation to $PaCO_2$ 30–35 mmHg

> Diuresis w/ mannitol & possibly furosemide

> Minimize anesthetic-induced cerebral vasodilation

• Limit volatile agent to 0.5 MAC, or

• d/c volatile agent & use propofol infusion w/ 100% oxygen

> Limit IVF (however, maintain euvolemia).

> Decrease $CMRO_2$ (mild hypothermia, barbiturates/propofol)

■ Bleeding

> Aggressive replacement w/ crystalloid, colloid, or blood products to maintain euvolemia w/ Hct approx 30

> Maintain platelets >100K.

> Maintain normal coag status.
> Check labs as needed.

POSTOP

Pain
- Mild to moderate
- Most pts have satisfactory analgesia w/ intermittent IV morphine postop, w/o need for PCA.

Complications
- Normal perfusion pressure breakthrough syndrome
  > Hyperperfusion syndrome that may occur after AVM resection
  > More common w/ large AVM
  > Associated w/ cerebral edema (hyperemia), increased ICP, intracerebral bleeding
  > Maintain BP within 20% of baseline MAP, especially in immediate postop period
- Postop intracerebral hemorrhage due to incomplete resection vs normal perfusion pressure breakthrough
- Neuro injury due to surgical-related trauma

SURGICAL PROCEDURE

Indications
- Presence of AVM
- If untreated, hemorrhage rate 3–4%/year w/ up to 30% mortality; therefore, AVMs are often resected in young pts

Procedure
- Craniotomy, positioning dictated by AVM location

Surgical Concerns
- Location & size of AVM will dictate operative approach
- Surgeon may use image-guided surgical system (eg, StealthStation)
- May use SSEP or MEP to monitor for neuro injury during resection
- Postop neurologic change, or delayed awakening from anesthesia
  > Pt may require emergent head CT to rule out hemorrhage, edema, or surgical trauma.

Typical EBL
- 300–500 cc but may be less for AVM after embolization

INTUBATION FOR EPIGLOTTITIS

JASON WIDRICH, MD

PREOP

Preop Considerations

- Epiglottitis is an acute infectious disease that can progress from sore throat to rapid airway obstruction.
  - Swelling occurs at the vallecula, epiglottis & arytenoids.
  - Most commonly occurs in children 2–6 years old.
- Diagnosis of epiglottitis is an emergency.
  - Most complications occur from delay in diagnosis or performing exam or laboratory studies that cause delays or agitate the child.
  - Consider calling for additional help w/ airway mgt, including an expert in surgical airway placement (eg, ENT surgeon).
- Most commonly caused by *H. influenzae* type B, *Staphylococcus aureus*, & beta-hemolytic streptococci. However, epidemiology is changing due to vaccination for *H. flu* type B.
- Differential diagnosis includes
  - Viral croup (usually younger pts)
  - Bacterial tracheitis
  - Foreign body

Physical Findings

- Classic findings
  - Sudden onset of fever
  - Drooling
  - Dysphagia
  - Preference for sitting & leaning forward
  - Muffled voice
- Important: Retractions, labored breathing, cyanosis indicate impending airway obstruction.

Workup

- Important: Suspicion or diagnosis of epiglottitis is an emergency. Do not delay airway mgt for diagnostic tests.
  - Characteristic signs of epiglottitis on lateral or AP x-ray include thumbprint or steeple shape to epiglottis.

Choice of Anesthesia

- Ideal pt mgt occurs in a setting w/ equipment for difficult airway mgt, cricothyrotomy, or tracheotomy & skilled personnel (eg, OR).
- Avoid examining the airway or performing painful procedures such as needle sticks or IV placement.
- Consider keeping the child w/ the parents if this will keep the child calm.
- GA. Begin an inhalation induction (halothane or sevoflurane) in the sitting position w/ ENT & difficult airway equipment available. In an adult w/ a functioning IV, can use a combination of IV & inhaled anesthetic.

INTRAOP

Monitors/Line Placement

- For the pt in distress, transport to OR immediately. Minimize stimulation or agitation of the child.
- If the pt is an adult or mature enough to accept an IV, then place it as soon as possible.
- Place ECG leads & an oxygen saturation monitor.
- Begin an inhalation induction (halothane or sevoflurane) in the sitting position w/ ENT surgeon & difficult airway equipment available.
  - ➤ In an adult w/ a functioning IV, can use a combination IV & inhaled anesthetic.

Intraop Concerns

- Important: Be prepared to perform (or ask ENT surgeon to perform) an emergent surgical airway if intubation attempts fail.
- For the pt w/ respiratory collapse & cyanosis
  - ➤ Attempt rapid oral intubation.
  - ➤ If unsuccessful, use a rigid bronchoscope, or perform cricothyrotomy or tracheotomy as necessary.
- Avoid preop medication. Apply a face mask w/ 100% O_2 or blow-by humidified oxygen.
- Although aspiration is a concern, it is not the overriding priority. Most of these children have been unable to eat or drink for some time before presentation. Prepare a suction w/ Yankauer tip in case of vomiting.
- When the child loses muscle tone, attempt to lay him or her supine. This may increase airway obstruction. Apply jaw thrust or maneuvers to optimize the mask airway. Positive airway pressure w/ the child still spontaneously breathing is the goal.

- If the airway can be maintained by mask, start an IV as soon as possible.
  - Then consider IV atropine or glycopyrrolate to decrease secretions & minimize bradycardia.
  - Start an IV fluid bolus of 10–20 cc/kg as these children are often dehydrated.
- Important: This inhalation induction w/o muscle relaxants can be slow & may require as long as 10–20 min for sufficient anesthetic depth to prevent reaction to airway manipulation. Continually assess airway patency w/ the mask & slight positive airway pressure.
- ETT selection & preparation
  - Because of airway swelling, prepare ETTs up to two sizes smaller than normal.
  - Consider extra-long ETT (eg, microlaryngeal tube).
  - Stylets may also be useful for added rigidity necessary to bypass swollen tissues.
- Consider squeezing the pt's chest during laryngoscopy to produce air bubbles & help identify the glottic opening.
- After airway is secured:
  - Meticulously tape ETT & consider use of restraints to minimize self-extubation.
  - Obtain blood cultures or other necessary lab tests.
  - Start IV antibiotics.

POSTOP

Pain
- Minimal

Complications
- Postobstructive pulmonary edema may occur; can be treated conservatively w/ diuretics & positive pressure ventilation.
- Extubation usually occurs within 36–72 h w/ resolution of swelling. Consider a leak test or visual examination of the larynx before attempting extubation to reduce chance of postextubation airway obstruction.

SURGICAL PROCEDURE

Indications
- Epiglottitis w/ airway obstruction

Procedure
- Airway mgt w/ tracheal intubation or surgical airway

Surgical Concerns
- Risk of complete airway obstruction & hypoxia

Typical EBL
- None

KNEE ARTHROSCOPY

KENNETH DRASNER, MD
MANUEL PARDO, JR., MD

PREOP

Preop Considerations
- Generally done as outpatient procedure in relatively healthy pts, often w/ sports injuries.

Physical Findings
- If pt has rheumatoid arthritis, look for c-spine involvement.

Workup
- Dependent on coexisting disease.

Choice of Anesthesia
- Can be performed under GA, spinal, epidural, or femoral/sciatic block. Some surgeons prefer to administer local anesthesia in selected pts.
- Choice of technique largely dependent upon anesthesia provider preference, duration of surgery, pt-related factors.
- High incidence of transient neuro symptoms (TNS) if performed under lidocaine spinal anesthesia.
  - ➤ Controversial, but positioning may produce stretch of lumbosacral nerve roots, resulting in decreased perfusion & enhanced lidocaine effect.
  - ➤ Low-dose lidocaine (25 mg) + fentanyl (25 mcg) may reduce risk.
  - ➤ Very low incidence of TNS w/ bupivacaine but may delay PACU stay even at low doses.

INTRAOP

Monitors/Line Placement
- One peripheral IV
- Routine monitors

Intraop Concerns
- Tourniquet pain may occur after 45–60 min; can be treated w/ narcotics or ketamine.

POSTOP

Pain
- Mild (eg, diagnostic arthroscopy) to moderate (eg, ACL repair), depending on extent of surgery.

Complications
- Serious complications are rare but can include infection, DVT, pulmonary embolism, peripheral nerve injury, fluid extravasation, or popliteal vascular injury.

SURGICAL PROCEDURE

Indications
- Variable; include arthritis, post-trauma assessment, ligament or cartilage repair.

Procedure
- Insertion of arthroscope, irrigation fluid. Surgery performed by placing instruments through additional incisions around knee.

Surgical Concerns
- Depend on type of surgery

Typical EBL
- Minimal

LABOR & VAGINAL DELIVERY

JOHN P. LEE, MD
SAM HUGHES, MD
MARK ROSEN, MD

PREOP

Preop Considerations
- Know gravida/para; expect nulliparous parturient to have a more protracted labor
- Souce of pain depends on stage of labor

➤ First-stage pain is mostly visceral from uterine contraction & cervical dilation (cervical plexus; sympathetics to T10-L1)
➤ Second-stage pain is somatic from stretching of vagina & perineum (pudendal nerve; S2–S4)

Physical Findings
■ Expect systolic ejection murmur
■ Anticipate possible difficult airway from weight gain of pregnancy & capillary engorgement

Workup
■ No labs necessary if history & physical normal

Choice of Anesthesia
■ For labor
  ➤ Lumbar epidural analgesia: Best analgesic: Segmental analgesia is titratable for all labor stages
    • Bupivacaine 0.03–0.25% w/ initial 8–12 mL bolus & infusion of 8–15 mL/h (or ropivacaine, L-bupivacaine, or other equianalgesic local anesthetics)
    • Fentanyl 50–100 mcg bolus & 2–5 mcg/mL can be added to enhance analgesia (particularly the lower local concentrations).
    • Additional bolus might be necessary to extend the block to include the sacral segments in second stage.
  ➤ Systemic opioid
    • 100 mcg fentanyl/h (no agent proven superior to another)
    • Minimally effective compared to regional analgesia
  ➤ Paracervical block (performed by obstetrical care provider)
    • Limited duration
    • Small risk of fetal bradycardia of unknown origin
    • 1% lidocaine, 10 mL each side
  ➤ Bilateral L2 sympathetic block
    • Limited duration
    • 1% lidocaine, 5–10 mL each side
    • Rarely performed
  ➤ Inhalational analgesia
    • 50% nitrous oxide, continuously or intermittently
    • Weakly analgesic
■ For delivery
  ➤ Low spinal anesthesia

- Administered immediately before vaginal delivery
- Bupivacaine 5–7.5 mg (±15–25 mcg fentanyl)

➤ Combined spinal-epidural
- Long (124-mm), small-gauge spinal needle passed through sited epidural needle
- Small dose of opioid (eg, 25 mcg fentanyl) and/or local anesthetic (eg, 2.5–5 mg isobaric bupivacaine)
- Very rapid onset

➤ Pudendal nerve block
- Administered by obstetrician for vaginal delivery (forceps, vacuum) or perineal repair
- Alternative to low spinal but less effective

➤ GA extremely rare
- Induce w/ rapid sequence induction

INTRAOP

Monitors/Line Placement

For labor:
- One peripheral IV
- BP monitoring
- Continuous fetal heart monitoring or q15min acceptable
- Monitoring of uterine contractions

For delivery: In addition to the above
- ASA monitors for GA or major regional block for operative vaginal delivery
- Resuscitation equipment immediately available for mother & baby

Intraop Concerns

- Maternal & fetal well-being
- Progress of labor
- Fever (infection)
- Bleeding
- Hypotension from regional blockade
- Total spinal w/ intended epidural local anesthetics
- IV local anesthetic toxicity (accidental IV bolus)

Intraop Therapies

- Ephedrine 5–10 mg IV for maternal hypotension from regional block
  ➤ May repeat w/ 15–25 mg

➤ If inadequate response to 5–10 mg IV ephedrine, phenylephrine is an alternative choice
- Oxytocin infusions for stimulating uterine activity

POSTOP

Pain
- Intrathecal (0.2–0.25 mg) or epidural morphine (4–5 mg) (recommended for third- or fourth-degree lacerations, mediolateral episiotomies)
- Consider ketorolac (15–30 mg IV/IM), NSAID, or opioid

Complications
- Postdural puncture headache
- Postpartum hemorrhage (uterine atony, cervical or vaginal lacerations, episiotomy)
- Nerve damage (obstetric palsy) from fetal compression in pelvis or malpositioning of mother during delivery (eg, prolonged lithotomy)

SURGICAL PROCEDURE

Indications
- Labor & delivery of newborn
- Postpartum repair of laceration, episiotomy or removal of retained placenta

Procedure
- First stage, latent phase (uterine contractions w/ cervical dilation to 4–5 cm)
- First stage, active phase (to complete cervical dilation)
- Second stage (complete cervical dilation to delivery)
- Third stage (delivery of baby to delivery of placenta)

Surgical Concerns
- Assessment of labor progress
- Assessment of fetal well-being (fetal heart rate, sono)
- Ensure hemostasis postdelivery w/ manual massage of uterus, repair of lacerations, & complete removal of placenta & membranes

Typical EBL
- 500 mL
- About 5% will have postpartum uterine atony & greater blood loss

LAPAROSCOPIC CHOLECYSTECTOMY

JASON WIDRICH, MD

PREOP

Preop Considerations
- Complications of gallstones
  - Biliary colic.
  - Acute cholecystitis.
  - Pancreatitis.
  - Bilioenteric fistula, including gallstone ileus.
- For pts w/ acute cholecystitis, laparoscopic cholecystectomy ("lap chole") is usually done after symptoms have subsided.
  - May also be done emergently for impending perforation.
  - Critically ill pt w/ sepsis might undergo percutaneous cholecystostomy instead of lap chole.
  - Open surgery more likely in pt w/ liver cirrhosis or pt w/ perforated gallbladder & peritonitis.
- Pt w/ severe respiratory & cardiovascular dysfunction may not tolerate intra-abdominal CO_2 insufflation.
- Previous abdominal surgery may make laparoscopic approach more difficult & may increase chance of conversion to open surgery.

Physical Findings
- May be none.
- Signs of acute cholecystitis including fever, right upper quadrant abdominal tenderness.

Workup
- CBC, LFTs, PT, PTT.
- ECG.

Choice of Anesthesia
- GA w/ ETT.
- If high likelihood of conversion to open surgery, consider thoracic epidural for postop pain control.

INTRAOP

Monitors/Line Placement
- Standard monitors
- One peripheral IV

■ NG or OG tube: reduces gastric distention, may improve surgeon's view

Intraop Concerns
■ See also Procedures chapter "Laparoscopic General Surgery."
■ Anticipate effects of intra-abdominal CO_2 insufflation.
  ➤ Pulmonary
    • Atelectasis, decreased FRC, decreased PaO_2, elevated PIP. Adjust ventilator settings accordingly.
    • Hypercarbia.
  ➤ Cardiac
    • Increased HR, SVR, BP.
    • Increased CVP, but may not reflect true volume status.
    • Increased intra-abdominal pressure & reverse Trendelenburg position will decrease lower extremity venous return.
■ Visceral, vascular or intra-abdominal organ injury can occur, especially w/ Veress needle or trocar insertion.
  ➤ Consider unrecognized hemorrhage as a cause of persistent hypotension or tachycardia.
■ CO_2 embolism is potentially fatal but rare complication.
  ➤ Can present w/ cardiovascular collapse from right heart failure.
  ➤ End-tidal CO_2 may exhibit a transient elevation followed by a decline.
  ➤ Can also have left-sided emboli through patent foramen ovale or pulmonary AV shunts
  ➤ May be more common in hypovolemic pt
■ Barotrauma
  ➤ Pneumothorax, including tension pneumothorax.
  ➤ Pneumomediastinum.
  ➤ Subcutaneous emphysema: can occur in neck & face; associated w/ large increases in pCO_2.
■ Surgeon may convert to open cholecystectomy for a variety of reasons, including hemorrhage, pneumothorax, bile leak or difficult exposure.

Intraop Therapies
■ Continue neuromuscular blockade to improve abdominal wall compliance & facilitate surgical exposure.
■ Avoid N_2O in long operations to minimize bowel distention.
■ Consider prophylactic antiemetics.

POSTOP

Pain
- Mild
- IV narcotics initially required in PACU, depending on intraop narcotic administration

Complications
- Nausea/vomiting
- Shoulder pain referred from diaphragmatic irritation
- Problems related to intraop laparoscopy may become manifest in PACU
  - Pneumothorax
  - Subcutaneous emphysema
  - Visceral, vascular or abdominal organ injury
  - Unrecognized hemorrhage
- Complications of gallstone disease
  - Sepsis
  - Gallstone ileus
  - Perforation of gallbladder
  - Pancreatitis

SURGICAL PROCEDURE

Indications
- Symptomatic cholelithiasis, including acute cholecystitis

Procedure
- Insert Veress needle & confirm intraperitoneal location
- Create CO_2 pneumoperitoneum
- Maintain pneumoperitoneum, usually with 10–15 mmHg pressure
- Place trocars for camera & surgical instruments
- Dissection of gallbladder from fossa beneath liver
- Identification of cystic duct & artery, which may require use of cholangiography
- Division & ligation of cystic duct & artery
- The gallbladder is separated from the inferior surface of the liver & placed in a bag.
- Gallbladder removed via one of the ports
- Ensure adequate hemostasis & inspect abdominal structures.
- Closure

Surgical Concerns
- Common bile duct injury

- Common bile duct stones
- Hemorrhage
- Infection
- Injury to bowel

Typical EBL
- Minimal

LAPAROSCOPIC ESOPHAGEAL FUNDOPLICATION (LAPAROSCOPIC NISSEN)

MARK T. GRABOVAC, MD

PREOP

Preop Considerations
- Indication for surgery is severe gastroesophageal reflux disease (GERD)
  - Pts w/ severe GERD considered at high risk for aspiration
  - Severe GERD may be complicated by chronic aspiration & reactive airway disease, chronic bronchitis or bronchiectasis
  - Severity of reflux can be partially assessed by
    - Control achieved by meds
    - Number of meds taken
    - Degree of orthopnea caused by reflux
    - Presence or absence of bilious material in mouth on awakening in morning
    - Frequency of nighttime awakening from reflux symptoms
  - Consider whether pain & symptoms are entirely from GERD (not cardiac ischemia) & whether orthopnea contributed to by CHF
- Common coexisting diseases
  - Obesity
  - Hiatal hernia
  - Reactive airway disease
  - Esophagitis
  - Esophageal cancer
- Pt w/ severe respiratory & cardiovascular dysfunction may not tolerate intra-abdominal CO_2 insufflation.
- Previous abdominal surgery may make laparoscopic approach more difficult & may increase chance of conversion to open surgery.

Physical Findings
- Obesity w/ predictors of difficult airway mgt
- Pulmonary exam for wheezing, signs of aspiration or rales

Workup
- CBC
- CXR if evidence of reactive airway disease, COPD or aspiration
- ECG & cardiac evaluation if etiology of pain is unclear

Choice of Anesthesia
- GA w/ ETT
- Little role for epidural unless open procedure is likely
  - If high likelihood of conversion to open surgery, consider thoracic epidural for postop pain control
- Use of N_2O may lead to bowel distention & difficulty w/ surgical exposure

INTRAOP

Monitors/Line Placement
- Standard monitors.
- Foley catheter (to decompress bladder & avoid surgical injury & for assessing urine output & fluid status).
- One large-bore peripheral IV.
- Consider arterial line for significant cardiac or pulmonary disease.
  - For instance, for $PaCO_2$ monitoring in COPD pt ($ETCO_2$ may be inaccurate).

Intraop Concerns
- See also Procedures chapter "Laparoscopic General Surgery."
- Anticipate effects of intra-abdominal CO_2 insufflation.
  - Pulmonary
    - Atelectasis, decreased FRC, decreased PaO_2, elevated PIP. Adjust ventilator settings accordingly.
    - Hypercarbia: $PaCO_2$ & $ETCO_2$ will increase from CO_2 insufflation, but other causes include airway obstruction, relative hypoventilation, bronchospasm, abdominal distention & decreased pulmonary compliance, pneumothorax, CO_2 embolus.
  - Cardiac
    - Increased HR, SVR, BP.
    - Increased CVP, but may not reflect true volume status.

- Increased intra-abdominal pressure & reverse Trendelenburg position will decrease lower extremity venous return.

■ Visceral, vascular or intra-abdominal organ injury can occur, especially w/ Veress needle or trocar insertion.
  ➤ Consider unrecognized hemorrhage as cause of persistent hypotension or tachycardia.
    - Bleeding may not be obvious (eg, confined to retroperitoneum).
    - Necessitates conversion to open procedure.
    - Need to obtain large-bore IV access & blood products.

■ CO_2 embolism is potentially fatal but rare complication.
  ➤ Can present w/ cardiovascular collapse from right heart failure.
  ➤ Can also have left-sided emboli through patent foramen ovale or pulmonary AV shunts.
  ➤ May be more common in hypovolemic pt.

■ Barotrauma
  ➤ Pneumothorax, including tension pneumothorax.
  ➤ Pneumomediastinum.
  ➤ Subcutaneous emphysema: can occur in neck & face; assoc w/ large increases in pCO_2, requiring large increase in minute ventilation.
  ➤ May need to relieve pneumoperitoneum for acutely unstable pt.

Intraop Therapies
■ Premed for aspiration
  ➤ Continue preop proton pump inhibitors or H2 blockers (consider additional dose).
  ➤ Consider metoclopramide 10 mg IV to stimulate gastric emptying 30 min prior to induction.
  ➤ Sodium citrate or Bicitra 15–30 mL PO immediately prior to induction.

■ Rapid sequence induction w/ cricoid pressure. Consider elevating head of bed to decrease risk of aspiration. Use succinylcholine for anticipated difficult airway or morbidly obese pt.

■ NG tube placed after induction/intubation to decompress stomach & decrease risk of aspiration. NG tube removed during placement of esophageal dilators & usually not replaced.

■ Large bougie dilators are passed to assist in both dilation & surgical wrap. Can cause esophageal perforation or dislodge ETT. Observe placement on video monitors.

- Continue neuromuscular blockade to improve abdominal wall compliance & facilitate surgical exposure.
- Increase minute ventilation during & after pneumoperitoneum to eliminate excess CO_2.
- Avoid N_2O.
- Consider prophylactic antiemetics.

POSTOP

Pain
- Mild.
- Treat w/ IV or oral narcotic, including PCA if needed.
- Consider ketorolac.

Complications
- Problems related to intraop laparoscopy may become manifest in PACU.
  - Pneumothorax
    - Needle thoracostomy may be necessary if tension pneumothorax occurs.
  - Subcutaneous emphysema
    - May be dramatic.
    - Crepitus over abdominal wall may extend to neck, face.
    - Rarely leads to airway compromise but assoc w/ pneumothorax & gas in mediastinum.
    - Rarely requires treatment when not associated w/ pneumothorax.
  - Visceral, vascular or abdominal organ injury.
  - Unrecognized hemorrhage.

SURGICAL PROCEDURE

Indications
- Not well defined
- Generally reserved for treatment of symptomatic GERD refractory to medical therapy, causing pulmonary complications or in pts who cannot tolerate medical treatment.

Procedure
- Insert Veress needle & confirm intraperitoneal location.
- Create CO_2 pneumoperitoneum.
- Maintain pneumoperitoneum, usually with 10–15 mmHg pressure.
- Place trocars for camera & surgical instruments.

- Involves surgical exposure of lower esophagus & upper stomach, w/ subsequent wrapping of upper stomach around the lower portion of the esophagus to create new lower esophageal sphincter & decrease GERD.
- Closure

Surgical Concerns
- May be technically difficult in obese pt or in pt w/ previous abdominal surgery
- Vascular or visceral injury

Typical EBL
- Minimal

LAPAROSCOPIC GENERAL SURGERY

RICHARD PAULSEN, MD

PREOP

Preop Considerations
- Pt w/ severe respiratory & cardiovascular dysfunction may not tolerate intra-abdominal CO_2 insufflation.
- Previous abdominal surgery may make laparoscopic approach more difficult & may increase chance of conversion to open surgery.

Workup
- CBC.
- Other labs dictated by coexisting disease.

Choice of Anesthesia
- GA w/ ETT.
- If high likelihood of conversion to open surgery, consider epidural for postop pain control.

INTRAOP

Monitors/Line Placement
- Standard ASA monitors.
- NG or OG tube: Reduces gastric distention, may improve surgeon's view

Intraop Concerns
- Anticipate effects of intra-abdominal CO_2 insufflation.

- Pulmonary
    - Atelectasis, decreased FRC, decreased PaO_2, elevated PIP. Adjust ventilator settings accordingly.
    - Hypercarbia: Usual 5–10 mmHg increase in pCO_2 w/ CO_2 insufflation.
    - Follow end-tidal CO_2 ($ETCO_2$) & increase minute ventilation as necessary. Pts w/ pulmonary disease may have poor correlation between $ETCO_2$ & pCO_2.
    - For large increase in $ETCO_2$ consider ABG to check pCO_2. This is more common w/ subcutaneous absorption of CO_2. May need to consider conversion to open surgery for persistent severe hypercarbia.
- Cardiac
    - Increased HR, SVR, BP.
    - Increased CVP, but may not reflect true volume status.
    - Increased intra-abdominal pressure & reverse Trendelenburg position will decrease lower extremity venous return.
- Visceral, vascular, or intra-abdominal organ injury, esp w/ Veress needle or trocar insertion.
    - Consider unrecognized hemorrhage as cause of persistent hypotension or tachycardia.
- CO_2 embolism is potentially fatal but rare complication.
    - Can present w/ cardiovascular collapse from right heart failure.
    - Can also have left-sided emboli through patent foramen ovale or pulmonary AV shunts.
    - May be more common in hypovolemic pt
- Barotrauma
    - Pneumothorax, including tension pneumothorax.
    - Pneumomediastinum.
    - Subcutaneous emphysema. Can occur in neck and face. Assoc w/ large increases in pCO_2.

Intraop Therapies
- Replace fluid deficit prior to insufflation & reverse Trendelenburg position.
- Continue neuromuscular blockade to improve abdominal wall compliance & facilitate surgical exposure.
- Avoid N_2O in long operations to minimize bowel distention.
- Consider prophylactic antiemetics.

POSTOP

Pain
- Minimal to moderate depending on type of surgery
- Right shoulder pain relatively common
- PCA transitioning to PO analgesics as tolerated
- Consider having surgeon infiltrate local anesthetic at port sites

Complications
- May detect problems in PACU that occurred intraop
  - Pneumothorax
  - Subcutaneous emphysema
  - Visceral, vascular, or abdominal organ injury
  - Unrecognized hemorrhage

SURGICAL PROCEDURE

Indications
- Varies by type of surgery
- Often preferred over open technique because of reduced morbidity, faster recovery times

Procedure
- Will vary w/ specific surgery, but general steps include
  - Create pneumoperitoneum. Usually done w/ Veress needle
  - Initiate CO_2 pneumoperitoneum
  - Maintain pneumoperitoneum, usually with 10–15 mmHg pressure
  - Place trocars for camera & surgical instruments.
  - Perform surgery
  - Closure

Surgical Concerns
- Maintain exposure w/ insufflation pressure <15 mmHg
- Proper trocar placement
- Consider need for conversion to open procedure
- Others as dictated by procedure performed

Typical EBL
- Generally minimal (25–100 cc) depending on site of surgery

LAPAROSCOPIC GYNECOLOGIC PROCEDURES

JASON WIDRICH, MD

PREOP

Preop Considerations
- A variety of gynecologic conditions may require laparoscopic surgery.
  - ➤ Determine implications of gynecologic disease (eg, pt w/ ruptured ectopic pregnancy may present w/ hypovolemic shock, requiring fluid resuscitation prior to induction of anesthesia).
- Pt w/ severe respiratory & cardiovascular dysfunction may not tolerate intra-abdominal CO_2 insufflation.
- Previous abdominal surgery may make laparoscopic approach more difficult & may increase chance of conversion to open surgery.

Physical Findings
- None typical

Workup
- CBC
- PT, PTT

Choice of Anesthesia
- GA w/ ETT

INTRAOP

Monitors/Line Placement
- Standard monitors.
- One or two peripheral IVs usually adequate.
- NG or OG tube: reduces gastric distention, may improve surgeon's view.

Intraop Concerns
- See also Procedures chapter "Laparoscopic General Surgery."
- Anticipate effects of intra-abdominal CO_2 insufflation.
  - ➤ Pulmonary
    - Atelectasis, decreased FRC, decreased PaO_2, elevated PIP. Adjust ventilator settings accordingly.
    - Hypercarbia: $PaCO_2$ & $ETCO_2$ will increase from CO_2 insufflation, but other causes include airway obstruction,

relative hypoventilation, bronchospasm, abdominal distention & decreased pulmonary compliance, pneumothorax, CO_2
embolus.

➤ Cardiac
  • Increased HR, SVR, BP.
  • Increased CVP, but may not reflect true volume status.
  • Increased intra-abdominal pressure will decrease lower
    extremity venous return.

■ Visceral, vascular or intra-abdominal organ injury can occur, especially w/ Veress needle or trocar insertion.

➤ Consider unrecognized hemorrhage as cause of persistent
hypotension or tachycardia.
  • Bleeding may not be obvious (eg, confined to retroperi-
    toneum).
  • Necessitates conversion to open procedure.
  • Need to obtain large-bore IV access & blood products.

■ CO_2 embolism is potentially fatal but rare complication.

➤ Can present w/ cardiovascular collapse from right heart
failure

➤ Can also have left-sided emboli through patent foramen ovale or
pulmonary AV shunts

➤ May be more common in hypovolemic pt

■ Barotrauma

➤ Pneumothorax, including tension pneumothorax.

➤ Pneumomediastinum.

➤ Subcutaneous emphysema: can occur in neck & face; assoc
w/ large increases in pCO_2, requiring large increase in minute
ventilation.

➤ May need to relieve pneumoperitoneum for acutely unstable pt.

■ Steep Trendelenburg position often used to facilitate surgical
exposure.

➤ Can lead to reduced lung volumes, reduced lung compliance,
right mainstem intubation.

Intraop Therapies

■ Continue neuromuscular blockade to improve abdominal wall compliance & facilitate surgical exposure.

■ Increase minute ventilation during & after pneumoperitoneum to
eliminate excess CO_2.

■ Avoid N_2O in long operations to minimize bowel distention.

■ Consider prophylactic antiemetics.

POSTOP

Pain
- Mild
- IV narcotics initially, then PO analgesics

Complications
- Problems related to intraop laparoscopy may become manifest in PACU.
  - Pneumothorax
    - Needle thoracostomy may be necessary if tension pneumothorax occurs.
  - Subcutaneous emphysema
    - May be dramatic
    - Crepitus over abdominal wall may extend to neck, face.
    - Rarely leads to airway compromise but assoc w/ pneumothorax & gas in mediastinum.
    - Rarely requires treatment when not assoc w/ pneumothorax.
  - Visceral, vascular or abdominal organ injury.
  - Unrecognized hemorrhage.

SURGICAL PROCEDURE

Indications
- Variety of gynecologic conditions may require laparoscopic surgery:
  - Pelvic pain
  - Endometriosis
  - Ectopic pregnancy
  - Uterine myoma
  - Laparoscopic-assisted vaginal hysterectomy
  - Oophorectomy
  - Tubal ligation

Procedure
- Insert Veress needle & confirm intraperitoneal location
- Create CO_2 pneumoperitoneum
- Maintain pneumoperitoneum, usually with 10–15 mmHg pressure
- Place trocars for camera & surgical instruments
- From this point, the procedure varies depending on the reason for laparoscopy
- Closure

Surgical Concerns
- Conversion to open procedure

- Hemorrhage
- Abdominal organ injury
- Urinary tract or uterine trauma

Typical EBL
- <200 mL

LARYNGECTOMY

ALISON G. CAMERON, MD

PREOP

Preop Considerations
- Pt likely to have significant smoking history, COPD.
  - ➢ Pt may also have significant alcohol use.
  - ➢ If tumor interferes with pt's ability to eat, pt may be severely malnourished, dehydrated, anemic.
  - ➢ Exercise tolerance may be significantly decreased; CAD is likely. Assess symptoms of CHF, angina.
  - ➢ Laryngeal cancer accounts for 2–3% of all cancers.
    - Tobacco, ETOH, HSV, radiotherapy are known risk factors. Males >50 years most highly affected.
  - ➢ Pt should be treated as having a difficult airway if any airway distortion or compromise is present. May need fiberoptic intubation/awake intubation under topical & transtracheal anesthesia.

Physical Findings
- Tracheal deviation
- Hoarseness
- Neck swelling

Workup
- ECG
- CXR
- Type & cross
- ABG to assess hypoxemia, CO_2 retention
- CT scan of neck for severity of obstruction/mass size

INTRAOP

Monitors/Line Placement
- Standard monitors.

- Two peripheral IVs.
- Arterial line.
- Foley.
- Depending on surgeon, neuromonitoring of facial nerve.

Intraop Concerns
- Decide whether pt at risk for difficult intubation. If so, consider awake intubation or tracheotomy.
- Bed may be turned 180 degrees so the pt's head is away from anesthesia provider.
  - ➢ Will need extensions for all tubing, including IVs & invasive lines.
- Head will be elevated 15–30 degrees.
- Sufficient padding of head/eyes is necessary because of surgeon's proximity to face.
- Neuromonitoring may be needed for facial nerve. If so, avoid muscle relaxants.
- Surgery may trigger vagal reflexes as well as dysrhythmias, prolonged Q-T interval (from effects on the carotid sinus & stellate ganglion).
- Venous air embolism is possible from large open veins in neck.
  - ➢ Monitor $ETCO_2$ (may also use precordial Doppler).
- The surgeon will request the ETT to be pulled back slowly as the incision for the tracheotomy is made. There is risk of airway fire at this point if electrocautery is used above the exposed ETT. Despite this, 100% oxygen should be used because of the possibility of desaturation.

POSTOP

Pain
- Moderate
- IV opioids
- PCA indicated

Complications
- Fistula formation (5–20%)
- Bleeding, hematoma
- Infection
- Nerve injury: facial n. (facial droop), phrenic n. (ipsilateral diaphragmatic paralysis)
- Parathyroid damage
- Pneumothorax
- Subcutaneous emphysema

SURGICAL PROCEDURE

Indications
- Airway obstruction due to tumor (eg, laryngeal cancer) or edema.
- Intractable aspiration.

Procedure
- Total laryngectomy includes excision from posterior third of tongue (or vallecula) to first or second tracheal rings.
- A tracheotomy is placed for surgery, but then the trachea is usually placed end to skin & the trach tube may no longer be needed.
- Thyroid gland is spared unless it is part of specimen.
- Supraglottic/hemi/near-total laryngectomies are all variations of the procedure.
- Frequently accompanied by neck dissection, pharyngectomy.

Surgical Concerns
- Case generally starts w/ ETT, which surgeon will manipulate & eventually remove when tracheotomy or tracheostomy is placed.
- There may be times when the ETT/trach is not in the pt.
  - ➤ This can last several minutes.
  - ➤ Vigilance is required as well as good communication w/ surgeon to prevent desaturation.

Typical EBL
- 200–1,000 mL depending on procedure & whether neck dissection is included.
- Can be massive if any large vessels are damaged.

LARYNGOSCOPY

ALISON G. CAMERON, MD

PREOP

Preop Considerations
- This chapter deals w/ direct laryngoscopy, as used for exam of the glottis & subglottic area.
- Laryngoscopy is often performed on a regular basis in pts w/ chronic conditions such as laryngeal papillomas.
- May be combined w/ esophagoscopy, bronchoscopy or nasal pharyngoscopy.
- High association w/ tobacco use, COPD, CAD, malnutrition.

Physical Findings

- Often none.
- Depending on lesion (tumors, viral papillomas, subglottic stenosis, vocal cord trauma, etc), may see masses on supra/subglottic pharyngeal surfaces via indirect laryngoscopy when placing ETT.
- Unrecognized airway compromise.
- Potential recurrent laryngeal nerve damage resulting in hoarseness & increased aspiration risk.

Workup

- Assess potential difficult airway (necessitating awake fiberoptic intubation or awake tracheostomy by surgeon).
- Dental assessment (pts are at risk for dental injury).

Choice of Anesthesia

- GA
  - ➤ Most techniques acceptable. Main considerations include
    - High level of surgical stimulation.
    - Quick cessation of stimulation (removal of laryngoscope).
    - Highly variable duration of surgery (minutes to hours).
    - Possible surgical requirement for apneic oxygenation or ventilating laryngoscope if ETT blocks access to surgical field.
  - ➤ Most significant implication of techniques w/o ETT is requirement for total IV anesthesia.
    - Short-acting anesthetics such as propofol & remifentanil are often appropriate choices.
- Local anesthesia
  - ➤ May be suitable for short procedures (eg, Teflon injection of vocal cords).
  - ➤ Topical anesthesia + glossopharyngeal nerve block may be needed to blunt gag reflex.
  - ➤ Disadvantages include lack of muscle relaxation & high stimulation level of procedure.

INTRAOP

Monitors/Line Placement

- Standard monitors.
- Small ETT (5.0–6.0) taped to the left side of mouth (surgeon's approach is usually from right).
- One peripheral IV.
- Peripheral nerve stimulator.

➤ Facial nerve stimulation may better correlate w/ neuromuscular blockade at vocal cords compared to ulnar nerve.
■ Table usually turned 90 degrees after GA induction.
➤ Use circuit extensions.

Intraop Concerns
■ Pt protection
➤ Dental guard
➤ Excellent padding of head/eyes necessary because of surgeon's proximity to facial structures & potential use of laser surgery.
■ Laser surgery considerations
➤ Laser surgery increases risk of airway fire.
➤ Follow airway fire precautions (see also Critical Events chapter "Airway Fire").
  • Metal tube or foil-wrapped tube
  • Saline-filled ETT cuff
  • Minimize inspired O_2% (<30%)
  • No N_2O
■ Maintain close communication w/ surgeon regarding airway manipulation, oxygenation, duration of case (often 5–10 minutes duration).
■ Considerations for airway papilloma surgery.
➤ Consider scavenging of aerosolized papilloma virus when papillomas are lasered.
➤ All OR personnel should wear masks to prevent inhalation of papilloma virus.
➤ Minimize coughing or "bucking" on the ETT as this may exacerbate pt's condition by spreading papilloma virus throughout the airway.

Intraop Therapies
■ Premedicate w/ antisialogogue.
■ GA maintenance w/ inhaled or IV anesthetic.
■ Pt may require steroids if significant edema is present or anticipated.
■ Paralysis w/ muscle relaxant is usually required for surgery on the vocal cords.
➤ Appropriate choices may include a short-acting nondepolarizing agent (eg, mivacurium) or a succinylcholine infusion.
■ Jet ventilation may be used via port on rigid laryngoscope (ventilating laryngoscope).
➤ Muscle relaxation helps to increase chest wall compliance & improve effectiveness of jet ventilation.

➤ Ensure that chest deflates after each ventilation to decrease risk of barotrauma.
➤ Typically, only 3–5 PSI inspiratory pressure is necessary.
■ Apneic oxygenation may also be used.

POSTOP

Pain
■ Minimal
■ Mild analgesics such as acetaminophen usually sufficient

Complications
■ Trauma to teeth, eyes, pharynx
■ Laryngospasm, bronchospasm
■ Aspiration
■ Pneumothorax w/ jet ventilation

SURGICAL PROCEDURE

Indications
■ Visualization of larynx, pharynx, hypopharynx.
■ Diagnosis & treatment of airway lesions including (but not limited to) foreign bodies, human papillomavirus, congenital webs/cysts, polyps, laryngomalacia, laryngeal atresia, post-traumatic stenosis, hemangioma.

Procedure
■ Surgeon will use rigid laryngoscope, which may be suspended from OR table.
■ Microscope may also be used for more delicate or precise surgery.
■ Surgeon may take biopsies or use laser w/ rigid laryngoscope in place.
■ Vocal cord surgery may include injection of Teflon, steroid, botulinum toxin.

Surgical Concerns
■ Airway fire during laser surgery.
■ Airway perforation.
■ Barotrauma (if using jet ventilation).
  ➤ Pneumothorax.
  ➤ Subcutaneous emphysema.
■ Facial trauma.
■ Bleeding.

Typical EBL
■ Minimal

LASER SURGERY OF THE AIRWAY

STEVEN YOUNGER, MD

PREOP

Preop Considerations
- Pt may have undergone multiple similar procedures in the past.
- Depending on diagnosis, pt may already have tracheotomy.
- For pts w/ laryngeal papillomas, airway secretions are potentially infectious.

Physical Findings
- Pt my have minimal findings, but possibilities include
  - Tracheotomy.
  - Stridor.
  - Vocal changes.

Workup
- CXR, ABGs, PFTs usually not necessary.

Choice of Anesthesia
- GA required.
- Pt immobility is paramount (particularly for laser surgery on the vocal cords).
- Plans for muscle relaxation must take into account the variable & often short duration of these cases. Options include
  - Frequent doses of short-acting nondepolarizing agent
    - W/ deep neuromuscular blockade, may take lengthy time to achieve adequate reversal w/ neostigmine
  - Succinylcholine infusion
    - Succinylcholine 600 mg in 100 cc NS.
    - Titrate to peripheral nerve stimulation.
    - Potential danger is development of phase II block if large cumulative doses are given.
- Airway mgt: Discuss ventilation options w/ surgeon. This may include:
  - ETT
    - Small size (eg, 4–5) needed for laryngeal laser surgery.
    - For pharyngeal laser surgery, can use larger ETT.
    - Use foil-wrapped ETT or a metal ETT designed for laser surgery.
    - Can also place via a tracheotomy (if present).

➤ Ventilating laryngoscope or bronchoscope, using either conventional positive-pressure ventilation or jet ventilation.
➤ Transtracheal catheter.
  • A long catheter passed between the vocal cords, combined w/ jet ventilation.
■ Keep FiO_2 <0.30 to minimize the chance of airway fire.
➤ Avoid N_2O because it supports combustion.
■ Consider using IV anesthesia, particularly if jet ventilation or apneic technique is required.
➤ One suggested combination: remifentanil, propofol & succinylcholine infusions.
➤ Deliver infusions as close to IV site as possible.

INTRAOP

Monitors/Line Placement
■ Standard monitors.
■ Peripheral nerve stimulator.

Intraop Concerns
■ Airway fire is the greatest concern during laser surgery (see also Critical Event chapter "Airway Fire").
➤ Fire requires fuel, oxidizer & ignition source.
➤ Mgt
  • Stop ventilation & gas flow through ETT.
  • Immediately remove ETT.
  • Perform laryngoscopy & reintubate the trachea.
  • Make sure fire is extinguished before administering oxygen.
  • Consider bronchoscopy to assess the extent of burn injury.
  • Follow blood gases to further assess gas exchange abnormalities.
■ Considerations for ventilating laryngoscope or bronchoscope use.
➤ Ventilation must be discontinued while the surgeon looks through the eyepiece so that airway contents are not blown into his/her face.
➤ Apnea may lead to hypoxemia & hypercarbia.
➤ Good communication is required to coordinate ventilation & operation.
■ ETT cuff can easily be damaged by the laser.
➤ Watch for development of cuff leak.
➤ May need to reintubate trachea if leak is severe.
■ Laser light reflected onto nonoperative surfaces can cause burns.

> Pt's eyes should be covered w/ pads to protect from injury from laser.
> OR personnel should wear eye protection when the laser is in use.
■ Consider "deep extubation."
> May minimize the risk of laryngospasm.
> Will minimize coughing on ETT w/ emergence.

POSTOP

Pain

■ Usually minimal for upper airway procedures

Complications

■ Airway edema
■ Airway obstruction & stridor
■ Airway burns
■ Postop airway bleeding
■ Laryngospasm

SURGICAL PROCEDURE

Indications

■ Airway laser surgery performed on lesions of the trachea, larynx, pharynx, hypopharynx
■ Lesions may include human papillomavirus, congenital webs/cysts, polyps, posttraumatic stenosis, hemangioma.

Procedure

■ Depends on location of lesion being treated w/ laser
■ Laryngeal
> Surgeon will use rigid laryngoscope, which may be suspended from OR table.
> Microscope may also be used for more delicate or precise surgery.
■ Tracheal
> May be performed w/ rigid bronchoscope or ventilating laryngoscope.
■ Pharyngeal or hypopharyngeal
> May not require laryngoscope for exposure.

Surgical Concerns

■ Need small ETT so that view of surgical field is not obscured
■ Airway fire
■ Airway perforation

- Barotrauma (if using jet ventilation)
  - ➤ Pneumothorax
  - ➤ Subcutaneous emphysema
- Tissue injury from laser

Typical EBL
- Minimal

LIPOSUCTION

JASON WIDRICH, MD

PREOP

Preop Considerations
- Most pts are obese, although morbid obesity is generally considered a contraindication for surgery.
  - ➤ See also Coexisting Disease chapter "Morbid Obesity."
- Preop evaluation must identify respiratory or cardiac disease, as physiology of liposuction may impose stress on these organ systems.
  - ➤ Respiratory
    - Pain or restrictive garments may compromise postop pulmonary function.
    - If required, prone positioning for surgery may impair ventilation.
  - ➤ Cardiac
    - Fluid shifts are common w/ liposuction; pts w/ heart failure, coronary disease or valvular disorders are more likely to develop complications.
    - The addition of local anesthetic solution w/ epinephrine may cause arrhythmias or affect cardiac function.
- Before the advent of tumescent therapy, blood loss requiring transfusion was common. Dilutional anemia is still possible for large-volume liposuction.

Physical Findings
- Many pts are obese.

Workup
- CBC.
- Other labs as indicated by coexisting disease.

Choice of Anesthesia
- Can be performed w/ GA, epidural anesthesia or MAC.
- Some terms specific to modern liposuction techniques.
  - ➤ "Wetting" refers to subcutaneous infiltration of fluid to distend fat cells.
  - ➤ "Tumescent anesthesia" refers to subcutaneous infiltration of epinephrine & local anesthetic-containing wetting solution.
    - Local anesthetic is usually dilute lidocaine (eg, 0.05–0.1%).

INTRAOP

Monitors/Line Placement
- Standard monitors.
- Foley catheter useful for large anticipated liposuction volumes.

Intraop Concerns
- Physiology of liposuction.
  - ➤ Subcutaneous infiltration of LR or NS w/ epinephrine & lidocaine.
    - Wetting distends fat cells.
    - Epinephrine provides vasoconstriction & reduces blood loss.
    - Lidocaine provides local anesthesia.
  - ➤ Cannula placed through small skin incisions & used to aspirate distended subcutaneous fat.
  - ➤ Cannula inevitably tears small feeder blood vessels & creates the equivalent of a subdermal burn injury.
  - ➤ Third-space fluid void created by tissue evacuation.
  - ➤ Fluid absorption of wetting solution occurs via hypodermoclysis.
- Lidocaine toxicity
  - ➤ Lidocaine dose w/ tumescent anesthesia is typically 35 mg/kg, though some surgeons administer 55 mg/kg or greater.
  - ➤ Pharmacokinetics of lidocaine at these doses for liposuction has not been well studied. Despite the large doses used, some studies have documented plasma lidocaine levels below "toxic" levels.
  - ➤ Lidocaine levels generally peak as late as 10–14 h.
- Positioning issues
  - ➤ Liposuction can be performed in a variety of positions (prone, lateral, supine).
  - ➤ Position may change during surgery.
  - ➤ Pt must be properly padded to prevent neuropathy.
- Complications of cannula insertion & manipulation

➤ Pneumothorax, vascular injury or abdominal viscus perforation possible.
➤ Air or fat emboli.
- Fluid overload & pulmonary edema
    ➤ Although the fluid infused for tumescent anesthesia is aspirated, up to 60–70% of the volume remains & can be absorbed by hypodermoclysis.
    ➤ Increased risk of fluid overload occurs when volume of fluid infused is greater than amount of fluid removed.
    ➤ "Large-volume" liposuction (>4–5 L aspirate, or removal of >1.5 L fat) is more likely to cause fluid mgt problems.
- Epinephrine toxicity
    ➤ Several mg of epinephrine may be infused as part of wetting solution, increasing the risk of hypertension or arrhythmias.
- Hypothermia from fluid infiltration.

Intraop Therapies
- Limit IV fluids to <1 L.
- Consider Foley catheter for closer evaluation of fluid status.
- ➤ For instance, prolonged surgery, multiple liters of tumescent fluid infusion or aspiration, hypotension, suspected fluid overload.
- Surgeon may request dexamethasone IV to decrease inflammation/swelling.
- Warming blanket or forced air warmer to prevent hypothermia.
- Consider IV furosemide for pts w/ a large positive fluid balance.
- Nausea/vomiting is common. Consider prophylactic antiemetics.

POSTOP

Pain
- Minimal to mild
- Pt usually has residual analgesia from local anesthetic infiltration
- Some pts require IV opiates in PACU

Complications
- DVT
- Pulmonary embolism
    ➤ Most common cause of death after liposuction.
    ➤ Consider intraop pneumatic compression device
    ➤ Fat embolism causing pulmonary occlusion rare, but fat globules can be seen in bloodstream

- Fluid overload or pulmonary edema
  - ➤ Pt may need a Foley catheter or IV furosemide to treat or prevent pulmonary edema
- Third-space fluid loss & hypotension
  - ➤ Initially fluid overload is the more common concern, although hours later in the postop course third-space fluid loss may occur & cause hypovolemia & hypotension. This has been implicated in some cases of postop death after liposuction
- Lidocaine toxicity may occur late in the postop period (4–12 h) due to the vasoconstrictive effect of the epinephrine & delay in absorption
- Epinephrine toxicity
- Cannula-related injury
  - ➤ Can include abdominal viscus perforation, vascular injury or pneumothorax
- Respiratory failure
  - ➤ Hypoxemia or hypoventilation from pain, narcotics or restrictive dressings
- Anemia requiring blood transfusion
- Hypothermia
- Garment restricting chest wall expansion or venous return
- Death (risk estimated at 1 in 5,000)
  - ➤ Risk factors for death
    - Multiple liters of wetting solution
    - Aspiration of large volumes of fat
    - Multiple cosmetic procedures at one sitting
    - Residual anesthesia or sedation impairing ventilation
    - Overly permissive postop discharge policies

SURGICAL PROCEDURE

Indications
- Obesity or localized fat deposits
- Cosmetic effect

Procedure
- Surgeon & pt decide the specific areas of treatment.
  - ➤ This may require drawing on the pt's skin in the preop period.
  - ➤ Surgeon may request that premedication be delayed until after this stage.
- GA, epidural anesthesia, or IV sedation
- Surgeon will create small incisions & inject SQ tumescent fluid.

➤ Sample wetting fluid: 1 L LR, 1 mg epinephrine, 200 mg lidocaine (35 mg/kg total lidocaine dose).
■ Adipose tissue can be removed w/ metal or ultrasonic suction cannula.
■ If tumescent fluid has been used, the surgeon will wait for 5–10 min after each area has been evacuated to ensure hemostasis.
■ The procedure is repeated until all targeted areas have been treated.
■ The entry points of incision are then closed.
■ Compressive garments are placed to reduce tissue dead space & reduce third-space fluid loss.

Surgical Concerns
■ Symmetry, desired cosmetic effect
■ Hematoma or seroma formation
■ Lidocaine toxicity
■ Fluid overload, pulmonary edema
■ Rarely, severe infection, necrotizing fasciitis
■ Other concerns noted in postop complications

Typical EBL
■ <1,000 mL

LUMBAR LAMINECTOMY

MICHELLE PARAISO, MD

PREOP

Preop Considerations
■ Pts often have chronic pain & may use opioids or NSAIDs.
■ Etiology of compression may be
  ➤ Degenerative (herniated disc or osteophyte).
  ➤ Congenital stenosis.
  ➤ Neoplasm.
  ➤ Trauma.
■ Pt may be sedentary due to pain.
  ➤ Pt may have unrecognized cardiac or pulmonary disease.
■ Anticipated EBL depends on
  ➤ Number of levels.
  ➤ Previous spine surgery.
  ➤ Extent of planned procedure (fusion, instrumentation, laminectomy, or laminotomy).

- Pt may have coexisting cervical spine dz.
  - ➤ Possible difficult intubation.

Physical Findings

- Cardiac & pulmonary exam to rule out undiagnosed disease
- Careful neuro exam to document preexisting deficits
  - ➤ Check upper extremity symptoms too (pain/numbness in hands or arms) assoc w/ extension of neck.
- Document preop blood pressure & vitals, esp in pts who will have deliberate hypotension.

Workup

- Most NSAIDs should be discontinued 10 days prior to surgery.
  - ➤ Periop use of COX-2 inhibitors remains controversial.
  - ➤ Opioids should be increased preop as NSAIDs are held.
- Blood work
  - ➤ CBC.
  - ➤ Type & screen for most laminectomies.
  - ➤ Type & cross for 1–3 units and/or autologous donation for multiple-level or redo laminectomy.
- If indicated by history/PE.
  - ➤ Electrolytes, BUN, Cr.
  - ➤ Glucose.
  - ➤ Coags.
  - ➤ ECG.

Choice of Anesthesia

- GA is most commonly used because
  - ➤ Pt comfort.
  - ➤ Airway controlled.
  - ➤ Allows neuromonitoring.
  - ➤ Facilitates deliberate hypotension.
- Regional anesthetic (spinal) sometimes used.
  - ➤ Advantage: Pt can position self & prevent injuries.
  - ➤ Disadvantage: Pt may be uncomfortable for long case in prone position.
    - Sedation difficult.
    - Unable to control airway.
    - May be impossible to assess neuro deficits in a timely fashion postop.

INTRAOP

- Standard ASA monitor
- Foley catheter for longer cases
- For single-level laminectomy or laminotomy
  - Single 18–16g IV
  - Arterial line, CVP if indicated by coexisting dz or if planned deliberate hypotension
- For multiple-level and/or redo laminectomy
  - Two 18–14g IVs
  - Arterial line needed for deliberate hypotension or extensive surgery
  - CVP indicated for coexisting dz & infusion of vasoactive meds for deliberate hypotension
- Neuromonitoring rarely required
  - EMG most frequently employed for lumbar laminectomy
- PA line rarely indicated; may be more difficult to use due to prone position

Intraop Concerns

- Intubation may be difficult if coexisting c-spine disease limits neck ROM
  - May require fiberoptic airway mgt
- Induction of GA done fully monitored on gurney
- Avoid sux if pt has significant myelopathy or neuro deficit
- May need to avoid hypotension/monitor w/ arterial line to provide adequate spinal cord perfusion pressure, esp in pts w/
  - Compromised cord
  - Spinal stenosis
  - Abnormal vascular supply
  - Myelopathy
- For multiple-level or redo laminectomy, cell saver & blood products should be available
  - Bleeding can occur from epidural veins or rarely from major vascular injury
- Pts are usually positioned prone.
  - Minimize period of "blackout" where vitals are not monitored during turn
  - Ventilate w/ 100% O_2 prior to & during turn
  - Establish the presence of adequate ventilation (ascultation/ $ETCO_2$), oxygenation, & BP ASAP after turn

- ➤ Need to check eyes & face after positioning & periodically throughout case w/ documentation
- ➤ Also need to check breasts, genitalia, neck position, & pressure points (elbows, knees, etc) after positioning
- Prone positioning can decrease venous return
  - ➤ Hypotension may be seen
- Pts in prone position for long cases or in cases w/ large blood loss & fluid replacement may have significant facial & airway edema
  - ➤ May require period of postop intubation w/ elevation of head to decrease swelling prior to extubation
  - ➤ Consider checking if pt can breathe around tube w/ cuff deflated prior to extubation
- Early neuro assessment critical
  - ➤ Pts should be awakened ASAP postop (even if they are to remain intubated) to allow for early neuro assessment
- Air embolus can cause hypotension & decrease in $ETCO_2$.

Intraop Therapies
- No muscle relaxant generally used for maintenance
  - ➤ Allows evaluation of nerve root stimulation by surgeon
  - ➤ Initial dose of nondepolarizing relaxant useful for intubation, positioning, & incision
- For multiple-level laminectomy consider
  - ➤ Hemodilution
  - ➤ Deliberate hypotension
  - ➤ Preop autologous blood donation

POSTOP

Pain
- Mild to moderate
  - ➤ Severe pain more likely in pts w/ chronic pain & opiate use
- Intrathecal/epidural morphine may be administered by surgeon
- PCA & oral narcotics are the mainstays of therapy

Complications
- Airway edema if in prone position for extended period or large fluid administration
  - ➤ Can delay extubation or cause difficult reintubation
- CSF leak from dural tear
- Nerve root injury
- Complications assoc w/ hypotension

➤ Retinal injury/blindness
➤ Stroke
➤ Myocardial ischemia
➤ ARF
■ Hemorrhage from major vascular injury possible
➤ Aorta, vena cava or iliacs can be injured
➤ Suspect esp if hypotensive or w/ decreasing Hct postop
■ Injuries assoc w/ prone positioning
➤ Blindness
➤ Brachial plexus injury
➤ Peripheral nerve injury
■ Spinal instability

SURGICAL PROCEDURE

Indications
■ Typical indications include treatment of
➤ Symptomatic degenerative disease.
➤ Spinal stenosis.
➤ Ruptured/herniated disc.
➤ Neoplasm.
➤ Cauda equina.
■ Laminectomy may also be performed to gain access to spinal canal for treatment of spinal AVM or tumor.

Procedure
Approached through posterior, midline incision
■ Laminectomy (piecemeal removal of posterior neural arch) is a complete removal of the lamina.
■ Laminotomy is a partial removal of the lamina.

Surgical Concerns
■ Early neuro assessment needs to be made.
➤ Significant deficits may require immediate return to OR.
■ Fusion may be required if laminectomy & decompression is extensive over several levels & instability results.

Typical EBL
■ Lumbar laminotomy: 25–500 mL
■ Lumbar laminectomy: 50–1,500 mL. More if
➤ Redo procedure
➤ Multiple levels involved
➤ Fusion required

LUNG TRANSPLANT

BETTY LEE-HOANG, MD

PREOP

Preop Considerations
- Pts are usually selected based on criteria including:
  - Advanced lung disease for which conventional therapies have failed
  - High risk for mortality within next few years
  - Severe functional limitations but able to ambulate
  - Age limits (55 years for heart-lung transplant, 60 years for bilateral lung transplant, 65 years for single-lung transplant)
- Some contraindications include:
  - Severe extrapulmonary organ dysfunction
  - Cancer that is active or has a high likelihood of recurrence
  - Active extrapulmonary infection such as HIV or hepatitis B or C
  - Active smoking
  - Active psychiatric illness
  - Severe malnutrition or obesity
- Must give immunosuppressants in the preop period, which are continued for the rest of the recipient's life. Usually cyclosporin or tacrolimus, azathioprine or mycophenolate mofetil, Solu-Medrol
- Broad-spectrum antibiotics & antifungals must be given prior to incision

Physical Findings
- Pts usually complain of severe dyspnea limiting their activities of daily living
- Pts w/ COPD are often O_2-dependent & CO_2 retainers
- Pts w/ cystic fibrosis will have chronic respiratory tract infections

Workup
- PFTs to assess severity of lung disease & to determine if pt can tolerate pneumonectomy (FVC >2 L, FEV_1 >800 cc, FEV_1/FVC >50% predicted)
- ABG to assess the degree of hypoxia & CO_2 retention
- Left & right heart catheterization & coronary artery angiography to rule out significant CAD & left & right heart failure
- Psychological assessment

Choice of Anesthesia
- GA
- Low dose of volatile agent
- No N_2O usually, to maintain high FiO_2 during one-lung ventilation
- Left-sided double-lumen tube
  - ➤ May need to withdraw double-lumen tube prior to a left pneumonectomy
- Preop spinal for intrathecal morphine
  - ➤ Thoracic epidurals are not used because there is a chance of requiring cardiopulmonary bypass (CPB)

INTRAOP

Monitors/Line Placement
- Standard monitors
- Arterial line, CVP catheter, PA catheter
  - ➤ Withdraw PA catheter prior to pneumonectomy.

Intraop Concerns
- Fluid replacement should be kept to a minimum, since the newly transplanted lung is susceptible to pulmonary edema.
- Maintain adequate PaO_2 & $PaCO_2$ during the institution of one-lung ventilation.
- When the pulmonary artery is clamped the PA pressures will increase. If this leads to acute RV failure, CPB may be needed.
- When the donor lung is perfused but not yet ventilated, a shunt may occur & again PaO_2 may decrease.
- Pts are usually kept intubated for 24 h, so the double-lumen tube will need to be changed to a single-lumen tube.
- After change to single-lumen tube, Integrity of suture lines in the bronchus of the donor lung will be verified w/ bronchoscopy.

Intraop Therapies
- If pt cannot tolerate one-lung ventilation or excessive increases in PA pressure, then CPB is instituted.
- If CPB is necessary for left thoracotomy, a femoral vein to femoral artery bypass may be used if there is difficulty accessing right atrium & aorta.
- For right thoracotomy or sternotomy, standard right atrium to aorta bypass is used.
- For excessive increases in pulmonary artery pressure, drugs w/ pulmonary vasodilatory activity (nitrates or hydralazine), inotropes (dopamine & norepinephrine), or diuretics may be used.

POSTOP

Pain

■ Moderate to severe, especially w/ thoracotomy incision.

■ If intrathecal morphine was used, pt should have analgesia for 24 h.

■ Pt may then receive a thoracic epidural catheter postop if coag status is normal.

Complications

■ Most common is mild transient pulmonary edema ("reperfusion or reimplantation pulmonary edema").

■ Complete dehiscence of the bronchial anastomosis requires immediate surgical correction, while partial dehiscence may be managed conservatively.

■ Infection: initially with "usual" organisms. With time, opportunistic infections become more common (eg, cytomegalovirus, Pneumocystis, Aspergillus).

■ Acute rejection: treated w/ steroids or other immunosuppression.

■ Chronic rejection: a fibroproliferative process that causes submucosal fibrosis & luminal obliteration (bronchiolitis obliterans). No definitive treatment.

SURGICAL PROCEDURE

Indication

■ End-stage pulmonary parenchymal disease or pulmonary hypertension

■ Single-lung transplant for COPD & other nonseptic pulmonary diseases

■ Double-lung transplant for infectious/vascular etiologies & bullous emphysema

■ Combined heart-lung transplant for Eisenmenger syndrome

Procedure

■ Procedure can be performed as
  ➤ Single-lung transplant
  ➤ Bilateral sequential lung transplant
  ➤ Bilateral "en-bloc" lung transplant
  ➤ As part of combined heart-lung transplant

■ Single-lung transplant is performed via posterolateral thoracotomy. Usual steps:
  ➤ After sufficient exposure, native lung is excised.
  ➤ Donor lung is placed in surgical field

> Bronchial anastomosis performed
> Pulmonary artery anastomosis performed
> Left atrial anastomosis (at confluence of pulmonary veins) performed
> Lung reinflated
> Perfusion re-established
> After satisfactory hemostasis, chest tubes are placed & chest is closed
■ Bilateral sequential lung transplant is usually performed via clamshell incision (bilateral thoracotomy w/ lower sternotomy)
> Steps are similar to single-lung transplant. The lung w/ poorer function is excised first
■ Bilateral "en-bloc" lung transplant & heart-lung transplant can be performed via standard median sternotomy or clamshell incision

Surgical Concerns
■ Proper size matching of donor organ
■ Integrity of vascular & bronchial anastomosis
■ Ischemia time of donor organ

Typical EBL
■ Varies markedly depending on pt's disease, amount of pleural scarring & other factors

---

MASTECTOMY

JASON WIDRICH, MD

PREOP

Preop Considerations
■ Pt w/ breast cancer typically presents for mastectomy after initial diagnosis, although pt may present w/ local or regional recurrence of breast cancer.
■ Mgt of the primary breast tumor may include
> Breast-conserving surgery (eg, lumpectomy, quadrantectomy, segmental mastectomy) + radiation therapy.
> Mastectomy + reconstruction (either immediate or delayed).
  • See also Procedures chapter "Breast Reconstruction."
> Mastectomy alone.
> Surgical staging of the axilla is typically done to determine prognosis & therapy.

- Additional therapy for breast cancer may include radiation therapy, chemotherapy or hormone therapy.
- Pt w/ metastatic breast cancer is usually treated w/ systemic therapy (hormonal or chemotherapy) or palliative radiation therapy.
  - Pt may require mastectomy for painful or fungating breast mass.
  - Pt w/ limited metastatic disease may undergo surgery.
- Metastatic breast cancer may involve
  - Brain, meninges or spinal cord: altered mental status or focal weakness.
  - Lung: pleural effusion.
  - Bone: pathologic fractures, vertebral involvement w/ spinal cord compression.
- Determine previous chemotherapy regimen & residual toxicities, including anemia or doxorubicin-induced cardiac toxicity.

Physical Findings
- Breast mass.

Workup
- CBC.
- Other workup based on coexisting disease.
- Determine prior workup for metastatic breast cancer.

Choice of Anesthesia
- GA or MAC, depending on extent of surgery.
  - Smaller excisions such as lumpectomy are most suitable for local anesthesia & MAC.
  - Larger resection, planned axillary dissection, or immediate breast reconstruction typically requires GA.

INTRAOP

Monitors/Line Placement
- Standard monitors.
- One peripheral IV usually adequate.

Intraop Concerns
- Do not place upper extremity peripheral IV on the side of the proposed mastectomy.
- For axillary dissection, avoid muscle relaxants after induction to allow identification of peripheral nerves.

Intraop Therapies
- Consider prophylactic antiemetics, as incidence of postop nausea/vomiting is relatively high.

POSTOP

Pain
- Mild to moderate, depending on size of resection & additional procedures performed (eg, axillary dissection, breast reconstruction)
  - For lumpectomy w/ local anesthesia, pt typically has minimal pain initially
    - PO analgesics usually adequate
  - For more extensive procedure, IV narcotics or PCA appropriate

Complications
- Nausea/vomiting
- Pneumothorax rare

SURGICAL PROCEDURE

Indications
- Breast cancer
  Procedure
- Variety of procedures include
  - Simple mastectomy: removal of breast tissue w/ no lymph node dissection
  - Surgical staging of axilla: standard lymph node dissection involves level I & II nodes. Level III axillary nodes medial to the pectoralis minor muscle are often not removed in standard evaluation. Minimum number of nodes sampled is typically 6–10
  - Lumpectomy: local excision of mass
  - Radical mastectomy: removal of breast, pectoral muscles, axillary lymph tissue
  - Modified radical mastectomy: removal of breast & axillary lymph nodes only
- Reconstruction can be accomplished w/ a prosthetic implant, rotational flap or free flap
- Axillary or pectoral drains may be placed prior to closure

Surgical Concerns
- Surgical margins free of tumor
- Lymphedema
- Bleeding

- Thoracodorsal & long thoracic nerve damage
- Wound infection
- Cosmetic effect & requirement for reconstruction

Typical EBL
- 150–500 mL

MEDIASTINOSCOPY

GIAC VU, MD

PREOP

Preop Considerations
- Determine why the mediastinoscopy is being done.
  - ➤ For example, does pt have a mediastinal mass or a lung tumor that has spread to the hilum or mediastinum?
- If a mediastinal mass is present, there is a potential for airway obstruction and/or hemodynamic compromise. See also Coexisting Disease chapter "Mediastinal Mass."

Physical Findings
- Depend on pathology present; some pts have few symptoms.
- If a mediastinal mass is present, there may be a difference in respiratory or cardiac signs & symptoms in the supine vs upright positions owing to compression of the mediastinum (including trachea, heart, pulmonary arteries) by the mass.
- In pts w/ a significant mediastinal mass, a superior vena cava syndrome may be present.
- Pts w/ lung tumors may have symptoms referable to their lung tumor (eg, cough).

Workup
- Dictated by the intrathoracic pathology. May include:
  - ➤ CT/MRI to define relationship of tumor to airway & other intrathoracic structures.
  - ➤ PFTs w/ flow-volume loops in upright & supine positions; may help show the degree of obstruction & whether an obstruction, if present, is intra- or extrathoracic.
  - ➤ An echocardiogram may be helpful if compression of the heart is suspected.

Choice of Anesthesia
- GA
  - ➤ Immobility is crucial during the surgical procedure to prevent mediastinal injury.

INTRAOP

Monitors/Line Placement
- BP cuff, preferably on the left arm.
  - ➤ Innominate artery compression by mediastinoscope may interfere w/ BP measurements on right.
- Consider arterial line if compression of the mediastinum by a mediastinal mass is significant.
- Pulse oximeter can be placed on right arm.

Intraop Concerns
- Pt position usually supine.
- Innominate artery compression w/ cerebral ischemia from diminished supply to right common carotid artery.
- Stretching of vagus nerve or trachea may cause bradycardia.
- Tracheal collapse possible.
  - ➤ Rarely, rigid bronchoscopy may be needed if this arises.
- Bleeding
  - ➤ Major bleeding may require exploration of the chest.
  - ➤ The pulmonary arteries are a relatively low-pressure system; application of pressure by the surgeon (via the incision made for mediastinoscopy) may suffice to stop bleeding from a pulmonary artery.

POSTOP

Pain
- Typically minimal

Complications
- Pneumothorax
- Damage to large airways
- Phrenic/recurrent laryngeal nerve damage
- Bleeding

SURGICAL PROCEDURE

Indications
- Staging of spread of pulmonary tumors
- Diagnosis of anterior mediastinal masses

Procedure
- After a small incision above the sternal notch, a short mediastinoscope is passed to the upper mediastinum. Nodes anterior & to the right of the trachea as well as carinal & sometimes subcarinal nodes can be sampled through this approach.
- Different approach (left anterior mediastinotomy in second interspace) may be required to biopsy left-sided nodes.

Surgical Concerns
- SVC obstruction or thoracic aneurysm increases risk of vessel injury by mediastinoscope.

Typical EBL
- Minimal

MITRAL VALVE REPLACEMENT OR REPAIR

LUNDY CAMPBELL, MD

PREOP

Preop Considerations
- Most common indications are severe mitral regurgitation or mitral stenosis.
  - See also Coexisting Disease chapters "Mitral Regurgitation" & "Mitral Stenosis."
  - Mitral stenosis creates a fixed obstruction to outflow. These pts are extremely sensitive to HR & preload & do not tolerate rapid reductions in SVR.
  - Mitral regurgitation can lead to pulmonary edema. Eventually the lesion progresses to right & left ventricular failure.
  - Both valvular lesions predispose the pt to CHF, w/ pulmonary edema, & pleural effusions.

Physical Findings
- Mitral stenosis: Opening snap & diastolic murmur best heard between apex & left sternal border. Atrial fibrillation quite common.
- Mitral regurgitation: May be acute (associated w/ MI or endocarditis) or chronic. Pansystolic murmur is loudest at the apex.

Workup
- CBC.

- Electrolytes, BUN, creatinine.
- LFTs, PT, PTT.
- ECG.
- Review results of cardiac workup:
    - ➤ Echocardiogram.
    - ➤ Left heart cath.
    - ➤ Possible coronary angiography.

Choice of Anesthesia
- GA.
- A variety of techniques are acceptable, as long as hemodynamic goals are maintained.
- Consider timing of postop extubation when determining narcotic dose.
- Consider use of intrathecal morphine for postop analgesia.

INTRAOP
Monitors/Line Placement
- Standard monitors.
- Arterial line.
- Central line.
- PA catheter may be useful, depending on pt disease & local practice patterns.
- TEE
    - ➤ Useful in assessing cardiac & valvular function.
    - ➤ See also Technique chapter "TEE Insertion and Basic Examination (Adult)."

Intraop Concerns
- Determine hemodynamic goals (see also Coexisting Disease chapters "Mitral Regurgitation" & "Mitral Stenosis").
    - ➤ Hemodynamic goals for mitral regurgitation
        - Maintain HR; avoid bradycardia.
        - Maintain an appropriate preload.
        - Avoid decreases in cardiac contractility.
        - Avoid sudden increases in SVR (afterload reduction improves forward flow).
    - ➤ Hemodynamic goals for mitral stenosis
        - Maintain sinus rhythm; avoid tachycardia or rapid atrial fibrillation (atrial kick contributes 20–35% of cardiac output in MS).

- Avoid sudden decreases in SVR.
- Avoid large increases in central blood volume.
- Avoid increases in pulmonary vascular resistance (eg, avoid acidosis, hypoxia, hypercarbia, pain, hypothermia, nitrous oxide).

■ Induction of anesthesia
- ➤ Maintain hemodynamic goals discussed above. Anticipate effects of anesthetic agents on hemodynamics.

■ Ensure baseline ACT is drawn.

■ Maintenance of anesthesia.
- ➤ Variety of techniques acceptable.
- ➤ Ensure adequate amnesia (eg, volatile agent, benzodiazepines).

■ Consider administration of hemostatic agent to reduce blood loss (eg, aprotinin, aminocaproic acid).

■ Administer heparin prior to beginning cardiopulmonary bypass (CPB).
- ➤ Confirm ACT >400 sec.

■ During CPB
- ➤ Ensure perfusionist maintains adequate MAP.
- ➤ Continue administration of amnestic agent (eg, volatile agent via CPB machine or IV benzodiazepines).

■ Weaning from CPB
- ➤ Inotropic agents may be necessary, especially in pts w/ cardiomyopathy.
- ➤ Monitor for signs of ischemia.
- ➤ Temporary pacing or mechanical support may be required.
- ➤ Treat any remaining coagulopathy aggressively.
  - Platelets that have circulated through the pump are usually dysfunctional, so platelets & any prebypass blood taken off should be given back to pt.
- ➤ After successful weaning, administer protamine & follow ACT.

■ Emergence
- ➤ Transport intubated pt to ICU w/ full monitoring.
- ➤ Maintain all inotropic agents.

Intraop Therapies
■ Pt w/ mitral stenosis
- ➤ Maintain hemodynamic goals.
- ➤ Maintain adequate MAP prior to valve repair.
- ➤ For hypotension, administer fluids cautiously to avoid pulmonary edema; consider use of phenylephrine to maintain SVR.

- Pt w/ mitral regurgitation
  - Maintain hemodynamic goals.
  - Inotropic agents may be indicated to maintain contractility.
  - Afterload reduction.
- Hemostatic agents may include aminocaproic acid, tranexamic acid, aprotinin.
- While weaning from bypass, inotropic agents may include dopamine, epinephrine, dobutamine, amrinone, milrinone.

POSTOP

Pain
- Moderate
- While intubated, sedation as needed
- For analgesia, IV narcotics needed initially, unless intrathecal narcotics administered

Complications
- Hemorrhage: may require re-exploration if severe or persistent, or if tamponade develops
- Tamponade: may require emergent bedside drainage or return to OR
  - See also Procedures chapter "Cardiac Surgery Re-Exploration."
- Cardiac failure: left ventricular assist devices or intra-aortic balloon pumps to assist a failing left ventricle
- Arrhythmias: correction of electrolyte abnormalities, antiarrhythmic agents (possible prophylactic use), cardioversion
- Heart block: temporary pacer placement
- Ischemia/myocardial infarction: avoid ventricular volume or pressure overload, administer beta blockade unless contraindicated

SURGICAL PROCEDURE

Indications
- Typical indications include NYHA class 3 or 4 CHF due to the mitral valve lesion.

Procedure
- Involves median sternotomy, aortic & venous cannula placement, initiation of CPB, cardioplegia & systemic hypothermia, repair of valve or placement of prosthetic valve, weaning from bypass, removal of cannula, closure.

Surgical Concerns

- Risk of air embolization is higher for open chamber surgery (vs CABG) & requires adequate air evacuation maneuvers when refilling heart.
- Perivalvular leaks may occur after valve is sewn in. TEE useful for detection & evaluation.
- For mitral valve repair, most consider TEE essential for evaluating adequacy of repair. Surgeon may elect to revise valve based on TEE findings.
- Weaning from bypass is critical time that may require placement of a mechanical left ventricle support device or return of pt to CPB.

Typical EBL

- Not usually recorded for CPB cases.

MYELOMENINGOCELE REPAIR

ATSUKO BABA, MD

PREOP

Preop Considerations

- Spina bifida is failure of closure of the caudal end of the neural tube.
- Myelomeningocele is a type of spina bifida characterized by a sac that contains neural elements.
- Lack of skin covering a myelomeningocele makes surgical closure within a few hours after birth a necessity to avoid infection.
- Incidence: 1/1,000 live births (male:female ratio approximately equal).

Physical Findings

- Varying degrees of motor & sensory deficits.
- Associated congenital anomalies: clubfoot, hydrocephalus, dislocation of the hips, extrophy of the bladder, prolapsed uterus, Klippel-Feil syndrome, Chiari II malformations, malrotation of the gut, craniofacial defects, scoliosis, cardiac defects (ASD/VSD).
- Myelomeningoceles vary in size; typically occur in the sacral or lumbar spine.

Workup

- Typically diagnosed before birth by high-resolution ultrasound and/or elevated maternal serum (Image not available on the Palm)-fetoprotein levels.
- Cardiac echo to rule out assoc congenital cardiac anomalies.
- If the patient is older, latex allergy can be documented w/ a radioallergosorbent test.

Choice of Anesthesia

- General endotracheal anesthesia.

INTRAOP

Monitors/Line Placement

- Well-functioning IV line
- Standard monitors

Intraop Concerns

- Intubation of the trachea in the lateral position to avoid injury to the exposed neural tissue.
- If induction of anesthesia is performed in the supine position, place the exposed neural tissue in the center of a doughnut pad to minimize injury to the myelomeningocele.
- Consider latex allergy precautions in this pt population w/ multiple mucous membrane exposures to latex products.
- Prone positioning is required for surgical repair of myelomeningocele; meticulous attention must be paid to positioning/padding.
- Maintain normothermia.
- Maintain near-normal BP to maintain perfusion to the spinal cord.
- Valsalva maneuver may be required intraop to ensure tight closure of the myelomeningocele sac to avoid postop CSF leak.

Intraop Therapies

- Continue dextrose-containing IV fluid at maintenance rate (4 cc/kg/h) intraop to avoid hypoglycemia.
- Although pts w/ myelomeningocele may have upper & lower motor neuron lesions, succinylcholine does NOT induce hyperkalemia.
- Long-acting muscle relaxants should be avoided in case nerve stimulation is required to identify functional neural tissue.

POSTOP

Pain

- Parenteral opioids.

- If pt has no baseline pulmonary dysfunction or intraop complications, extubate at the end of the case when extubation criteria are met.
- Prone positioning should be continued postop.

Complications
- CSF leak.
- Hydrocephalus; monitor head circumference.
- Meningitis/ventriculitis.
- Wound infection.
- Mortality is approaching zero.

SURGICAL PROCEDURE

Indications
- Open dural sac & skin defect typically over the lumbar/sacral spine.

Procedure
- Goal of surgery is complete skin closure, reconstitution of normal intrathecal environment, preservation of neural tissue.

Surgical Concerns
- Complete skin closure may require a rotational skin flap.
- Approx 15% of pts w/ myelomeningocele have hydrocephalus at birth; ventriculoperitoneal shunt may be need to be placed simultaneously at the time of the myelomeningocele repair.

Typical EBL
- Negligible; 25 cc.

MYRINGOTOMY & TYMPANOSTOMY

ATSUKO BABA, MD

PREOP

Preop Considerations
- Pts who require myringotomy & tympanostomy have a higher incidence of URIs; consider rescheduling a case if symptoms indicative of lower respiratory involvement (fever, productive cough) are present.
- Pts w/ cleft palate have a higher incidence of recurrent/chronic otitis media requiring myringotomy & tympanostomy.

Physical Findings
■ Chronic serous otitis media or recurrent acute otitis media.
■ Decreased mobility of the tympanic membrane.
■ Often accompanied by hypertrophied tonsils & adenoids.

Workup
■ No additional workup is usually necessary.

Choice of Anesthesia
■ Usually performed under mask GA.
■ An inhalational induction is effective but some pts require premed w/ oral midazolam or IM ketamine.
■ Nitrous oxide may be used safely in the induction of anesthesia.

INTRAOP

Monitors/Line Placement
■ Standard monitoring
■ If pt is otherwise healthy & surgical time is minimal, it is not necessary to start an IV line; it is prudent to have succinylcholine & atropine available for IM or sublingual injection.

Intraop Concerns
■ This pt population is at higher risk of intraop laryngospasm secondary to their higher incidence of URIs.
■ Since these pts are not routinely intubated, when the head is turned for the procedure, make certain a patent airway can be maintained prior to incision.
■ Occasionally, the otolaryngologist will manually examine the adenoids, which will require a significantly deeper level of anesthesia for the increased stimulation.
■ Intraop Therapies
■ Give postop pain meds immediately after induction of anesthesia to ensure a more comfortable emergence & a shorter recovery room stay.

POSTOP

Pain
■ Usually minimal, requiring only acetaminophen (up to 40 mg/kg per rectum given immediately after induction of anesthesia; oral acetaminophen can be given in the recovery room to older pts)
■ Alternative method of postop pain control: intranasal fentanyl 1–2 mcg/kg given immediately after induction of anesthesia

Complications
- Periop laryngospasm

SURGICAL PROCEDURE

Indications
- Chronic serous otitis media for >3 mo, >6 episodes of acute otitis media within a year, or an acute otitis media episode unresponsive to antibiotics.

Procedure
- An operating microscope is used to examine the ear canal w/ a speculum, remove excess cerumen, make a small incision in the tympanic membrane & place a tympanostomy tube.

Surgical Concerns
- Pts w/ small ear canals (Down's syndrome) may require a longer surgical time.
- Postop bleeding.

Typical EBL
- None to minimal.

NEPHRECTOMY (RADICAL & DONOR)

JASON WIDRICH, MD

PREOP

Preop Considerations
- Types of nephrectomy
  - ➤ Simple
    - Removal of kidney. May be done for irreversible renal damage from infection, obstruction, calculus, trauma, congenital disease, renovascular HTN.
  - ➤ Partial
    - Can be done for renal cell carcinoma ("nephron-sparing surgery") or benign disease.
  - ➤ Radical
    - Done for renal cell carcinoma.
  - ➤ Donor
    - Living donation for renal transplant.
  - ➤ Laparoscopic-assisted surgery increasingly used for some types of nephrectomy.

- Considerations for renal cell cancer
  - Tumor may spread to IVC or right atrium, causing tumor thrombus.
  - May present w/ mets, although some tumors are detected early.
  - Renal cell cancer involving heart may require cardiopulmonary bypass for resection of tumor.
- Note baseline renal function, since nephrectomy can lead to renal insufficiency or renal failure requiring dialysis.
- Pts scheduled for donor nephrectomy are generally healthy, or w/ mild or well-treated systemic disease.
- Note adequacy of BP control in pt w/ renovascular HTN.

Physical Findings
- None typical.

Workup
- CBC, PT, PTT, electrolytes, BUN, creatinine.
- ECG.
- For renal cell carcinoma pt.
  - Echo, MRI, or CT to evaluate tumor size, spread & IVC or cardiac tumor thrombus.
  - Metastatic workup.
- Renal angiography usually done for donor nephrectomy pt

Choice of Anesthesia
- GA.
- Thoracic epidural can be used as GA adjunct & for postop analgesia.
  - Avoid epidural in pt w/ renal cell cancer w/ IVC & cardiac extension who may require cardiopulmonary bypass.
  - Relative contraindication for regional anesthesia is metastasis to spine.
- Epidural analgesia not needed for laparoscopic surgery.

INTRAOP
Monitors/Line Placement
- Standard monitors.
- One or two large-bore peripheral IVs.
- Foley catheter.
- Arterial line or central line depending on coexisting disease & extent of planned resection.
  - Not usually needed for donor nephrectomy or simple nephrectomy.

➤ For radical nephrectomy w/ IVC extension, consider both arterial & central line.

Intraop Concerns
■ Position may be supine or lateral.
   ➤ Proper exposure may require flexion of table or use of kidney rest.
■ Blood loss may occur from damage to renal vessels, aorta, IVC.
■ Laparoscopic procedure may require conversion to open procedure for a variety of indications, including bleeding.
   ➤ See also Procedures chapter "Laparoscopic General Surgery."
■ Pneumothorax may occur.

Intraop Therapies
■ For donor nephrectomy pt
   ➤ Significant volume expansion w/ crystalloid (typically 4–6 L in adult).
   ➤ Mannitol & furosemide often used to promote diuresis (urine output >1.5 mL/kg/h).
   ➤ Heparin is given prior to cross-clamp of renal vessels, w/ protamine for reversal.
■ Surgeon may request indigo carmine or methylene blue to rule out a urine leak.
■ Compression stockings for DVT prophylaxis.

POSTOP

Pain
■ Mild to severe, depending on incision & extent of resection
   ➤ Laparoscopic approaches have least pain
   ➤ Subcostal incision is generally more painful
■ PCA
■ Epidural analgesia useful for open procedures

Complications
■ Intraop injury to GI tract
■ Hemorrhage from renal vessels, IVC, aorta
■ DVT, pulmonary embolism
■ Pneumothorax
■ Renal failure

SURGICAL PROCEDURE

Indications
■ Renal cell carcinoma.

- Renovascular HTN.
- Renal damage from infection, obstruction, calculus, trauma, congenital disease.

Procedure
- Pt is placed in either the supine or lateral position.
- Incision may be midline, subcostal, flank, thoracoabdominal or laparoscopic.
- Approach may be extraperitoneal or intraperitoneal.
- The kidney & its hilum are identified through the perinephric fat & the vascular supply is ligated.
- The ureter is identified, clamped & ligated.
- The kidney can now be mobilized & resected.
- Radical nephrectomy may involve ipsilateral adrenalectomy & regional lymph node dissection.
- For donor nephrectomy, renal vessels are not clamped until immediately prior to nephrectomy, to minimize ischemia time.
- Adequate hemostasis is achieved.
- Closure.

Surgical Concerns
- Hemorrhage.
- Pneumothorax from pleural perforation.
- Infection.
- Urinary fistula or leak.
- Renal failure.

Typical EBL
- Minimal for laparoscopic approach.
- 500 mL for simple or radical nephrectomy.
- 1,000–1,500 mL for partial nephrectomy.

NONEMERGENT CESAREAN SECTION

JOHN P. LEE, MD
SAM HUGHES, MD
MARK ROSEN, MD

PREOP

Preop Considerations
- Anesthetic implications of physiologic changes of pregnancy

➤ Need for left uterine displacement
➤ Presence of decreased FRC
➤ Requirement for full stomach precautions: administer nonparticulate antacid (eg, bicarbonate) preop; metoclopramide and/or ranitidine optional

■ Pt may suffer considerable blood loss, particularly if nonelective procedure.
■ Volume load (give 10–20 mL/kg crystalloid, particularly before regional anesthesia & in fasted pts)
■ Consider prophylactic ephedrine (15 mg IV) before regional anesthetic.
■ Prepare ephedrine for potential hypotension.
■ Consider awake fiberoptic intubation for difficult airway.

Physical Findings
■ Possible difficult airway from weight gain of pregnancy & capillary engorgement.
■ Expect systolic murmur.

Workup
■ CBC, blood type & screen; consider coags.
■ Work up any preexisting pregnancy-related complications.
■ Confirm fetal heart rate & reason for cesarean section to help select anesthetic choice & timing.

Choice of Anesthesia
■ Spinal anesthesia, T4-S4 dermatomes must be anesthetized.
    ➤ 12.5–15 mg hyperbaric bupivacaine common.
    ➤ Addition of 0.15–0.25 mg morphine common (for postop analgesia).
    ➤ Addition of 15–20 mcg fentanyl may improve intraop block.
■ Lumbar epidural anesthesia, T4-S4
    ➤ 20 mL (after test dose & administered in divided doses) of: 2% lidocaine w/ epinephrine 1:200,000 (2 mL 8.4% bicarbonate optional to speed onset), or
    ➤ 3% chloroprocaine (fast onset), or
    ➤ 0.5% bupivacaine (slow onset, longer duration)
    ➤ 4–5 mg morphine for postop analgesia
    ➤ 50–100 mcg fentanyl may improve intraop block
■ General anesthesia
    ➤ Before birth
        • Rapid sequence induction (thiopental 4–5 mg/kg—succinylcholine 1.5 mg/kg)

- 50% nitrous oxide in oxygen, and
- 0.5 MAC volatile agent
➤ After birth
- 70% nitrous oxide
- 0.25 MAC volatile agent, and
- Opioids (150–250 mcg fentanyl)
- May add benzodiazepine
- Neuromuscular blockade helpful
- Awake extubation

INTRAOP

Monitors/Line Placement
■ Fetal heart rate on arrival in OR
■ Large-bore venous access

Intraop Concerns
■ Failed intubation
■ Aspiration
■ Hemorrhage
■ Hypotension
■ Seizure from accidental rapid injection of local anesthetic IV
■ Rare: air or amniotic fluid embolus
■ Uterine exteriorization often causes nausea

Intraop Therapies
■ Aspiration and/or failed intubation: Maintain cricoid pressure, ventilate by mask or LMA, & awaken pt for fiberoptic intubation.
■ Inadequate ventilation by mask or LMA: consider cricothyrotomy, otherwise awaken mother & consider regional anesthetic (continuous spinal).
■ Maternal hypotension w/ regional anesthesia is common. Rx w/ left uterine displacement, fluids, & ephedrine 10–25 mg IV or 10–50 mcg phenylephrine (if ephedrine unsuccessful after 3 doses).
■ Patchy block can be supplemented by additional local anesthetic (epidural) or conscious sedation (IV fentanyl, midazolam, propofol, and/or ketamine, 0.25 mg/kg).
■ Uterine atony & hemorrhage: Observe uterine tone after placenta delivered for indication of possible hemorrhage. Rx is:
  ➤ Uterine massage.
  ➤ Oxytocin administered after placenta delivered: 20–40 IU in 1 L by rapid infusion, not IV push (hypotension, cardiac arrest reported).

➤ Methylergonovine (Methergine) 0.2 mg IM or prostaglandin F2-alpha (Hemabate) 0.25 mg IM if atony unresponsive to oxytocin alone. Doses may be repeated.

➤ Consider fluid resuscitation w/ colloid, additional IV access, & call for blood if bleeding persists or profound.

POSTOP

Pain

- Intrathecal (0.15–0.2 mg) or epidural morphine (4–5 mg) for postop pain control.
- Consider ketorolac (15–30 mg IV/IM) for synergism.
- Narcotics via PCA.
- Continuous epidural infusion of dilute local anesthetic; rarely indicated.

Complications

- Postpartum hemorrhage from uterine atony, genital tract disruption, retained placenta & membranes (may require manual removal of placenta, D&C, reoperation [hysterectomy])

SURGICAL PROCEDURE

Indications

- Failure to progress
- Cephalopelvic disproportion
- Failure to descend
- Breech presentation
- Malpresentation
- Multiple gestation
- Previous C-section

Procedure

- Involves incision through the uterus, delivery of the baby, exteriorization of the uterus, repair of the uterine incision, manual massage of the uterus to promote a contracted uterus.

Surgical Concerns

- Ensure hemostasis w/ manual massage of the uterus, repair of any lacerations, & complete removal of placenta & membranes
- Persistent bleeding may require cross-clamp of uterine arteries or even hysterectomy.
- Identification & preservation of ureters.

Typical EBL

■ 1,000 mL (more if maternal hemorrhage is the indication for procedure)

OFF-PUMP CABG (OPCAB)

ERIC M. BROUCH, MD
MARTIN J. LONDON, MD

PREOP

Preop Considerations

■ Preop evaluation
  ➤ Current pt selection for OPCAB may vary dramatically between surgeon/center. Some surgeons select only "high-risk" pts w/ appropriate anatomy to avoid deleterious effects of CPB, while others may select lower-risk groups (faster recovery, smaller incision, earlier extubation, etc).
  ➤ OPCAB may be particularly advantageous in those w/ significant cerebrovascular disease, renal insufficiency/failure, or COPD.
■ Preop meds
  ➤ Give all antianginals & antihypertensives (particularly beta blockers) as close to normal dosing as possible.
  ➤ Provide appropriate anxiolysis & analgesia for the immediate preop period as ischemia on arrival in OR is well documented. For same-day admits, oral diazepam 5–10 mg PO is an option w/ IV supplementation during IV placement. For inpts, consider IM morphine 0.1–0.15 mg/kg w/ lorazepam 1–2 mg IM depending on age & medical status on call to OR.
  ➤ Avoid oversedation in the elderly.
  ➤ Ensure supplemental oxygen is administered following premedication.
  ➤ Orders for discontinuation of heparin must be discussed w/ the surgeon as practice varies.
    • Pts w/ "stable" unstable angina will usually have heparin discontinued 2–4 h preop.
    • Those w/ ongoing chest pain or critical left main disease may be continued until arrival in OR.

Physical Findings
- Careful airway exam & identification of a potentially difficult airway is crucial to avoid the "stress" of hypoxemia or hypercarbia w/ attendant catecholamine release & hemodynamic stimulation, which may precipitate ischemia.
  - Consider awake fiberoptic intubation in high-risk cases w/ appropriate attention to avoiding stress (consider esmolol, remifentanil, or other short-acting agents to control hemodynamics).
- Carefully evaluate pt's daily range of BP & HR; usually strive to maintain values within 20% of these values intraop to avoid cardiac or cerebral ischemia. This is especially important for OPCAB w/ the absence of CPB & cardioplegia, which markedly reduce myocardial oxygen demand.
  - Evaluation of BP may be difficult in outpts, but other physical signs (LVH, renal insufficiency, known carotid disease) imply higher resting blood pressure.
- Evaluate carefully for signs of CHF.
- Evaluate for evidence of occlusive carotid disease.

Workup
- Extensive evaluation frequently includes but not limited to
  - Cardiac catheterization
  - Echocardiogram
  - CXR
  - Carotid duplex ultrasound
  - Pulmonary function tests
- Coronary anatomy: The following are particularly relevant:
  - Degree of coronary artery disease.
  - Presence of significant left main disease.
  - Presence of collateral circulation & the ejection fraction.
  - Cardiac catheterization findings are particularly important as certain vessels are more feasible to graft (ie, LAD) w/o major vertical displacement of the heart.
- Cardiac function: Know the following:
  - Concurrent valvular disease, particularly ischemic mitral regurgitation & aortic insufficiency.
  - Systolic function & amount of viable myocardium downstream of vessels to be bypassed.
    - Unlike pump cases, regions of myocardium may be temporarily ischemic at physiologic temperatures & decrement in function, at least temporarily, may occur.

Choice of Anesthesia

- GA w/ controlled ventilation is required.
  - Any combination of opioid (fentanyl, sufentanil, remifentanil, etc), volatile agent (isoflurane, sevoflurane, or desflurane) & IV adjuvant (midazolam, propofol) can be used as long as hemodynamics are appropriately managed.
  - Your comfort level w/ the potential hemodynamic side effects of a particular anesthetic agent should be your guide.
  - Many centers use fentanyl (10–20 mcg/kg), midazolam (0.05–0.10 mg/kg) and/or propofol infusion w/ volatile agent supplementation because of cost considerations.
  - Avoid nitrous oxide given risk of hypoxemia & potential hazards of coronary or cerebral air embolus.
- Avoid tachycardia, which is the most common response to surgical stimulation in the underanesthetized pt & the key factor precipitating ischemia in the heart room.
- Most centers practice "fast tracking" in which pts are extubated 3–6 h postop (or as soon as they meet criteria in older or more complicated pts), as opposed to older practices of mandatory overnight ventilation.
  - OPCAB pts may be better candidates for early extubation (including in the OR) given absence of CPB, although this is markedly influenced by the speed of surgery, change in body temp, or provocation of ischemia during the case.
- Regional anesthesia may be useful in some pts, particularly those undergoing thoracotomy incision (used primarily in redo procedures).
  - A single-shot spinal (ie, morphine 0.1 mg/kg) or even thoracic epidurals (infrequent) are used in some centers.
  - A thoracic epidural, if used, is usually placed the night before surgery.

INTRAOP

Monitors/Line Placement

- Prior to induction
  - At least one large-bore peripheral IV
  - Radial arterial line
- Central access, most commonly via the RIJ, should be established in all pts for monitoring at least CVP & administering heparin.
- PA catheter use depends on surgeon & center.

➤ OPCAB pt selection, availability & expertise of clinicians w/ TEE, the presence of other comorbidities & the postop recovery facilities should guide choice of catheter.

➤ Ejection fraction & associated valvular disease are the key factors guiding timing of PAC placement (pre or postinduction).

➤ Many centers have significantly decreased use of PAC for cost reasons & concern over possible PA catheter risks & OR efficiency.

■ TEE may be helpful, although it is not commonly used in many private centers for either CABG or OPCAB (especially in low- and moderate-risk pts).

➤ Ensure pt is adequately anesthetized prior to probe insertion.

➤ Decompress the stomach w/ an OG tube before & after TEE use.

➤ TEE imaging during the actual period of the surgical anastomosis is often not helpful due to vertical retraction of the heart away from the esophagus, as well as tethering of the myocardium by the suction immobilizer, which causes a "pseudo" wall motion abnormality. However, the presence of new or worsened mitral regurgitation (presumably ischemic in origin) or SWMAs in adjacent or at-risk segments can be clinically useful.

■ A device to measure the activated clotting time is required to manage heparin dosing & reversal.

Intraop Concerns

■ A perfusionist & the cardiac surgeon should be available prior to induction.

➤ The bypass machine is usually set up "dry" (tubing assembled but not primed).

■ Primary goals for induction include

➤ Avoiding hemodynamic instability & maintaining MAP & HR within 20% of baseline.

➤ Always have vasopressors prepared to treat hypotension following induction (usually caused by vasodilation in the setting of mild hypovolemia, but occasionally significant depression of myocardial contractility may occur, especially if ischemia occurs).

➤ Avoid sodium thiopental in pts w/ impaired ventricular function.

➤ Use low-dose opioids and/or short-acting beta blocker (esmolol) to blunt response to direct laryngoscopy & intubation.

➤ Early neuromuscular blockade is useful to offset muscle rigidity from opioids & should be maintained throughout the case.

■ After induction obtain

> Baseline ACT.
> ABG.
> Cardiac output if a PAC is being used.
> TEE basic exam for contractile function, valvular lesions, aortic arch atheromatous disease.

■ Sternotomy is highly stimulating & requires adequate anesthesia to avoid hemodynamic changes.
> Remember to deflate the lungs.

■ After sternotomy
> The IMA, saphenous veins, or radial artery is harvested.
> The pericardium is opened & the heart & aortic arch are exposed.
> Packing is placed under the heart to vertically elevate it, which exposes the left ventricle, which is posterior to the right ventricle in the chest.
> The circumflex & the right coronary branches require the greatest amount of displacement, which may cause significant compression of the right or left atrium, impeding ventricular filling & ejection w/ resultant hypotension.
  • Phenylephrine or other pressors & judicious volume loading may be required at this point.
> The patient is placed in Trendelenburg to facilitate surgical exposure as well as increase venous return.
> A suction immobilizer is placed on the myocardium adjacent to the coronary artery being grafted.
> The combination of ventricular displacement & ischemia (if it occurs) may markedly depress ventricular function & cardiac output, requiring inotropes.
  • Usually the surgeon will first release the vertical displacement & retraction (if possible), which should normalize hemodynamics quickly.
  • Although nitroglycerin is the obvious choice of drug for treating ischemia, it may be difficult to use in this setting w/ cardiac displacement & impaired filling.
  • CVP measurement may not be helpful due to distortion of the atria.
  • TEE may be more useful, particularly the midesophageal four-chamber view.

■ Heparin is administered & the ACT obtained prior to manipulation of coronary arteries.
> The heparin dose may vary w/ surgeon, w/ some using a low-dose regimen of 100 U/kg to maintain an ACT of 2x baseline,

while most prefer a standard dose of 300 U/kg to obtain an ACT >450 sec.

- Prophylactic antiarrhythmic drugs to treat possible reperfusion ventricular dysrhythmias are frequently used for off-pump cases & include
  - $MgSO_4$ 1–2 mg IV and/or
  - Lidocaine 1–4 mg/min after bolus of 1–1.5 mg/kg
- After dissection of the diseased vessel but prior to performing the distal anastomosis, the surgeon may use ischemic preconditioning:
  - The coronary artery is occluded for 5 min while observing the ECG, TEE & other monitors (PAC pressures) for evidence of ischemia.
  - After this period, the vessel is released & reperfusion is allowed for a similar time period prior to reclamping for distal anastomosis.
  - W/ the introduction & increasing use of coronary shunts, many surgeons no longer consider preconditioning necessary since the period of ischemia may be only 2–3 min, in contrast to approximately 10–12 min per vessel w/o shunting.
- ACT should be repeated q20–30min w/ additional heparin administered to maintain the target ACT.
  - During normothermia heparin will be metabolized much quicker than w/ hypothermic bypass.
- The proximal anastomoses are usually performed in a similar manner to routine CABG, using a side-biting partial occlusion clamp on the aorta.
  - Even by avoiding CPB w/ OPCAB, there is still significant risk in selected pts for stroke due to aortic arch atheromatous disease.
- After completion of grafts
  - Cardiac function should be assessed by TEE/cardiac output, etc, & blood pressure stabilized prior to discontinuing arterial cannula & reversing heparin.
  - Heparin is reversed w/ protamine.
  - Antiarrhythmics may be weaned if rhythm has been stable.
- Maintaining normothermia during OPCAB is critical, particularly to prevent coagulopathy, but can be a challenge.
  - Forced air warming techniques are recommended if possible.
  - Skin prep may be prewarmed to avoid excessive cooling.
  - A heating blanket under the pt is helpful, as are low gas flows & airway humidification.
  - When planning intraop extubation, normothermia is critical.
- Serial hematocrits should be checked & fluid/blood replacement optimized prior to transfer to ICU.

- Monitor invasive BP, HR, ECG & O_2 saturation during ICU transport & bring medications to treat BP, HR, ischemia, arrhythmias.

Intraop Therapies
- Multiple vasopressors & inotropes should be available, particularly during manipulation of heart & anastomoses. These include but are not limited to
  - Phenylephrine
  - Ephedrine
  - Epinephrine
  - Calcium
  - Dopamine
  - Norepinephrine
  - Amrinone/milrinone
- Vasodilators such as sodium nitroprusside & nitroglycerine should also be readily available.

POSTOP

Pain
- Fast tracking & early extubation should not preclude adequate pain control.
- Consider pt's specific postop pain mgt needs along with your center's unique practices in tailoring your anesthetic.
  - Some centers avoid or prefer IV opioids or NSAIDs (ie. ketorolac).
  - Usually small doses of IV morphine are well tolerated even in pts w/ early extubation.
  - Some centers prefer ketorolac IV or by suppository.
- IMA dissection is associated w/ greater postop pain than saphenous vein or radial artery alone.

Complications
- Bleeding is most common cause of return to OR. Manifested as continued output from chest tubes, frequently w/ hypotension & need for blood products & fluid resuscitation.
  - Coagulopathy & thrombocytopenia are less common w/ OPCAB than after CABG but still may occur.
  - Surgical bleeding from anastomoses occurs w/ similar or perhaps greater frequency than w/ CBP due to a less ideal surgical field.
- Heart failure and/or fluid overload are uncommon but may occur, particularly if significant ischemia has occurred.
- Hypertension

➢ May be unresponsive to sedation or narcotics.
➢ Nitroprusside and/or nitroglycerin infusions may be required.
- CVA. Although avoidance of CPB would be expected to reduce the incidence of CVA, it has not eliminated it, given the need for proximal anastomoses on the ascending aorta. Use of alternate sites (subclavian artery) may reduce it, but these are technically difficult.

SURGICAL PROCEDURE

Indications
- Typical indications include multivessel coronary artery disease.
- Left main coronary artery disease is a contraindication.
- Although grafting the circumflex & right coronary arteries is significantly more difficult than the LAD, the use of multivessel OPCAB is increasing dramatically & in many practices is performed in well over 50% of pts.

Procedure
- Involves sternotomy, followed by dissection of grafts & anastomosis to diseased vessels & the aorta w/o the use of CPB & ischemic arrest

Surgical Concerns
- Sewing grafts on an actively beating heart is technically difficult & may cause hemodynamic instability or arrhythmias from the manipulation.
- In addition, certain regions of myocardium will be ischemic while these grafts are placed.

Typical EBL
- Should be substantially less than w/ the use of CPB (less blood lost w/o cannulation or the varying degree of coagulopathy assoc w/ CPB)
- However, w/ sternotomy & dissection, an EBL of 300–500 mL can be expected.

OMPHALOCELE REPAIR

ATSUKO BABA, MD

PREOP

Preop Considerations
- Incidence: 1/5,000–10,000 live births, male predominance
- 75% incidence of other congenital defects

- Cardiac anomalies (20%)
- Trisomy 13/18/21
- Beckwith-Wiedemann syndrome (macroglossia, organomegaly, gigantism, symptomatic hypoglycemia)
- Pentalogy of Cantrell (omphalocele, sternal, diaphragmatic, pericardial & cardiac anomalies)
- Exstrophy cloaca (omphalocele, exstrophy bladder, imperforate anus)
- Renal anomalies

- 33% are preterm
- Cover exposed viscera w/ moist dressings & a plastic bowel bag & maintain neutral thermal environment to decrease fluid & heat loss
- Decompress stomach w/ orogastric tube to decrease risk of regurgitation & pulmonary aspiration
- Maintain adequate hydration (6–12 cc/kg/h); protein-containing solutions should constitute 25% of replacement fluids to compensate for the protein loss & third-space translocation
- Mortality is 28%

Physical Findings
- External herniation of abdominal viscera through the base of the umbilical cord covered by an intact hernia sac

Workup
- Diagnosed in the first trimester of pregnancy by fetal ultrasound
- Hypovolemia evidenced by hemoconcentration & metabolic acidosis
- Appropriate workup to detect assoc conditions

Choice of Anesthesia
- General endotracheal anesthesia w/ possible awake intubation after decompression of the stomach

INTRAOP
Monitors/Line Placement
- Two peripheral IVs.
- Arterial line is helpful for BP monitoring & ABGs.

Intraop Concerns/Therapies
- Because of coexisting hypovolemia, anesthetics must be titrated slowly to avoid hypotension.
- Opioids and/or volatile anesthetics can be used.

- Nitrous oxide may cause intestinal distention, interfering w/ the return of viscera into the abdomen.
- A tight surgical abdominal closure can lead to
  - ➤ Compression of the inferior vena cava, leading to hypotension.
  - ➤ Compression of the diaphragm w/ decreased pulmonary compliance.
  - ➤ Compression of perfusing vessels to abdominal organs.
- Preterm neonates are vulnerable to retinopathy of prematurity w/ high oxygen concentrations.
- When primary surgical abdominal closure is not possible, the herniated viscera is temporarily covered with a Dacron-reinforced Silastic silo, w/ the contents being slowly reduced over 1–2 wks.
- Maintain body temp & continue replacement fluids.

POSTOP

Pain
- Use narcotics judiciously if pt is extubated.

Complications
- Mechanical ventilation postop is usually indicated for 24–48 h w/ monitoring in the NICU.
- May require TPN.
- A tight surgical closure may lead to hemodynamic, pulmonary & abdominal organ dysfunction.
- Infection.

SURGICAL PROCEDURE

Indications
- Abdominal wall defect w/ the goal of safely replacing herniated viscera into the abdomen.

Procedure
- Safely replace herniated viscera into the abdominal cavity w/ primary surgical closure or staged repair w/ a Silastic silo & definitive closure in 10–14 days.
- Surgical Concerns
- Impaired ventilation & venous return will result from overaggressive attempts at closure.

Typical EBL
- 5–10 cc/kg.

OPEN CHOLECYSTECTOMY

JASON WIDRICH, MD

PREOP

Preop Considerations
- Most often performed in pts for whom laparoscopic surgery cannot be tolerated or completed.
  - ➤ See also Procedures chapter "Laparoscopic Cholecystectomy."
- Abdominal pain may cause splinting & decreased FRC.
- Pt may have sepsis if cholangitis is indication for surgery.

Physical Findings
- RUQ abdominal pain, fever, chills, jaundice, Murphy's sign.

Workup
- CBC.
- CXR.
- ECG.
- LFTs.
- PT, PTT.

Choice of Anesthesia
- GA.
- Consider thoracic epidural catheter for postop analgesia.

INTRAOP

Monitors/Line Placement
- Standard ASA monitors.
- One peripheral IV usually adequate.

Intraop Concerns
- Rapid sequence induction if pt at risk for aspiration.
- Reverse Trendelenburg, which may be required for surgical exposure, may decrease venous return.
- Narcotics can cause spasm of the sphincter of Oddi & interfere w/ cholangiography.

Intraop Therapies
- Although controversial, meperidine may cause less sphincter of Oddi spasm than morphine or fentanyl.
- Naloxone 40 mcg in repeated doses can break spasm as well.

POSTOP

Pain
- Moderate to severe
    - PCA
    - Thoracic epidural analgesia

Complications
- Nausea/vomiting
- Postop atelectasis, splinting, respiratory insufficiency
- Shoulder pain referred from diaphragmatic irritation

SURGICAL PROCEDURE

Indications
- Symptomatic cholelithiasis, acute cholecystitis, choledocholithiasis.

Procedure
- Right subcostal incision or midline incision.
- Gallbladder, cystic duct & artery are identified on inferior surface of the liver.
- Cholangiography can be used to identify the biliary tree.
- Cystic duct & artery are divided & the gallbladder is taken off the surface of the liver.
- Occasionally the ducts are explored for extraction of stones.

Surgical Concerns
- Clear delineation of cystic duct & artery.
- Biliary injury, including biliary leak.

Typical EBL
- 200 mL.

ORGAN HARVEST

JOSEPH COTTEN, MD, PHD

PREOP

Preop Considerations
- Performed in pt who has suffered brain death
- Contraindications (some are relative)
    - Age >65–70
    - Untreated sepsis

- ➤ Extracranial malignancy
- ➤ Transmissible disease (eg, hepatitis, HIV)
- ■ Respiratory dysfunction may be present from
  - ➤ Trauma (hemo- or pneumothorax)
  - ➤ Aspiration
  - ➤ Atelectasis
  - ➤ Pneumonia
  - ➤ Pulmonary edema
- ■ Hypotension may be present due to
  - ➤ Neurogenic shock
  - ➤ Hypovolemia
  - ➤ Hypothermia
  - ➤ Cardiac dysfunction
- ■ Hypovolemia, if present, may result from
  - ➤ Diabetes insipidus
  - ➤ Hemorrhage
  - ➤ Hyperglycemia
  - ➤ Mannitol therapy
- ■ Hypothermia may be present because brain-dead pts cannot regulate their core temp
- ■ Dysrhythmias are common & atropine-resistant; potential causes:
  - ➤ Hypothermia
  - ➤ Myocardial ischemia or contusion
  - ➤ Inotropic infusions
  - ➤ Electrolyte/blood gas abnormalities
  - ➤ All brain-dead individuals undergo terminal arrhythmias resistant to therapy
- ■ Diabetes insipidus is common. Loss of ADH production causes
  - ➤ Hypotonic diuresis
  - ➤ Hypovolemia
  - ➤ Hyperosmolality
  - ➤ Hypernatremia
  - ➤ Hypomagnesemia
  - ➤ Hypokalemia
  - ➤ Hypophosphatemia
  - ➤ Hypocalcemia
- ■ Coagulopathy & DIC are possible hematologic complications
- ■ Local transplant donor network may already be involved w/ pt's care in the ICU. To optimize organ perfusion, therapy for the following conditions may be in place:
  - ➤ Fluid replacement

- D5 0.25% NS w/ 20 mEq KCl at 150 mL/h
- Blood products to correct coagulopathy & maintain hematocrit at 25–30
➤ Hypotension
  - Normal saline bolus
  - Dopamine up to 20 mcg/kg/min to maintain SBP >90 or MAP >70 mmHg
  - Phenylephrine, norepinephrine, or epinephrine
➤ Diabetes insipidus
  - For urine output >300–500 mL/h & serum sodium >150, DDAVP 0.1 mcg/kg IV
➤ Hypothermia
➤ Warming or cooling blankets as necessary to maintain core temp 36.5–37.5 degrees C

Physical Findings
■ Signs of brain death

Workup
■ Declaration of brain death by physicians not involved in organ procurement must be documented
■ Identify & treat electrolyte & hematologic abnormalities

Choice of Anesthesia
■ GA
■ The goal of anesthesia is to maintain optimal organ perfusion & cellular oxygenation while blunting the remaining spinal, cardiovascular & adrenal medullary reflexes
■ Muscle relaxation is useful to prevent movement & to facilitate surgery
  ➤ Long-acting muscle relaxants are appropriate (eg, pancuronium)

INTRAOP

Monitor/Line Placement
■ Arterial line to monitor BP, blood counts, ABGs, lytes
■ Central line to assess volume status
■ Foley catheter required to decompress bladder; also helps assess renal perfusion & volume status

Intraop Concerns
■ Maintain "rule of 100s" to optimize organ perfusion:
  ➤ Keep systolic BP >100 mmHg (MAP >70).

- Urine output >100 mL/h
- PaO_2 >100 mmHg
- Other recommended goals
  - Hgb >10 mg/L
  - CVP in normal range
  - $PaCO_2$ 40 mmHg
- For lung donors
  - Consider decreasing FiO_2 to minimize oxygen toxicity
  - Lung perfusate may contain prostaglandin E1, which can cause profound hypotension
  - Pleural & tracheal dissection may cause ventilation & oxygenation difficulties
  - Following lung perfusion, ventilation is continued at 4 breaths/min, then stopped; the trachea is then suctioned, extubated
- Note time of aortic cross-clamping, which signals start of cold ischemia time
- Anesthetic care is stopped after aortic cross-clamp

Intraop Therapies
- Inotropic support
  - Dopamine (first choice)
  - Phenylephrine
  - Norepinephrine
  - Epinephrine
    - Consider dopamine 3 mcg/kg/min during norepinephrine or epinephrine therapy for renal vasodilation
- Arrhythmia therapy
  - Treat ventricular arrhythmias w/ lidocaine
  - Treat bradycardia w/ isoproterenol (bradycardia is atropine-resistant)
  - Have defibrillator available
- Diabetes insipidus
  - Administer DDAVP 0.1 mcg/kg IV when urine output is 300–500 mL/h or greater
- Maintain temp above 36.5–37.5 degrees C
  - Warm OR environment
  - Heating or forced air warming blanket
  - Fluid warmer
- Administer heparin (typically 300 U/kg) prior to cross-clamping & cardioplegia

POSTOP

Pain
- Not applicable

Complications
- Not applicable

SURGICAL PROCEDURE

Indications
- For procurement of kidneys, liver, heart, lungs, pancreas, bowel.

Procedure
- Local surgeons or a traveling team of surgeons may perform the procedure.
- Following dissection, organs are cooled & perfused in situ via cannulas & cross-clamps w/ preservative solution & harvested *en bloc* through a midline incision (suprasternal notch to pubis) & sternotomy.
- Vessels cannulated: distal aorta (for GI organs & kidney perfusion), ascending aorta (for cardioplegic administration), inferior mesenteric vein (for liver perfusion), main pulmonary artery (for lung perfusion if to be harvested), IVC (for bleedout)
- Cross-clamping: SVC & aorta (proximal to innominate artery & at diaphragm)
- Following cardioplegia, all organs are perfused simultaneously w/ cold preservative.

Surgical Concerns
- Adequacy of organs for transplant.

Typical EBL
- Anticipate transfusing 2 U PRBCs.

ORIF OF HIP

MARK T. GRABOVAC, MD

PREOP

Preop Considerations
- Cause of fracture

➤ In elderly pt, fractures of femoral neck/head usually secondary to mechanical fall
  • Etiology of fall in elderly may be related to significant cerebrovascular disease, valvular heart disease, alcohol use, GI bleed w/ anemia or CAD.
  • Elderly pt may have multiple coexisting diseases: COPD, DM, CAD, dementia (see also Coexisting Disease chapter "The Elderly Patient").
➤ In younger pt, fracture may be related to trauma, avascular necrosis or tumor.
  • ORIF of acetabulum usually due to trauma in younger pt; frequently associated w/ other injuries.
■ Pt may have anemia or hypovolemia.
■ Pt may have pre-existing DVT from immobility.
  ➤ Determine if pt is receiving anticoagulant therapy (eg, Coumadin, LMWH).
  ➤ Consider risk of anticoagulant w/ regional anesthesia.
■ Pt may have decreased gastric emptying due to pain & trauma.
■ Severe pain may limit ability to cooperate w/ positioning.

Physical Findings
■ Signs of hypovolemia (increased HR, decreased BP).
■ Evaluate for significant cardiac, pulmonary & CNS disease, particularly in elderly pt.
  ➤ Cardiac: CHF, murmurs secondary to valvular disease (especially AS).
  ➤ Pulmonary: COPD, pneumonia, pulmonary edema.
  ➤ Neuro: CNS disease may be etiology of fall.
    • Look for signs of stroke, carotid bruit, altered mental status, dementia.
    • Altered mental status may preclude use of regional anesthesia.
■ Extremities: assess for DVT, decreased pulses or edema.

Workup
■ CBC, electrolytes, BUN, creatinine, glucose.
■ ECG.
■ Further cardiac evaluation & other workup as indicated from history & physical.
■ Type & cross-match for at least 2 units for femoral head or acetabular fractures.

■ Trauma pts need thorough evaluation of associated injuries, including possibility of cervical spine injury.
  ➤ Unstable hemodynamic status from trauma may require fluid & blood resuscitation prior to ORIF of hip.

Choice of Anesthesia
■ For percutaneous pinning of femoral neck, either GA or regional block is an appropriate choice.
■ For ORIF of acetabulum or femoral head replacement, consider use of GA due to possible large blood loss & increased length of procedure.
  ➤ Regional block may be used to supplement GA.
■ Epidural or spinal
  ➤ May be technically difficult due to pt's inability to assume lateral or seated position due to pain.
  ➤ Pt may have significant DJD or other spine disease, making neuraxial block more difficult.
    • Consider paramedian approach.
    • Single injection spinal may be technically easier than epidural.
  ➤ If pt will receive postop anticoagulation, epidural may not offer distinct advantage over spinal, since epidural catheter should be removed prior to anticoagulation.
■ Lumbar plexus block
  ➤ Can be used to supplement GA.
  ➤ Can place catheter to administer additional local anesthetic.
  ➤ Same difficulty with positioning as for SAB or epidural.

INTRAOP
Monitors/Line Placement
■ Standard monitors
■ Foley catheter.
■ For percutaneous pinning of femoral neck.
  ➤ One peripheral IV acceptable.
  ➤ Consider arterial line, depending on coexisting disease.
■ For replacement of femoral head or ORIF of acetabulum
  ➤ Two large-bore IVs required.
  ➤ Consider arterial line & central line because of increased blood loss potential.
  ➤ Consider PA line only for severe coexisting cardiac disease (pulmonary HTN, severe MR, CHF, cardiomyopathy).

Intraop Concerns

- Correct hypovolemia & anemia prior to induction of GA or placement of regional block.
- Pinning of femoral neck
  - Generally well tolerated even by relatively sick pts.
  - For pinning procedures, special fracture table may be used.
- Femoral head replacement or ORIF acetabulum
  - Consider cell saver.
  - Anticipate large volume of blood loss.
- Elderly pt
  - Minimize sedation when regional anesthetic used due to potential for postop delirium.

Intraop Therapies

- Pinning of femoral neck
  - Stimulation level from percutaneous pinning is relatively low compared to open surgery.
- Femoral head replacement or ORIF acetabulum
  - To reduce blood loss or transfusion requirement, consider controlled hypotension or isovolemic hemodilution in suitable pt (should not be used routinely in elderly pts).
- Regional block considerations
  - Small, divided doses of ketamine (eg, 10–20 mg IV) may be useful to facilitate positioning.
    - Regional anesthetics may require small doses of phenylephrine or ephedrine to maintain BP in chronically hypertensive pt w/ cerebrovascular disease.
  - If a spinal is used, intrathecal morphine can be administered for postop analgesia.
- Consider beta blockade in pt who has had adequate volume resuscitation & who has known CAD or risk factors for CAD.

POSTOP

Pain

- Moderate to severe
  - Pain is usually improved after percutaneous pinning of femoral neck fracture but may still be substantial.
  - Pain is greater after replacement of femoral head (similar to total hip arthroplasty) or ORIF of acetabular fracture.
- Epidural analgesia

> Need to remove epidural catheter prior to starting postop anti-coagulation because of risk of epidural hematoma.
> Consider epidural morphine prior to removal of catheter.
- Lumbar plexus block
  > Continuous infusion through lumbar plexus catheter w/ mixture of local anesthetic & narcotic can be used for postop analgesia.
- PCA narcotic generally provides satisfactory analgesia in pt w/o regional block.

Complications
- Delirium
  > In elderly pt, postop delirium can result from sensitivity to narcotics & other meds.
- DVT & pulmonary emboli.
- Fat embolism.
- Pulmonary edema, CHF.
  > More likely in elderly pt with pre-existing LV dysfunction or valvular disease.
- Complications of massive transfusion (more likely w/ ORIF acetabular fracture).

SURGICAL PROCEDURE

Indications
- Repair/stabilization of fracture of femoral neck, head or acetabulum.

Procedure
- Femoral neck fracture generally corrected by percutaneous pin fixation under fluoroscopy.
- Severe fracture involving the femoral head is uncommon but may require replacement of femoral head w/ cemented prosthesis (similar to hemiarthroplasty).
- ORIF of acetabular fracture is an extensive procedure involving large amount of hardware & large incision to repair.
  > Typically, young trauma pt who is placed in traction prior to repair.

Surgical Concerns
- Treatment of fractures w/ traction in elderly population is assoc w/ high morbidity & mortality due to pulmonary emboli, pneumonia, sepsis.
- Early treatment associated w/ better functional recovery & fewer complications.

- ORIF acetabular fracture is a challenging & often lengthy procedure.
- Sciatic nerve injury.

Typical EBL
- For percutaneous pinning: minimal, but hematoma may contain 500–1,000 cc blood.
- For replacement of femoral head: 500–1,600 cc.
- For ORIF of acetabulum: >1,000 cc but can be >1 blood volume.

ORTHOTOPIC LIVER TRANSPLANT

CLAUS NIEMANN, MD

PREOP

Preop Considerations
- See also Coexisting Disease chapters "Chronic Liver Disease and Liver Cirrhosis" and "Acute Liver Failure."
- Spectrum of diseases causing liver failure include
  - ➤ Chronic liver failure
    - Hepatitis B, C
    - Alcoholic liver disease
    - Cryptogenic disease
    - Primary sclerosing cholangitis
    - Primary biliary cirrhosis
    - Wilson's disease
  - ➤ Acute liver failure
    - *Amanita* mushroom toxicity
    - Hepatitis A
    - Drug-induced
    - Wilson's disease
- Severity of chronic liver disease is determined by the modified Child-Pugh classification & the model for end-stage liver disease (MELD)
- Evaluate for multiple organ system manifestations of liver failure:
  - ➤ CNS
    - Hepatic encephalopathy
    - For pt w/ acute liver failure: evaluate for increased ICP. Cerebral edema & herniation are significant risks. Head CT & ICP monitoring may be needed & specific treatment (hyperventilation, mannitol) may be required
  - ➤ Cardiac

- Hyperdynamic circulation
- Cirrhotic cardiomyopathy
- Coronary artery disease
➤ Respiratory
  - Hepatopulmonary syndrome (PaO_2 <70 mmHg, or A-a O_2 gradient >20 mmHg from intrapulmonary vascular dilatation)
  - Portopulmonary hypertension (precapillary/arteriolar pulmonary hypertension, mean PA pressure >25 mmHg at rest, w/ other causes of pulmonary hypertension excluded)
➤ GI
  - Portal hypertension w/ esophageal varices & upper GI bleed
  - Ascites
➤ Hematologic
  - Anemia
  - Thrombocytopenia (from splenic sequestration)
  - Prolonged PT/PTT
  - Decreased fibrinogen
➤ Renal
  - Hepatorenal syndrome
  - Acute renal failure
  - Electrolyte disturbances
➤ Miscellaneous
  - Infection
  - Malnutrition, cachexia

Physical Findings
- Clinical findings are those of end-stage liver disease: ascites, malnutrition, jaundice, edema, spider angiomas, asterixis (described also in Coexisting Disease chapter "Chronic Liver Disease and Liver Cirrhosis")

Workup
- Pts w/ liver failure receive workup of hepatic & extrahepatic disease prior to listing for liver transplant.
- Cardiac workup is important, since liver transplant is associated w/ many sources of cardiovascular stress, including
  ➤ Potential for massive hemorrhage, hypovolemia, anemia
  ➤ Large fluid shifts & blood product requirements
  ➤ Marked lability in BP & HR, w/ significant hypotension, bradycardia & cardiac arrest possible upon liver reperfusion
  ➤ Frequent development of electrolyte abnormalities

- Cardiac workup includes
  - ➤ Echocardiogram
    - Typical pattern is hyperdynamic LV function; suspect primary cardiac dysfunction if this is not present.
    - Pts w/ hemochromatosis more likely to develop cardiac dysfunction
    - Echo used to estimate PA systolic pressure
  - ➤ CXR
  - ➤ ECG
  - ➤ Right heart cath for suspected PA hypertension
  - ➤ For pts w/ higher likelihood of coronary artery disease (eg, advancing age, diabetes), further tests may include
    - Pharmacologic stress thallium
    - Dobutamine stress echo
    - Coronary angiography & left heart cath
  - ➤ Important: months may have elapsed since initial eval; consider whether additional or repeat cardiac eval is needed.
- Repeat key studies immediately prior to transplant (ECG, CXR, CBC, electrolytes, BUN, creatinine, LFTs, PT, PTT, fibrinogen)
- Anticipate large transfusion requirements
  - ➤ Coordinate blood product requirements w/ blood bank
  - ➤ Typical blood products at start of case: 10 units PRBCs, 10 units FFP
  - ➤ Involve intraop cell salvage personnel
  - ➤ Consider use of rapid transfusion device

Choice of Anesthesia
- GA required
  - ➤ Rapid sequence induction due to risk factors for aspiration
  - ➤ Avoid nitrous oxide administration
  - ➤ Most anesthetic agents acceptable; avoid drugs primarily dependent on hepatic metabolism
  - ➤ Epidural anesthesia not used due to coagulopathy & relatively low postop narcotic requirements

INTRAOP

Monitors/Line Placement
- Standard monitors
- Arterial line
- Central line (consider large-bore introducer)
- PA line

➤ Assess cardiac output, filling pressure
➤ Evaluate PA pressure
■ Peripheral IVs
  ➤ Two or three large-bore IVs
  ➤ Consider rapid infusion catheter (7 or 8.5 Fr)
■ Foley catheter
■ Nasogastric or orogastric tube
  ➤ Consider risk of nosebleed due to coagulopathy & bleeding from esophageal varices.
■ TEE
  ➤ Consider use for LV function monitoring or detection of air embolus, pulmonary embolus or myocardial ischemia.

Intraop Concerns
■ Specific concerns vary during phase of case. Three phases of liver transplant:
  ➤ Phase 1: dissection
  ➤ Phase 2: anhepatic
  ➤ Phase 3: reperfusion
■ General concerns
  ➤ Hemodynamic instability
    • Hypovolemia from hemorrhage, massive fluid shifts
    • Decreased venous return from liver manipulation (temporary obstruction of vena cava) or application of vena cava cross-clamp
    • Cardiac dysfunction (eg, myocardial ischemia)
    • Ionized hypocalcemia can contribute to hypotension
  ➤ Severe coagulopathy & hemorrhage
    • Pre-existing coagulopathy or thrombocytopenia predisposes to bleeding
    • Portosystemic collaterals lead to increased bleeding during dissection
    • Consumption of coagulation factors from hemorrhage
    • Dilution of coagulation factors
    • Citrate toxicity & hypocalcemia
    • Treat w/ PRBCs, FFP, cryoprecipitate, platelets as needed
    • Consider hemostatic agent to reduce blood loss (eg, aminocaproic acid, aprotinin)
    • Consider octreotide infusion (100-mcg bolus, 100-mcg/h infusion) to reduce splanchnic blood flow & reduce risk of variceal hemorrhage

> Electrolyte/glucose abnormalities
  • Monitor labs frequently (q30–60min); correct as necessary.
> Renal dysfunction
  • Maintain adequate preload
  • Consider loop diuretic, mannitol infusion
  • For anuric renal failure, consider need for intraop continuous venovenous hemofiltration (CVVH). This may be preferable to continuous arteriovenous hemofiltration (CAVH)
> Respiratory compromise
  • Can occur from a variety of causes, including pulmonary edema
> Hypothermia is common due to abdominal exposure, large fluid & blood requirements & placement of cold liver graft. Prevention may include
  • Forced air warmer
  • Fluid warmers
  • Breathing circuit humidification or low fresh gas flow rate
  • Warm irrigation to abdominal cavity
■ Dissection phase
> Observe general concerns discussed above
> Correct coagulopathy to minimize bleeding during reperfusion phase
> At the end of the dissection phase, prepare for the anhepatic phase by a technique of volume loading in anticipation of a significant decrease in preload after vena cava clamps are applied
■ Anhepatic phase
> Begins after clamping of major vessels (portal vein, hepatic artery, vena cava)
> Biggest hemodynamic change w/ complete caval cross clamp is 40–60% decrease in preload, w/ corresponding decrease in cardiac output & filling pressures
  • Fluid loading is required before cross-clamp
  • Excess fluid administration during the anhepatic phase may produce hepatic congestion from fluid overload after reperfusion
> Can be managed w/ or w/o the use of venovenous bypass (VVB)
  • VVB requires venous cannula placement above & below IVC
  • With VVB, requirement for fluid loading is generally less
> Consider renal protection strategy during this phase (eg, VVB, dopamine, loop diuretic, mannitol)

➤ "Piggyback" surgical technique refers to partial occlusion of the vena cava, w/ an end-to-side anastomosis, instead of insertion of donor vena cava. Decrease in preload is usually less than w/ complete cross-clamp of vena cava

➤ Anticipate worsening metabolic acidosis & increased coagulation factor requirements

➤ Anhepatic phase ends w/ unclamping of the portal vein

■ Reperfusion phase

➤ Pt is at risk for profound cardiovascular compromise for the first few minutes after reperfusion. Although preload will increase after release of vena cava cross-clamps, hypotension can occur from profound vasodilation, metabolic acidosis, hypothermia, hyperkalemic preservative solution, vasoactive peptides or sudden atrial stretch

• The "postreperfusion syndrome" consists of arrhythmias (atrial, ventricular, severe bradycardia) & profound hypotension

• Cardiac arrest can occur from hyperkalemia (3–5% incidence) or other causes

• Other causes of hypotension at this time include air embolism, fat embolism, myocardial ischemia

➤ Treatment of hypotension will depend on suspected causes, but vasopressor treatment may be required (eg, epinephrine 10 mcg to >1 mg, norepinephrine, phenylephrine)

➤ Bleeding may occur from anastomosis suture sites.

➤ Fibrinolysis can occur & cause increased bleeding

• May require treatment w/ aminocaproic acid (75-mg/kg load, 15-mg/kg/h infusion)

➤ Assess function of new liver. These signs include

• Bile production

• Improvement in PT

• Improvement of metabolic acidosis (eg, improved base deficit on ABG)

• Rise in serum glucose

➤ Consider potential for postop extubation based on intraop course & degree of encephalopathy

➤ Prepare for transport & postop care in the ICU

Intraop Therapies

■ Immunosuppression & prophylactic antibiotics per surgeon's protocol

- Blood products for hemorrhage or coagulopathy
- Calcium chloride for ionized hypocalcemia
- Hemostatic agent (aminocaproic acid or aprotinin) to reduce bleeding
- Octreotide to reduce splanchnic blood flow
- Balloon tube tamponade (eg, Minnesota or Blakemore tube) for recent or ongoing esophageal variceal bleeding
- Antifibrinolytic agent (eg, aminocaproic acid)
- Renal protection agents (dopamine, furosemide, mannitol)
- CVVH for anuric renal failure
- Specific treatment for hyperkalemia (see Critical Event chapter "Hyperkalemia")
- Vasopressors for hypotension (epinephrine, phenylephrine, norepinephrine)

POSTOP

Pain
- Mild to moderate
- Relatively low postop pain levels despite large upper abdominal incision
- Pts usually do not require PCA
- Epidural catheter not usually placed

Complications
- Bleeding
  - May cause hemodynamic instability
  - May require re-exploration
- Respiratory failure
  - Can occur from a variety of causes, including pulmonary edema from fluid overload, transfusion-related acute lung injury or ARDS
- Biliary leakage
  - May lead to sepsis
  - May require revision of biliary anastomosis
- Delayed liver graft function
  - Primary nonfunction requires immediate relisting for transplantation

SURGICAL PROCEDURE

Indications
- End-stage liver disease.

- Acute liver failure.
- Hepatocellular carcinoma.

Procedure
- Types of donor livers include
  - ➤ Full-size cadaver liver to adult or child.
  - ➤ "Split" adult cadaver liver to two adults.
  - ➤ Pared-down segments from cadaver donor to adult or child.
  - ➤ Living donor.
    - Left lateral segment to child.
    - Right or left lobe to adult.
- Operation proceeds in three phases
  - ➤ Dissection phase.
    - Chevron incision typically used.
    - Free adhesions.
    - Mobilize vascular structures around liver (portal vein, hepatic artery, infrahepatic vena cava, suprahepatic vena cava).
    - Isolate common bile duct.
    - Ligate hepatic artery.
    - Dissection phase ends w/ placement of cross-clamps on portal vein, suprahepatic & infrahepatic vena cava.
    - "Piggyback" technique refers to partial occlusion of the IVC, w/ an end-to-side anastomosis, instead of insertion of donor IVC.
  - ➤ Anhepatic phase
    - Period of time when liver is not in the circulation.
    - Three anastomoses are completed: suprahepatic vena cava, infrahepatic vena cava, portal vein.
    - After completion of anastomoses, cross-clamps are released.
    - Anhepatic phase ends w/ unclamping of the portal vein.
  - ➤ Reperfusion phase
    - Begins w/ vascular reperfusion of the liver graft & continues until procedure ends.
    - After unclamping, assess integrity of anastomoses & correct if necessary.
    - Complete hepatic artery anastomosis.
    - Perform cholecystectomy on liver graft.
    - Perform biliary drainage procedure, either choledochocholedochostomy or choledochojejunostomy w/ Roux-en-Y loop.
    - Ensure hemostasis.
    - Close.

Surgical Concerns
- Hemorrhage.
- Coagulopathy.
- Quality & integrity of anastomoses.
- Size of donor organ vs pt size.
- Graft function.
- Postop thrombosis of hepatic artery & portal vein.
  - ➤ Thrombosis of the hepatic artery requires relisting for transplantation.

Typical EBL
- Highly variable, from <1,000 mL to multiple (>10) blood volumes.

OVUM RETRIEVAL

RENÉE J. ROBERTS, MD

PREOP

Preop Considerations
- Performed for in vitro fertilization (IVF) & other forms of assisted reproductive technology
- Must be performed within a narrow time window, established by the timing of hormonal stimulation protocol

Physical Findings
- Procedure is performed in women of child-bearing age, usually healthy

Workup
- No special considerations

Choice of Anesthesia
- Conscious sedation or MAC, GA, or spinal anesthesia
- GA
  - ➤ There is concern that anesthesia meds administered during ovum retrieval may influence success rates w/ IVF
  - ➤ Anesthetic drugs can be detected in follicular fluid
  - ➤ Nitrous oxide has been implicated as a factor contributing to decreased IVF success rate, but this is controversial
- Spinal anesthesia

➤ Can be performed w/ low-dose bupivacaine (eg, 4 mg) & fentanyl 25 mcg
➤ Risk of postdural puncture headache is highest in this age group
■ MAC
➤ Increasingly used to minimize exposure to general anesthetics
➤ One suggested regimen
  • Fentanyl 100 mcg & midazolam 2 mg after IV start
  • Position pt, then begin propofol infusion at 30–100 mcg/kg/min
  • Propofol 50–100 mg IV bolus as needed for additional sedation
  • If still painful, ketamine 10 mg IV as needed
➤ Other techniques acceptable, including use of short-acting opioids remifentanil or alfentanil

INTRAOP

Monitors/Line Placement
■ Standard monitors.
■ One peripheral IV.

Intraop Concerns
■ Most painful part of procedure is puncture of vaginal wall & ovaries.
■ For procedure under MAC, watch for airway obstruction or respiratory depression.
■ Avoid antihistamines, as they may reduce implantation rate of IVF.

POSTOP

Pain
■ Minimal; cramping may be treated w/ oral narcotics or non-narcotic meds.

Complications
■ Vaginal bleeding, usually minimal.
■ Multiple transvaginal needle punctures can cause unrecognized intra-abdominal or retroperitoneal hemorrhage.
➤ Consider hemorrhage for pt w/ unexplained drop in Hct, hypotension, tachycardia, or signs of peritoneal irritation.

SURGICAL PROCEDURE

Indications
■ Infertility
■ Volunteer ovum donor

Procedure
- Ovarian hyperstimulation induced by hormonal therapy
- Procedure performed in lithotomy position
- Transvaginal puncture of ova guided by vaginal ultrasound probe
- Usually performed on bilateral ova
- Procedure occasionally done via abdominal approach w/ abdominal ultrasound, depending on position of uterus

Surgical Concerns
- Quantity of oocytes retrieved
- Factors that may affect fertilization rate
  - Pt age
  - Assisted reproduction indication
  - Needle gauge & suction pressure used for aspiration
  - Oocyte culture medium
- Inadvertent injury to bowel or other structures, leading to hemorrhage

Typical EBL
- Minimal

PACEMAKER PROCEDURES

ART WALLACE, PHD, MD

PREOP

Preop Considerations
- Preop rhythm: Is the pt pacemaker-dependent at present?
- If in third-degree block.
  - Pt must be monitored 100% of the time.
  - Place an arterial line to ensure adequate perfusion during case.
  - If pt is having pacemaker replacement, a temporary pacing wire may need to be placed to maintain rhythm while pacemaker is disconnected.
  - Treat pts w/ third-degree block as if their life depends on the device: IT DOES.

Pacemaker codes (North American Society for Pacing & Electrophysiology [NASPE] / British Pacing & Electrophysiology Group)
- First letter denotes chamber paced:
  - O: None
  - A: Atrium

- ➤ V: Ventricle
- ➤ D: Dual (A+V)
- ➤ S: Single
- ■ Second letter denotes chamber sensed:
  - ➤ O: None
  - ➤ A: Atrium
  - ➤ V: Ventricle
  - ➤ D: Dual (A+V)
  - ➤ S: Single
- ■ Third letter denotes response to sensed event:
  - ➤ O: None
  - ➤ I: Inhibited
  - ➤ T: Triggered
  - ➤ D: (I+T)
- ■ Fourth letter denotes programmability/rate response:
  - ➤ O: None
  - ➤ R: Adaptive rate
  - ➤ P: Simple programmable
  - ➤ M: Multiprogrammable
  - ➤ C: Communicating
- ■ Fifth letter denotes antitachycardia functions:
  - ➤ O: None
  - ➤ P: Antitachycardia pacing
  - ➤ S: Shock
  - ➤ D: Dual (P+S)

  Modes, actions, typical indications
- ■ Mode AOO
  - ➤ Atrium: paced but not sensed
  - ➤ Ventricle: ignored
  - ➤ Inhibited: asynchronous
  - ➤ Indication: intact conduction system w/ bradycardia, high electrical noise (OR use only)
- ■ Mode AAI
  - ➤ Atrium: paced & sensed
  - ➤ Ventricle: ignored
  - ➤ Inhibited: synchronous
  - ➤ Indication: intact conduction system w/ bradycardia: sick sinus syndrome
- ■ Mode VOO
  - ➤ Atrium: ignored
  - ➤ Ventricle: paced but not sensed

➤ Inhibited: asynchronous
➤ Indication: afib w/ high-grade block (II or III), high electrical noise (OR use only)

■ Mode VVI
➤ Atrium: ignored
➤ Ventricle: paced & sensed
➤ Inhibited: synchronous
➤ Indication: afib w/ high-grade block (II or III)

■ Mode DOO
➤ Atrium: paced but not sensed
➤ Ventricle: paced but not sensed
➤ Inhibited: asynchronous
➤ Indication: third-degree block in high electrical noise (OR use only)

■ Mode DVI
➤ Atrium: paced but not sensed
➤ Ventricle: paced & sensed
➤ Inhibited: synchronous
➤ Indication: third-degree block

■ Mode DDD
➤ Atrium: paced & sensed
➤ Ventricle: paced & sensed
➤ Inhibited: synchronous
➤ Indication: third-degree block

Physical Findings
■ Usually nothing until ECG is examined

Workup
■ What is the rhythm disturbance?
➤ First-degree AVB, second-degree AVB, third-degree AVB, other?
■ What is the planned operation?
➤ Pacemaker (one, two, or three leads?)
➤ Implantable cardioverter-defibrillator (ICD): see Procedure chapter "ICD Placement"
➤ ICD + pacemaker
■ Is this pacemaker a three-lead device being placed for CHF mgt?
➤ Placement of these devices requires a coronary sinus lead, which may take multiple hours to place
➤ These pts are in heart failure & may not tolerate extensive time on the catheterization table w/o intubation

Choice of Anesthesia
- MAC if possible
- For three-lead pacemakers for CHF, pt symptoms (orthopnea) & duration of case are critical to decision

INTRAOP

Monitors/Line Placement
- Standard monitors
- Arterial line if pt has third-degree block
- Arterial line if ICD device is being placed
- Arterial line if pt has CHF

Intraop Concerns
- For pt dependent on pacemaker (eg, third-degree block), loss of pacemaker capture can lead to severe bradycardia or asystole.
  - Prepare transcutaneous pacemaker.
  - Consider medical therapy for bradycardia.
    - Atropine.
    - Dopamine.
    - Epinephrine.
    - Isoproterenol.
  - DO NOT administer lidocaine for ventricular escape rhythm, as this can be lethal.

POSTOP

Pain
- Small incision assoc w/ minimal pain.
- Local infiltration w/ bupivacaine after pacemaker placement is excellent.

Complications/Concerns
- Do not pace in VOO or DOO mode unless you are constantly monitoring pt as ventricular tachycardia or fibrillation will result from R-on-T phenomenon.
- Monitoring is essential for a period of time.
- CXR for lead placement & to rule out pneumothorax
- Cardiac injury from lead placement: tamponade, etc.
- Infection.

SURGICAL PROCEDURE

Indications
- Second- or third-degree AVB block w/ symptoms
- Asymptomatic third-degree AVB

- Asymptomatic Mobitz II second-degree AVB
- Asymptomatic Mobitz II second-degree AVB at or below His bundle
- First-degree AVB w/ symptoms of low cardiac output relieved by pacing
- First-degree AVB in pt w/ CHF
- Three-lead pacemaker: severe CHF
- ICD: ventricular fibrillation or tachycardia

Procedure
- Small incision under clavicle
- Subclavian cannulation
- Fluoroscopic guidance of lead placement
- Pocket development for device
- Testing of device function
- Closure

Surgical Concerns
- Bleeding, infection, proper lead placement

Typical EBL
- Minimal

PANCREAS TRANSPLANT

BETTY LEE-HOANG, MD
MANUEL PARDO, JR., MD

PREOP

Preop Considerations
- Pt is typically an insulin-dependent diabetic w/ diabetic nephropathy & renal insufficiency.
- Procedure is usually performed as a simultaneous kidney & pancreas transplant, although it may be performed as a solitary procedure.
- Complications of diabetes include ketoacidosis, neuropathy, gastroparesis, autonomic dysfunction, atherosclerosis, coronary artery disease, microangiopathies, increased risk of infection, delayed wound healing & renal disease. See also Coexisting Disease chapter "Diabetes Mellitus."
- Drug therapy issues
  - ➣ Determine insulin & oral hypoglycemic agent dosing.
  - ➣ Pts should continue all their cardiovascular meds preop.

Physical Findings
- Pt may have manifestations of advanced diabetes (see above).

Workup
- Most of pt workup is completed prior to listing for transplant. This may include
  - CBC.
  - CXR.
  - Electrolytes, BUN, creatinine.
  - Immunologic evaluation.
  - Blood & HLA typing.
  - HIV, HTLV, CMV testing.
  - Cardiac evaluation.
    - ECG.
    - Echocardiogram.
    - May include noninvasive eval or cardiac cath.
  - Other components of workup may include GI, peripheral vascular disease, cerebrovascular disease, urologic eval.
- Because of long waiting times on transplant list, pts are periodically re-evaluated.
- Once scheduled for the procedure, pt is admitted to the hospital & the following eval occurs:
  - Repeat history & physical.
  - Repeat key lab studies.
  - CXR.
  - ECG.
  - Because of the urgent nature of transplant surgery, there is little time to pursue extensive further workup. If pt's medical conditions have worsened, pt may be bypassed as a transplant candidate & another pt scheduled instead.
- For the anesthesia provider, it is most important to focus on the cardiac workup, since pts are at increased risk of significant CAD.
- Most pts having pancreas transplant also undergo simultaneous kidney transplant; therefore, need to evaluate the pt's history of chronic renal failure, including frequency & method of dialysis. See also Coexisting Disease chapter "Chronic Renal Failure" & Procedures chapter "Renal Transplant."

Choice of Anesthesia
- GA w/ endotracheal intubation

➤ Because of the risk of aspiration from gastroparesis, pts should receive Bicitra & possibly metoclopramide before induction.

➤ Rapid sequence induction of GA is appropriate.

➤ Consider avoiding sevoflurane because of renal toxicity of metabolites.

➤ Maintain muscle relaxation.

INTRAOP

Monitors/Line Placement

■ Standard ASA monitors.

■ Arterial line recommended for BP control & for frequent blood sampling to check glucose, electrolytes, ABGs.

■ Central venous line useful for CVP monitoring & for continuous drips such as insulin or dopamine.

■ Peripheral IV access adequate for possible blood transfusion & rapid fluid delivery.

■ A glucometer should be available to monitor serum glucose.

■ Foley catheter.

Intraop Concerns

■ Discuss antibiotic & immunosuppressive meds w/ the transplant surgeon.

➤ Antibiotics typically ceftriaxone & fluconazole.

➤ Immunosuppression may include methylprednisolone & thymoglobulin.

■ Serum potassium levels may increase during the operation & may require treatment.

■ Surgeon may prefer colloid (eg, albumin) for fluid therapy because swelling & edema of graft may be less than w/ crystalloid fluid only.

■ Pt is usually extubated at end of surgery & taken to the ICU because of the complexity of postop nursing care.

Intraop Therapies

■ Insulin, glucose mgt

➤ Monitor serum glucose closely during the operation.

• Prior to unclamp of pancreas, hourly glucose check is adequate.

• After unclamping, monitor glucose q30min. Typical decrease in glucose is 50 mg/dL/h.

➤ If initial serum glucose is >200 mg/dL, consider regular insulin infusion.

➤ Stop insulin drip (if used) prior to pancreas reperfusion, as drop in glucose is used as a sign of graft endocrine function.

➤ If serum glucose is <100 mg/dL, start a 5% dextrose infusion.

■ Surgeon may request heparin bolus & infusion during anastomosis to reduce risk of thrombosis.

POSTOP

Pain

■ Moderate

■ IV narcotics including fentanyl and/or morphine, commonly administered via PCA

Complications

■ Bleeding requiring re-exploration

■ Graft loss from thrombosis

■ Intra-abdominal infection, abscess

■ Leak or problem w/ exocrine drainage

■ Graft rejection

■ Long-term complications of immunosuppression, including infection & malignancy

SURGICAL PROCEDURE

Indications

■ Insulin-dependent diabetes.

■ Typically, pt is expected to develop diabetic complications that exceed the risks of the transplant surgery & long-term immunosuppression.

Procedure

■ Prior to implantation, graft is prepared by transplant team.

■ Pancreatic graft usually placed in right iliac fossa.

■ Exploration & mobilization of iliac vessels.

■ Anastomosis of donor portal vein to recipient external iliac vein.

■ Anastomosis of donor superior mesenteric artery & splenic artery to recipient external iliac artery.

■ Exocrine drainage of pancreas. Two options:

➤ Enteric drainage: anastomose donor duodenum to recipient small bowel loop.

➤ Bladder drainage: anastomose donor duodenum to recipient bladder.

■ The recipient's native pancreas is left in place.

■ Kidney transplant (if performed simultaneously) is done after implantation of pancreas.

Surgical Concerns
■ Thrombosis of arterial supply or venous drainage.
■ Complications of exocrine drainage.
  ➤ Enteric drainage: anastomotic breakdown, abscess formation, graft loss.
  ➤ Bladder drainage: fluid, electrolyte (esp bicarbonate) loss, leak, urinary tract problems.

Typical EBL
■ 200–400 cc.

PANCREATICODUODENECTOMY (WHIPPLE PROCEDURE)

JAMES BRANDES, MD

PREOP

Preop Considerations
■ Whipple procedure involves resection of the head of the pancreas & surrounding structures for cancer.
■ Gastric outlet obstruction is common, increasing aspiration risk.
■ If pancreatic mass is an endocrine tumor, there is the possibility of MEN syndrome.
  ➤ Insulinoma is the most common pancreatic endocrine tumor.
■ Pt may be dehydrated secondary to bowel prep.

Physical Findings
■ May have jaundice & nontender palpable gallbladder (Courvoisier's sign).
■ May have DVT or migratory thrombophlebitis (Trousseau's syndrome) due to cancer-related hypercoagulable state.

Workup
■ CBC, electrolytes, BUN, creatinine, glucose, PT, PTT, LFTs.
■ ECG.
■ Surgeon typically orders abdominal CT scan.
  ➤ Determine proximity of tumor to the portal vein, as this may indicate an increased chance of hemorrhage.

- If tumor is insulinoma or other endocrine tumor, consider the possibility of concurrent pheochromocytoma & pursue appropriate workup.
- Type & cross 4 units PRBCs.

Choice of Anesthesia
- GA required.
- Thoracic epidural useful as GA adjunct & for postop analgesia.
- Rapid sequence induction.
- Avoid nitrous oxide to limit bowel distention, as surgery may be lengthy.
- Premed to reduce aspiration risk (eg, Bicitra, H2 blocker).

INTRAOP

Monitors/Line Placement
- Standard monitors
- Arterial line
- Central line may be helpful to monitor fluid status, as third-space losses can be extensive & surgery may be lengthy
- Two large-bore peripheral IVs
- Foley catheter

Intraop Concerns
- Hemorrhage
  - ➤ May be sudden & extensive during dissection near portal vein, mesenteric blood vessels, vena cava
- Hypothermia due to lengthy surgery w/ large exposure of the viscera
- Fluid shifts
  - ➤ Large third-space losses, typically 10–20 mL/kg/h
- Procedure may be shorter than expected if surgeon does not perform Whipple (eg, if tumor is deemed unresectable)

Intraop Therapies
- Blood transfusion as necessary
- Forced air warmer, fluid warmers

POSTOP

Pain
- Moderate to severe
  - ➤ Thoracic epidural
  - ➤ PCA if no epidural

Complications
- Hypothermia
- Anemia
- Hypovolemia
- Hyperglycemia

SURGICAL PROCEDURE

Indications
- Cancer of the head of the pancreas, common bile duct, ampulla of Vater or duodenum

Procedure
- Resection of the head of the pancreas, duodenum & common bile duct
- Often the pylorus is spared
- A Roux-en-Y loop of jejunum is mobilized & anastomosed to the stomach, common bile duct & pancreas

Surgical Concerns
- Resectability of tumor
  - As many as 80% of pts who undergo a laparotomy for a Whipple will have unresectable disease
  - However, many of these pts will have a gastrojejunostomy and/or choledochojejunostomy as palliative procedures
- Bleeding from the portal vein or IVC is a major concern, as the portal vein travels directly behind the head of the pancreas

Typical EBL
- 500–800 mL typical, but the potential exists for rapid massive hemorrhage

---

PARATHYROIDECTOMY

ANNEMARIE THOMPSON, MD

PREOP

Preop Considerations
- Parathyroidectomy indicated for
  - Primary hyperparathyroidism

- Some pts w/ asymptomatic mild hypercalcemia are followed w/ medical therapy.
  ➢ Parathyroid carcinoma is a very rare indication for surgery.
- Awareness of symptoms of hypercalcemia & preop treatment important.
- Primary hyperparathyroidism most commonly caused by parathyroid adenoma (75–85%) or parathyroid hyperplasia.
- Secondary hyperparathyroidism is related to hypocalcemia & occurs most commonly w/ chronic renal failure, intestinal malabsorption.
- Tertiary hyperparathyroidism refers to pt w/ secondary hyperparathyroidism who subsequently develops "autonomous" function of hyperplastic parathyroid glands.
- Potential coexisting diseases: Renal failure, multiple endocrine neoplasia (types 1, 2a, 2b).
- Symptoms & signs
  ➢ Hypercalcemia usually asymptomatic, detected by routine screening.
  ➢ Symptoms of hypercalcemia can include
    - "Bones": Demineralization, arthralgias, bone pain.
    - "Stones": Kidney stones w/ renal colic. Other renal findings can include polyuria, dehydration, renal insufficiency.
    - "Abdominal moans": Constipation/nausea.
    - "Psychic groans": Mild depression.
    - "Fatigue overtones": Weakness, fatigue.
- Pt may require treatment of hypercalcemia prior to surgery.
  ➢ Consider hydration prior to induction of anesthesia.
  ➢ Hydration w/ NS & diuresis w/ furosemide will decrease calcium levels by 1.6–2.4 mg/dL.
  ➢ Do not use calcium-containing IV fluids.
  ➢ Other pharmacologic therapies include. bisphosphonates, glucocorticoids, plicamycin, calcitonin.

Workup
- Serum calcium level >10.5 mg/dL
  ➢ May need to correct for albumin level.
  ➢ Can also obtain ionized calcium.
- Other electrolytes
  ➢ Phosphate decreased in primary hyperparathyroidism, increased in secondary/tertiary hyperparathyroidism.
  ➢ Chloride elevated.

- Immunoassay to detect elevated parathyroid hormone levels.
- Pt may have a preop MIBI scan to detect parathyroid function.
- ECG.
  - ➤ Findings include shortened QT interval from hypercalcemia.

Choice of Anesthesia
- GA most commonly used.
- Superficial cervical plexus block can supplement GA.

INTRAOP
Monitors/Line Placement
- Standard monitors.
- One peripheral IV adequate.

Intraop Concerns
- Watch for hypertension or cardiac arrhythmias due to hypercalcemia (esp ventricular dysrhythmias).
- Maintain adequate minute ventilation, as hypercarbia may lead to acidosis & increased ionized calcium.
- Closely monitor neuromuscular function: Pts w/ hyperparathyroidism may have unpredictable response to nondepolarizing muscle relaxants.
- Pts w/ hypercalcemia complicated by osteoporosis may be more susceptible to fractures/compression fractures during transfer & laryngoscopy.
- With emergence, take steps to minimize coughing to reduce venous bleeding at operative site.
- Surgeon will likely request blood draw for parathyroid hormone level after clipping of veins draining parathyroid gland.
  - ➤ Parathyroid hormone has a half-life of minutes & may show a reduction intraop.

POSTOP
Pain
- Typically minimal

Complications
- Airway, respiratory complications
  - ➤ Bleeding, neck hematoma can cause life-threatening airway compromise.
  - ➤ Mgt of airway compromise from neck hematoma

- Notify surgeon & OR immediately.
- Consider immediate removal of neck sutures at the bedside to decompress airway.
- Anticipate difficulty w/ intubation from airway edema, neck swelling, tracheal deviation.
- Prepare difficult airway equipment; consider obtaining extra help w/ airway mgt.
- Prepare equipment & personnel for surgical airway: tracheostomy, cricothyrotomy
  - ➤ Other causes of respiratory distress
    - Recurrent laryngeal nerve injury (either unilateral, resulting in hoarseness, or bilateral, which can result in aphonia & stridor).
    - Pneumothorax.
- ■ Hypocalcemia
  - ➤ Serum calcium will decrease within 24 h after parathyroidectomy, nadir within 3–7 days.
  - ➤ If pt has significant preop bone demineralization, "hungry bone syndrome" may occur & calcium level may drop precipitously.

SURGICAL PROCEDURE

Indications
- ■ Primary hyperparathyroidism, including some asymptomatic pts

Procedure
- ■ Neck exploration to identify all four parathyroid glands
- ■ For reoperation, median sternotomy may be required to identify parathyroid
- ■ Removal of 3 to 3.5 glands for parathyroid hyperplasia
- ■ Removal of affected gland for parathyroid adenoma
- ■ Surgeon may send intraop frozen section to identify parathyroid tissue

Surgical Concerns
- ■ Periop dehydration due to hypercalcemia
- ■ Postop hypocalcemia
- ■ Recurrent laryngeal nerve injury
- ■ Postop bleeding

Typical EBL
- ■ <50 mL

PATENT DUCTUS ARTERIOSUS (PDA) LIGATION

LYDIA CASSORLA, MD

PREOP

Preop Considerations
- Prematurity often present
- Pts may be extremely small (<500 g).
- CHF due to excessive pulmonary blood flow usually present.
- Inadequate systemic blood flow & failure to thrive often present.
- Moving premature infants has considerable risk; surgery is often performed in the nursery.
- Systemic air embolus is a risk if air enters venous circulation; meticulous air bubble prevention is indicated.
- Pulmonary vascular changes & high pulmonary vascular resistance may develop if PDA untreated.

Physical Findings
- Bounding pulses w/ a pulse pressure >30 mmHg suggests a hemodynamically significant ductus.
- CHF is usually present in surgical pts, with a gallop rhythm common. Murmur may be systolic, continuous, diastolic, or minimal depending on size of ductus & relative resistances in the aorta & pulmonary artery.
- Pulmonary: tachypnea, decreased PaO_2, increased $PaCO_2$.
- Failure to thrive may be present if systemic cardiac output or feeding compromised.
- Differential O_2 saturation in upper vs lower body indicates right-to-left shunting across ductus.

Workup
- Diagnosis by echocardiography in nearly all cases.
- Assess pulmonary function.
- CXR: findings of respiratory distress syndrome may mimic or mask those of PDA
- Measure O_2 saturation above & below ductus.
- Review blood gas, hemoglobin, coagulation, electrolyte studies.
- Many nursery pts are already intubated. If so, assess tube for air leak to ensure ability to ventilate w/ open chest.
- Have blood immediately available for transfusion prior to procedure.

Choice of Anesthesia

- GA required.
- If anesthesia performed in ICU, fentanyl + midazolam + relaxant is typical.
- For older pts who have aorta patched, eliminate N_2O due to risk of expansion of intravascular air.

INTRAOP

Monitors/Line Placement

- Pt nearly always in RLD position as ductus nearly always on L regardless of L or R aortic arch.
- Monitor BP & SpO_2 in right upper quadrant, as surgeon may occlude the descending aorta & left subclavian if difficulties occur.
- Second monitor of SpO_2 & BP in lower extremity for early detection of inadvertent occlusion of descending aorta.
- Assess need for arterial line individually. If placed for procedure, R arm is preferred location (see above).
- Adequate IV access for blood transfusion required.
- Maintain access to ETT at all times.
- Have hand ventilation setup ready w/ air/O_2 blender if surgery performed outside OR.
- Have appropriately sized suction catheters, laryngoscope & mask available at all times.
- Continuous temp monitoring is indicated.
- Use CO_2 monitoring if available for surgeries outside OR.
- Extubation at end of procedure desired for pts not intubated preop.

Intraop Concerns

Infants

- Be extremely careful about volume administration in tiny pts. Blood volume no more than 10% of weight in premature infants; often <100 cc! Minimize IV dead space & administer drugs as close to pt as possible.
- Dilute all meds appropriately for small pts prior to onset of procedure (it is very brief).
- Temp control is a major challenge for premature infants. Keep them warm.
- Maintain HR as cardiac output is highly dependent upon HR (heart is volume loaded due to L-to-R shunt).
- Fentanyl w/o vagolytic, surgical stimulation, or concurrent inotrope may cause undesirable bradycardia. Pancuronium prior to fentanyl is usually adequate for prevention.

■ Inotropes are commonly administered preop; minimize intraop bradycardia.

■ Administer anesthesia just prior to incision, as pts may not tolerate sedation w/o surgical stimulation.

■ Maintain lowest appropriate FIO_2 for premature infants. Anticipate need to increase FIO_2 during procedure to maintain SpO_2 during lung retraction.

■ Lung compliance decreases during lung retraction; higher airway pressures may be temporarily necessary. Follow CO_2 if available.

■ When ductus is ligated, watch for increase in diastolic BP & immediately assess circulation in lower extremity to rule out inadvertent ligation of descending aorta.

Children

■ Usually stable & tolerate procedure well.

Adults

■ Ductus often calcified, complicating surgery. Aorta usually requires patch & surgery may require aortic cross-clamp during repair.

■ One-lung ventilation appropriate if tolerated.

Intraop Therapies

■ Treat bradycardia aggressively if not immediately resolved by cessation of surgical manipulation.

■ If pharmacologic treatment of hypotension indicated for infants, use agent w/ positive chronotropic effect (eg, epinephrine or ephedrine) rather than phenylephrine.

■ Be prepared to increase ventilatory pressures & FIO_2 as needed during procedure. If using ICU ventilator, know how to operate equipment or have appropriate help present.

■ Hand ventilation often helpful to re-expand lung at end of procedure as chest tube usually not placed.

POSTOP

Pain

■ Intercostal block, caudal & epidural may be considered as indicated by pt age & size

■ Pain minimized if no chest tube or drain

Complications

■ Rupture of ductus

■ Ligation of descending aorta

- Ligation of anomalous great vessel
- Ligation of pulmonary artery
- Ligation of bronchus
- Damage to pulmonary vein or artery
- Damage to recurrent laryngeal nerve
- Pneumothorax
- Hemothorax
- Increased postop ventilatory support requirements

SURGICAL PROCEDURE

Indications
- PDA w/ CHF in infancy
- Persistent PDA in childhood or adulthood
- Decreased O_2 saturation in lower body in older child or adult indicates high pulmonary vascular resistance & significant risk if ductus closed

Procedure
- Device closure in cardiac cath lab
- Thoracoscopic surgery
- Open thoracotomy
- Thoracotomy w/ aortic cross-clamp in selected older pts

Surgical Concerns
- Proximity of recurrent laryngeal nerve
- Fragility of ductus tissue & potential for rupture in infants
- Calcification of ductus in adults
- Proximity of vital structures
- Potential for air embolus if aorta opened

Typical EBL
- Minimal if no complication occurs

PELVIC EXENTERATION

JASON WIDRICH, MD

PREOP

Preop Considerations
- Performed for gynecologic malignancies that have spread locally; surgery involves resection of pelvic tissue.

- Considerations by organ system depend on coexisting diseases & potential toxic side effects of chemotherapy.
- Bowel prep may result in electrolyte or volume status changes.

Physical Findings
- Palpable pelvic mass.
- Uterine, bladder, vaginal or rectal bleeding.

Workup
- CBC, electrolytes, BUN, creatinine, LFTs, glucose, PT, PTT.
- Type & cross-match >2 units PRBCs.
  - ➤ More blood may be needed if pt starts w/ a lower hematocrit or if large blood loss is anticipated (eg, from tumor eroding into pelvis).
- Workup for metastatic disease performed prior to surgery.
- Further workup based on history & physical.

Choice of Anesthesia
- Usually done w/ GA due to extent of resection & length of surgery.
- Epidural anesthesia can be used as adjunct to GA or for postop pain control.

INTRAOP

Monitors/Line Placement
- Standard monitors.
- Two large-bore peripheral IVs.
- Arterial line.
- Foley catheter.
- Other monitors as indicated by coexisting diseases.

Intraop Concerns
- Large blood loss may cause hemodynamic instability.
- Coagulopathy.
- Hypothermia.
- Nerve injury to peroneal nerve from lithotomy position.
- Infection.
- Deep venous thrombosis.

Intraop Therapies
- Third-space fluid requirement 10–15 mL/kg/h.
- Consider upper body forced air warmer, fluid warmers, humidified circuit, intra-abdominal lavage w/ warm saline to keep pt warm.
- Platelets & FFP in addition to packed red cells may be needed.

- Use compression stockings for DVT prophylaxis.
- Antibiotics should cover gram-positive, gram-negative & anaerobic bacteria.
- Surgery can be lengthy; duration depends on processing of pathologic samples & difficulty of reconstruction.

POSTOP

Pain
- Moderate to severe
- IV narcotics or an epidural will be needed to treat pain following this major resection

Complications
- Bleeding
- Hypothermia
- Deep venous thrombosis or pulmonary embolus
- Wound infection
- Pyelonephritis
- Ureteral fistula
- Ileus
- Small bowel obstruction

SURGICAL PROCEDURE

Indications
- Cervical & vaginal carcinoma that is locally invasive.

Procedure
- Pt is placed in either supine or lithotomy position.
- Midline abdominal incision w/ identification of the uterus, vagina, cervix, bladder, rectum.
- Liver, peritoneum, diaphragm are inspected.
- Samples from lymph node dissections are examined by pathology.
- Resection is undertaken only if metastasis has not spread outside the pelvis.
- Sections of the omentum & bowel will be used for reconstruction.
- The descending colon can either be reanastomosed to the distal anus/rectum or turned into an ileostomy.
- Resection may extend into perineum; an ileostomy may be necessary.
- The stented ureters can be reanastomosed to another section of the descending colon that has been fashioned into a neobladder.

- Reconstruction of the vaginal vault is performed w/ omental tissue or myocutaneous muscle flaps.
- The resections may be partial & limited to uterus, bladder & vagina (anterior) or uterus, vagina & rectum (posterior).

Surgical Concerns
- Metastasis: multiple samples are sent to pathology throughout the resection.
- Adequacy of bowel prep.
- Hemorrhage.

Typical EBL
- 1,200–4,000 mL.

PERICARDIAL WINDOW

MICHAEL J. YANAKAKIS, MD

PREOP

Preop Considerations
- Hemodynamic instability in the setting of pericardial effusion
- Physiology assoc w/ cardiac tamponade or constrictive pericarditis
  - ➤ Impaired diastolic filling of heart
  - ➤ Decreased cardiac output from reduced stroke volume w/ an increased CVP
  - ➤ Equalization of diastolic pressures in the absence of severe LV dysfunction (RAP = RVEDP = LAP = LVEDP)
  - ➤ Stroke volume is relatively fixed — cardiac output dependent on heart rate

Physical Findings
- Jugular venous distention
- Hypotension
- Tachycardia
- Narrowed arterial pulse pressure
- Pulsus paradoxus (tamponade)
- Kussmaul's sign (constrictive pericarditis)
- Muffled heart sounds
- Normal or enlarged cardiac silhouette in tamponade & pericardial calcifications w/ pericarditis

- Nonspecific decreased voltage on ECG w/ generalized ST-segment elevation in pts w/ a component of pericarditis
  - Abolished y-descent as a result of impaired diastolic filling in tamponade & a possibly accentuated y-descent as a result of early diastolic filling in constrictive pericarditis
  - Normal or accentuated x-descent in tamponade

Workup
- Echocardiography is crucial in the diagnosis of pericardial effusion as well as estimating the volume of the effusion
- Surgical treatment is often appropriate for traumatic, postop, & recurrent effusions. Etiology of recurrent effusions is most commonly:
  - Malignant
  - Uremic
  - Autoimmune
  - Infectious/tubercular
  - Radiation-induced

Choice of Anesthesia
- GA (local anesthesia can be used for pts for simple drainage via a subxiphoid approach)
  - Do not induce until pt is prepped & surgeon is ready to start
- Induction w/ ketamine or etomidate
- Avoid cardiac depression, bradycardia, vasodilation
- Consider pretreatment w/ atropine
- Consider pancuronium (vagolytic) if nondepolarizing agent used

INTRAOP
Monitors/Line Placement
- Large-bore IV access essential.
- Arterial line & CVP monitoring, but the placement of these monitors should not delay urgent drainage in the unstable pt.

Intraop Concerns
- Avoid cardiac depression, bradycardia, vasodilation.
- Pts may continue to be hypotensive even after effective evacuation of the effusion; this may be related to underlying coronary artery disease.
- Avoid high mean airway pressures that can compromise venous return.
- Atrial arrhythmias (potential role for prophylactic digoxin)

- Pulmonary edema post-drainage as a result of increased right ventricular output.

Intraop Therapies
- No evidence that use of inotropic agents alters the hemodynamics of tamponade physiology prior to drainage.

POSTOP

Pain
- Depends on whether sternotomy, thoracotomy, or subxiphoid incision employed
- Consider intrathecal narcotic or postop use of thoracic epidural if incision is more extensive

Complications
- More likely in catheter drainage than w/ subxiphoid incision
- Coronary artery laceration
- Myocardial perforation
- Pneumothorax

SURGICAL PROCEDURE

Indications
- Cardiac tamponade or constrictive pericarditis w/ hemodynamic instability
- Recurrent pericardial effusions
- Traumatic postop cardiac tamponade
- Technical difficulty or complication w/ simple drainage technique

Procedure
- Subxiphoid pericardial window: Entire chest is prepped for potential sternotomy, & a midline incision is made over the xiphoid process & epigastrium. The xiphoid is elevated or excised. The pericardium is opened between two stay sutures & examined for the presence of blood. If blood is found, definitive repair should ensue without delay

Surgical Concerns
- Extensive manipulation of the heart that impairs cardiac filling
- Frequent arrhythmias
- Potential cardiac perforation

Typical EBL
- Significant in the event of cardiac perforation
- Greater if CPB used

PHEOCHROMOCYTOMA RESECTION

MERLIN LARSON, MD

PREOP

Preop Considerations
- Determine adequacy of sympathetic blockade. Check for:
  - Alpha blockade (BP).
  - Beta blockade (HR).
- Ask pt about symptoms:
  - Palpitations.
  - Tachycardia.
  - Headache.
  - Flushing.
- Check orthostatic signs
  - Blood volume may be deficient.

Physical Findings
- Flushing, tachycardia

Workup
- Check urinary excretion of catecholamine metabolites.
  - Endocrinologist usually is consulted preop & does this.
- Evaluate myocardial strain & adequacy of sympathetic blockade.
  - Cardiologist may do this in preop consultation.

Choice of Anesthesia
- GA can be used for both laparoscopic & open procedures.
  - 90% oxygen w/ vapor or propofol may improve wound healing & decrease nausea & vomiting.
  - Some surgeons request avoidance of nitrous oxide during laparoscopic procedures.
- For open procedure, may use epidural
  - Epidural should be low thoracic.
  - Epidural does not prevent catecholamine surges during procedure.

INTRAOP

Monitors/Line Placement
- Arterial line is essential.
- CVP useful.
- Pulmonary artery catheter optional if pt has history of ischemic heart disease.

Intraop Concerns
- Catecholamine surges from surgical manipulation can produce dramatic hemodynamic alterations in BP & HR.
- Arrhythmias may occur.
- Vasopressors or fluids may be required to support BP after tumor is removed.
- Relative hypovolemia may be present after tumor is removed.
  - CVP may reveal this.

Intraop Therapies
- Drug infusions should be ready & primed before the case begins; multiple simultaneous infusions may be required:
  - Nitroprusside
  - Phenylephrine
  - Esmolol

POSTOP
Pain
- Laparoscopic procedures require minimal analgesics.
- Epidural is beneficial if the procedure is open.

Complications
- Secondary to epinephrine release during the procedure
  - MI.
  - Stroke.
  - Ventricular tachycardia or fibrillation.

SURGICAL PROCEDURE
Indications
- Catecholamine-producing tumors of adrenal gland or extra-adrenal chromaffin tissue

Procedure
- Position
  - Open midline incision
  - Full lateral position for laparoscopic procedure

Surgical Concerns
- Bleeding from major vessels
- Hemodynamic instability in periop period

Typical EBL
- 500 mL

PYLORIC STENOSIS REPAIR

LEI WANG, MD

PREOP

Preop Considerations
- Pyloric stenosis is caused by thickening of the circular muscle fibers at the lesser curvature of the stomach and pylorus. Etiology is unknown.
- Incidence: 1.5–3/1,000 Caucasian births, lower in African Americans & Asians.
- Predominantly occurs in males (M:F > 4:1).
- Tends to run in family.
- Higher incidence in first-born child.
- Hypovolemia & electrolyte abnormalities should be corrected before surgery.
- NG tube should be inserted to prevent aspiration.
- Pyloric stenosis is a medical emergency but not a surgical emergency.
- Pt usually presents w/ hypokalemic, hypochloremic metabolic alkalosis.

Physical Findings
- Pt presents w/ projectile, bile-free vomiting after every feed at 3–6 wks of age.
- Physical exam reveals an olive-sized, palpable mass at midepigastric area.
- Infant is usually lethargic & dehydrated (poor skin turgor, dry mucous membranes, sunken fontanelles, sunken eyes, decreased BP, increased pulse, decreased urine output, weight loss).

Workup
- Diagnosis confirmed w/ ultrasound & barium swallow.
- CBC.
- Electrolytes.
- BUN, Cr.

Choice of Anesthesia
- GA.

INTRAOP
- Stomach should be emptied w/ large-bore NG tube before induction.
- Standard monitors.

- Rapid sequence IV induction is most commonly used. However, inhalation induction w/ cricoid pressure is also used.
- Anesthetic is maintained w/ volatile agents. Muscle relaxation is not required for the procedure.
- Rectal Tylenol & local anesthetics injected by surgeon are adequate for postop pain control.
- Minimize narcotics because they may prolong awakening.
- Extubate pt awake.

POSTOP

Pain
- Typically minimal

Complications
- Postop respiratory depression & apnea not uncommon secondary to metabolic alkalosis & GA.
- Hypoglycemia may occur 2–3 h after surgery secondary to depletion of liver glycogen store.
- Small feeds can begin 4–6 h postop.

SURGICAL PROCEDURE

Indications
- Pyloric stenosis

Procedure
- Pyloromyotomy is performed through a small right transverse incision or right paramedian incision

Surgical Concerns
- Duodenal perforation

Typical EBL
- Minimal

RADICAL NECK DISSECTION

JASON WIDRICH, MD

PREOP

Preop Considerations
- Radical neck dissection is performed for pts w/ head & neck cancer.
  - ➤ May be part of a more extensive procedure for cancer: eg, panendoscopy (laryngoscopy, esophagoscopy, bronchoscopy),

tumor resection, plastic surgery reconstruction including free flap.
- Many pts have smoking histories & diseases assoc w/ tobacco or alcohol use.
- Airway
  - Tracheal deviation or airway compromise may be present from tumor or edema.
  - Previous radiotherapy may make tissues more friable & prone to bleeding & less compliant ("woody" in texture).
  - Pts may have tracheostomy.
- Respiratory
  - COPD common.
  - Shortness of breath or cough may be present.
- Cardiovascular
  - HTN, CAD common.
  - Consider benefits of periop beta blockade in reducing cardiac morbidity.
- Hematologic
  - Anemia/coagulopathy may be present as a result of neoplastic disease or as a result of myelosuppression from chemotherapy.

Physical Findings
- Airway: check for factors predicting difficult intubation
  - Stridor.
  - Visible tumor on mouth, neck, tongue.
  - Limited range of neck motion.
  - Hoarseness.
- Cardiopulmonary
  - Check for bruits, murmurs.
  - Shortness of breath, decreased breath sounds, wheezes, or crackles suggestive of COPD.
- Hematologic
  - Note bruising, spontaneous bleeding, epistaxis.

Workup
- Check CBC, electrolytes, BUN, creatinine, glucose, PT, PTT.
- Type & screen.
- Airway exam is particularly important. Consider additional tests to supplement clinical exam:
  - X-ray or CT of neck.
  - Indirect or direct laryngoscopy or fiberoptic airway exam.

- Cardiac workup as indicated by history.
- CXR & ABG if severe COPD is suspected.

Choice of Anesthesia

- GA required.
- Airway mgt considerations.
  - Alterations in head and neck anatomy related to cancer & treatment such as radiation therapy may lead to difficulty w/ tracheal intubation.
  - Difficulty w/ airway mgt will depend on the extent to which tumor involves or impinges on the airway.
  - If severe airway obstruction or narrowing is present, consider tracheotomy under local anesthesia prior to induction of GA.
  - Consider awake direct laryngoscopy ("awake look") under topical anesthesia to evaluate airway structures prior to induction.
  - Consider awake fiberoptic intubation for anticipated difficulty (eg, immobile or friable tissues).
  - If a difficult airway is anticipated, the surgeon should be present during induction w/ equipment for emergency surgical airway (eg, tracheotomy or cricothyrotomy).

INTRAOP

Monitors/Line Placement

- Standard monitors.
- Two peripheral IVs usually adequate.
- Foley catheter.
- Arterial line useful to assess hemodynamics.
  - Dissection near carotid can produce baroreflex-mediated hypotension, hypertension, arrhythmias.
  - Pts commonly have CAD & may benefit from close BP monitoring.
  - Extensive or lengthy surgery may be assoc w/ increased potential for blood loss.
  - Anticipated free flap for reconstruction may require close attention to BP to maintain perfusion of flap.
- Central access is not usually necessary & may interfere w/ the surgical field.
  - If central access is required, the line may be placed on the non-operative side of the neck (IJ or subclavian) or via a femoral approach.

Intraop Concerns

■ Many of these pts have significant cardiac disease. Maintain hemo-dynamics closely, especially during induction.

■ Airway mgt may change during the case.
  ➤ If the resection will involve the tongue, larynx, mandible, or both sides of the neck, a tracheotomy or tracheostomy may be placed intraop.
  ➤ A sterile tracheotomy tube, ETT & breathing circuit extension may be required to connect to the breathing circuit.

■ Stimulation of the carotid body can cause various arrhythmias, most often bradycardia.

■ Avoid muscle relaxation if surgeons are monitoring & preserving motor nerves (eg, facial nerve).

■ Potential for blood loss.
  ➤ Particularly during dissection around the internal jugular vein & carotid artery

■ Venous air embolism is a risk, given location of surgical field above level of heart.
  ➤ See also Critical Event chapter "Venous Air Embolism."

■ If free flap is required as part of plastic surgery reconstruction, need to maintain perfusion of free flap.
  ➤ See also Procedures chapter "Free Flap."

Intraop Therapies

■ Consider reducing blood loss by
  ➤ Elevating head of bed.
  ➤ Achieving mild controlled hypotension (unless contraindicated by significant end-organ disease).

■ Maintain normothermia, particularly if free flaps are used for recon-struction.

■ If carotid manipulation results in bradycardia or arrhythmias.
  ➤ Ask surgeon to stop stimulation.
  ➤ Administer 1–7 mcg/kg atropine IV if bradycardia persists.
  ➤ Consider increase in depth of anesthesia.
  ➤ Ask surgeon to infiltrate local anesthesia to decrease vagal response to stimulation.

■ Consider potential benefits of postop ICU care:
  ➤ If pt will remain intubated (eg, secondary to airway edema & potential for airway obstruction).
  ➤ If pt had free flap as part of reconstruction.

➤ If intraop course was marked by significant hemodynamic instability, esp in pt w/ significant cardiovascular disease.

POSTOP

Pain
- Mild to moderate, depending on extent of resection
- IV narcotics or PCA usually adequate

Complications
- Nausea/vomiting
- Anemia
- Hemorrhage
- Pneumothorax
- Airway edema, airway obstruction after extubation
  - ➤ See also Critical Event chapter "Airway Obstruction."
- Air embolism
- Nerve injury
  - ➤ Facial nerve
  - ➤ Phrenic nerve (diaphragmatic paralysis)
  - ➤ Recurrent laryngeal nerve (vocal cord paralysis if unilateral, stridor if bilateral)
- Alcohol withdrawal in pts w/ alcohol abuse
- Compromise of tissue grafts (due to hypertension, hypotension or thrombosis)

SURGICAL PROCEDURE

indications
- Certain head & neck cancers.

Procedure
- Functional neck dissection is limited to cervical lymph nodes.
- Modified neck dissection is a functional dissection + dissection of anterior & posterior neck & omohyoid muscles.
- Radical neck dissection is a modified dissection that involves the sternocleidomastoid (SCM), internal jugular vein & cranial nerve XI.
  - ➤ Incision is made from mandible to clavicle.
  - ➤ Transection of SCM.
  - ➤ Ligation of IJ.
  - ➤ Inferiorly, identification & preservation of brachial plexus, phrenic, vagus, carotid.
  - ➤ Superiorly, identification of hypoglossal, lingual, facial nerves, w/ preservation if possible.

> Tumor, lymph tissue or any involved structures are dissected & removed (eg, submental tissues, tongue, mandible, larynx, pharyngeal tissues).

> Large resections that do not allow for wound closure may require reconstruction w/ a rotational pectoral flap or a free flap.

Surgical Concerns

- Bleeding
  > Erosion of tumor into carotid artery.
- Hematoma requiring evacuation.
- Compromise of tissue flap.
- Nerve injury.
- Wound infection.
- Airway obstruction.

Typical EBL

- 150 mL for functional dissection to >1,500 mL for radical dissection w/ plastic surgery reconstruction.

RADICAL RETROPUBIC PROSTATECTOMY

JASON WIDRICH, MD

PREOP

Preop Considerations

- Prostate cancer occurs most commonly in elderly population
  > Rise in incidence of prostate cancer may be related to increased use of prostate-specific antigen (PSA) & earlier diagnosis at an asymptomatic stage
- See also Coexisting Disease chapter "The Elderly Patient."

Physical Findings

- None typical, except on prostate exam

Workup

- CBC
- PT/PTT
- Electrolytes, BUN, creatinine
- ECG
- Type & cross-match

Choice of Anesthesia
- GA most common, although can use spinal or epidural anesthesia

INTRAOP

Monitors/Line Placement
- Standard monitors
- At least one large-bore peripheral IV
- Foley catheter (also used by urologist in the surgical anastomosis)
- Arterial line or central line may be useful in pts w/ significant cardiac disease

Intraop Concerns
- Positioning: lithotomy position
- Bleeding may occur during dissection of prostate

Intraop Therapies
- Vagal stimulation from bladder manipulation can cause bradycardia
  - ➤ Treat by halting the stimulus, increasing depth of anesthesia
  - ➤ IV glycopyrrolate or atropine if bradycardia persists
- Surgeon may request IV indigo carmine or methylene blue to help identify urine leak or ureteral openings in bladder
  - ➤ SpO_2 will drop temporarily w/ dye administration.

POSTOP

Pain
- Mild to moderate
- IV narcotics or PCA
- Ketorolac IV

Complications
- Anemia or hemorrhage: follow postop Hct
- Bowel injury
- Peroneal nerve injury
- DVT, pulmonary embolism

SURGICAL PROCEDURE

Indications
- Prostate cancer

Procedure
- Midline infraumbilical incision
- Pelvic lymph nodes may be removed for staging
- Prostate gland is dissected

- Blood loss typically occurs from the prostatic dorsal vein complex, which ultimately drains into the internal iliac veins
- Prostate gland removed along w/ seminal vesicles & ampullae of the vas deferens
- Urinary tract continuity re-established by vesicourethral anastomosis, using Foley catheter as a guide
- Most surgeons attempt a "nerve-sparing procedure" to preserve potency by sparing the neurovascular bundle on either side of the prostate

Surgical Concerns
- Margins free of tumor
- Rectal damage
- Urinary incontinence
- Impotence
- Bleeding
- Wound infection

Typical EBL
- 1,500 mL

REDO CABG WITH CARDIOPULMONARY BYPASS (CPB)

ERIC M. BROUCH, MD
MARTIN J. LONDON, MD

PREOP

Preop Considerations
- Premeds
  - ➤ Order all antianginals & antihypertensives to be given prior to surgery.
  - ➤ Provide adequate anxiolysis & analgesia using premeds to minimize ischemia on OR arrival.
    - Outpts: consider oral diazepam 5–10 mg PO w/ IV midazolam (1–2 mg) and/or low-dose fentanyl.
    - Inpts: consider IM morphine 0.1–0.15 mg/kg w/ lorazepam 1–2 mg IM on call to OR.
  - ➤ Order supplemental oxygen w/ premedication. Avoid oversedation in the elderly.
- For unstable angina pt on IV heparin, discuss d/c orders w/ surgeon.

➤ Can usually stop heparin 4 h preop in pts w/o chest pain or left main disease
■ Prophylactic antibiotics: cefazolin 1 g or vancomycin 1 g most common.

Physical Findings

■ Airway exam & ID of difficult airway is crucial to avoid hypoxemia, hypercarbia, catecholamine release, which may cause ischemia.
➤ Consider awake fiberoptic intubation in high-risk pt, using esmolol, remifentanil, or other short-acting agents to control hemodynamics.
■ Evaluate pt's daily range of BP & HR & maintain intraop values w/in 20% to minimize cardiac, cerebral, or renal ischemia.
■ Evaluate for CHF.
■ Evaluate for occlusive carotid disease.

Workup

■ Evaluation includes
➤ Cardiac catheterization
➤ Echocardiogram
➤ CXR
➤ Carotid duplex ultrasound
➤ Pulmonary function tests
■ Need to know from cardiac evaluation
➤ Number of diseased vessels
➤ Presence of significant left main disease
➤ Status of collateral circulation
➤ Ejection fraction
■ Redo CABG requires attention to
➤ Status of previous grafts (usually one or more are occluded, placing the pt at high risk for intraop ischemia).
➤ Surgical plans for new bypass conduits (ie, radial artery may be required).
➤ Also consider anatomic factors that may indicate increased risk of repeat median sternotomy, such as enlarged RV, dilated aortic root, or patent vein graft to right coronary artery.
■ Look for
➤ Concurrent valvular disease, particularly ischemic mitral regurgitation (may require annuloplasty).
➤ Aortic stenosis (propensity for subendocardial ischemia).

➤ Aortic insufficiency (anterograde cardioplegia via the aortic root may distend the ventricle).

Choice of Anesthesia

- General anesthesia w/ controlled ventilation is required.
- Most centers practice "fast tracking": pt is extubated as soon after surgery as he or she meets criteria (responsive, intact neuro status, stable hemodynamics & cardiac rhythm, normothermic, minimal bleeding).
- Provided hemodynamics are carefully managed (note that tachycardia is the key factor precipitating pre-CPB ischemia), can use any combination of
  ➤ Opioid (eg, fentanyl, sufentanil, remifentanil)
  ➤ Volatile agent (eg, isoflurane, sevoflurane, desflurane)
  ➤ IV adjuvant (midazolam, propofol)
- Typical regimen
  ➤ Fentanyl (10–20 mcg/kg).
  ➤ Midazolam (0.05–0.10 mg/kg).
  ➤ And/or propofol infusion w/ volatile agent supplementation.
  ➤ Avoid nitrous, given risk of hypoxemia & potential hazards of coronary or cerebral air embolus.
- Regional used in some pts, especially w/ thoracotomy incision
  ➤ A single-shot spinal (morphine 0.01 mg/kg) is most common, although thoracic epidurals are also used.
  ➤ Place epidural night before surgery, given bleeding concerns w/ anticoagulation for CPB.

INTRAOP

Monitors/Line Placement

- Place 14g or 16g IV & radial arterial line prior to induction.
- Central access, usually via RIJ, needed for all pts for central pressure monitoring & administration of IV heparin.
- PA catheter use depends on surgeon & center.
  ➤ Availability & expertise w/ TEE, the presence of comorbidities & postop recovery facilities guide CVP vs PA catheter choice.
  ➤ Consider preinduction PA catheter if pt has poor ejection fraction and/or associated valvular disease.
- TEE can be helpful for evaluation of regional wall motion, global contractility, valvular lesions & aortic arch atheromatous disease.
  ➤ Ensure pt is well anesthetized prior to probe insertion.
  ➤ Decompress the stomach w/ an OG tube before & after TEE use.

■ Activated clotting time measurement is required to manage heparin dosing & reversal.
■ Measure core temp (bladder or rectal) & surrogate of cerebral temp (nasopharyngeal) to manage cooling & rewarming from CPB.
  ➤ Avoid increasing core to cerebral temp gradient (associated w/ jugular venous desaturation).

Intraop Concerns
■ Perfusionist & cardiac surgeon should be available prior to induction.
■ Sternotomy for redo CABG involves removal of existing wires, use of an oscillating saw to enter the outer table of the sternum & dissection w/ a surgical scissor to penetrate the inner table of the sternum.
  ➤ 2 units PRBCs should be immediately available in the room during this period.
  ➤ Laceration of the ventricle (usually the right ventricle as it is anterior in the chest) or transection of an existing graft can occur at this time & during subsequent dissection to remove the heart from the pericardium.
  ➤ Ventricular fibrillation may be the first & only presenting sign of ventricular laceration. External defibrillator pads should be placed on entry to the OR, although they may not be effective if a severe laceration or graft transection occurs.
  ➤ Some surgeons prefer to expose the femoral vessels in high-risk pts prior to sternotomy for potential cannulation should laceration occur.
    • Usually, CPB will be converted to normal aortic cannulation once the pt is stabilized.
■ During induction
  ➤ Avoid hemodynamic instability & maintain MAP & HR w/in 20% of baseline.
  ➤ Avoid pentothal in pt w/ impaired LV function.
  ➤ Use low-dose opioids, volatile anesthesia and/or short-acting beta blockers (eg, esmolol) to blunt response to laryngoscopy & intubation.
  ➤ Consider early nondepolarizing muscle relaxant to offset muscle rigidity from opioids & maintain throughout case.
  ➤ Alternate strategy: "light" or no relaxation to monitor for light anesthesia.
■ After induction obtain
  ➤ Baseline ACT & ABG

- ➤ Cardiac output if a PA catheter is being used
- ➤ TEE basic exam
- Antifibrinolytics are commonly used (epsilon-aminocaproic acid, tranexamic acid), esp in pts undergoing repeat sternotomy or those who refuse blood products.
  - ➤ Common regimen: single IV bolus of aminocaproic acid 5 g administered w/ heparin & after protamine or by constant infusion starting prior to sternotomy.
- For redo CABG, the serine protease inhibitor aprotinin has been shown to significantly reduce blood loss & is commonly used.
  - ➤ A 1-mL test dose should be initially administered, carefully observing for anaphylaxis (which is very rare w/ first-time use).
  - ➤ Usual dosing includes a loading dose of 2 million KIU after induction, an additional 2 million KIU added to the CPB pump prime & a continuous infusion of 500,000 KIU per hour during surgery.
  - ➤ ACT monitoring should be performed using kaolin activator (do not use Celite). ACTs are an inaccurate reflection of heparin levels. A value of 750 sec is recommended prior to CPB.
  - ➤ Other antifibrinolytic agents SHOULD NOT be used w/ aprotinin to avoid a prothrombotic state, which could cause acute graft occlusion.
- Consider prebypass phlebotomy in pt w/ adequate Hct to prevent platelet degranulation during CPB.
  - ➤ Sequester blood gradually during IMA harvesting via the central line, or have perfusionist drain via venous cannula just prior to CPB.
  - ➤ In a high-risk redo case, the risk of precipitating ischemia by overly aggressive phlebotomy prior to CPB can outweigh the small infectious risks of transfusion.
- Saphenous vein & radial artery harvest may begin prior to sternotomy.
- After sternotomy, the left IMA is usually harvested, the pericardium is opened & the heart & aortic arch are exposed.
- Manipulation of the heart & existing vein grafts can cause sudden & intractable ischemia in the prebypass period.
  - ➤ Atheromatous disease in vein grafts is sandy & very friable & can easily embolize distally to the myocardium.
  - ➤ Careful attention to the ECG, TEE & filling pressures is mandatory.
- Prior to aortic cannulation
  - ➤ Give heparin (300–400 U/kg).

- An ACT of 450–500 sec is required prior to initiation of CPB (in presence of aprotinin, higher ACTs are usually recommended).
- ➤ Heparin resistance usually due to prolonged preop heparin use w/ depletion of antithrombin III substrate can occur.
  - Treat heparin resistance w/ 1 unit FFP or synthetic recombinant AT-III.
- ■ Cannulation
  - ➤ Surgeon places aortic cannula first. Perfusionist can use this to transfuse from CPB machine prior to bypass.
  - ➤ Keep systolic blood pressure <110 mmHg during cannulation to decrease chance of aortic dissection.
  - ➤ Venous cannula is placed into the IVC via the RA appendage.
  - ➤ A cannula is often placed in the coronary sinus through the RA for retrograde cardioplegia.
  - ➤ LV vent may be placed via the right superior pulmonary vein to prevent LV distention during CPB.
- ■ Prior to CPB, PA catheter should be withdrawn 3–5 cm to avoid wedging.
  - ➤ Can use TEE to visualize PAC tip, usually in the right pulmonary artery just above the transverse aortic valve view in the upper esophagus.
- ■ After testing the venous & arterial cannulas, CPB is started.
  - ➤ Stop ventilation when full flow is confirmed by perfusionist.
- ■ Myocardial preservation during CPB
  - ➤ Exclude heart from circulation (aortic cross-clamping).
  - ➤ Arrest heart w/ high-potassium cardioplegia.
  - ➤ Induce regional hypothermia w/ cold cardioplegia.
  - ➤ Other strategies can also be used.
- ■ During CPB: assess adequacy of tissue perfusion by
  - ➤ Online arterial & venous oxygen saturation monitoring.
  - ➤ Serial ABG/Hct determinations.
  - ➤ Arterial blood pressure monitoring.
    - Maintain MAP >50 mmHg (65 mmHg or greater in pt w/ CVD or renal insufficiency).
  - ➤ Urine output
- ■ Monitor ACT & give additional heparin as needed.
- ■ Keep Hct >20–22% w/ PRBCs.
- ■ Considerations prior to weaning from bypass
  - ➤ Rewarm.
  - ➤ Establish stable rhythm & rate.
  - ➤ Prepare for pacing.

➤ Reestablish ventilation.
➤ Optimize lab values (esp pH, hematocrit, potassium & calcium).
➤ Plan for maintaining adequate cardiac output & systolic blood pressure.
  • Pre-CPB LV function & cross-clamp time are major determinants of need for inotropic support post-CPB.
  • Use PA catheter-derived CO & SVR & TEE LV function to guide therapy.
■ Wean CPB gradually by occluding venous return to the pump, increasing preload, allow ventricle to eject & override the arterial flow. Then reduce pump flow & stop CPB.
■ Protamine
  ➤ Give 1-cc test dose of protamine & observe for hypotension, anaphylaxis, or PA hypertension.
  ➤ Give standard protamine dose of 1–1.3 mg per 100 units of heparin over at least 5 min.
  ➤ Confirm ACT returns to baseline, giving additional protamine if needed.
  ➤ Watch for rise in ACT if heparin-rich blood from the CPB circuit is reinfused.
■ Notify surgeon when protamine is started. Surgeon will d/c venous cannula & perfusionist will drain residual blood for reinfusion. Can give blood to pt in 100-cc increments, guided by PA diastolic pressure and/or LV end-diastolic area on TEE transgastric short-axis view. Use reverse Trendelenburg position to facilitate volume administration.
■ ICU transport
  ➤ Optimize fluid/blood therapy prior to ICU transfer.
  ➤ Monitor invasive BP, HR, ECG & O_2 saturation during transport.
  ➤ Bring meds to treat BP, HR, ischemia & arrhythmias.

Intraop Therapies
■ Keep bolus doses of vasopressors (phenylephrine, ephedrine & epinephrine) ready to treat hypotension due to vasodilation, hypovolemia, or impaired contractility. Surgical manipulation of the heart causes hypotension but is transient. Closely watch the surgical field & communicate w/ surgeon about BP/HR changes.
■ Dual-channel pacemaker must be immediately available.
  ➤ Ischemia & impaired AV conduction due to potassium cardioplegia commonly cause AV block & bradycardia.
  ➤ Maintain HR 80–90 bpm for several hours after CPB to avoid LV/RV distention.

- Calcium chloride (1 g incrementally) commonly used during weaning from CPB.
- May need infusion of catecholamines (dopamine, epinephrine, dobutamine) or phosphodiesterase inhibitors (amrinone, milrinone) to wean from CPB, esp if pt has impaired LV function.
- Use intra-aortic balloon counterpulsation when inotropic support alone is inadequate (systemic hypotension, cardiac index <2.0 $L/min/m^2$, high filling pressures) to augment diastolic coronary perfusion & forward flow.
  - Aortic insufficiency is a relative contraindication to IABP.
  - Can use TEE to check position of IABP (must be placed below the level of the left subclavian & carotid vessels).

POSTOP

Pain

- "Fast tracking" & early extubation should not preclude adequate pain control. Options:
  - IV short-acting opioids
  - IV NSAID (eg, ketorolac)
  - Avoid NSAIDs in pt w/ renal insufficiency.
- CABG w/ IMA dissection is more painful than CABG w/ saphenous vein harvest alone.

Complications

- Hypertension is a common problem, often unresponsive to sedation or narcotics. May need nitroprusside or nitroglycerin infusions or careful use of beta blockers (esmolol, metoprolol).
- Bleeding is most common cause of return to OR. Manifestations:
  - Continued output from chest tubes
  - Hypotension
  - Need for of fluid & blood products
- Coagulopathy is common.
  - Usually from impaired platelet function.
  - Platelet count also declines, usually by 50%.
  - Coagulation factor dilution occurs but is rarely severe enough to cause bleeding.
  - Hypothermia after CPB enhances bleeding.
    - Treat w/ forced air rewarming in the ICU.
  - Cardiac tamponade may occur if excessive blood accumulates in mediastinum.
- Atrial fibrillation

➤ Occurs in 20–40% of pts, most commonly on POD 2–3.

➤ Can be associated w/ hypotension.

➤ A more serious complication is stroke due to thrombus & embolization.

➤ Useful therapies include diltiazem, amiodarone, procainamide, beta blockers and/or digoxin. Synchronized cardioversion may be required.

■ Low cardiac output syndrome

➤ Most common in pt w/ poor preop LV function and/or

➤ Pt w/ inadequate myocardial preservation on CPB, or

➤ Technically poor revascularization (eg, small distal targets, excessive calcification, intramyocardial vessels)

➤ IABP usually required for LV failure.

➤ RV failure is less common & more difficult to treat & may require insertion of a PA balloon (technically difficult).

➤ If CO remains low despite IABP, consider placement of ventricular assist device.

■ Stroke/neuropsychological changes

➤ Overt CVA may occur in 1–3% of pts but is most common in the elderly, diabetics, females, pt w/ prior CVA, pt w/ aortic arch atheroma and/or concurrent carotid disease.

➤ Subtle degrees of dysfunction & cognitive disturbances are common.

➤ A complete TEE & epiaortic evaluation of the aortic arch & potential cannulation site for evidence of aortic atheroma (w/ mobile components imparting the greatest degree of risk) should be performed in high-risk pts.

SURGICAL PROCEDURE

Indications

■ Typical indications include multivessel CAD or significant left main CAD.

■ Procedure

■ Involves sternotomy, dissection of new grafts (saphenous veins, left or right internal mammary artery, radial artery or other arteries) w/ anastomoses to vessels distal to obstructing lesions & occluded existing conduits after initiation of CPB & ischemic arrest.

Surgical Concerns

■ Adequate conduits are essential for performing multiple anastomoses. This can be problematic in a redo pt.

- Adequate surgical exposure for cannulating the heart & aorta. Exposure of the heart due to previous adhesions is substantially more complex & risky in redo pts.
- Avoidance of ischemia due to mechanical effects altering existing graft flow or embolization of loose atheromatous disease in diseased vein grafts is important.
- Performing distal anastomoses on a nonbeating, well-protected heart is the primary reason for performing CABG on bypass. Long-term graft patency may be optimized using this approach. Other approaches: off-pump CABG.

Typical EBL
- Highly variable & surgeon-specific.
- Exact EBL is difficult to quantitate & rarely done.
- 2–4 units of blood loss common.
- Redo cases are usually associated w/ increased blood loss & blood product usage, although use of aprotinin can at times markedly diminish requirements.

RENAL TRANSPLANT

HSIUPEI CHEN, MD
MICHAEL GROPPER, MD, PHD

PREOP

Preop Considerations
- Establish volume status. Factors include:
  - Whether pt is anuric or oliguric
  - Most recent dialysis session
  - Type of dialysis: Hemodialysis more prone to cause hypovolemia than CAPD
- Determine whether pt is prone to hyperkalemia.
- Determine dialysis access site (peritoneal vs hemodialysis).
  - Dialysis catheter can be used for venous access. Withdraw any heparin from line before using.
  - Document thrill in AV fistula, & avoid placing IV lines in that extremity.
- Common coexisting diseases: HTN, CAD, DM, anemia, electrolyte abnormalities (hyperkalemia most lethal)

Physical Findings
- AV fistula, central line, or peritoneal access for dialysis
- Baseline BP, MAP. Will need to maintain BP near baseline when renal vessels unclamped.
- Chest exam for evidence of CHF or fluid overload

Workup
- Check dialysis schedule, last dialysis done, volume status.
- Electrolytes (esp K+), Hct
- ECG: Look for evidence of ischemia or hyperkalemia

Choice of Anesthesia
- GA most common

INTRAOP
Monitors/Line Placement
- CVP for assessing volume status & administering pressors; triple-lumen catheter preferred, given multiple infusions required postop.
- Caution: Do not place BP cuff or IV in limb w/ AV fistula.

Intraop Concerns
- Maintain normal perfusion pressure, generally using low concentrations of inhalational agents.
- Fluids: Most surgeons request loading 2–4 L crystalloid prior to reperfusion of new kidney. Use 0.9% NaCl (avoid K+ in LR).
- BP: To maintain near-normal MAP, use minimum concentration of inhaled anesthetic necessary for amnesia. Most surgeons discourage phenylephrine because of potential renal artery vasoconstriction.
- Muscle relaxant: Maintain muscle relaxation, especially during anastomosis of renal vessels. This facilitates exposure & ensures lack of movement w/ low concentrations of anesthetics. Consider nonrenally cleared relaxant (eg, cisatracurium).
- If pt has functioning AV fistula, position the extremity carefully to minimize risk of thrombosis. Check for thrill periodically intraop.

Intraop Therapies
- Administer immunosuppressive agents requested by surgeon (eg, 1 g IV methylprednisolone [Solu-Medrol]).
- Measures to promote renal perfusion after anastomosis.
    - ➤ IV fluid to maintain CVP 10–15 mm Hg.
    - ➤ Furosemide (Lasix) & mannitol (usually administered over 30 min during vascular anastomoses).

➤ Maintain normal MAP. Surgeon may request higher BP if urine output appears inadequate. Inotrope/vasopressor to maintain MAP: mixed beta & alpha agonists (ie, ephedrine) preferred over pure alpha agonist.

➤ Dopamine infusion (usually 3 mcg/kg/min) & Lasix infusion (usually 10 mg/h) initiated at completion of vascular anastomoses.

POSTOP

Pain

■ Moderate, given size of abdominal incision & lower abdominal location. Consider infiltration of local anesthetic in wound, as well as postop PCA for 1–2 days.

Complications

■ Hyperkalemia following release of vascular clamp after completion of the arterial anastomosis or release of potassium from preservative.

SURGICAL PROCEDURE

Indications

■ End-stage renal disease

Procedure

■ Donor kidney placed in iliac fossa, renal artery anastomosed to iliac a., renal vein anastomosed to iliac vein. Bladder filled w/ irrigation using 3-way Foley catheter, then ureter anastomosed to bladder.

Surgical Concerns

■ Quality of anastomoses, perfusion of kidney

Typical EBL

■ 100–300 cc

REPAIR OF ATRIAL SEPTAL DEFECT (ASD)

KATHRYN ROUINE-RAPP, MD

PREOP

Preop Considerations

■ Most common type is a secundum ASD, located in the region of the fossa ovalis. Associated abnormalities include mitral valve prolapse & mitral regurgitation.

- Less common types are located in the inferior portion of the interatrial septum (primum ASD) or adjacent to the entrance of the superior or inferior vena cavae & associated w/ anomalous pulmonary venous connections (sinus venosus ASD).
- Physiologic consequences of the defect are determined by defect size, ventricular compliance & pulmonary artery pressures.
  - ➤ Large defect & substantial flow from the left to right atrium (shunt) can lead to atrial enlargement, dilatation of the right ventricle & pulmonary arteries & pulmonary hypertension.
- Atrial arrhythmias may occur, especially after the third decade of life.
- Symptoms may include fatigue, dyspnea, palpitations.
- Surgical mortality risk is greater in pts who undergo surgical repair after age 24 & in whom pulmonary artery pressure exceeds 40 mmHg.
- Repair can be performed as percutaneous procedure in cardiac cath lab or in OR w/ cardiopulmonary bypass (CPB), both discussed below.

Workup
- Echocardiogram can
  - ➤ Define defect type, size & location
  - ➤ Detect mitral valve abnormalities
  - ➤ Determine cardiac chamber size
  - ➤ Describe pulmonary venous connections
  - ➤ Assess ventricular function
- Cardiac catheterization may be performed to measure pulmonary artery pressures or define pulmonary venous connections.
  - ➤ 100% FiO_2 challenge can discriminate between "reversible" & "irreversible" pulmonary hypertension.

Choice of Anesthesia
- General anesthesia usually chosen for repair in cardiac cath lab & in OR w/ sternotomy.

INTRAOP
Monitors/Line Placement
- Repair in cardiac cath lab
  - ➤ Use large-bore peripheral IV.
  - ➤ Cardiologist will place vascular sheaths for access as well.
- Repair in OR
  - ➤ Use arterial line & large-bore IV access during surgical repair of ASD.

➤ Place a central line or measure pulmonary artery pressures in any pt w/ depressed myocardial function or pulmonary hypertension.

Intraop Concerns
■ Remove air from all IV tubing & syringes.
  ➤ These pts are at risk of paradoxical embolus.
■ Repair in the cardiac cath lab (selected secundum defects) is accomplished via a closure device placed percutaneously, then guided by fluoroscopy & transesophageal echocardiography.
  ➤ Some cardiologists ask to limit IV fluids to prevent stretch of the atria.
  ➤ Near the start of the procedure, the cardiologist will determine cardiac chamber saturations. During sample acquisition, ventilate pt using room air & provide normocarbia.
  ➤ Expect to give cefazolin 25 mg/kg or 1 g in patients >40 kg before the device is placed.
  ➤ Pt will receive IV heparin titrated to keep the ACT >200.
  ➤ When the cardiologist uses lateral cameras to image the heart, he/she will ask you to abduct the pt's arms to an overhead position. Ask older pts to try this position while awake & check for symptoms of brachial plexus stretch.
  ➤ Rarely, a catheter can puncture the myocardium & cause tamponade.
  ➤ Near the end of the procedure, ask the cardiologist to inject the percutaneous cannulation site (usually the groin) w/ a long-acting local anesthetic.
  ➤ Consider tracheal extubation during the 15 min the cardiologist is holding pressure on the percutaneous cannulation site after sheath removal.
■ Repair in the OR requires a sternotomy, submammary incision or thoracotomy & CPB.
  ➤ Administer intrathecal or IV narcotics for postop pain control.
  ➤ Before draping, place defibrillation pads on the pt if the incision is going to be a limited sternotomy, submammary, or thoracotomy.
  ➤ Transesophageal echocardiography can be used to detect intracardiac air, determine adequacy of repair & assess ventricular & mitral valve function.
  ➤ CPB
    • Check ACT before CPB. It should be >480 sec.

- The period of CPB is usually <30 min.
- Give additional anesthetic & muscle relaxant immediately before CPB so the pt will not breathe spontaneously while the left heart is open to air.
- If you placed a pulmonary artery catheter, pull it back to 15 cm before CPB.
➣ Surgical concerns include
  - Removal of air from the left atrium before the heart is allowed to beat & eject blood (you will be asked to ventilate pt to increase pulmonary venous return, fill the left heart, & deair the left atrium. You also will be asked to place the pt in steep head-down position before removal of the fibrillator or aortic cross-clamp).
➣ Most pts do not need inotrope therapy to separate from CPB.
➣ After CPB
  - Look for intracardiac air or residual defects & assess ventricular function using transesophageal echocardiography.
  - Some pts may be ready for tracheal extubation before leaving the OR. Some surgeons prefer extubation after a postoperative CXR is completed & reviewed.

POSTOP

Pain
- For CPB approach, can be managed effectively by intrathecal or IV narcotics
- Pts who undergo percutaneous placement of a closure device tend to have minimal postop pain.

Complications
- Substantial mediastinal drainage is unusual in pts after ASD repair.
- Air in the left-heart chambers can lead to stroke, but this is very unusual.
- Pts who have atrial arrhythmias preop are at increased risk to have them postop.
- For cath lab approach
  ➣ The closure device can migrate during or after placement, usually to the pulmonary artery (this is a rare complication).
    - Pts have a CXR before hospital discharge to look for the device.
    - If the device migrates, pts are given the option to return to the cath lab or OR for device removal & ASD closure.

SURGICAL PROCEDURE

Indications
- ASD

Procedure
- Repair in the cardiac cath lab (selected secundum defects) is accomplished via a closure device placed percutaneously, then guided by fluoroscopy & transesophageal echocardiography
- Repair in the OR requires a sternotomy, submammary incision, or thoracotomy & CPB
  - Procedure involves
    - Venous cannulation via the inferior & superior vena cavae
    - Either placement of a fibrillator directly on the heart or aortic cross-clamp application followed by cardioplegia to arrest the heart
    - Use of the pericardium as a patch
    - A right atriotomy surgical approach
    - Suture or patch placement to close the defect

Surgical Concerns
- W/ CPB
  - Removal of intracardiac air prior to weaning from CPB
  - Residual defects
  - Minimal exposure to homologous blood products
- W/ cath lab approach
  - Migration of device
  - Risk of cardiac perforation, tamponade

Typical EBL
- Minimal w/ cath lab approach
- Transfusion often not required w/ CPB approach; depends on patient size & preop hematocrit

---

REPAIR OPEN GLOBE

JASON WIDRICH, MD

PREOP

Preop Considerations
- Intraocular pressure (IOP) must be controlled as much as possible to prevent further injury to the globe or blindness.

- Movement, straining, coughing, hypercarbia, HTN, airway instrumentation may all increase IOP.
- Pts often have full stomachs & are at risk of aspiration.

Workup
- Labs should be ordered as indicated by H & P.
- If the open globe injury was secondary to trauma, suspect craniofacial & C-spine injury & address in the pt workup.

Choice of Anesthesia
- GA is the method of choice because it provides less opportunity for IOP elevation during induction & throughout surgery, which may be lengthy.

INTRAOP

Monitors/Line Placement
- Standard ASA monitors.
- Monitoring for neuromuscular blockade.

Intraop Concerns
- Premed w/ benzodiazepines to reduce anxiety will be useful, but narcotic premed should be given carefully because it may lead to nausea or emesis.
- Aspiration precautions (eg, 10 mg metoclopramide IV, ranitidine 50 mg IV, 15–30 mL sodium citrate PO) should be followed in pts who are not NPO.
- Fasciculation from succinylcholine is undesirable because it may increase pressure on the eye. A plan for cricoid pressure during induction, or gentle positive-pressure ventilation through cricoid pressure, needs to be made on a case-by-case basis.
- For children, an inhaled induction through cricoid pressure before an IV can be placed may be the only way to prevent further agitation & IOP changes.
- Positioning to prevent nerve injury & protection of the unaffected eye is still a priority.

Intraop Therapies
- Maintain neuromuscular blockade until the globe is closed.
- Avoid hypercapnia, HTN.
- Oculocardiac reflex

➤ A trigeminal-vagal reflex resulting from tension on ocular structures.

➤ Can cause various arrhythmias but most often bradycardia & a concurrent fall in BP.

➤ Treated by stopping the stimulus & giving glycopyrrolate (in incremental doses, 0.2 mg at a time) as needed.

■ If liquid vitreous substitutes are needed to replace a vitreous leak, avoid nitrous oxide during the procedure. It can expand & cause increases in IOP that may compromise flow from the retinal artery.

■ Prior to emergence, suction pharynx & stomach.

■ Administer prophylactic antiemetics.

■ Lidocaine (1–1.5 mg/kg) or narcotics can assist w/ emergence & a smooth awake extubation by blunting cough reflexes.

POSTOP

Pain

■ Treat w/ acetaminophen and/or opiates.

Complications

■ Nausea/vomiting.
■ Corneal abrasion.
■ Aspiration.
■ Diplopia.
■ Photophobia.

SURGICAL PROCEDURE

Indications

■ Ruptured or lacerated globe

Procedure

■ Layered repair of sclera, cornea, assoc structures. May need to incise conjunctiva or extraocular muscles to gain adequate exposure

Surgical Concerns

■ IOP, coughing or movement, infection, loss of ocular contents w/ visual loss

Typical EBL

■ Minimal

RESECTION OF CARCINOID TUMOR

JASON WIDRICH, MD

PREOP

Preop Considerations

- Carcinoid syndrome is present in approx 2–5% of pts w/ carcinoid tumors. Carcinoid syndrome is caused by overproduction of vasoactive substances by a carcinoid tumor.
  - ➤ Best-characterized substance is serotonin, but others include histamine, corticotropin, dopamine, kallikrein, neurotensin, prostaglandins, substance P.
  - ➤ Tumor usually occurs in GI tract but may also occur in lungs & bronchi.
- Signs & symptoms usually present only in pt w/ liver mets, or if tumor releases vasoactive substances outside of portal circulation.
- Pt w/ carcinoid syndrome will likely be receiving the somatostatin analog octreotide.
  - ➤ Octreotide is highly effective in reducing symptoms. Mechanism involves binding to somatostatin receptor on tumor.
  - ➤ Typical dose 150 mcg SC TID.

Physical Findings

- Typically none in the absence of carcinoid syndrome.
  - ➤ Manifestations of carcinoid syndrome include
    - Episodic flushing
    - Wheezing
    - Diarrhea
    - Right-sided valvular disease
- Cardiac valve lesions include
  - ➤ Tricuspid regurgitation & stenosis
  - ➤ Pulmonic regurgitation & stenosis
  - ➤ Left-sided valve disease less common

Workup

- Evaluate for symptoms of carcinoid syndrome.
  - ➤ Consider echo to evaluate for tricuspid regurgitation & pulmonic stenosis.
  - ➤ Urinalysis for 5-HIAA (breakdown product of serotonin) is used in diagnosis.
- CBC, electrolytes, BUN, Cr, glucose.

- PT, PTT for pts w/ liver mets.
- Surgeon may order abdominal CT scan.
  - ➤ Check for tumor location/multiplicity.

Choice of Anesthesia
- GA.
- Epidural anesthesia useful for postop pain control in intra-abdominal & intrathoracic resections.

INTRAOP
Monitors/Line Placement
- Standard monitors
  - ➤ 1 or 2 peripheral IVs.
  - ➤ Consider arterial line.
  - ➤ Consider TEE or PA catheter for pts w/ severe right-sided valvular pathology.

Intraop Concerns
- Surgery is most often intra-abdominal.
  - ➤ Thoracic resection may require double-lumen ETT for exposure.
- Significant blood loss may occur during tumor resection if resection includes metastatic disease to the liver.
- Vasoactive substances may be released from tumor manipulation, causing intraop carcinoid crisis.

Intraop Therapies
- Give octreotide IV (50 mcg) & SQ (50 mcg) prior to tumor manipulation to help block hemodynamic effects.
- Pts at risk for carcinoid crisis: flushing associated w/ bronchospasm, severe hypotension & cardiovascular collapse.
  - ➤ Additional IV bolus of octreotide 50 mcg may be helpful to manage carcinoid crisis.
- Avoid drugs that may cause histamine release.
- Catecholamines may increase release of substances from tumor & worsen symptoms.
  - ➤ Avoid catecholamine administration if possible.
- Rarely, a hypertensive carcinoid crisis may occur (eg, from tumor manipulation); may respond to IV octreotide as well as vasodilator therapy.

POSTOP

Pain
- Moderate to severe
- Depends on location of incision, extent of surgery
- PCA or epidural

Complications
- Carcinoid crisis
  - ➤ Watch for continued signs of carcinoid syndrome or crisis.
  - ➤ Surgical resection of carcinoid tumor may not eliminate all metastatic lesions, so hemodynamic changes may persist.
  - ➤ Consider continuation of octreotide therapy.

SURGICAL PROCEDURE

Indications
- Tumor causing local irritation, pain, bleeding, obstruction (GI or pulmonary).
- Symptoms from carcinoid syndrome increasing in frequency or severity.

Procedure
- Surgical technique varies considerably depending on location of tumor (lung, liver, GI tract, ovary). See other Procedures chapters for tumor removal from intrathoracic or intra-abdominal location.

Surgical Concerns
- Significant bleeding from tumor resection.
- Mediator release w/ manipulation of tumor.

Typical EBL
- 200–1,000 mL.
- Blood loss varies depending on vascular supply to tumor & adjacent structures (liver, GI tract, pulmonary vessels).

RETINAL SURGERY (SCLERAL BUCKLE & VITRECTOMY)

JASON WIDRICH, MD

PREOP

Preop Considerations
- Variety of indications for retinal surgery

➤ Diabetic retinopathy w/ vitreous hemorrhage or retinal detachment
➤ Retinal detachment may require a variety of procedures
  • Laser therapy
  • Intraocular gas tamponade (pneumatic retinopexy)
  • Scleral buckle
  • Vitrectomy
➤ Epiretinal membrane (macular pucker)
➤ Macular hole
▨ Pt may be receiving acetazolamide, which decreases aqueous humor production but can also affect electrolyte status (low K, Low Na)

Physical Findings
▨ None typical

Workup
▨ Stop aspirin or anticoagulant drugs.
▨ Electrolytes, BUN, creatinine for pt on acetazolamide
▨ Additional workup based on coexisting disease (eg, diabetes)

Choice of Anesthesia
▨ GA or MAC w/ regional block
  ➤ Although GA is most common, surgeon may have preference for regional block
  ➤ Regional anesthetic may be unsuitable for pt who is uncooperative, has a chronic cough, or cannot lie flat

INTRAOP

Monitors/Line Placement
▨ Standard monitors.
▨ One peripheral IV.

Intraop Concerns
▨ Minimize pt movement during surgery.
▨ Oculocardiac reflex can result from tension on ocular structures, causing bradycardia & other arrhythmias.
▨ Avoid nitrous oxide for the following conditions:
  ➤ If liquid vitreous substitutes are needed to replace a vitreous leak.
  ➤ If pt will have a gas bubble injected to stabilize the retina.
  ➤ N_2O can cause IOP increases.

➤ Discontinue N_2O at least 10 min prior to gas injection & avoid for the next 4–6 wks.
■ For GA, minimize coughing on emergence.

Intraop Therapies
■ Oculocardiac reflex is treated by halting the stimulus, increasing depth of anesthesia & administering IV glycopyrrolate or atropine if bradycardia persists.
■ Consider prophylactic antiemetics.
■ Mannitol therapy may be requested to reduce IOP.
➤ Foley catheter should be in place.

POSTOP

Pain
■ Mild
■ PO analgesics

Complications
■ Nausea/vomiting
■ Corneal abrasion

SURGICAL PROCEDURE

Indications
■ Variety of indications, including
➤ Diabetic retinopathy
➤ Vitreous hemorrhage
➤ Retinal detachment
➤ Epiretinal membrane (macular pucker)
➤ Macular hole
➤ Effects of previous ocular surgery

Procedure
■ Varies depending on specific procedure performed
■ Scleral incision
■ Insertion of microsurgical instruments
■ Surgery
■ Closure

Surgical Concerns
■ Hemorrhage
■ Vitreous loss

Typical EBL
- Minimal

ROTATIONAL & FREE FLAPS

DHANESH K. GUPTA, MD

PREOP

Preop Considerations
Preop considerations focus on coexisting diseases:
- Cancer pts: coexisting disease assoc w/ age (HTN, CAD, COPD, diabetes mellitus)
- Trauma pts: coexisting disease assoc w/ previous injuries
- Pressure ulcers: diabetes or spinal cord injury/stroke leading to skin breakdown
- Nonhealing wounds: diabetes or vascular disease

Physical Findings
- If head & neck cancer, abnormal airway anatomy

Workup
- Ischemic heart disease workup in at-risk pts

Choice of Anesthesia
- GA indicated for control of airway in lengthy procedures that may involve the head or neck
- Regional anesthesia can be used in many cases & may also provide for postop analgesia in some cases

INTRAOP

Monitors/Line Placement
- For free flaps, arterial line useful for aggressive monitoring of BP, which reflects flap perfusion pressure
- Consider volume status monitors (Foley catheter, possible CVP).

Intraop Concerns
- Flap perfusion: maintain euvolemia & normotension, avoid vasoconstrictors.
- Keep pt warm to prevent hypothermia-associated coagulopathy & vasoconstriction.

- Maintain Hct at approx 30 to ensure optimal oxygen delivery to the flap.
- Muscle relaxation may assist surgical flap dissection.
- Autonomic hyperreflexia may be a concern if spinal cord injury is present.

Intraop Therapies
- Fluid therapy for euvolemia (consider colloid).
- Forced air warming & fluid warmers to maintain core temp.
- Avoid vasoconstrictors that may compromise flap perfusion.

POSTOP

Pain
- Moderate.
- Regional technique for analgesia may be associated w/ significant hypotension that compromises flap perfusion.

Complications
- Flap failure (vascular thrombosis) requires emergent re-exploration.
  - ➤ On reinduction of anesthesia, watch for hypotension that can worsen flap perfusion.

SURGICAL PROCEDURE

Indications
- Large wound exposing bone, vasculature, and/or infected tissues
- Large surgical resections for cancer (esp head/neck & orthopedic)
- Poorly healing traumatic or diabetic wounds

Procedure
- Position variable
- Free flap can be lengthy procedure (6–12 h)
- Dissection of muscle (possibly w/ overlying skin) & identification of feeding arteries & veins
- Transfer of flap to wound (either rotation or free transfer) & reanastomosis of vascular pedicle

Surgical Concerns
- Flap perfusion: hypotension, hypovolemia, hypothermia, vasoconstrictors may decrease flap perfusion or promote vessel thrombosis
- Muscle relaxation may assist flap resection

Typical EBL
- 500 mL

ROTATOR CUFF SURGERY

DAVID SHIMABUKURO, MDCM

PREOP

Preop Considerations
- Often performed in relatively young, healthy pt
- Injury may be related to a sports or job-related injury

Physical Findings
- Document any neuro deficits.

Workup
- As appropriate for pt's age & comorbidities

Choice of Anesthesia
- Can be performed w/ regional block (eg, interscalene), GA or both
- Interscalene block (see also Technique chapter "Interscalene Brachial Plexus Block")
  - Blocks C4, C5, C6 nerve roots
  - Local anesthetics appropriate for this surgery include
    - Mepivacaine 2%, L-Bupivacaine 0.5% (mixed 1:1) 20 mL for surgery
    - L-Bupivacaine 0.5% or 0.75% 20 mL + 40 mg tetracaine + epinephrine 1:200,000 for postop pain control
  - Does not anesthetize overlying skin & subcutaneous tissue (may require local supplementation by surgeon)
  - Complications: ipsilateral paralysis of diaphragm, pneumothorax, Horner's syndrome
- Regional & combined techniques can provide postop pain control

INTRAOP

Monitors/Line Placement
- Standard monitors
- Arm on affected side will be prepped into surgical field.
  - Do not put IV or BP cuff on this arm
- One peripheral IV adequate

Intraop Concerns
- Normally done in "beach chair" position w/ no immediate access to airway

■ Air embolus is extremely rare but possible, as operative site is above the level of the heart

Intraop Therapies
■ Adequate muscle relaxation, either from muscle relaxant or interscalene block

POSTOP

Pain
■ Moderate to severe
  ➤ Extremely painful during immediate postop period
■ Pain control: interscalene block, PCA, or PRN analgesics
  ➤ In pts w/ pre-existing neuro deficits, regional anesthesia should be carefully discussed

Complications
■ None specific to this procedure

SURGICAL PROCEDURE

Indications
■ Injury to the rotator cuff of the shoulder

Procedure
■ Open repair of the injury

Surgical Concerns
■ Generally considered a low-risk procedure
■ Risk of nerve injury

Typical EBL
■ Minimal

SKIN GRAFT

DHANESH K. GUPTA, MD

PREOP

Preop Considerations
■ Wide variety of pts require skin graft.
  ➤ Pt may be critically ill (eg, burn, major trauma).
  ➤ Skin graft may be small & a relatively minor part of surgery.

■ For burn & trauma pts: large third-space loss, difficult IV access, coexisting diseases associated w/ burns (lung injury, sepsis, denervation injury, etc).

Physical Findings
■ Depend on indication for skin graft.

Workup
■ Dictated by coexisting disease.

Choice of Anesthesia
■ Local anesthesia possible if limited skin flap harvest site.
■ Regional may also be useful for postop pain mgt.
■ GA may be preferable if multiple position changes required (eg, skin from posterior leg harvested for face).

INTRAOP

Monitors/Line Placement
■ Standard monitors plus those required by coexisting disease.
■ Consider arterial line for large skin grafts (eg, for burn pt).

Intraop Concerns
■ Large doses of local anesthetic w/ epinephrine may be employed at harvest site, w/ risk of local anesthetic overdose or systemic absorption of epinephrine.
■ Blood loss may be deceptive from multiple skin harvest sites.
■ Large surface area may be uncovered, leading to hypothermia.

Intraop Therapies
■ Forced air warmers, humidified circuits, warmed fluids, warmed ambient temp of OR.

POSTOP

Pain
■ Harvest site extremely painful
■ Pts having repeated skin grafts may be narcotic-tolerant
■ Consider regional analgesia for larger grafts

Complications
■ Bleeding
■ Local anesthetic toxicity
■ Hypertension/tachycardia from absorption of epinephrine-containing local anesthetic solutions

SURGICAL PROCEDURE

Indications
- Re-epithelization of burns or noninfected partial-thickness wounds

Procedure
- Skin graft harvested w/ dermatome & sutured to recipient site

Surgical Concerns
- Hypothermia from large exposed surface area

Typical EBL
- 200 mL or greater, depending on size of graft

SPINAL FUSION

JASON WIDRICH, MD

PREOP

Preop Considerations
- Considerations & risks vary based on coexisting disease, etiology of spine disease, location of fusion (cervical, thoracic, lumbar), number of levels involved.
  - May have high intraop blood loss (multiple blood volumes), resulting in hypovolemia & anemia.
  - Pts are at risk for vital organ ischemia (eg, heart, brain, spinal cord).
- Predictors of blood loss include
  - Large number of spinal levels requiring fusion.
  - Revision of previous spine surgery.
  - Severe scoliosis.
  - Tumors.
  - Abscesses.
  - AVMs.
  - Neuromuscular disease.
- Surgery may involve combined anterior & posterior fusions, or a staged procedure.
- consider potential coexisting disease in this pt population.
  - Pulmonary
    - Severe kyphosis or scoliosis (>30 degrees) at T-spine level may cause restrictive lung disease (see also Coexisting Disease chapter "Kyphoscoliosis").

- Severe pulmonary disease may limit pt's ability to tolerate one-lung ventilation w/ thoracic anterior spinal fusion.
- ➤ Cardiac
  - Coronary artery disease is more likely in older pts & may provide a contraindication to controlled hypotension or severe anemia.
  - Restrictive pulmonary disease can lead to right heart failure (cor pulmonale).
- ➤ Neuro
  - Chronic opiate use from chronic pain may result in tolerance.
  - Sensory or motor deficits may be present.
  - Pts who are paralyzed preop (eg, after acute trauma) may be at risk for spinal shock or autonomic hyperreflexia, depending on timing of spinal injury.
- ➤ Musculoskeletal
  - Pt requiring fusion secondary to trauma may have unstable thoracic, lumbar, or cervical spine. Pt may also have other injuries: rib, leg, or pelvic fracture, or closed head injury.

Physical Findings
- Depend on severity & type of spinal pathology & impact on other organ systems.
- Document all preop neuro deficits.

Workup
- CBC, PT, PTT, electrolytes, BUN, creatinine.
- Type & cross-match for PRBC or whole blood.
- For cervical spinal fusion, determine stability of cervical. spine, range of motion & symptoms w/ neck movement. Assess likelihood of difficult airway mgt.
- Further workup based on coexisting disease.

Choice of Anesthesia
- GA usually used, although spinal anesthesia can be performed for small, uncomplicated fusion at lumbar level.
- For cervical spine fusion, decide whether pt w/ anticipated difficult airway will require awake intubation.
- If neuro monitoring is planned, anesthetic choices may require modification to minimize interference (see below).
- Wake-up test (movement of all extremities to command) may be required during the procedure to assess integrity of spinal motor pathways.

➤ If intraop wake-up test is planned to evaluate neuro function, discuss in detail w/ pt prior to procedure.

➤ To facilitate wake-up, use short-acting anesthetics & narcotics.

■ Muscle relaxants are not required intraop & may interfere w/ some types of neuro monitoring (eg, EMG, motor evoked potentials, wake-up test).

INTRAOP

Monitors/Line Placement

■ Standard monitors.

■ At least two large-bore peripheral IVs.

■ An arterial line & central line are useful if significant blood loss anticipated.

➤ If central line used, obtain CVP before & after position changes to establish trends in filling pressures.

■ Specialized neuro monitoring

➤ Wake-up test can assess adequacy of motor tracts (perfusion to anterior spinal cord).

➤ Somatosensory evoked potentials (SSEPs) may be used to monitor for posterior spinal cord ischemia.

➤ Motor evoked potentials (MEPs) may be used to monitor for anterior spinal cord ischemia.

➤ Electromyography (EMG) may be used to monitor for nerve root compression.

➤ MEP & SSEP are gaining support for use as a monitor of spinal cord ischemia in lieu of a wake-up test.

■ Discuss w/ neuro monitoring staff regarding possible anesthetic interference w/ monitoring. Typical considerations:

➤ SSEPs

• Avoid volatile anesthetics or keep <0.5 MAC.

• Propofol, narcotics, muscle relaxants do not interfere w/ SSEP.

➤ MEPs

• Avoid volatile anesthetics or keep <0.5 MAC.

• Avoid muscle relaxants.

• Propofol, narcotics do not interfere w/ signal.

➤ EMG

• Avoid muscle relaxants.

➤ Baseline SSEP/MEP can be obtained to determine whether anesthetics are interfering w/ the signal.

Intraop Concerns

■ Postop airway edema & airway obstruction
  ➤ Of greatest concern in prolonged posterior fusion w/ large fluid requirement because of dependent airway structures.
  ➤ Also a concern w/ cervical spine fusion because of proximity to airway.
■ Postop mechanical ventilation
  ➤ Simple laminectomy, diskectomy with one- or two-level fusion not likely to require postop ventilation.
  ➤ Factors increasing need for postop mechanical ventilation.
    • Combined, multiple-level anterior & posterior fusion.
    • Pre-existing pulmonary disease, especially w/ thoracotomy for anterior fusion.
    • Cervical spine fusion with C3-C5 involvement (potential phrenic nerve & diaphragmatic dysfunction).
    • Large anticipated analgesic requirements.
■ Hemorrhage & hypovolemia major concerns during spinal fusion.
  ➤ Bleeding can begin during dissection into the erector spinous muscles & dissection of muscle attachments to bone.
  ➤ Vertebrectomy also assoc w/ increased blood loss
  ➤ Risk of bleeding is particularly high in revisions of prior spine surgery because of excess scar tissue & adhesions obscuring anatomy.
  ➤ Use arterial line & CVP to assist w/ clinical monitoring of adequate volume status.
  ➤ Attempt to maintain urine output >0.5 mL/kg/h.
  ➤ Concerns w/ massive hemorrhage (see also Critical Events chapter "Hemorrhage").
  ➤ Consider point-of-care hemoglobin testing.
■ In addition to overt hemorrhage, specific causes of hypotension during spinal fusion include
  ➤ Venous air embolism w/ entrapment of air into the epidural veins.
  ➤ Fat embolism.
  ➤ Hemorrhage from unrecognized vascular injury (see below).
■ Specific concerns for posterior spinal fusion in the prone position.
  ➤ Increased risk of endotracheal tube dislodgement, kinking or obstruction from secretions.
  ➤ Increased risk of airway edema.
  ➤ Risk of compression of vascular structures at hips & upper extremities.

➤ Risk of rhabdomyolysis w/ prolonged pressure on dependent tissue.

➤ Brachial plexus, ulnar or peroneal neuropathies.

➤ Risk of pressure on eyes leading to postop visual loss or corneal abrasion.

➤ Risk of excess neck extension or flexion.

➤ If abdomen not properly suspended, intra-abdominal pressure will increase, w/ increased epidural venous pressure leading to increased bleeding.

■ Specific concerns for cervical procedures.

➤ If cervical spine is damaged from acute traumatic injury, spinal shock can occur.

➤ Pt w/ unstable cervical spine will require either require awake intubation or induction w/ in-line stabilization of head & neck.

➤ Surgical injury to vertebral arteries, carotid artery, jugular vein or vagus nerve possible.

■ Specific concerns for thoracic procedures.

➤ After anterior fusion, pt will have decreased lung volumes & atelectasis.

➤ W/ anterior approach, risk of damage to thoracic vessels, esophagus, lung & brachial plexus.

➤ Collapse of lung or one-lung ventilation may further compromise respiratory function.

➤ Surgery at lower thoracic levels may require dissection into diaphragm.

■ Specific concerns for lumbar or lower thoracic procedures.

➤ Anterior approach may be associated w/ bowel manipulation, injury to aorta, vena cava, iliac vessels or ureters.

➤ Profuse bleeding can occur from injury to major vessels.

■ Decision regarding postop care will depend on coexisting disease, stress of proposed surgery, intraop course. Common indications for ICU care include

➤ Postop respiratory failure or airway edema.

➤ High analgesic requirements.

➤ Hemodynamic instability.

➤ Persistent hypovolemia or anemia requiring continued fluid or blood resuscitation.

➤ Other intraop complication.

Intraop Therapies

■ Blood products as needed to replace red cells, platelets or coagulation factors.

- Consider strategy to reduce intraop blood loss or reduce transfusion requirement.
  - Preop autologous donation.
  - Intraop cell salvage.
  - Hemodilution.
  - Low transfusion threshold.
    - Actual transfusion trigger is based on coexisting disease & risk of end-organ ischemia.
  - Controlled hypotension
    - In general, avoid the combination of hypotension & severe anemia, especially in pt w/ significant end-organ disease.
- For combined anterior & posterior fusion, use of a rotating bed frame may eliminate the need for "flipping" the pt onto another OR table, allowing easy positioning for anterior & posterior dissections.
- Neuromonitoring issues: approach to loss of SSEP or MEP signal.
  - Goal should be to return mean BP to baseline or slightly above baseline (by infusion of IV fluids or blood, or by pharmacologic means).
  - Rule out anesthesia drug-related effect on monitoring signals.
  - Surgeon may consider supplemental test of neuro function (eg, wake-up test).
  - Surgeon may release surgical traction likely contributing to neuro impairment.
- Emergence
  - Minimize excessive coughing, especially if spine is unstable.
  - Consider moving pt off OR table onto hospital bed before emergence.
  - If a repair is staged or incomplete, pt may be placed in a brace to prevent movement w/ an unstable spine.
    - Check if brace will cause pressure ulcers or limit respiratory function.

POSTOP

Pain
- Moderate to severe
- Severe pain more likely w/ surgery involving multiple levels, especially in pt w/ preop chronic pain & chronic narcotic use
- IV narcotics via PCA are the mainstay of therapy
- Intraop, surgeon may inject intrathecal morphine (5–8 mcg/kg) under direct vision. This can provide analgesia for approximately 24 h
  - Intrathecal fentanyl (25–50 mcg in adult) can also be added.

Complications
- Hematologic
  - Persistent bleeding
  - Thrombocytopenia
- Respiratory
  - Upper airway edema from transfusions or neck dissection
  - Pneumothorax
  - Transfusion-associated acute lung injury
  - Respiratory failure from other causes
  - DVT, pulmonary embolism
  - Fat embolism
- CNS
  - Dural tear
  - Spinal cord ischemia, new neuro deficits
- Cardiac
  - Persistent hypovolemia
  - Hemodynamic instability
- Sepsis

SURGICAL PROCEDURE

Indications
- Scoliosis or kyphosis
  - >60 degrees (absolute indication).
  - >40 degrees (relative indication).
- Neuromuscular disorders (cerebral palsy, muscular dystrophy).
- Instability.
- Osteomyelitis.
- Tumor.

Procedure
- Posterior approaches.
  - Prone position.
  - Dissection down to the lamina & spinal processes through the paraspinous & erector spinae muscles of the back.
- Anterior approaches
  - An anterior cervicothoracic approach for high T-spine procedures will involve resection of clavicle & part of first rib to gain exposure to spine. This approach will also involve collapse of the lung on the operative side to gain access to the spine through the pleural space.

➤ A transthoracic approach for mid T-spine procedures is accomplished through a thoracotomy incision w/ pt in lateral position. There is a risk of damage to lung parenchyma & vascular structures that may necessitate rib removal & lung deflation on the operative side.

➤ An anterior transdiaphragmatic approach for lower T-spine procedures requires an incision to free the diaphragm on one side of the body to allow entrance into the thoracic & the retroperitoneal regions.

➤ Anterior abdominal approaches (T- & L-spine procedures) are classified as transperitoneal (done in supine position) or retroperitoneal (lateral position). The retroperitoneal surgery requires less bowel manipulation.

■ From a variety of different positions, dissection is performed to get to the level of the spine.

■ Anterior fusions require removal of the vertebrae & disks.

■ Posterior fusions involve removal of the lamina & processes surrounding the spinal cord.

■ Great care is taken to avoid damaging structures in the surgical field. These structures vary depending on the approach, but can include

➤ Dura, spinal cord.

➤ Nerve roots.

➤ Blood vessels.

➤ Ureters.

➤ Major abdominal & thoracic organs.

➤ Major structures in the neck.

■ Decortication of bone & dissection near the epidural veins are high-risk areas for blood loss & air or fat emboli.

■ Once the spinal cord is exposed, grafts, rods, and/or screws will be used to re-establish the structure & continuity of the spine.

■ When reconstruction & fusion are complete, the layers of tissue are closed.

■ If there is still a question of instability, pt may be placed in a brace for the postop period to allow for healing, or as a bridge to a future procedure (staged repair).

Surgical Concerns

■ Hemorrhage.

➤ Significant blood loss occurs during resection of vertebrae & scraping muscle & tissues off the spine.

➤ Massive bleeding can occur from damage to epidural veins, spinal arteries or larger vascular structures that need to be circumvented during resection (aorta, iliac, renal vessels).
- Neuro injury
  ➤ Spinal cord ischemia from direct damage or surgical retraction, especially when vertebrae have been removed & the cord is unprotected.

Typical EBL
- 200–5,000 mL or higher, depending on pathology & extent of surgery.
- Blood loss can increase to multiple blood volumes.

SPLENECTOMY

JASON WIDRICH, MD

PREOP

Preop Considerations
- Indications for splenectomy include diverse conditions.
  ➤ Hematologic.
    - Immune thrombocytopenia.
    - Spherocytosis.
    - Beta-thalassemia.
    - Sickle cell disease.
    - Autoimmune hemolytic anemia.
  ➤ Malignancy.
    - Leukemia.
    - Lymphoma (Hodgkin's & non-Hodgkin's).
  ➤ Trauma.
  ➤ Splenic disease.
    - Abscess
    - Cyst
    - Aneurysm
- Note underlying disease process & any systemic manifestations.
  ➤ For instance, effects of prior chemotherapy for malignancy.
- For trauma, may be part of laparotomy for intra-abdominal bleeding.
  ➤ Pt may have other injuries secondary to blunt or penetrating trauma.
- Procedure may be performed laparoscopically, especially if spleen is normal size.

Physical Findings
- Potential splenomegaly.
- Bruising, bleeding or petechiae related to thrombocytopenia.

Workup
- CBC, PT, PTT.
- Other workup based on coexisting disease.
- Pneumococcal vaccine to prevent overwhelming sepsis.
- Type & cross-match for PRBCs.
- Consider platelet transfusion for thrombocytopenia.

Choice of Anesthesia
- GA.
- For open procedure, consider thoracic epidural catheter for analgesia.
  - Assess coag status & risk of epidural hematoma before proceeding w/ regional anesthesia.
  - Thrombocytopenia is common in pts requiring splenectomy.

INTRAOP

Monitors/Line Placement
- Standard monitors.
- One or two large-bore peripheral IVs.
- Arterial line & central line depending on coexisting disease & setting of splenectomy (eg, trauma pt w/ bleeding vs elective laparoscopic surgery).

Intraop Concerns
- Incision may be midline, subcostal or laparoscopic.
  - See also Procedures chapter "Laparoscopic General Surgery."
- Position may be supine or lateral.
- Trauma pt
  - Blood loss could be much greater if splenic repair is planned rather than splenectomy.
  - Approx 25% of all traumatic splenic injuries require splenectomy.
- Surgeon may convert a laparoscopic approach to open procedure for a variety of reasons, including hemorrhage, bowel perforation or difficult exposure.
- Muscle relaxation & controlled ventilation preferable for both open abdominal & laparoscopic procedures.
- Pneumothorax.

Intraop Therapies
- Platelet transfusion may be required after splenic resection.
  - Prior to splenectomy, platelet transfusion may result in minimal increase in platelet count.
- Consider antiemetic prophylaxis.

POSTOP

Pain
- Mild to moderate
  - Laparoscopic approach less painful than open surgery
- PCA
- Epidural analgesia for open procedures

Complications
- Postop atelectasis, splinting, respiratory failure
- Shoulder pain referred from diaphragmatic irritation
- Bleeding
- DVT, pulmonary embolism
- Thrombocytopenia
- Injury to pancreas, stomach or colon
- Sepsis
- Subphrenic abscess
- Pneumothorax

SURGICAL PROCEDURE

Indications
- Hematologic
  - Immune thrombocytopenia
  - Spherocytosis
  - Beta-thalassemia
  - Sickle cell disease
  - Autoimmune hemolytic anemia
- Malignancy
  - Leukemia
  - Lymphoma (Hodgkin's & non-Hodgkin's)
- Trauma
- Splenic disease
  - Abscess
  - Cyst
  - Aneurysm

Procedure
- Skin incision or laparoscopic port placement
- Colon is mobilized
- Accessory splenic tissue is identified
- Short gastric vessels are ligated
- Spleen is mobilized
- Splenic artery & vein are isolated & ligated
- Spleen is resected
  - ➤ For laparoscopic procedure, spleen may be morselized & removed through laparoscopic port, or additional incision may be made
- Adequate hemostasis is achieved.
- Closure

Surgical Concerns
- Hemorrhage
- Infection/sepsis related to encapsulated bacteria
- Injury to colon, stomach or pancreas
- Subphrenic abscess
- Portal vein thrombosis (rare but potentially fatal)
- Pneumothorax

Typical EBL
- Laparoscopic: <500 mL
- Open procedures: 500–1,000 mL or greater, depending on setting

---

STRABISMUS SURGERY

ATSUKO BABA, MD

PREOP

Preop Considerations
- Malalignment of the visual axis can be congenital or acquired
- Assoc w/
  - ➤ Myelomeningocele
  - ➤ Traumatic cranial nerve palsies
  - ➤ Congenital myopathy
  - ➤ Congenital syndromes (Apert, Crouzon, Down)
- Virtually all require surgery for correction
- Outcome is improved w/ early intervention

- Incidence of malignant hyperthermia is increased in pts undergoing strabismus repair; take a thorough personal/family history of malignant hyperthermia susceptibility
- Strabismus is relatively common (5% of population); male:female incidence is approx equal

Physical Findings
- Ocular malalignment

Workup
- Testing for malignant hyperthermia is controversial. The most accurate test is the in vitro halothane/caffeine contracture test, but this is performed in less than 20 U.S. centers. Serum creatinine phosphokinase can be used as a screening test but is normal in 30% of susceptible pts
- ECG & echo may be indicated in pts w/ associated myopathies to rule out coexisting cardiac dysfunction

Choice of Anesthesia
- General endotracheal anesthesia

INTRAOP

Monitors/Line Placement
- Standard monitoring.
- IV access can be obtained after a mask induction, if mask induction is not contraindicated.
- Monitor vigilantly for signs of malignant hyperthermia:
  - Unexplained tachycardia.
  - Increased end-tidal CO_2.
  - Muscular rigidity.
  - Masseter spasm.
  - Increased temp (a late finding).

Intraop Concerns
- Phenylephrine 1–10% may be used to induce mydriasis & hemostasis; minimal amounts of 1–2.5% phenylephrine will avoid significant systemic HTN.
- Alternative agents that induce mydriasis but do not induce systemic HTN are cyclopentolate 0.5% & tropicamide 0.5%.
- Traction on the extraocular muscles can cause vagal stimulation via the trigeminal-vagal reflex, typically causing sinus bradycardia, but can also cause other dysrhythmias; HR increases rapidly when traction is released.

- The oculocardiac reflex may diminish as the surgery proceeds secondary to fatigue.
- Succinylcholine use can cause extraocular muscle contraction rather than paralysis for up to 15 min; this can alter the results of the forced duction test performed by the ophthalmologist to estimate any restriction in movement of the extraocular muscles.

Intraop Therapies

- Bradycardia caused by the oculocardiac reflex usually resolves w/ release of tension on the extraocular muscles, but if the bradycardia is severe or does not resolve, treatment is required: atropine for bradycardia & lidocaine for other dysrhythmias.
- The oculocardiac reflex is prevented by a retrobulbar block via the afferent limb of the trigeminal-vagal reflex.
- Dantrolene should be readily available to treat an episode of malignant hyperthermia.

POSTOP

Pain

- Acetaminophen and/or opioids (intraop/postop opioids may increase postop nausea/vomiting)

Complications

- Postop nausea/vomiting common (50–80%); no one antiemetic has been shown to consistently decrease postop nausea/vomiting in this population

SURGICAL PROCEDURE

Indications

- Strabismus

Procedure

- Shortening/lengthening of extraocular muscles to straighten the eyes cosmetically & to allow binocular vision

Surgical Concerns

- Adjustable suture approach can be used in adults & cooperative older children; an adjustable suture is tied in the extraocular muscles to allow shortening/lengthening postop.
- Continued malalignment in 30%
- Infection

Typical EBL

- Minimal

TETRALOGY OF FALLOT (TOF) REPAIR

KIM SKIDMORE, MD

PREOP

Preop Considerations

■ Most common cyanotic congenital heart disease
■ Incidence: 0.3/1,000 live births
■ The four components of TOF are:
➤ Right ventricular outflow tract obstruction (RVOTO)
  • Usually infundibular (ie, subvalvar) but also can be valvar and/or supravalvar
➤ Right ventricular hypertrophy
➤ VSD w/ R-to-L shunt when cyanotic (& L-to-R shunt often)
➤ Overriding aorta
■ Common coexisting cardiac conditions
➤ 11% chance of persistent left superior vena cava (may require cannulation during bypass if large; drains into the coronary sinus, making it always enlarged)
➤ 25% chance of right aortic arch
➤ 8% chance of abnormal coronary arteries
■ Pt probably has "tet spells" (ie, hypercyanotic spells when agitated).
➤ Pt may not have hypoxemia (aka "pink tet") if right ventricular outflow tract obstruction is minimal.

Workup

■ CXR
➤ Boot-shaped heart from right ventricular hypertrophy
■ ECG
➤ Right ventricular hypertrophy
➤ Right atrial dilation
➤ Right bundle branch block
■ Echo
➤ For evaluation of pulmonic valve, coronary arteries, VSD

Choice of Anesthesia

■ Premed
➤ If >12 mo of age, may give 0.5–1 mg/kg PO Versed, not to exceed 20 mg
➤ If pt refuses oral premed, consider ketamine 1 mg/kg IV or 4 mg/kg IM
■ GA can be induced by either inhaled or IV route

INTRAOP

Monitors/Line Placement
- Two peripheral IVs.
- Arterial line.
- ACT to manage heparin dosing.
- TEE.

Intraop Concerns
- Bleeding is more likely if the procedure is a reoperation.
- Surgeon will ligate patent ductus arteriosis (PDA) or Blalock Taussig shunt upon initiation of bypass to minimize shunting & hypoperfusion.
  - Under stress a PDA may reopen up to age 1 year, so many centers elect to ligate the PDA during all cardiac operations in infants, even if a preop echo does not reveal a PDA.
- For significant hypoxemia during case
  - Increase SVR w/
    - Neo-Synephrine 3 mcg/kg.
    - Ketamine 1 mg/kg IV.
    - Direct abdominal pressure.
    - Elevation of legs.
  - Less helpful but may work: decrease PVR w/ hyperventilation & increased FIO_2.
  - If desaturation persists, decrease RVOTO by IV fluids, decreased inotropy, decreased HR (eg, halothane or esmolol).
- If there is right ventricular dysfunction postbypass, a patent foramen ovale may be created as a pressure pop-off.
- If there is poor ventricular function, the chest may be left open for a few days.

POSTOP

Pain
- Moderate
- Pts usually remain intubated after procedure & receive IV opiates

Complications
- Complete heart block
  - May resolve as edema disappears within 7 days
  - Permanent pacemaker may be placed to intraop epicardial leads
- Residual VSD
- Aortic regurgitation or tricuspid regurgitation
  - May develop if VSD patch closure changed cusps or flow pattern

- Right ventricular dysfunction
  - Likely if pulmonary hypertension is severe, or if ventriculotomy was required to resect significant amounts of infundibulum
  - Pulmonic regurgitation & right ventricular dysfunction are very common several years after repair, especially when repaired by transannular patch
- Residual right ventricular outflow tract obstruction
- Ventricular tachycardia
  - Late mortality may occur from ventricular tachycardia, especially if repair was late in life & the right ventricle developed more abnormally
- Pulmonary hypertension
- Pulmonic stenosis
  - May occur w/ cryopreserved conduit material, because it does not grow as the child grows

SURGICAL PROCEDURE

Indications
- TOF

Procedure
- Goals of total repair include
  - Close the VSD
  - Open the RV outflow obstruction
  - Repair any pulmonary artery stenosis
- Specific steps may include
  - Pulmonic valve commissurotomy involves repair of the pulmonic valve, desirable when it is not too dysplastic
  - Transannular patch placement
  - Conduit of homograft material from right ventricle to pulmonary artery, including a valve
  - VSD patch
  - Resection of excessive muscle in the right ventricle outflow tract

Surgical Concerns
- Residual VSD
- AV block
- Residual RV outflow tract subpulmonic, pulmonic, or branch stenosis or regurgitation at the valve

Typical EBL
- Infants require blood to prime the cardiopulmonary bypass machine
- Postbypass, blood not always required

THORACOSCOPY

LYDIA CASSORLA, MD

PREOP

Preop Considerations
- Wide range of pt conditions: end-stage lung disease to healthy pts w/ spontaneous pneumothorax or pulmonary nodule.
- Assess pt's ability to tolerate one-lung ventilation (OLV).
- Anemia or low cardiac output will reduce SpO_2 if an intrapulmonary shunt is present during OLV.

Physical Findings
- Depend on pt condition.

Workup
- Assess pulmonary function; evaluation depends on lung disease present (see Procedure chapter "Thoracotomy & Lung Resection").
- Hemoglobin.
- CXR.
- Look for signs or findings of pulmonary hypertension as OLV is less well tolerated when pulmonary hypertension is present (see Coexisting Disease chapter "Pulmonary Hypertension").

Choice of Anesthesia
- GA
- OLV
    - ➤ Any technique acceptable; however, double-lumen ETT often results in more rapid lung collapse than bronchial blocker or UNIVENT tube due to larger lumen for gas to escape nonventilated lung.
    - ➤ CPAP is not possible with bronchial blocker; choose another technique for compromised pts.
- Muscle relaxation not required.
- Consider regional anesthesia or regional narcotics if chest tube placed at end of procedure.
- Extubation at end of procedure is desired.

INTRAOP

Monitors/Line Placement
- Monitor pulse in dependent arm to detect axillary compression.

■ Arterial line: useful in management of OLV in pts at risk of desaturation; in healthier pts an arterial line may not be required.

Intraop Concerns
■ Procedure requires OLV; be prepared for CPAP O_2 to nonventilated lung if persistent perfusion results in significant desaturation.
■ Despite successful OLV, the nonventilated lung may collapse very slowly or incompletely when severe lung disease is present; prepare the surgeon!
■ Thoracoscopic procedures often take more time than equivalent open procedures.
■ In pts w/ global lung disease or desaturation, blood gas determination during OLV may assist in mgt.

Intraop Therapies
■ Be prepared for CPAP if OLV not tolerated. Surgical exposure may be compromised by CPAP, however.
■ Expand lungs & maintain 30 cm H_2O inspiratory pressure during final closure of chest if no chest tube is placed.
■ Consider use of local anesthesia for dermatomes w/ incisions.

POSTOP

Pain
■ Incisional pain minimal if thorax not opened
■ Chest tubes add to discomfort significantly if used

Complications
■ Failure to achieve surgical goals w/o open thoracotomy
■ Bronchopleural fistula
■ Damage to pulmonary artery or vein
■ Pneumothorax
■ Hemothorax
■ Damage to intercostal vessel or nerve

SURGICAL PROCEDURE

Indications
■ Expanding. Include need for tissue diagnosis of pulmonary disease, pulmonary bleb, pulmonary nodule, severe COPD (lung volume reduction surgery), patent ductus arteriosus, pneumothorax, esophageal disease.

Procedure
- A wide variety of procedures are performed, including surgery for lung biopsy, pulmonary bleb resection, pulmonary nodule resection, lung volume reduction, patent ductus arteriosus, pleurodesis, esophageal resection.

Surgical Concerns
- Proximity of great vessels, heart, lungs, major airways.

Typical EBL
- Minimal unless complication occurs.

THORACOTOMY & LUNG RESECTION

JAMES JUSTICE, MD
LYDIA CASSORLA, MD

PREOP

Preop Considerations
- Pts are at high risk for pulmonary complications due to site of surgery
- Coexisting pulmonary diseases may include
  - COPD
  - Regional lung disease & atelectasis
  - Tumors w/ large blood flow that may cause significant right-to-left shunt
  - Reactive airway disease
  - Pneumonia
  - Pleural effusion
  - Empyema
- Coexisting cardiovascular diseases may include
  - CAD
  - HTN
  - Pulmonary HTN
  - Right ventricular hypertrophy or failure
  - SVT
- For pts w/ lung cancer, look for paraneoplastic syndromes (Cushing's, Eaton-Lambert, hypercalcemia, hyponatremia).
- Optimize preop pulmonary function
  - Stop smoking
  - Consider/continue bronchodilation
  - Consider/continue antibiotics or steroids

➤ Ensure adequate pulmonary toilet
  - Hydrate & clear secretions
  - Consider mucolytics & expectorants
  - Administer chest PT if appropriate
■ Optimize & stabilize other medical problems
■ Discuss & educate patient about postop incentive spirometer use & provide motivation for postop respiratory care

Physical Findings
■ May be minimal depending on the diagnosis, but possible findings include
  ➤ Hoarseness
  ➤ Tracheal deviation
  ➤ Abnormal oxygen saturation or cyanosis
  ➤ Tachypnea
  ➤ Prolonged expiratory phase of respiration
  ➤ Decreased breath sounds, rales, ronchi, wheezing
  ➤ Decreased heart tones, cardiac murmurs, irregular heartbeat, signs of elevated right-sided pressures or pulmonary HTN (precordial heave, loud or unsplit P2, S4 or S3, distended neck veins, hepatic congestion, edema)
  ➤ Horner's syndrome
  ➤ Superior vena cava syndrome (face & upper extremity flushing, edema, poor tracheal air movement)

Workup
■ Assess exercise tolerance
■ Assess pulmonary function: preop pulmonary function is highly predictive of postop success
■ Important risk factors for lobectomy
  ➤ Stair climbing <3 flights
  ➤ Predicted postoperative FEV_1 <1 L or 40–50% predicted
  ➤ Significant hypercapnia ($PaCO_2$ >45 on room air)
  ➤ Maximum oxygen consumption <10–15 mL/kg/min
  ➤ RV/TLC >50%
  ➤ Predicted postop FEV_1 >40–50% acceptable for lobectomy
■ For pneumonectomy
  ➤ Stair climbing <5 flights
  ➤ Hypercapnia on room air
  ➤ FEV_1 <2 L or 50% predicted or 50% of FVC
  ➤ $FEF_{25-75\%}$ <50% predicted

- ➤ Predicted postop DLCO <40%
- ➤ Predicted postop FEV_2 0.85L or <70% blood flow to remaining lung
- ➤ Max oxygen consumption <10–15 mL/kg/min
- ➤ Unilateral balloon occlusion of pulmonary artery or mainstem bronchus on operative side results in mean PAP >40 mmHg, severe dyspnea, $PaCO_2$ >60 mmHg, or PaO_2 <45 mmHg
- ■ Review history for bronchoscopy findings of intrabronchial lesion; may affect ability to place double-lumen ETT (DLET)
- ■ Look for signs or history of pulmonary hypertension, as one-lung ventilation (OLV) less well tolerated.
- ■ Cardiac workup as indicated
    - ➤ Echocardiogram can assess right & left heart function
    - ➤ PA systolic pressure can usually be estimated by echo
- ■ CXR
    - ➤ Assess tracheobronchial tree
    - ➤ Look for bullae
    - ➤ Look for signs of pulmonary hypertension (enlarged, redistributed vascular markings)
- ■ ECG: look for RVH, RAE, RAD, ischemia, supraventricular arrhythmia
- ■ ABG if indicated by findings
- ■ CBC, BUN, Cr
- ■ CT or MRI can identify compromised tracheal lumen or lung bullae

Choice of Anesthesia
- ■ Consider thoracic (T6) or lumber epidural for postop pain control. Spinal narcotic a second choice if epidural not possible
- ■ GA w/ controlled ventilation required, usually w/ OLV
- ■ Combined regional/general techniques w/ excellent postop analgesia ideal for rapid extubation & optimal pulmonary function
- ■ IV or inhalational techniques acceptable
    - ➤ Inhalation agents usually do not inhibit hypoxic pulmonary vasoconstriction (HPV) or increase shunting clinically & may enhance bronchodilation
    - ➤ Narcotic-based techniques must not depend upon N2O for amnesia, as high FIO2 required during OLV
- ■ Advantages of OLV include optimal surgical exposure & lung isolation from secretions & blood. Strongest indications are:
    - ➤ Pneumonectomy & upper lobectomy
    - ➤ Posterior thoracic procedures (eg, involving aorta or spine)
    - ➤ Large bronchopleural fistula

> Prevention of spillage of blood, pus, or fluid from one lung to another
> See also Technique chapter "Double-Lumen Endobronchial Tube Placement."
- Major risks of OLV
  > Difficulty w/ DLET or bronchial blocker insertion or positioning
  > Potential for hypoxia
  > Difficulties related to reduced airway diameter
- Contraindications to instrumenting a mainstem bronchus w/ a double-lumen tube or bronchial blocker include a mass in the bronchus
  > Consider DLET on the contralateral side

INTRAOP

Monitors/Line Placement
- Multiple large-bore peripheral IV access needed to treat rapid hemorrhage if pulmonary artery or vein inadvertently disrupted.
- Arterial line for BP & ABG monitoring.
- CVP monitor if indicated by pt condition, or if lobectomy or larger resection planned.
  > Limitations include COPD & lateral position, which render absolute values less useful than trends.
  > Placement on side of thoracotomy prevents risk of pneumothorax on nonsurgical side.
- Pulmonary artery (PA) catheter may be useful for certain pts (eg, if pneumonectomy planned) or left heart disease, right heart failure, or pulmonary HTN present.
  > Pts are at high risk for pulmonary artery rupture from PA catheter.
    • Float into wedge position if measurement desired; otherwise keep catheter just past pulmonary valve, especially during lung manipulation.
- Fluid warmer.
- Forced air warmer for lower body.

Intraop Concerns
- Proper placement of DLET (see Technique chapter "Double-Lumen Endobronchial Tube Placement").
- Choice of DLET or bronchial blocker, including UNIVENT, according to clinical indications & expertise.

- ➤ If DLET is chosen, left-sided tube preferred for all procedures unless contraindicated by left mainstem bronchial mass or narrowing.
- ➤ CPAP is not possible with bronchial blocker; choose another technique for compromised pts.
- ➤ Check DLET or bronchial blocker placement w/ fiberscope before & after lateral positioning. CXR a possible alternative to confirm positioning if fiberscope not available.
- ■ Avoid light anesthesia to minimize risk of bronchospasm or pulmonary HTN. Muscle relaxants, narcotics & volatile anesthetics may reduce bronchospasm & enhance ventilation.
- ■ Muscle relaxation ideal to facilitate intercostal incision but may not be necessary during thoracotomy w/ a chest retractor.
- ■ High risk of positioning complications (eg, brachial plexus, dependent ear & eye).
  - ➤ Verify proper arm support frequently during surgery, as incision alters structural integrity of support.
- ■ Assess PO2 & relationship of end-tidal to arterial CO2 after positioning & after initiation of OLV.
- ■ Pts w/ COPD or bronchospasm are at high risk for lung hyperinflation w/ potential for hemodynamic compromise (dynamic hyperinflation).
  - ➤ Maximize expiratory time & consider intentional hypoventilation, especially during OLV.
- ■ Use N2O w/ caution due to risk of expansion of pneumothorax & potential for pulmonary hypertension. 100% oxygen often required during OLV.
- ■ In healthy pts, tidal volume may be maintained w/ OLV; however, if COPD is present, reductions may be indicated. Keep PIP <30–35 cm H_2O to minimize risk of pneumothorax in dependent lung.
- ■ Hypoxia early in course of OLV usually due to persistent perfusion of nonventilated lung. Treatment options include
  - ➤ CPAP to nondependent lung.
  - ➤ Intermittent collapsed lung hand ventilation.
  - ➤ PEEP to dependent lung (only after CPAP to nondependent lung).
  - ➤ Anesthetic management to minimize PA pressure.
  - ➤ Hypoxia can be eliminated if surgeon clamps PA; however, not all pts will tolerate this, so watch for signs of pulmonary HTN or right heart failure.
- ■ Desaturation after 10–15 min of OLV usually due to shunt in ventilated lung.

- ➤ Verify DLET or bronchial blocker position.
- ➤ Clear secretions or blood.
- ➤ Adjust ventilatory parameters.
- Pneumonectomy
  - ➤ If PAC in place, pull back to main PA.
  - ➤ Assess pulmonary pressure & right heart function w/ trial clamping of pulmonary artery. Adjust anesthetic and/or vasoactive drug therapy appropriately.
  - ➤ If left pneumonectomy, may require reposition of DLET when bronchus ligated.
  - ➤ Avoid hyperinflation of remaining lung. Consider intentional hypoventilation if necessary to avoid this.
  - ➤ Do not connect drain to suction, as negative intrapleural pressure on operative side may cause mediastinal shift & hemodynamic compromise.
- Hand ventilate & observe lung when re-expanding OLV-induced atelectasis.
- Minimize coughing on emergence & plan for earliest possible extubation to minimize risk of bronchopleural fistula or other barotrauma.
  - ➤ Consider IV or tracheal lidocaine, narcotics.
  - ➤ Suction trachea to remove secretions prior to extubation.
- If postop intubation desired, convert to single-lumen ETT whenever possible. Use tube changer if difficult intubation.

POSTOP

Pain

- Typically severe due to incision & chest tubes.
- Epidural narcotic and/or local anesthetic most effective. Intrapleural catheter & intercostal nerve blocks less effective.
- Pain predisposes to pulmonary complications.

Complications

- Atelectasis results from pain & splinting, retained secretions or blood.
  - ➤ Suctioning, upright position, deep breathing, cough may improve atelectasis. Bronchoscopy may be indicated.
- Bronchopleural fistula common & may compromise ventilation.
  - ➤ Usually results from poor integrity of suture/staple line of bronchial stump & resolves in a few days.

- Risk of pneumothorax if chest tube not functioning or recurrent bronchopleural fistula after D/C of chest tube.
- Postop pulmonary infections occur w/ prolonged intubation or chest tube placement.
  - ➤ Proactive pain control & pulmonary toilet indicated.
- Cardiac dysrhythmias are common.
- Left recurrent laryngeal nerve injury may result in vocal cord palsy. Does not usually result in stridor or airway obstruction.
- Phrenic nerve injury will result in paralysis & elevation of hemidiaphragm & possible respiratory compromise.
- Considerations for pneumonectomy
  - ➤ If pericardium opened (intrapericardial pneumonectomy) & not adequately repaired, heart may herniate into operative side of chest, esp if drain connected to suction. Usually results in decreased preload from kinked cavae, MI, or death. This is an acute surgical emergency. Have high suspicion if arrhythmia, elevated peak airway pressures, or cardiac arrest occurs postop.

SURGICAL PROCEDURE
Indications
- Tumor, infection, bronchiectasis, bullae, COPD, pneumothorax, lung transplant, descending aortic surgery, thoracic spine surgery, hemoptysis.

Procedure
- Lateral decubitus position.
- Posterolateral intercostal incision, usually T4-T8. Partial rib resection may be necessary for exposure.
- OLV or compression of lung necessary.
- Diseased segment, lobe, or whole lung isolated w/ control of bronchus, artery & vein prior to excision. Chest tube placed following lobectomy but contraindicated after pneumonectomy. (Drain is placed & should not be connected to suction.)

Surgical Concerns
- Pts w/ previous pulmonary disease or radiation may have scarring & significant bleeding from dissection.
- All pts at risk for inadvertent tear of pulmonary vein or artery.
- Surgeon may compress heart, vena cavae, great vessels or cause arrhythmia.
- Trauma to lung tissue & airways.

- Systemic air embolus from open pulmonary vein.
- All pericardial defects should be closed, using prosthetic material if necessary, to prevent cardiac herniation.
- Bronchopulmonary fistula.

Typical EBL
- 150–300 mL for uncomplicated lobectomy.
- Pneumonectomy or tumor resection may result in large blood loss.

THYROIDECTOMY

ANNEMARIE THOMPSON, MD

PREOP

Preop Considerations
- Euthyroid state is preferred for elective surgery
  - Mild/moderate hypothyroidism has not been assoc w/ adverse surgical outcomes
  - If pt has myxedema coma, thyroid replacement is indicated preop
- If pt is hyperthyroid & needs thyroidectomy urgently/emergently, be ready to manage excessive sympathetic activity/thyroid storm (see below).
- Potential coexisting diseases
  - Myopathies
  - Myasthenia gravis
  - Other autoimmune diseases
- Physical exam: Ask about positional dyspnea, stridor, hoarseness

Workup
- Preop thyroid function tests
  - TSH
  - Free T4
- CXR and/or chest CT if thyroid mass extends into mediastinum to look for airway narrowing
- Flow-volume loops if intrathoracic mass w/ uncharacterized obstruction

Choice of Anesthesia
- GA most commonly used

INTRAOP

Monitors/Line Placement

- Peripheral IV & other monitors as indicated by pt's periop medical problems
- If large thyroid/thyroid mass is present, be aware of potential altered airway anatomy
  - ➤ May need fiberoptic intubation
- If thyroid mass extends into mediastinum w/ tracheal/mainstem bronchus compression, refer to chapter on "Mediastinal Mass."

Intraop Concerns

- Thyroid storm is a potential life-threatening complication in pts w/ a history of hyperthyroidism. Treatment includes
  - ➤ Propranolol/esmolol
  - ➤ IV fluids
  - ➤ Sodium iodide 250 mg IV q6h
  - ➤ Propylthiouracil 200–400 PO/NGT 6 h
  - ➤ Hydrocortisone 100 mg IV q6h
  - ➤ Consider antipyretics & external cooling for fever

POSTOP

Pain

- Typically minimal

Complications

- Bleeding & neck hematoma causing life-threatening airway compromise due to neck swelling & tracheal deviation.
  - ➤ Mgt
    - Notify surgeon & OR immediately because hematoma can enlarge rapidly.
    - Prepare equipment for difficult airway mgt prior to intubation attempts. Consider tracheal intubation before development of stridor.
    - If pt has airway obstruction or respiratory symptoms that could be related to neck hematoma, remove neck sutures at pt's bedside to decompress the hematoma. This may improve mask ventilation & ease of direct laryngoscopy.
    - Ask surgeon to prepare equip for tracheotomy or cricothyrotomy in case of failed intubation.
- Recurrent laryngeal nerve injury (either unilateral, resulting in hoarseness, or bilateral, which can result in aphonia & stridor).

- Pneumothorax.
- Hypocalcemia/hypoparathyroidism.
  - Unintentional removal of parathyroid glands will cause serum calcium to decrease within 24 h, nadir within 3–7 days.
  - Pt may develop signs of hypocalcemia, including laryngeal spasm.
  - Treatment is calcium chloride or calcium gluconate.

SURGICAL PROCEDURE

Indications
- Large toxic multinodular goiters
- Solitary toxic adenomas
- Thyroid nodules suspicious for cancer

Procedure
- Neck exploration w/ subtotal thyroidectomy/mediasternotomy (if thyroid mass extends into thorax)

Surgical Concerns
- Postop bleeding
- Recurrent laryngeal nerve injury
- Postop hypocalcemia
- Pneumothorax

Typical EBL
- <50 mL

TONSILLECTOMY & ADENOIDECTOMY

RENÉE J. ROBERTS, MD

PREOP

Preop Considerations
- Pt may have associated URI.
- Indication for surgery may include airway obstructive symptoms or acute peritonsillar abscess.

Physical Findings
- May include
  - Chronic nasal obstruction.
  - Poor feeding.
  - Obstructive sleep apnea.

- CO_2 retention.
- Pts w/ craniofacial abnormalities may have pre-existing difficult airways.

Workup
- Make sure there are no pre-existing bleeding disorders.
- Obstructive sleep apnea from tonsillar hypertrophy may lead to pulmonary HTN & RV failure; if suspected this should be evaluated.

Choice of Anesthesia
- GA.
  - Inhaled induction is used in children who will not tolerate IV.
- Oral RAE ETT is usually used for intubation.

INTRAOP

Monitors/Line Placement
- One peripheral IV.
- Standard monitors.

Intraop Concerns
- Pt may have difficult mask ventilation or intubation due to tonsillar swelling or hypertrophy.
- Placement of oral retractor by surgeon may cause ETT obstruction, w/ increased peak airway pressure.
  - After removal of retractor, examine tongue for swelling.

Intraop Therapies
- Consider antiemetic.
  - Occasionally Decadron 0.25 mg/kg is used to reduce swelling.
  - In children 40 mg/kg Tylenol PR for pain control, in addition to narcotics.

POSTOP

Pain
- Mild to moderate
- Visual analog scale pain score 3–4 after adenoidectomy, 7–9 after tonsillectomy

Complications
- Bleeding
  - In severe cases, this may require re-exploration. This may pose an anesthetic challenge because of

- Hypovolemia from bleeding (more susceptible to hypotension on induction)
- Full stomach from swallowed blood
- Potential for aspiration of blood
  - ➤ Lack of pt cooperation increases difficulty of mgt
- Airway obstruction
- Apnea
- Nausea/vomiting

SURGICAL PROCEDURE

Indications
- Recurrent infections
- Obstruction from hypertrophic tonsils

Procedure
- Local infiltration of tonsillar bed w/ local anesthetic w/ epinephrine
- Placement of throat pack
- Dissection & removal of tonsils
- Hemostasis
- NG suction after throat packs removed

Surgical Concerns
- Excessive bleeding
- Removal of throat pack

Typical EBL
- Variable; blood loss can be occult because blood may be swallowed during or after the procedure

---

TOTAL ABDOMINAL HYSTERECTOMY

JASON WIDRICH, MD

PREOP

Preop Considerations
- Hysterectomy can be performed through abdominal or vaginal approach.
  - ➤ Abdominal hysterectomy is used for pts w/ previous surgeries, larger resections, large uterus, or decreased pelvic inlet.

- Abdominal hysterectomy may be combined w/ bilateral salpingo-oophorectomy & extensive lymph node dissection as part of surgery for cancer.
- Pulmonary involvement or pleural effusion may be present in pts w/ cancer.
- Hypovolemia or anemia may be present if indication for surgery is severe uterine bleeding.
- Pt may have abnormal coagulation because of cancer or chemotherapy.
- Pt will likely have bowel prep the evening before surgery.

Physical Findings
- None typical. May have palpable mass in lower abdomen.

Workup
- CBC.
- Further workup based on coexisting disease.
- Consider type & screen.

Choice of Anesthesia
- GA is most often performed, especially for pts requiring larger or prolonged resections.
- Spinal or epidural may also be acceptable; should cover to T4–6 level.
    - ➤ Pt w/ obesity or pulmonary disease may not tolerate steep Trendelenburg position often used during surgery.

INTRAOP
Monitors/Line Placement
- Standard monitors.
- At least one large-bore peripheral IV.
- Foley catheter.
- Consider arterial line & central line for pts who require larger or more extensive resections & those whose cardiovascular status requires more intensive monitoring.

Intraop Concerns
- Blood loss: transfusion may be necessary, especially in anemic pts.
- Muscle relaxation or epidural local anesthetic may be needed to improve surgical exposure.

Intraop Therapies
- Blood loss & IV fluids may cause dilutional coagulopathy.

- Vagal stimulation from grasping the cervix can cause arrhythmias, most often bradycardia.
  - ➤ Treat by stopping the stimulus, increasing anesthetic depth & giving IV glycopyrrolate if bradycardia persists.
- Ephedrine or vasopressin may be injected locally by surgeon to decrease blood loss. HTN or dysrhythmias may result.
- Consider prophylactic antiemetics, as incidence of nausea & vomiting is increased.

POSTOP

Pain
- Moderate
  - ➤ Increased pain more likely in pt w/ extensive dissection
- IV narcotics via PCA, or epidural analgesia

Complications
- Nausea/vomiting (common): can be treated w/ antiemetics
- Anemia or hemorrhage: monitor by following postop Hct & transfuse as needed
- Femoral nerve injury
- Wound infection

SURGICAL PROCEDURE

Indications
- Myomas, endometriosis, dysmenorrhea, GYN cancers.

Procedure
- Pfannenstiel or midline incision
- Uterus is dissected from round, broad & ovarian ligaments.
- Uterine vessels are clamped & tied.
- Uterosacral & cardinal ligaments are ligated.
- Vagina is entered & cervix is removed, at which time uterus may be removed.
- A vaginal cuff is created from the remaining tissue.
- The peritoneum is reapproximated & the abdomen is closed.
- In women in the later stages of child-bearing age, a bilateral salpingo-oophorectomy may be performed as well.

Surgical Concerns
- Bleeding, femoral nerve damage, wound infection.

Typical EBL
- Varies w/ procedure & pathology.
- Ranges from a few hundred milliliters to >1 L.

TOTAL HIP ARTHROPLASTY

HSIUPEI CHEN, MD
MICHAEL GROPPER, MD, PHD

PREOP

Preop Considerations
- If fracture is present, possible preop complications include:
  - Occult blood loss.
  - Dehydration.
  - Hypoxia due to fat embolism (triad of dyspnea, confusion, & petechiae usually present within 72 h of fracture).
  - Thromboembolism.
- Common coexisting diseases in this usually elderly population.
  - Osteoarthritis.
  - Rheumatoid arthritis (RA).
    - In pts w/ severe RA requiring steroids or methotrexate, get lateral c-spine radiograph to assess for atlantoaxial subluxation & need for fiberoptic intubation.
    - For preop steroid use, consider stress-dose steroids; pt may have glucose intolerance, fragile skin, easy bruising.
  - Coronary artery disease.
  - Cerebral vascular disease.
  - COPD.
  - Diabetes.
- If pt has severe pulmonary disease, discuss w/ surgeon need for cemented prosthesis (which may increase pulmonary complications).
- Look for coagulopathy.
  - Surgery assoc w/ high blood loss potential.
  - Correct coagulopathy preop.
  - Consider aprotinin for high-risk bleeding cases.
  - Consider intraop red cell salvage.

Physical Findings
- Pts w/ arthritis may have limited joint mobility in neck & extremities.

■ Most pts (esp elderly) will have limited exercise tolerance because of hip, making cardiopulmonary status more difficult to assess.

Workup
■ CBC.
■ ABG if pt hypoxic & suspected to have fat embolism.
■ Preop EKG to establish risk & baseline.

Choice of Anesthesia
■ GA
  ➤ Advisable in obese pt or arthritic pt w/ anticipated difficult airway.
  ➤ Consider in redo total hip arthroplasty (THA), which is assoc w/ increased blood loss & longer operative times.
  ➤ May be combined w/ spinal or epidural.
■ Spinal anesthesia
  ➤ Consider isobaric local anesthetic to limit cephalad spread & sympathectomy (compared to hyperbaric solution).
  ➤ If pt unable to sit, may administer hypobaric solution w/ pt in lateral decub position.
  ➤ Can administer intrathecal morphine to provide analgesia for up to 24 h.
■ Epidural anesthesia
  ➤ Offers benefit of postop analgesia.
  ➤ Communicate w/ surgeon regarding timing of postop anticoagulation. Remove epidural catheter prior to initiation of anticoagulant therapy to reduce risk of epidural hematoma.
■ Important: Avoid neuraxial blockade in pts receiving preop anticoagulation because of increased risk of epidural hematoma.
■ Neuraxial blockade assoc w/ reduction in blood loss by 30–50%.
■ Hypotensive or regional anesthesia that lowers MAP to ~55 mmHg effective in reducing blood loss.
  ➤ Ensure pt's other organ systems can tolerate this.
  ➤ May want to avoid hypotensive technique in pt w/ significant cardiovascular or cerebrovascular disease.

INTRAOP
Monitors/Line Placement
■ Routine monitors.

- Consider arterial line, which may be useful for close BP monitoring & blood draws.
  - BP often drops during cementing & hardware implantation.
- Central line optional
  - Consider introducer sheath if pt has poor peripheral veins.
  - Consider for pt w/ significant cardiac disease (eg, CHF).
- Adequate peripheral IV access required for fluid resuscitation & blood transfusion.
- Anesthesia usually induced on gurney, especially if pt has significant pain.
- Foley catheter placed after induction.

Intraop Concerns
- Fat embolism syndrome.
  - Clinical triad of dyspnea, confusion, petechiae.
  - Under GA, can present w/ hypotension, petechiae, hypoxemia.
  - Most common during insertion of femoral prosthesis.
  - Mgt includes supportive care, oxygen administration, mechanical ventilation, repair of fracture.
- Bone cement implantation syndrome.
  - Methylmethacrylate cement implicated as cause, although pressurization of cement into femoral canal, as well as surgical manipulation of femoral canal w/ rasps, etc, may be contributing factors.
  - Manifestations include hypoxia, hypotension, dysrhythmias, pulmonary HTN, decreased cardiac output.
  - Most common during insertion of femoral prosthesis
  - Consider prophylaxis w/ increased FiO_2 & maintenance of adequate volume status.
  - Surgeons may place vent in distal femur to decrease intramedullary pressure or perform high-pressure lavage of femoral shaft to remove debris.
  - Mgt includes supportive care (eg, increased oxygen, vasopressors or inotropes).
- Pulmonary embolism
  - May represent a spectrum of fat embolism or cement implantation syndrome.
  - Findings can include hypoxemia & hypotension.
  - Mgt includes supportive care.
  - See also Critical Event chapter "Pulmonary Embolism."

- Hemorrhage
  - Usually visible from operative field, although bleeding into thigh can contribute 500–1,000 ml to EBL.
  - Red cell salvage may be useful in minimizing allogeneic blood transfusion.
- Positioning issues
  - Pt in lateral decubitus, w/ upper arm suspended.
  - Consider axillary roll.
  - Keep spine straight, especially c-spine.
  - Pad & position pt carefully to minimize chance of peripheral nerve injury.

Intraop Therapies
- Consider controlled hypotension to MAP of 55 mmHg if pt does not have significant cardiovascular or cerebrovascular disease.

POSTOP

Pain
- Moderate to severe.
- Consider intrathecal or epidural morphine. Watch for respiratory depression, esp in elderly pts.
- Consider PCA if pt did not receive epidural or spinal analgesia.

Complications
- Postop hemorrhage usually monitored by following drain output. Some surgeons use postop cell salvage from drain.
- Pts at high risk of DVT & pulmonary embolism. Pts usually receive DVT prophylaxis with low-molecular-weight heparin, & possibly compression stockings or intermittent pneumatic compression device.

SURGICAL PROCEDURE

Indications
- Osteoarthritis, pathologic fractures of femoral neck, prosthesis failure, trauma.

Procedure
- Total hip arthroplasty refers to replacement of femoral & acetabular components of hip joint.
- Hemi-arthroplasty refers to replacement of only one component.

- Bipolar or unipolar refers to the engineering of the femoral component (bipolar more common because it allows greater range of motion).
- Some prostheses do not require cement & may therefore have reduced chance for hypotension.
- Basic steps of procedure
  - Hip is exposed via lateral incision.
  - Femoral head is removed.
  - Intramedullary canal is reamed.
  - Prosthesis is measured & then hammered into place (this is when embolization may occur).
  - Acetabular component is placed in pelvis.

Surgical Concerns
- Blood loss
  - EBL during hip revisions can be considerable. Consider arranging autologous donation or providing intraop cell salvage.
- Sciatic nerve injury

Typical EBL
- 500–3,000 cc.
- Anticipate higher blood loss for repeat surgery.

TOTAL KNEE ARTHROPLASTY

MARC SCHROEDER, MD

PREOP

Preop Considerations
- High incidence of periop DVT.
  - Consider DVT prophylaxis (w/o prophylaxis ~50% incidence of DVT, w/ prophylaxis ~10–20%).
- Risk of procedure increases w/ increased age/comorbidities.
- Common coexisting diseases
  - Osteoarthritis.
  - Seropositive/seronegative rheumatoid arthritis.
  - Hemophilia.
  - Pt may be obese.

Physical Findings
- Airway/neck

- If pt is obese airway, mgt may be more difficult.
- Jaw/cervical arthritis can lead to decreased range of motion of those joints.
- In pts w/ arthritis, look for limitations of c-spine extension.

Workup
- Depends on coexisting disease
  - Consider restrictive pulmonary disease in rheumatoid pts.
- Assess knee range of motion: chronic knee pain may make pt positioning difficult.

Choice of Anesthesia
- GA vs regional: no preference.
- Potential advantages of regional: may decrease blood loss, may decrease incidence of DVT, results in minimal respiratory impairment, provides postop pain control (favors early mobilization). However, it may be technically difficult in elderly pts w/ arthritic changes in their spines or scoliosis.
- Need T12-S2 anesthesia (T8 if tourniquet is used) for regional techniques.
- Epidural anesthesia has increased risk of epidural hematoma in pts who are anticoagulated for DVT/PE prophylaxis.

INTRAOP

Monitors/Line Placement
- Consider invasive monitors for increased age/comorbidities as indicated by those comorbidities (also helpful during periods of hemodynamic instability, such as tourniquet release).
- One or two peripheral IVs adequate.

Intraop Concerns
- Pulmonary embolism in 1–7% of patients (after tourniquet release, watch for rare severe pulmonary embolism or cardiovascular collapse).
- Prolonged use of tourniquet may result in elevated BP.
  - Attempt to limit tourniquet time to 2 h.
  - Tourniquet should be inflated to 100 mmHg above systolic pressure.
  - After tourniquet deflation, prepare for hypotension, tachycardia & possible pulmonary emboli (cement, thrombi, bone marrow, debris) w/ hypoxia & possible cardiac arrest.
  - Pt may have lactic acidosis after tourniquet release: ensure adequate ventilation.

Intraop Therapies
- DVT prophylaxis (eg, compression stockings, anticoagulant regimens).
  - ➤ Prior to tourniquet release, ensure adequate hydration & have vasopressors ready.
- Treat comorbid conditions.

POSTOP

Pain
- Moderate to severe
- PCA, epidural, spinal opiates, peripheral nerve block (single shot or by catheter) are all appropriate

Complications
- DVT, thromboembolization
  - ➤ Consider early postop ambulation to prevent DVT
- Fat embolism syndrome: hypoxia, axillary/subconjunctival petechiae, mental status changes, pulmonary edema, tachycardia, fever, thrombocytopenia, leukocytosis
- Postop bleeding
- Overall mortality <1%

SURGICAL PROCEDURE

Indications
- Various forms of degenerative joint disease, including osteoarthritis, post-traumatic arthritis, knee arthropathy from hemophilia, rheumatoid arthritis

Procedure
- Replacement of both tibial & femoral portions of the knee joint w/ metallic & plastic components (these implants may or may not be cemented w/ methylmethacrylate)

Surgical Concerns
- Position: supine
- Prophylactic broad-spectrum antibiotic (eg, cephalosporin)
- Surgical time 2–3 h
- Peroneal nerve injury
- Intraop femoral bone fractures

Typical EBL
- 300–500 mL

TRACHEAL RESECTION

JAMES MITCHELL, MBBS

PREOP

Preop Considerations
- Uncommon major surgery
- Airway is shared by anesthesia provider & surgeon
  - ➤ Often poses significant difficulty in maintaining ventilation while allowing surgical access: initially due to disease, then surgical disruption, then fragile reconstructed airway w/ awkward positioning
- Mgt requires close communication w/ surgeon

Physical Findings
- Pt may have minimal findings, but must assess:
  - ➤ Degree of obstruction to airflow
  - ➤ Ability to lie supine
  - ➤ Ability to cough & clear secretions

Workup
- Careful evaluation of airway
- Usual assessment of comorbidities (often pts are smokers w/ coronary disease)
- Delineation of lesion by x-ray, tomography, fluoroscopy, CT, or MRI
- Imaging of adjacent structures: barium swallow, angiography
- Respiratory function testing: characteristic flow-volume loop
- Bronchoscopy, biopsy
- Not all lesions are resectable: palliation w/ dilatation, stent or laser
- Detailed plan for airway mgt must be discussed & agreed on w/ the surgeon

Choice of Anesthesia
- GA
  - ➤ Decide airway mgt plan before surgery. Plan for mgt may include
    - Intermittent positive-pressure ventilation (IPPV)
    - High-frequency positive-pressure ventilation
    - Jet ventilation
    - Spontaneous ventilation
    - Cardiopulmonary bypass
    - Combination of above techniques
- Epidural placement for postop analgesia if a thoracotomy is planned

■ Preop sedation is used w/ great caution or not at all in pts w/ incipient obstruction

INTRAOP

Monitors/Line Placement
■ Routine monitors
■ Large-bore peripheral IVs
■ Arterial line indicated (on left for right thoracotomy)
■ Central line or PA catheter not generally needed unless pt has severe cardiac disease
■ Prepare sterile breathing circuit
■ Prepare broad selection of ETTs, including
  ➤ Small-diameter ETT
  ➤ Armored ETT
  ➤ Extra-long ETT (eg, microlaryngeal tube)
■ High-frequency or jet ventilator if use is being considered
■ Cardiopulmonary bypass machine primed & ready if use is planned

Intraop Concerns
■ Possibility of airway obstruction on induction
  ➤ Have assistance & surgeon present w/ rigid bronchoscopes available
  ➤ Induction w/ preservation of spontaneous ventilation may be safest (eg, gentle inhaled induction)
  ➤ Alternatively, awake fiberoptic-guided intubation after topical anesthesia to the airway if rigid bronchoscopy is not planned
  ➤ Technique that permits use of 100% oxygen is desirable
■ Significant airway manipulation required intraop
■ Neck may be secured in flexion at end of surgery.

Intraop Therapies
■ Ventilation strategies during tracheal resection include
  ➤ Jet ventilator catheter passed through ETT (which is above resection) for manual or high-frequency jet ventilation
  ➤ Positive-pressure ventilation through sterile ETT inserted by surgeon into trachea below resection (intermittent extubation while sewing anastomosis)
  ➤ For low lesions, bronchial intubation by the surgeon & positive-pressure ventilation to one lung or both separately
  ➤ Spontaneous ventilation (may be complicated by hypercarbia, coughing, possible airway soiling)

> Cardiopulmonary bypass (has complications of systemic anticoagulation)

■ After anastomosis, airway pressures must be minimized: spontaneous ventilation or low tidal volume positive-pressure ventilation

■ Plan for extubation at end of surgery to minimize exposure of anastomosis to positive airway pressure

■ Reintubation will be difficult (head flexed, edematous airway) & will require a fiberoptic bronchoscope both for intubation & to verify the tube tip is not touching the anastomosis

POSTOP

Pain

■ Mild to moderate, depending on access to trachea.
> Thoracotomy route is most painful.

■ Treat w/ carefully titrated narcotics or epidural infusion.

Complications

■ Anastomotic dehiscence assoc w/ poor outcome.
> Greater risk of dehiscence w/ postop ventilation, steroids, infection, extensive tracheal disease.
> Reduced risk of dehiscence w/ use of vascularized flap covering anastomosis.
> Minimize tracheal tension w/ head flexion (maintained postop w/ a suture from chin to anterior chest for several days).

■ Head flexion may cause cervical spinal cord compression.

SURGICAL PROCEDURE

Indications

■ Uncommon surgery; performed for tumor, fistula, stenosis or trauma
■ Tumor must not be invading mediastinum.
■ Likely postop ventilation is a relative contraindication.

Procedure

■ Cervical or sternotomy approach to high lesions.
> Initially head is extended & a roll is placed between scapulae.
> Repositioning required for anastomosis w/ head flexed & roll deflated or removed.

■ Right thoracotomy, head flexed approach to low or carinal lesions.

Surgical Concerns

■ Tracheal mobilization to allow anastomosis w/o tension.
■ Maintaining tracheal blood supply.

Typical EBL
- Highly variable: generally lowest for cervical approach w/o sternotomy.

TRACHEOESOPHAGEAL FISTULA (TEF) REPAIR

CLAIRE M. BRETT, MD

PREOP

Preop Considerations
- TEF results from incomplete formation of the tracheoesophageal septum.
- Variety of anatomic lesions are seen. Gross's classification:
  - Type A: esophageal atresia w/o fistula (7–9% of cases).
  - Type B: esophageal atresia w/ proximal fistula.
  - Type C: esophageal atresia w/ distal fistula (80–90% of cases).
  - Type D: esophageal atresia w/ proximal & distal fistula.
  - Type E: tracheoesophageal fistula w/o atresia (H type).
  - Type F: esophageal stenosis.

Physical Findings
- Morbidity in the perinatal period is usually related to cardiorespiratory function & anomalies, which must be carefully evaluated.
- Cardiovascular.
  - Cardiac disease is seen in ~30–40% of infants w/ TEF.
  - An isolated ventricular defect is most common.
  - Other lesions include tetralogy of Fallot, patent ductus arteriosus, atrial septal defect, coarctation of the aorta.
- Pulmonary
  - Aspiration of feeds (proximal fistula) or stomach contents (distal fistula) may occur.
  - Degree of pulmonary insult associated w/ TEF is related to:
    - Degree of aspiration/size of the fistula.
    - Underlying pulmonary function (prematurity, pulmonary hypertension, infection, associated anomalies).
    - Significance of abdominal distention.
    - Presence of musculoskeletal abnormalities (weakness).
    - In addition, inherent abnormalities of the trachea are common, especially tracheomalacia.
- Other findings

➤ GI anomalies are common (∼20%), including midgut malrotation, annular pancreas, duodenal atresia.

➤ Genitourinary anomalies are less common (∼10%) & except for renal agenesis will not lead to symptoms in the neonatal period (hydronephrosis, renal lobules).

➤ Musculoskeletal anomalies (vertebral abnormalities, radial aplasia, polydactyly, knee abnormalities) are common (∼30%) & may be the first hint to the clinician to consider whether other anomalies are present.

Workup

■ Preop eval should focus on assessment of the severity & course of pulmonary dysfunction & recognition of associated anomalies, particularly cardiovascular.

■ Assess respiratory compromise.

➤ Aspiration of gastric secretions or feeds.

➤ Gastric distention.

➤ Other pulmonary dysfunction (eg, from prematurity).

■ Review chest/abdominal x-ray & ABGs.

➤ Examining the trends in these studies is vital to prepare for supportive care in the OR.

➤ Examination of the abdominal films is important to ensure that surgery beyond the repair of esophageal atresia & ligation of a fistula is not necessary.

■ Electrolytes (including calcium, glucose, pH) may be abnormal, since these infants may be premature, are NPO & may develop sepsis, especially in the setting of aspiration/pneumonia.

■ Type & cross-match blood.

■ Consultation w/ a pediatric cardiologist is common & advisable.

➤ Cardiac lesions may be difficult to detect & assess; as a result, echocardiography is routine in the preop assessment of a newborn w/ TEF.

➤ Defining the anatomy of the aortic arch (if not apparent on CXR) is important for the surgeon, since L thoracotomy is necessary if there is a R aortic arch.

➤ In the absence of evidence of heart disease, if the expertise to perform & analyze an echocardiogram is not readily available, & if the infant is clearly in need of ligation of the fistula, surgery should proceed.

■ Infant should remain NPO preop, w/ the head slightly elevated to decrease the chance of reflux of stomach contents to the fistula. A tube should remain in place to keep the proximal esophageal pouch suctioned. Monitoring & respiratory support need to be tailored to pt's clinical status.

Choice of Anesthesia

- Intubation may be performed safely either in the spontaneously breathing child or after muscle relaxant is administered.
- The choice of inhaled or IV agents before, during, or after intubation depends on the cardiovascular response of the infant to the initial agent & the expertise/choice of the anesthesia provider.
- One logical approach to induction/intubation is:
  - Attempt an awake intubation w/ or w/o a small dose of an IV agent (fentanyl 1–2 mcg/kg), monitoring oxygenation.
    - If the trachea is intubated after 1–2 attempts, proceed w/ IV or inhaled anesthesia or a combination.
  - If the awake intubation is traumatic or unsuccessful after ~2 attempts, deliver an IV bolus of fentanyl, propofol, or thiopental; proceed to intubate the trachea.
  - If the trachea cannot be intubated after delivery of IV or inhaled agents, but ventilation w/ a mask is easy, consider giving a muscle relaxant.
  - If the abdomen becomes overly distended (or is so at presentation to the OR), discuss gastrostomy placement (possibly under local anesthesia) w/ the surgeon.
  - In all scenarios, because the fistula is usually just proximal to the carina in the posterior trachea, the ETT has to be advanced deeper than in other surgical procedures to avoid ventilating the gut.
    - Advance the tube to the right mainstem, then withdraw it to the point where breath sounds are heard bilaterally.
    - It is important to auscultate the lungs before intubation, because differential breath sounds may be present (eg, from infiltration, atelectasis).
    - In all scenarios, ventilation should be w/ the lowest peak airway possible to minimize gas passing through the fistula into the gut.
- Rotation of the ETT so that the bevel faces posteriorly to avoid ventilating the fistula can be attempted.
  - However, given the likelihood of movement of the ETT w/ pt positioning, the benefit of meticulous attention to the position of the ETT should be balanced w/ delaying surgery when

cardiorespiratory status is acceptable. The precise location of the fistula is seldom known during the induction of anesthesia.

➤ Gentle positive-pressure ventilation w/ the ETT in any position in the trachea is probably all that is necessary.

■ Selection of the anesthetic does not have to include plans to return to spontaneous ventilation at the end of surgery.

➤ The overwhelming majority of infants will require postop ventilatory support.

INTRAOP

Monitors/Line Placement

■ Arterial line

➤ In the majority of cases, an arterial line is of use in monitoring cardiorespiratory status both intraop & postop.

■ CVP

➤ Consider placement of a central venous catheter.

➤ Many infants will require postop IV alimentation (especially if a primary esophageal anastomosis is performed).

➤ A central venous catheter may be of benefit for delivery of fluids & blood products in the OR.

➤ If two peripheral IV catheters are functional, the risks of placing a central venous catheter in a newborn must be justified.

Intraop Concerns

■ Until the fistula is ligated, ventilation of the gut can be a problem, requiring repositioning of the ETT.

■ Airway obstruction secondary to surgical manipulation is a major risk, since retraction of the easily compressible neonatal trachea is repeatedly necessary.

➤ The incidence of tracheomalacia in these infants w/ TEF is not insignificant, predisposing to airway compression.

■ Compression of the lung in the surgical field is necessary, so close observation of the surgical field is essential. Communicate w/ the surgeon about oxygenation, ventilation, cardiovascular status.

■ The 2.5- to 3.5-mm ETT can be obstructed secondary to blood or mucous deposits, especially in this type of thoracotomy.

➤ Warming & humidifying the inspired gases may help.

➤ Suctioning the ETT may be necessary, since intraop airway secretions can be copious.

➤ Displacement of the ETT is more likely in this type of surgery.

- Avoid hyperoxia.
  - In the setting of prematurity, adjust the FIO_2 to maintain oxygen saturation at ~90–95%.
- Ventilation of premature infants is complicated by the need to balance the poor pulmonary compliance that accompanies respiratory distress syndrome (less common since the introduction of surfactant therapy) & other pulmonary disorders vs the increased risk of air leak (pneumothorax/pneumomediastinum) during positive-pressure ventilation.

Intraop Therapies

- A bougie (or other tube) may need to be manipulated in the proximal pouch if the surgeon undertakes a primary reanastomosis of the esophagus.
  - This can compress the trachea or great vessels or dislodge the ETT.
- Airway suctioning may require frequent interruption of the procedure.
- Rarely, the surgeon will request endoscopy (esophageal and/or tracheal) at the completion of the procedure.

POSTOP

Pain

- Pain can be treated aggressively because the neonate will be ventilated postop.
- Weaning of ventilatory support is primarily related to the status of the esophageal anastomosis in vigorous term infants w/ no other anomalies or intraop complications.
- In some cases where there had been a long gap esophageal atresia but a primary anastomosis was performed, the surgeon often advises that the infant remain deeply sedated & ventilated for as long as 5–7 days to allow for healing & stabilization of the esophageal surgery.
- Infants w/ associated congenital heart disease, genitourinary anomalies & musculoskeletal problems may require other surgery, but usually not in the neonatal period.
  - These anomalies may complicate fluid & ventilatory support.
- Premature infants also have their postop course defined by a variety of medical scenarios beyond their TEF.

Complications

■ Esophageal motility abnormalities w/ gastroesophageal reflux & feeding problems.

■ Esophageal stricture.

■ Esophageal rupture/leak causing mediastinitis/sepsis.

■ Tracheomalacia associated w/ cyanotic & apneic episodes that may eventually require tracheostomy.

■ Recurrent aspiration pneumonia, at least in part caused by esophageal dysmotility & aspiration.

SURGICAL PROCEDURE

Indications

■ Procedure is dictated by the anatomy of the lesion. The goals are to:
➤ Ligate the connection between the GI & respiratory tracts.
➤ Correct esophageal atresia.

Procedure

■ TEF is ligated either via L or R thoracotomy or thoracoscopic procedure.
➤ If the aortic arch is the typical left-sided structure, the approach to the fistula is from the right & vice versa.

■ After the fistula is ligated, the surgeon typically defines the anatomy of the esophagus to determine if a primary anastomosis is possible.
➤ With most cases of the common type of lesion (type C), this is possible.
➤ In isolated esophageal atresia, the gap between the proximal & distal esophagus usually is long (>2 vertebral bodies), so primary repair is impossible.

■ The surgeon may request placement of a variety of dilating bougies or other devices into the proximal pouch to facilitate identifying the anatomy.
➤ This may lead to tracheal compression or distortion, ETT movement, compression of the lung, and/or compression of major blood vessels.
➤ Meticulous attention to ventilation, oxygenation & hemodynamics as well as the surgical field is essential during these maneuvers.

■ If a primary anastomosis is not attempted, a gastrostomy is placed.
➤ A gastrostomy may also be placed if the infant has other anomalies that are assoc w/ failure to thrive or feeding problems (eg, cyanotic heart disease, major neuro malformation, prematurity, chromosomal abnormalities).

- At the completion of the operative procedure, the surgeon may attempt endoscopy of the esophagus and/or the trachea, but this is rare.
- Thoracoscopic approach to repair of type C TEF in infants >3 kg is routine at a number of pediatric centers. The concerns for this approach are related to
  - Insufflation of carbon dioxide & hypercarbia.
  - Compression of intrathoracic structures.
  - Unappreciated blood loss.

Surgical Concerns
- Identifying the TEF involves locating other structures intimately related to the fistula, such as the azygous vein & the vagus nerve, whether the procedure is via thoracotomy or thoracoscopy. A primary esophageal anastomosis is almost always possible in the setting of type C TEF but in contrast is rarely possible in isolated esophageal atresia. Long gap esophageal atresia is defined as >2 vertebral bodies between the proximal & distal pouches.
- The risks of a thoracotomy in a newborn are primarily defined by the ease of compression of the intrathoracic structures, including the trachea, lungs & major blood vessels.
  - Dramatic cardiovascular & respiratory compromise may occur suddenly & repeatedly during this surgery.
  - Profuse secretions & blood in the trachea may interfere w/ ventilation & oxygenation repeatedly & require suctioning of the ETT during the surgery.
- Anastomotic leak
  - Routinely, the infant undergoes a barium swallow ~7 days postop.
  - W/o evidence of leak, the infant is fed.
  - The swallow is repeated at ~6 weeks postop to evaluate for stricture.
  - Dilatation of a stricture may be necessary.
    - Approx 30% of these pts subsequently require a fundoplication to treat significant reflux.
    - Reflux is treated aggressively to avoid exacerbating stricturing of the esophagus & pulmonary aspiration.

Typical EBL
- Not usually significant, but in the setting of thoracotomy blood loss is always a risk.

TRACHEOTOMY

ANDREW CHUNG, MD
MANUEL PARDO, JR., MD

PREOP

Preop Considerations
- Determine whether pt is scheduled for tracheotomy or tracheostomy.
  - ➤ A tracheotomy is a surgical opening made into the trachea for airway management. This is more common.
  - ➤ A tracheostomy is the surgical creation of a stoma from the trachea to the overlying skin. This is most commonly done as part of surgery for cancer resection.
- Emergency tracheotomy is one of the surgical airway techniques in a pt w/ a difficult airway.
- Elective tracheotomy often done for ICU pts who are dependent on mechanical ventilation.
- Elective tracheotomy may be the best intubation choice for:
  - ➤ Airway trauma (laryngeal fracture or disruption).
  - ➤ Upper airway obstructions (abscesses, tumor, or sleep apnea).
  - ➤ Facial trauma (basilar skull fractures w/ CSF leak or nasal fractures).

Physical Findings
- Examine airway carefully.
- If pt is on mechanical ventilator, note the ventilator settings. If PEEP >10 cm H_2O or minute ventilation >15 L/m, pt may desaturate during transport & may require ICU ventilator intraop.

Workup
- None.

Choice of Anesthesia
- GA w/ ETT.
- Tracheotomy may be performed under local anesthesia in pt w/ difficult airway.

INTRAOP

Monitors/Line Placement
- Standard.

Intraop Concerns

- May need an ICU ventilator for transport & intraop to maintain a high minute ventilation & PEEP. Consider calling respiratory therapist to prepare ICU ventilator.
- Tracheal stimulation may cause pt to cough.
- ETT cuff can be punctured during the incision of trachea, causing air leak & ineffective ventilation. Can often re-establish an air-tight seal by packing pharynx w/ gauze.
- Surgeon will ask for withdrawal of ETT prior to placing tracheotomy tube. Only withdraw by a short distance so that ETT can be advanced back into trachea if there is difficulty placing tracheotomy tube.
- After surgeon places tracheotomy tube, check for end-tidal CO_2 & bilateral breath sounds.
- Types of tracheotomy tubes
  - Metal (Jackson) or plastic (Shiley, Portex).
  - Single cannula or double cannula.
  - Cuffed or uncuffed.
  - Fenestrated (for speaking) or nonfenestrated.

POSTOP

Pain

- Minimal.

Complications

- Dislodgement of tracheotomy tube into subcutaneous tissue.
  - This is most likely during first few days postop, until a tract forms.
  - If tracheotomy tube dislodged in early postop period, consider face mask ventilation until ENT surgeon available to replace.
  - Fiberoptic bronchoscope can confirm proper positioning.
  - After tract forms, replacement of tracheotomy tube is usually straightforward.
  - Some surgeons leave sutures around tracheal rings. Pulling on the sutures will bring the trachea close to the skin & facilitate replacement of the tracheotomy tube.
  - With tracheostomy, the large stomal opening allows easy placement of an ETT.
- Barotrauma causing pneumothorax, subcutaneous & mediastinal emphysema: Can occur from positive-pressure ventilation through misplaced tracheotomy tube.

■ Hemorrhage: Not common w/ fresh tracheotomy. With long-term tracheotomy, risk of tracheo-innominate artery fistula increases. In that rare condition, pt may need urgent surgery for repair.

SURGICAL PROCEDURE

Indications
■ Typical indications: Difficult intubation, airway trauma, airway obstruction, long-term artificial airway

Procedure
■ Involves dissection of vessels, nerves, & thyroid isthmus. Incision is usually made in third or fourth tracheal ring.
■ Some surgeons leave sutures around tracheal rings.

Surgical Concerns
■ False passage can be created in pts w/ prior surgeries (eg, cancer resection).

Typical EBL
■ Minimal

TRANSHIATAL ESOPHAGECTOMY

MERLIN LARSON, MD

PREOP

Preop Considerations
■ Pt often has reflux; consider rapid sequence induction.
■ Consider thoracic epidural, T7-T8 for postop analgesia.
■ Before the case begins, ask surgical team if they prefer overnight intubation.
■ No need for double-lumen tube.

Physical Findings
■ Listen to chest for rales or wheezes as respiratory status may change during surgery.
■ Examine neck carefully because the esophageal anastomosis will be on the left w/ the CVP on the right.
■ Examine pt for possible nutritional deficiencies.

Workup
■ Pulmonary

- CXR
- Consider PFTs.
- Consider ABGs.
- Cardiac procedure is a high-stress procedure.
  - Evaluate EKG.
  - Consider echocardiogram.
- Check electrolytes.
- Check albumin for nutritional status.
- Starting digitalis prophylactically before surgery is controversial. It is considered because atrial fibrillation can occur perioperatively.

Choice of Anesthesia
- GA required, but may use epidural intermittently w/ local anesthetics & opioids

INTRAOP

Monitors/Line Placement
- Standard monitors.
- Arterial line essential because of hemodynamic changes during mediastinal dissection.
- CVP useful for assessing fluid status.

Intraop Concerns
- Passing stomach through the mediastinum produces hemodynamic instability.
- Hemodynamic changes during mediastinal dissection may require vasopressors and/or fluids.
- Uncontrolled bleeding during blunt mediastinal dissection necessitates opening the chest. This will require rapid placement of a double-lumen tube & fluid resuscitation.
- If extubation is planned, use epidural at the end of case to ensure comfortable emergence.
- 90% oxygen w/ vapor or propofol during the case may improve wound healing & decrease nausea/vomiting.
  - Some surgeons request avoidance of nitrous oxide.
- Take special care during placement of esophageal stethoscope & NG tube. Ask surgeon before advancing NG tube.

Intraop Therapies
- Vasopressors, maintenance of fluid status
- Maintain urine output but avoid overhydration: pleural effusions are common postop.

POSTOP

Pain
- Moderate to severe
- Epidural or PCA required
  - ➤ Epidural infusion will not provide analgesia for neck incision. Additional parenteral opioids may be required

Complications
- Cardiovascular collapse during mediastinal dissection
- Respiratory failure in postop period
- Breakdown of anastomosis, which can result in mediastinitis & sepsis

SURGICAL PROCEDURE

Indications
- Carcinoma or high-grade stricture of the esophagus

Procedure
- Involves abdominal incision, then passing stomach through the mediastinum w/ blunt dissection. Anastomosis is in the neck

Surgical Concerns
- Uncontrolled bleeding
- Anastomotic breakdown

Typical EBL
- 1,000 mL

TRANSJUGULAR INTRAHEPATIC PORTOSYSTEMIC SHUNT (TIPS)

LINDA LIU, MD

PREOP

Preop Considerations
- Altered mental status from encephalopathy
- Full stomach considerations due to ascites or GI bleeding
- Poor drug clearance due to hepatic failure
- Coexisting diseases: coagulopathy, renal insufficiency, anemia

Physical Findings
- Jaundice

- Ascites
- Asterixis
- Bruising
- Petechiae

Workup
- Labs: hematocrit, platelet count, PT/PTT, liver function tests, electrolytes (BUN/Cr)
- Documentation of portal hypertension

Choice of Anesthesia
- Often done w/ conscious sedation by interventional radiologists
- Anesthesia may be required if pt is actively bleeding or has very altered mental status

INTRAOP
Monitors/Line Placement
- Adequate IV access
- Arterial line if pt actively bleeding & hemodynamically unstable

Intraop Concerns
- Proper lead protection for physicians due to x-rays

Intraop Therapies
- Minimize sedatives due to poor liver & often poor renal function

POSTOP
Pain
- Minimal to none

Complications
- Hepatic encephalopathy, decline in liver function.
  - ➤ Monitor for change in mental status. Keep sedatives postop to a minimum.
- Stents may occlude immediately or over a period of time: stents are evaluated for patency w/ ultrasound the next morning & whenever signs of portal hypertension return.
- Bleeding: serial hematocrits are obtained for 24 hours as well as monitoring for change in abdominal girth & blood pressure. If severe, transfusions & return to the OR are possibilities.
- Pts are usually kept in the ICU overnight for monitoring.
- Independent predictors of short-term mortality.

> ➤ Need for emergent TIPS.
> ➤ ALT >1,000.
> ➤ Bilirubin >3.
> ➤ Encephalopathy pre-TIPS

SURGICAL PROCEDURE

Indications
■ Complications of portal hypertension
> ➤ Variceal hemorrhage
> ➤ Refractory ascites
> ➤ Hepatic hydrothorax

Procedure
■ Using a percutaneous approach & angiographic guidance, a communication via an expandable stent is created between the hepatic & portal veins through the liver.

Surgical Concerns
■ Postop bleeding due to the blind passages that are made in the liver
■ Usually a catheter is left in the internal jugular vein. It can be used for volume resuscitation if pt bleeds postprocedure or for repeat TIPS if ultrasound shows an occluded shunt the next day.

Typical EBL
■ Minimal

TRANSSPHENOIDAL HYPOPHYSECTOMY

SUSAN RYAN, PHD, MD

PREOP

Preop Considerations
■ Determine if the pituitary tumor is hormone-secreting.
> ➤ Three most common syndromes:
> • Acromegaly (growth hormone [GH])
> • Cushing's disease (ACTH)
> • Prolactin-secreting tumors
■ Pt may also have symptoms from a large pituitary tumor:
> ➤ Visual disturbances
> ➤ Impaired posterior pituitary function (thirst & orthostasis from diabetes insipidus [DI])

Physical Findings

- Depend in part on hormone secretion
- GH-secreting tumor (acromegaly)
  - Bone & soft tissue enlargement
  - Large mandible
  - Large tongue
  - Redundant hypopharyngeal tissue
  - Hoarseness
  - Tracheal stenosis
  - Vocal cord paralysis
  - Hypertension
  - LVH
  - Cardiomegaly
  - CHF
  - Cervical compression
  - Lumbar stenosis
  - Carpal tunnel syndrome
  - Proximal myopathy & weakness
  - Paresthesias
- ACTH-secreting tumor (Cushing's disease)
  - Cushingoid appearance
  - HTN
  - Glucose intolerance
  - Truncal obesity w/ cervical fat pads
  - Myopathy
  - Osteoporosis
  - Adrenal hyperplasia
- Prolactin-secreting tumor
  - Osteoporosis
  - Galactorrhea
  - Gynecomastia

Workup

- Appropriate endocrine panel
- Electrolytes, creatinine, CBC, PT, PTT, glucose
- EKG (even in young pt if GH-secreting)
- CXR (if GH-secreting & clinically indicated)
- If DI suspected: Serum osmolality, urine specific gravity & osmolality

Choice of Anesthesia

- GA

INTRAOP

Monitors/Line Placement
- Standard monitors usually adequate.
- If pt has Cushing's or acromegaly, place an arterial line to facilitate BP & glucose monitoring.

Intraop Concerns
- Airway: Acromegalic pts can be very difficult to intubate, even when they appear to have only a large mandible.
  - Anticipate possible distorted anatomy or redundant hypopharyngeal tissues.
  - For a direct laryngoscopy, larger than usual laryngoscope blades and/or smaller tubes may be needed.
  - Have emergency equipment available, such as an LMA, fiberoptic scope, & surgical airway equipment.
  - Consider an awake fiberoptic intubation.
- HTN & tachycardia
  - Afrin or phenylephrine is applied to the nares in the nasal approach.
  - Epinephrine is injected into the nose in the sublabial approach.
- DI
  - May cause intraop hypernatremia, hyperosmolality, hypovolemia, hypotension.
- Bleeding in airway & esophagus
- Venous air embolism
  - Pt at risk because of sitting position, but overall risk is lower than craniotomy in sitting position.
  - Concern may be decreased if pt's head is turned to the side & held in pins, because venous pressure stays higher.
- Venous hypertension: Common problem causing bleeding

Intraop Therapies
- Hypertension & tachycardia
  - Usually occurs briefly & episodically from agents applied to the nares.
  - Often responds to propofol bolus.
  - May require use of esmolol or nitrates if severe.
  - Labetalol appropriate for continued hypertension.
- DI
  - Replete free water.
  - Avoid high sodium-containing solutions.

➤ Consult w/ surgeon on dose of vasopressin. May begin w/ 2 mcg IV DDAVP & then observe response. Usual dose is 2 mcg IV bid. Lysine vasopressin dose: 5–10 units SC q4h.

■ Bleeding in airway & esophagus
➤ Place OG tube & throat pack.

■ Venous hypertension resulting in bleeding
➤ Decrease intrathoracic pressure.
➤ Lower tidal volumes.
➤ Increase muscle relaxation.
➤ Hand ventilation
➤ Treat arterial hypertension.
➤ Relieve gastric distention by OG tube suction.

■ Airway concerns w/ emergence
➤ Pt must be awake & able to protect airway prior to extubation.
➤ Some bleeding will continue postop, & pt must be able to protect airway.
➤ Consider brief postop intubation on T-piece or ventilator for acromegalic pts, particularly if pt was difficult to intubate.
➤ Reintubation is more difficult following this procedure than following many others due to bleeding in the pharynx & hypopharynx.

POSTOP

Pain

■ Usually mild. Usually requires IV pain med for first 24 h.

Complications

■ Airway obstruction & aspiration
➤ Mild airway obstruction & aspiration from bleeding in many pts.
➤ More severe obstruction from relaxed & redundant hypopharyngeal tissue in acromegalics.
➤ Acromegalics may have sleep apnea at baseline, & require postop intubation or close postop observation w/ monitoring.

■ Electrolyte imbalance
➤ Pts may develop DI, cerebral salt wasting, or SIADH.
➤ Begin close monitoring of electrolytes & urine output in the PACU.

■ Postdural puncture headache
➤ Pt may require a blood patch.

■ Nerve injury or hematoma requiring emergent reoperation.

SURGICAL PROCEDURE

Indications
- Pituitary mass

Procedure
Lumbar drain may be placed at beginning of procedure to provide the ability to extract CSF or deliver fluid, facilitating visualization & surgical excision of the mass.
- Fluoroscopy used to guide speculum placement.
- Abdominal incision made to harvest small amount of fat.
- Pituitary mass removed by one of two approaches: incision & speculum below the upper lip (sublabial) or speculum & incision intra-nares.

Surgical Concerns
- CSF leak, meningitis, surgical damage to optic nerve, bleeding from carotid or cavernous sinus, continued bleeding requiring packing w/ possibility of neurologic injury

Typical EBL
- 50–300 cc

TRANSURETHRAL RESECTION OF BLADDER TUMOR (TURBT)

SAMIR DZANKIC, MD
JASON WIDRICH, MD

PREOP

Preop Considerations
- Bladder tumor is usually seen in older populations who may have pre-existing medical problems.
- Pt may have hematuria, painful urination, or urinary frequency.

Workup
- Other findings & workup dictated by the presence of coexisting disease.

Choice of Anesthesia
- GA may be indicated in pts who require ventilatory or hemodynamic support during procedure.

➤ Maintenance of GA.
  • Muscle relaxation is not necessary but may be considered in lateral wall resections, where there is a risk of stimulating the obturator nerve.
  • Perforation of the bladder can occur from the rigid cystoscope during unexpected motor activity.
  • Minimize narcotics since postop pain is usually minimal.
■ Regional anesthesia: spinal (need coverage to T9–10 level). Possible advantages: may be easier to recognize possible complications, such as bladder perforation.

INTRAOP

Monitors/Line Placement
■ Standard monitors.
■ One peripheral IV usually adequate.

Intraop Concerns
■ Carefully pad pressure points since pt will be in lithotomy position during the procedure.
  ➤ High concern for peroneal nerve compression at lateral fibular head.
■ Bladder perforation.
  ➤ Extraperitoneal perforation results in pain in the periumbilical, inguinal or suprapubic regions, pallor, sweating, abdominal rigidity, nausea, vomiting, hypotension; urologist may notice irregular return of irrigation fluid.
  ➤ Intraperitoneal perforation is manifested as back pain, abdominal pain or shoulder pain.
■ Bleeding.
■ Stimulation of obturator nerve.
  ➤ Nerve passes next to the lateral bladder wall, bladder neck & lateral prostatic urethra.
  ➤ Stimulation of the obturator nerve by electrocautery may cause the thigh muscles to contract violently, leading to bladder perforation.
  ➤ This reflex may be eliminated by either blocking neuromuscular transmission w/ a muscle relaxant during GA or w/ regional anesthesia.

Intraop Therapies

- Possible hypotension upon return from lithotomy position. Typical Rx:
  - ➤ Volume (250–500 cc of NS/LR) or
  - ➤ Ephedrine/phenylephrine.
- Perforation of the bladder. Mgt includes
  - ➤ Stop surgery.
  - ➤ Perform cystourethrogram to locate perforation & treat appropriately.

POSTOP

Pain

- Typically minimal.

Complications

- Intraop complications such as bladder perforation or hemorrhage may not become evident until postop period.

SURGICAL PROCEDURE

Indications

- The most common type of tumor is transitional cell carcinoma, followed by squamous cell carcinoma & adenocarcinoma.

Procedure

- W/ pt in lithotomy position.
- Cystoscope or resectoscope is introduced under direct vision into the bladder.
- The tumor is identified & resected using cutting current of the electrode of the resectoscope.
- Coagulating current is used to cauterize the base of the tumor.
- Typical duration of procedure: around 1 h.

Surgical Concerns

- Perforation of the bladder w/ intraperitoneal extravasation of irrigating fluid.
  - ➤ The surgeon will likely terminate surgery as quickly as possible.
  - ➤ Small perforations are generally treated via tamponade w/ placement of Foley catheter, diuretics & occasionally ureteral stents.
  - ➤ Larger perforation might need exploration & repair.

Typical EBL

- 100 mL.

TRANSURETHRAL RESECTION OF THE PROSTATE (TURP)

MICHAEL J. YANAKAKIS, MD

PREOP

Preop Considerations

■ Pts who present for TURP are typically elderly males who may have a variety of coexisting medical diseases. Preop evaluation should be directed toward the detection & treatment of these conditions prior to anesthesia.

Physical Findings

■ Enlarged prostate gland.

Workup

■ ECG.
■ CBC w/ platelets.
■ Electrolytes.
■ PT/PTT if regional anesthesia considered.

Choice of Anesthesia

■ Regional may be preferred over GA.
  ➤ Risk: Incidence of postdural puncture headache is quite low in this population (<1%).
  ➤ Benefit: Regional anesthesia allows for evaluation of mental status, which is important in the assessment of TURP syndrome.

INTRAOP

Monitors/Line Placement

■ Standard monitors
■ Invasive monitoring only if indicated from history & physical exam

Intraop Concerns

■ Absorption of irrigation solution, leading to TURP syndrome
  ➤ Dilutional hyponatremia
  ➤ Volume overload
■ Intraop bleeding
■ Bladder perforation, which can be more easily detected under regional anesthesia in that pts may present w/ shoulder pain
  ➤ Lithotomy position may give rise to peroneal nerve compression
  ➤ Lithotomy also a risk factor for transient neuro symptoms (TNS) (see "Spinal Anesthesia" chapter). Pts at greatest risk are those

receiving lidocaine or tetracaine w/ vasoconstrictor, making bupivacaine an attractive option

Intraop Therapies
- EBL can be significant if venous sinuses are entered
- Treat TURP syndrome (volume overload, hyponatremia, hypotonicity secondary to absorption of irrigant) w/
  - ➤ Administration of hypertonic saline
  - ➤ Diuresis
  - ➤ Restoration of serum sodium to >120

POSTOP

Pain
- Usually not significant

Complications
- Postop bleeding
- TURP syndrome
- Bladder perforation
- Hypothermia
- Bacteremia

SURGICAL PROCEDURE

Indications
- TURP is performed to relieve bladder obstruction from an enlarging prostate gland.
- The size of the enlarged prostate or adenoma must be carefully assessed preop to determine if the resection can be completed in <2 h. Exceeding 2 h may lead to excessive absorption of irrigation fluid.

Procedure
- A resectoscope is introduced via the urethra into the bladder.
  - ➤ Tissue protruding into the prostatic urethra is resected in small pieces.
  - ➤ Bleeding is controlled w/ the coagulating current.
  - ➤ The resection is performed w/ the use of continuous irrigation using a near-isotonic solution such as sorbitol 2.7% w/ mannitol 0.54% or glycine 1.5%.
  - ➤ After the prostatic tissue is resected & the bleeding controlled, the small pieces of tissue are irrigated from the bladder & the resectoscope is removed.

Surgical Concerns

■ TURP syndrome: Hyponatremia, volume overload, hypotonicity
  ➤ Seizures.
  ➤ Mental status changes and/or coma.
  ➤ Visual disturbances.
  ➤ Cardiovascular dysfunction.
  ➤ Nausea/vomiting.
■ Do not exceed 2 h to minimize likelihood of TURP syndrome.
■ Infection: May be prudent to provide prophylaxis w/ gentamicin.
■ Bleeding.
■ Bladder perforation.

Typical EBL

■ Minimal in most cases.
■ Intraop & postop bleeding has been reported in a small percentage of pts.

TRICUSPID VALVE REPAIR OR REPLACEMENT

JOAN J. CHEN, MD

PREOP

Preop Considerations

■ Most common reason for surgery is tricuspid regurgitation (TR), although pt may have combined tricuspid stenosis (TS) and TR.
■ TR (see also Coexisting Disease chapter "Tricuspid Regurgitation").
  ➤ Usually occurs secondary to right ventricular dilatation caused by left-sided valvular heart failure, congestive heart failure or chronic cor pulmonale.
  ➤ Other etiologies include rheumatic heart disease, infective endocarditis, chest trauma, carcinoid syndrome, Marfan's syndrome, right-sided myocardial infarction, thyrotoxicosis, congenital Ebstein's anomaly.
■ TR is usually well tolerated unless assoc w/ biventricular failure.
  ➤ Symptoms include fatigue, dyspnea.
  ➤ Other manifestations include pulmonary edema, pleural effusions, prerenal failure, hepatic congestion w/ impairment of synthetic function & ascites.
■ If etiology of TR is rheumatic heart disease, other valvular involvement is usually present.

■ Because TR is usually related to LV failure or left-sided valve lesion, medical mgt is directed at treating those conditions.

Physical Findings

■ Jugular venous contour w/ large v-wave & rapid y-descent.
■ Right ventricular lift assoc w/ RVH.
■ Holosystolic murmur best heard along the lower left sternal border, which may increase w/ inspiration.
■ Pulsatile, enlarged liver.
■ Peripheral edema.

Workup

■ CBC, electrolytes, BUN, creatinine, LFTs, PT, PTT.
■ ECG may reveal right atrial & ventricular enlargement or atrial fibrillation.
■ Review results of cardiac evaluation.
   ➤ Echocardiography may show right atrial & ventricular enlargement, dilation of hepatic veins, IVC & coronary sinus.
      • Echo can also identify other valve lesions or myocardial dysfunction.

Choice of Anesthesia

■ GA
   ➤ Consider intrathecal morphine at start of surgery for postop pain control.
■ Anesthesia mgt includes treating existing pulmonary HTN, which will decrease right ventricular pressure & the degree of tricuspid regurgitation.
■ Many anesthetic drugs acceptable, as long as hemodynamic effects are anticipated & treated appropriately.
   ➤ Consider avoiding nitrous oxide, as it may increase pulmonary vascular resistance.

INTRAOP

Monitors/Line Placement

■ Standard monitors.
■ Two large-bore peripheral IVs.
■ Arterial line.
■ Central line.
   ➤ CVP elevations may not accurately reflect intravascular volume.
■ PA catheter.

➤ May be useful in mgt of volume status, pulmonary HTN, cardiac output.
➤ May be difficult to place & needs to be withdrawn during repair or replacement of the valve.

■ TEE.
➤ May be useful in assessing valve repair postbypass.
➤ Can also be used to evaluate LV & RV function & presence of intracardiac air.

■ Foley catheter.

INTRAOP CONCERNS

■ Standard preparation for cardiopulmonary bypass (CPB), including heparin to maintain ACT >400 sec.
■ Hemodynamic goals for TR include.
➤ Maintain high preload.
  • IV fluids as necessary to attain euvolemic or mild hypervolemic state; helps to maintain RV stroke volume.
➤ Maintain elevated HR.
➤ Maintain NSR if possible.
➤ Minimize negative inotropes.
  • Consider need for inotropic support, even before induction of GA.
➤ Maintain SVR.
  • Changes in SVR usually do not affect TR unless pt has concomitant left-sided valve lesion.
➤ Avoid increasing pulmonary vascular resistance.
  • Maintain pulmonary vascular resistance in the normal to decreased range.
  • Helps prevent increased RV workload & subsequent increased regurgitant volume.
  • Start therapy to decrease PVR if significant pulmonary HTN is present.
■ If >1 valve lesion is present, adjust hemodynamic goals to reflect the dominant valve pathology.

Intraop Therapies

■ Therapy of pulmonary HTN.
➤ Avoid further increases in PVR by
  • Correcting hypercarbia, hypoxemia, acidosis or light anesthesia.

- Stopping nitrous oxide, alpha agonists or overinflation of lungs w/ high mean airway pressures.
➤ Consider pharmacologic options to decrease PVR:
  - Inotropic support (eg, dobutamine, isoproterenol, amrinone).
  - Pulmonary vasodilators (eg, nitric oxide, prostaglandin E1 [epoprostenol, Flolan], nitroglycerin, sodium nitroprusside).
■ Upon weaning from bypass, consider need for inotropic support based on observation of heart, filling pressures & TEE findings.
■ Reverse heparin w/ protamine & follow ACT.

POSTOP

Pain
■ Moderate.
■ IV sedatives to tolerate mechanical ventilation.
■ IV narcotics for analgesia.
■ Consider need for PCA after extubation.
■ Intrathecal morphine typically provides 24 h of analgesia.

Complications
■ Hemorrhage, cardiac tamponade.
  ➤ May require emergent surgery.
  ➤ Notify surgeons & OR staff immediately for return to OR.
  ➤ See also Procedures chapter "Cardiac Surgery Re-Exploration."
■ Coagulopathy.
  ➤ Esp w/ long CPB time.
  ➤ Treat w/ FFP, platelets.
  ➤ Ensure adequate reversal of heparin w/ protamine.
■ RV failure.
  ➤ Often related to pulmonary HTN.
  ➤ Treat w/ inotropes & pulmonary vasodilators as listed above.
■ Arrhythmias or heart block.
  ➤ Antiarrhythmics or cardioversion as needed.
  ➤ For third-degree heart block, activate temporary pacer.
■ Stroke.
  ➤ Possibly from microembolic events on CPB.
  ➤ Evaluate w/ head CT.
■ Methemoglobinemia if nitric oxide used.
  ➤ Treat w/ methylene blue or ascorbic acid.
■ Renal failure.
  ➤ May require hemodialysis.

SURGICAL PROCEDURE

Indications

- Tricuspid replacement is decreasing as most surgeons favor repair of valve if possible.
  - ➤ Accurate assessment of tricuspid valve function can be difficult in the preop period.
  - ➤ The decision for repair vs replacement is sometimes made during direct examination of the tricuspid valve during surgical correction of left-sided valvular lesions.
- Options for tricuspid repair include
  - ➤ Annuloplasty w/ ring insertion.
  - ➤ Suture plication.
  - ➤ Commissurotomy.

Procedure

- Median sternotomy.
- Aortic & bicaval cannulation for CPB.
- Procedure can be performed either w/ the heart fibrillating or w/ aortic cross-clamping & diastolic arrest.
- An incision through the right atrium exposes the tricuspid valve.
- Following tricuspid repair or replacement, the atrial wall is closed & air is vented from the heart.
  - ➤ For secondary functional TR or ruptured chordae tendineae, repair w/ simple annuloplasty is performed more often.
  - ➤ For TR w/ an organic origin, wide commissurotomy followed by annuloplasty is the preferred operation.
  - ➤ In isolated TR from infective endocarditis, the valve is sometimes resected w/o replacement to decrease the risk for reinfection in high-risk pts (eg, IVDU).
  - ➤ When valve replacement is the only option, the porcine valve is the preferred prosthesis.
- After adequate myocardial resuscitation, pt is weaned from CPB.
- Chest is closed.

Surgical Concerns

- Heart block
  - ➤ Injury to AV node & His bundle can occur because of their proximity to the tricuspid annulus.
  - ➤ This can cause complete heart block, requiring temporary pacemaker.
    - Temporary pacing wires are usually placed intraop.

Typical EBL
- Not usually estimated for CPB cases

TUBAL LIGATION

JASON WIDRICH, MD

PREOP

Preop Considerations
- Often performed postpartum but may be done electively at other times.
- If performed postpartum, the following considerations may apply:
  - ➤ Pt may already be receiving an anesthetic or have an epidural catheter left in place after delivery specifically for this procedure.
  - ➤ Cardiac: blood volume does not return to normal for several days postpartum.
  - ➤ Pulmonary: functional residual capacity improves after delivery.
  - ➤ GI: reflux continues into the postpartum period.
  - ➤ Heme: pt may still be at risk for hemorrhage, coagulation disorders.
  - ➤ Tubal ligation may not be indicated in the face of severe pre-eclampsia or eclampsia.

Workup
- Airway assessment, particularly for soft tissue edema postpartum.
- CBC w/ platelets.
- Other coagulation studies are influenced by the anesthetic technique & pt's current health status.
- Order a urine pregnancy test if the procedure is being performed electively a significant period after a delivery or abortion.
- Further cardiopulmonary workup dictated by pt's medical history.
- If the procedure occurs postpartum, determine the blood loss that occurred during delivery & assess pt's volume status.

Choice of Anesthesia
- Spinal or epidural anesthetic can be used in the postpartum period or continued after C-section. GA is felt to carry a slightly increased risk because of airway edema & the possibility of reflux.
- If GA is chosen, a rapid sequence induction should be used in postpartum pts.

INTRAOP

Monitors/Line Placement
- One 18g IV
- Foley catheter
- Standard monitors

Intraop Concerns
- Hypotension w/ induction of regional anesthesia
- Difficult airway & soft tissue swelling
- Aspiration prophylaxis
- Postpartum hemorrhage

Intraop Therapies
- Sodium citrate PO or IV metoclopramide to decrease risk of aspiration
- Trendelenburg position to remove bowel from surgical field of vision
- Foley catheter to decompress bladder & improve visualization
- 1 L fluid bolus to prevent hypotension secondary to initiation of regional anesthetic

POSTOP

Pain
- Mild to moderate
- Controlled w/ spinal/epidural narcotics postpartum, or IV/PO narcotics

Complications
- Aspiration pneumonitis

SURGICAL PROCEDURE

Indications
- Elective sterilization.

Procedure
- After vaginal deliveries, infraumbilical incision is made down to the parietal peritoneum & the fallopian tubes are located. An avascular portion of the mesosalpinx/tube is located & ligated.
- Tubal ligation can also be performed at the end of a C-section by identification & ligation of the fallopian tubes.

Surgical Concerns
- Hemorrhage.
- Ectopic pregnancy in the future.

Typical EBL
- Minimal

UPPER EXTREMITY AV FISTULA PLACEMENT

JASON WIDRICH, MD

PREOP

Preop Considerations
- Pts present w/ end-stage renal disease (ESRD) requiring access for hemodialysis.
- Pts may have a previous failed or thrombosed graft; this will influence location of next graft & may affect anesthetic plan, especially regional block options.
- Chronic renal failure can affect many organ systems (see also Coexisting Disease chapter "Chronic Renal Failure"). Findings may include
  - Pulmonary
    - Pulmonary edema from fluid overload, CHF, pleuritis
  - Cardiac
    - HTN
    - CHF
    - CAD
    - Pericardial effusion secondary to uremia
    - Hypotension secondary to excessive removal of fluid in hemodialysis prior to operation
  - GI
    - Peptic ulcer disease
    - GI bleed
    - Delayed gastric emptying
  - Hematologic
    - Anemia
    - Impaired platelet function
  - Neurologic
    - Neuropathy
    - Altered mental status
    - Seizures
    - Autonomic dysfunction
  - Metabolic
    - Renal drug clearance & elimination are affected

> Electrolyte abnormalities
  • Hyperkalemia is most important to detect, as it can cause life-threatening arrhythmias
  • Other: phosphorus, calcium, potassium, sodium, magnesium disorders
> Immune
  • Pts are more prone to infections & sepsis
■ Etiologies of renal failure include
  > HTN
  > Diabetes
  > Glomerulonephritis
  > Pyelonephritis
  > Connective tissue diseases (eg, systemic lupus erythematosus)
■ Most important information to determine
  > Etiology of renal failure
    • Cause of renal failure may be a multisystem disease like diabetes mellitus, w/ particular anesthetic considerations such as gastroparesis
  > Urine output
    • Pts w/ oliguria or anuria are more likely to develop volume overload w/ excess fluid administration.
  > Current dialysis method (if already dialyzed)
    • Type (peritoneal vs hemodialysis)
    • Frequency (usually 3x per week for hemodialysis, continuous for peritoneal)
    • Access route for hemodialysis (fistula, graft, or central vein dialysis catheter)
  > Current volume status
    • For instance, evidence of CHF or pulmonary edema
  > Coexisting cardiovascular disease
    • Pts w/ renal failure have higher incidence of CAD

Physical Findings
■ May be minimal. It is most important to look for signs of uremia & volume overload, including pulmonary edema
  > Pulmonary: rales, SOB, decreased breath sounds (from effusion)
  > Cardiac: orthopnea, increased JVD, irregular rhythm, chest pain, HTN, friction rub on auscultation (from pericarditis)
  > Neurologic: altered mental status, somnolence, neuropathy, autonomic dysfunction

Workup
- CBC
- ECG
- Electrolytes
  - Check electrolytes & know when they were drawn in relation to most recent dialysis.
  - Hyperkalemia is most important abnormality to detect. Some pts have chronic hyperkalemia despite dialysis. Correlate w/ ECG, since hyperkalemic changes (peaked T waves, etc) may or may not be present.
- Consider checking coagulation (PT, PTT) for regional block.
- Other tests as indicated by H & P (eg, glucose in diabetic pt).
- Assess previous grafts for thrill or bruit.

Choice of Anesthesia
- Effect of premed may be exaggerated in pts w/ ESRD.
- MAC w/ local anesthesia may be sufficient for many fistulas, especially at the wrist.
- Regional anesthesia
  - Axillary, interscalene, or supraclavicular block may be used for surgical block.
  - Choice of block depends on proposed location of AV fistula.
- General anesthesia
  - May be the method of choice if site for fistula is not amenable to local or regional block (eg, proximal location in arm), or if long operative time is expected

INTRAOP

Monitors/Line Placement
- One peripheral IV.
- Standard monitors.
- Refrain from placing lines or blood pressure cuffs in extremities w/ grafts or on the proposed operative side.
- Pt may already have central dialysis access, which can be used.
  - Dialysis line may contain concentrated heparin solution.
  - Remove heparin before using line.

Intraop Concerns
- For induction of GA in pt w/ gastroparesis (eg, diabetic gastropathy), use rapid sequence intubation. Also consider:
  - Bicitra 30 mL PO in the preop period for aspiration prophylaxis.

> Metoclopramide, an H2 blocker, or a proton pump inhibitor in the preop period.
- Succinylcholine is contraindicated for ESRD pts who are hyperkalemic (eg, [K+] >5.5 mEq/L) or those exhibiting symptoms of hyperkalemia (peaked T waves).
- Minimize fluids to avoid fluid overload, as EBL is usually minimal.

Intraop Therapies
- Surgeon may request IV heparin prior to arterial clamping.
  > Protamine may be required after unclamping of fistula.

POSTOP

Pain
- Usually minimal
- Pain is usually easily managed w/ IV/PO narcotics
- Pt may have residual analgesia from regional block

Complications
- Thrombosis
- Graft failure
- CHF/pulmonary edema from fluid overload
- Arterial steal
- Infection
- Hyper/hypokalemia
- Myocardial ischemia (silent ischemia common in diabetic pt)

SURGICAL PROCEDURE

Indications
- ESRD

Procedure
- A skin incision is made over the areas from which the venous & arterial access is to be obtained.
- Fistula locations include
  > Anastomosis of cephalic vein to radial artery at the level of the wrist.
  > Radial or ulnar artery to the antebrachial vein.
  > Brachial artery to the axillary or basilic vein.
  > If the veins cannot be grafted, an artificial Teflon graft may be used to complete the vascular anastomosis.
    - Procedures involve a cutdown to the vessel & tunneling the graft under the skin to the artery.

- When the connection is completed & flow has been established, the skin incisions are closed.

Surgical Concerns
- Thrombosis (20%)
- Graft failure (10%)
- Infection
- Arterial steal
- Seroma

Typical EBL
- 25–50 mL

VAGINAL HYSTERECTOMY

JASON WIDRICH, MD

PREOP

Preop Considerations
- Hysterectomy can be performed through abdominal or vaginal approach (see also Procedures chapter "Total Abdominal Hysterectomy")
- Indication for surgery more likely to be uterine prolapse; not likely to be GYN cancer
- Vaginal approach assoc w/ significantly less morbidity & mortality

Physical Findings
- None typical

Workup
- CBC
- Type & screen
- Further workup based on coexisting disease

Choice of Anesthesia
- GA, epidural, or spinal appropriate

INTRAOP

Monitors/Line Placement
- Standard monitors
- One peripheral IV usually adequate

Intraop Concerns
- Possibility of blood loss or requirement for conversion to abdominal hysterectomy
- Trendelenburg position may be used to facilitate surgical exposure

Intraop Therapies
- Third-space fluid loss relatively low (eg, 4–6 mL/kg/h)
- Vagal stimulation from grasping the cervix can cause bradycardia.
  - ➣ Treat by halting the stimulus, increasing depth of anesthesia & giving glycopyrrolate or atropine if bradycardia persists.
- Antiemetic prophylaxis

POSTOP

Pain
- Mild to moderate
- Intermittent IV narcotics or PCA

Complications
- Nausea/vomiting
- Anemia or hemorrhage
- Peroneal nerve injury from positioning
- Bladder injury
- Wound infection

SURGICAL PROCEDURE

Indications
- Myomas, endometriosis, dysmenorrhea

Procedure
- Pt placed in lithotomy position
- Peritoneum is entered through paracervical incision
- Identification & ligation of uterosacral ligaments, cardinal ligaments, uterine vessels
- Uterus is removed through the incision. Peritoneum & vaginal cuff are reapproximated
- Procedure sometimes done as laparoscopy-assisted vaginal hysterectomy
  - ➣ Laparoscopy may be useful for diagnostic reasons, to remove adhesions or to assist with salpingo-oophorectomy

Surgical Concerns
- Bleeding, wound infection, bladder damage

Typical EBL
■ <500 mL

VENTRICULAR SEPTAL DEFECT (VSD) REPAIR

BETTY LEE-HOANG, MD

PREOP

Preop Considerations
■ VSD is the most common congenital cardiac malformation.
  ➤ The most frequent location of the opening in the ventricular sep-
    tum is the perimembranous region, in the upper section near the
    valves.
  ➤ Other sites: muscular septum, infundibulum.
■ Blood is shunted left to right through the VSD, causing increased
  pulmonary blood flow.
■ Pt may go on to develop pulmonary hypertension.
■ Amount of shunt is calculated by the pulmonary blood flow to systemic blood flow ratio. Amount of shunt depends on the relative
  compliance of the receiving chamber, the PVR, the SVR & somewhat
  on the size of the defect. Restrictive defects are those w/ a pressure
  gradient of <64 mmHg across the defect. Small defects are less than
  a third of the size of the aortic annulus.
■ Surgery to close congenital VSD is usually done during the first year
  of life.

Physical Findings
■ VSD size affects the severity of symptoms.
■ Large VSD may present w/ respiratory failure due to the high
  pulmonary blood flow, which reduces pulmonary compliance &
  increases work of breathing.
■ Symptoms include fatigue, labored breathing, failure to thrive.
■ VSD is often diagnosed by a heart murmur & then confirmed through
  echocardiogram or cardiac cath.

Workup
■ Medical treatment for CHF should be initiated prior to surgery,
  including digoxin & diuretics.
■ Pt's nutritional status should be optimized.

Choice of Anesthesia
- Premed recommended w/ midazolam to prevent crying or struggling, which may stress the circulatory system.
- Anesthesia can be induced w/ an inhaled anesthetic if pt has good myocardial function; otherwise ketamine or an opioid can be used.

INTRAOP

Monitors/Line Placement
- Standard ASA monitors, arterial line, large IV access
- TEE recommended for intraop monitoring of cardiac function; can also be used to confirm success of surgical repair

Intraop Concerns
- Efforts must be made to maintain or increase PVR to decrease pulmonary blood flow
- All bubbles must be removed from the IV & arterial lines to prevent air embolus

Intraop Therapy
- Therapy to increase PVR includes
  - Reducing inspired O_2
  - Preventing hyperventilation
  - Permitting hypercapnea
  - Acidosis
  - High mean airway pressure
  - Sympathetic stimulation
  - Hypervolemia
- Pt should receive antibiotic prophylaxis against bacterial endocarditis

POSTOP

Pain
- Moderate.
- Managed w/ IV narcotics.

Complications
- Pt may need inotropic support to wean from cardiopulmonary bypass.
- Arrhythmias & heart block can occur from damage to the conduction system postop; may require medical treatment & external pacing.

> If the rhythm is not normalized after 1 week postop, when swelling is expected to have resolved, a permanent pacemaker is often required.
- Bleeding may occur & should be monitored through chest tube drainage.

SURGICAL PROCEDURE

Indications
- Indicated for pts w/ symptoms to prevent long-term pulmonary damage & pulmonary HTN

Procedure
- Performed w/ cardiopulmonary bypass; the VSD is closed w/ a patch

Surgical Concerns
- May be residual VSD along the edge of the patch postop
  > If >4 mm, return to bypass is often indicated
  > Additional VSDs in other locations may be more visible w/ color flow Doppler after closure of the large VSD

Typical EBL
- Varies depending on pt size but should be minimal

VENTRICULOPERITONEAL SHUNT

DHANESH K. GUPTA, MD

PREOP

Preop Considerations
- If pt is s/p subarachnoid hemorrhage (SAH), external ventricular drain may be present

Physical Findings
- If increased ICP
  > Nausea/vomiting
  > Confusion
  > Obtundation
- If s/p peritoneal craniotomy for aneurysm clipping
  > Many pts will have limited mouth opening due to TMJ pain
  > A few pts may have TMJ dysfunction
- Note pt's preop neuro deficit, including level of consciousness

■ Note baseline BP if s/p SAH to prevent worsening ischemia due to hypotension

Workup
■ None specific

Choice of Anesthesia
■ GA usually indicated to control airway w/ head movement & protect from aspiration

INTRAOP

Monitors/Line Placement
■ Consider PIV in arm opposite of VP shunt to allow accessibility during procedure.

Intraop Concerns
■ Possible need for rapid sequence induction due to nausea/vomiting.
■ Minimal use of premeds if poor mental status preop.
■ 90-degree bed turn w/ side to be worked on away from anesthesiologist.
■ Field includes side of head, face, neck, chest, & abdomen.
    ➤ Tape tube securely on side opposite of surgical incision.
    ➤ Protect eyes from Betadine prep by covering w/ Tegaderm.
■ Sudden increase in surgical stimulation w/ catheter tunneling may occur (<1–3 min duration).
    ➤ Can treat w/ short-acting hypnotic.
■ Possible pneumothorax w/ rigid tunneling.

Intraop Therapies
■ If pt on chronic anticonvulsant therapy, duration of action of muscle relaxants may be shortened.

POSTOP

Pain
■ Mild, esp if local anesthetic used in abdominal wound

Complications
■ Delayed awakening

SURGICAL PROCEDURE

Indications
■ Increased +ICP (chronic)

Procedure

■ A connection is made between the cerebral ventricles & peritoneum via a tunneled, subcutaneous catheter to permit drainage of CSF.

Surgical Concerns

■ Muscle relaxant may assist in peritoneal shunt placement.

Typical EBL

■ <100 mL

PART THREE

Critical Events

ACIDOSIS

WILLIAM RHOADS, MD

DESCRIPTION

- Definitions
  - Acidemia: pH <7.35
  - Acidosis: process that lowers the pH
  - Metabolic acidosis: reduction in plasma bicarbonate. Can be caused by bicarbonate loss, buffering of a noncarbonic acid (eg, lactic acid), or retention of diet-generated acid (eg, sulfuric acid in renal failure).
    - Compensation involves stimulation of ventilation, w/ decrease in pCO_2.
    - Plasma anion gap $= Na - Cl - HCO_3$ (normal 10–14)
    - Metabolic acidosis classified as anion gap or non-anion gap acidosis
  - Respiratory acidosis: increased pCO_2 from decreased alveolar ventilation.
    - Compensation involves renal hydrogen ion excretion, which takes 3–5 days for maximum response.
- Metabolic acidosis
  - Common causes of anion gap acidosis
    - Ketoacidosis (related to diabetes, starvation, alcohol)
    - Lactic acidosis (assoc w/ hypotension, shock, cardiac arrest, tissue ischemia, tonic-clonic seizure)
    - Renal failure
    - Rhabdomyolysis
    - Ingestion of salicylate, methanol, ethylene glycol, paraldehyde
  - Common causes of non-anion gap acidosis
    - GI HCO_3 loss: diarrhea, pancreatic fistula, biliary drainage
    - Renal tubular acidosis
    - Carbonic anhydrase inhibitors or potassium-sparing diuretics
    - Dilutional (vigorous resuscitation w/ saline)
    - Hypoaldosteronism
- Respiratory acidosis
  - Common causes of acute respiratory acidosis
    - Drug therapy: opiates, sedative-hypnotics, IV & inhaled anesthetics, muscle relaxants

- Muscle weakness (related to drug therapy or neuromuscular disease)
- Upper airway obstruction
- Acute pulmonary process (eg, pulmonary edema, bronchospasm, pneumonia, pneumothorax, hemothorax)
- Acute exacerbation of chronic lung disease (eg, asthma, COPD)
- Acute CNS process (eg, stroke, intracranial hemorrhage)
  - ➤ Causes of chronic respiratory acidosis
    - Obesity-hypoventilation syndrome
    - Neuromuscular disease (eg, myasthenia gravis, polio, amyotrophic lateral sclerosis, multiple sclerosis, Guillain-Barre syndrome)
    - Chronic lung disease (COPD, chronic bronchitis, emphysema)
    - For pt w/ minimal primary medical care, periop presentation of respiratory acidosis may represent a chronic process.

DIAGNOSIS
- Clinical history may suggest underlying cause of acidosis.
  - ➤ Conditions w/ increased risk of periop metabolic acidosis
    - Surgical procedure assoc w/ extreme blood or fluid loss, sepsis
    - Pts w/ hepatic or bowel ischemia, renal failure
- ABG: for measurement of pH, pO_2, pCO_2. Calculated values include base excess, bicarbonate.
- Electrolytes: measure to evaluate anion gap & electrolyte abnormalities
- BUN/Cr: if elevated, supports volume depletion as contributing factor
- Signs & symptoms of metabolic acidosis
  - ➤ Respiratory: dyspnea on exertion
  - ➤ Cardiac: ventricular arrhythmias, hypotension (related to reduced contractility), diminished effect of inotropes
  - ➤ Neuro: lethargy & coma possible but more common w/ respiratory acidosis
- Signs & symptoms of respiratory acidosis
  - ➤ Overall, symptoms much more common w/ acute respiratory acidosis
  - ➤ Neuro: headache, blurred vision, restlessness, anxiety, delirium, somnolence
  - ➤ Cardiac: arrhythmias, hypotension
- Other manifestations of acidosis

➤ Impaired uptake of oxygen by Hgb
➤ Multiple effects on drug handling, including decreased protein binding of anesthetic drugs (eg, thiopental)
➤ Decreased efficacy of local anesthetics due to decreased ionization
➤ Prolonged action of some nondepolarizing neuromuscular blockers (vecuronium, pancuronium, atracurium)

MANAGEMENT
■ Review clinical history for clues to underlying processes.
■ Obtain ABG, electrolytes, BUN, Cr.
■ Diagnose primary acid-base disorder. Primary disorder causes pH to shift in that direction.
■ Determine if compensation is appropriate & consider additional primary disorder.
■ Treat underlying disease process discovered.
■ Other supportive measures
  ➤ For mechanically ventilated pt, increase minute ventilation to facilitate respiratory compensation.
  ➤ Administer oxygen to pt w/ possible tissue ischemia.
  ➤ Treat hypovolemia & low cardiac output.
  ➤ Treat hyperkalemia if present.
  ➤ Bicarbonate replacement may be indicated in some situations (eg, most non-gap acidoses, pH <7.0).
    • Bicarbonate therapy rarely indicated for lactic acidosis or diabetic ketoacidosis

ACLS ALGORITHMS: ASYSTOLE

CHRISTINE A. WU, MD

DESCRIPTION
■ Definition: Cardiac standstill; flatline on EKG

DIAGNOSIS
■ ECG monitor & pulse check. Confirm asystole on 2 leads to differentiate fine VF.

MANAGEMENT
■ CPR until asystole confirmed in 2 or more leads.

- Rapid scene survey for any evidence personnel should stop resuscitation.
- IV, intubate.
- Consider causes: hypoxia, hyperkalemia, hypokalemia, acidosis, drug OD, hypothermia.
- Consider immediate transcutaneous pacing (TCP).
- Epinephrine 1 mg IV/ET q3–5min.
- Atropine 1 mg IV/ET, repeat in 3–5 min to a total of 0.03–0.04 mg/kg.
- Consider termination of efforts again.

ACLS ALGORITHMS: BRADYCARDIA

CHRISTINE A. WU, MD

DESCRIPTION
- Definition
  - Absolute bradycardia: HR <60 in adults
  - Relative bradycardia: Inadequate HR leading to serious signs or symptoms (CP, SOB, altered mental status, hypotension, shock, CHF, MI)

DIAGNOSIS
- ECG monitor & pulse check

MANAGEMENT
- Assess ABCs.
- Secure airway, IV access, give O_2.
- Attach monitors (pulse ox, BP, EKG).
  If serious signs or symptoms (chest pain, SOB, AMS, hypotension, shock, CHF, MI):
- Atropine 0.5–1 mg IVP
- Transcutaneous pacing (eg, Zoll pads)
- Dopamine 5–20 mcg/kg/min IV
- Epinephrine 2–10 mcg/min IV
- If secondary to beta blocker OD, glucagon 5–10 mg IV bolus/ 1–5 mg/h
- For asymptomatic Mobitz II or third-degree block
  - Prepare for transvenous pacing.
  - May use transcutaneous pacemaker if symptoms develop prior to transvenous pacer placed.

For asymptomatic sinus, junctional, or Mobitz I bradycardia, observe.

ACLS ALGORITHMS: PULSELESS ELECTRICAL ACTIVITY (PEA)

CHRISTINE A. WU, MD

DESCRIPTION
- Definition: Rhythms that do not generate a pulse yet have electrical activity or
  - Electromechanical dissociation (EMD)
  - Pseudo-EMD
  - Idioventricular rhythms
  - Ventricular escape rhythms
  - Bradyasystolic rhythms
  - Post-defibrillation idioventricular rhythms
- Most importantly, these rhythms are often assoc w/ specific clinical states that can be reversed when identified early & treated appropriately.

DIAGNOSIS
- ECG monitor & pulse check

MANAGEMENT
- Start CPR, IV, intubate.
- Consider causes & treat appropriately:
  - Hypovolemia
  - Tablets (drugs)
  - Hypoxia
  - Tamponade (cardiac)
  - Hydrogen ion (acidosis)
  - Tension pneumothorax
  - Hyper/hypokalemia
  - Thrombosis (coronary)
  - Hypothermia
  - Thrombosis (pulm. emboli)
- Epinephrine 1 mg IV/ET q3–5min
- Atropine 1 mg IV/ET if HR <60 bpm. Repeat q3–5min to a total of 0.03–0.04 mg/kg.

ACLS ALGORITHMS: TACHYCARDIA

CHRISTINE A. WU, MD
LINDA LIU, MD

DESCRIPTION
■ Definition: Abnormally rapid HR (HR >100) that is symptomatic & needs immediate evaluation; mgt depends on diagnosis & underlying source.

DIAGNOSIS
■ Assess if pt is stable or unstable (ie, symptoms of CP, SOB, SBP <90, CHF, ischemia, MI).
■ If stable, then determine if ventricular (wide complex) or atrial (usually narrow complex).
   ➤ Wide complex can also result from atrial tachycardia w/ aberrancy.
■ Then assess whether pt has preserved heart function or poor ejection fraction (EF) in order to determine treatment.

MANAGEMENT
■ Unstable (symptoms of CP, dyspnea, SBP <90, CHF, ischemia/infarct)
   ➤ Prepare for immediate cardioversion.
   ➤ O_2 by face mask
   ➤ Ensure airway, IV access.
   ➤ Consider sedation unless pt hemodynamically unstable (hypotensive, pulmonary edema, unconscious).
   ➤ Synchronized cardioversion
■ Stable ventricular tachycardia
   ➤ O_2 by face mask; ensure airway, IV access
   ➤ Determine whether VT is monomorphic or polymorphic.
   ➤ If monomorphic VT, then determine cardiac function.
   ➤ Preserved heart function: acceptable treatments:
      • Procainamide
      • Sotalol
      • Amiodarone
      • Lidocaine
   ➤ Poor EF (<40%): acceptable treatments:
      • Amiodarone (150 mg IV over 10 min)

- Lidocaine (0.5–0.75 mg/kg IV push)
- Synchronized cardioversion
■ If polymorphic VT, then check QT interval.
  ➤ Normal baseline QT interval:
    - Treat ischemia.
    - Correct electrolytes.
    - Meds (choose one):
    - Beta blockers
    - Lidocaine
    - Amiodarone
    - Procainamide
  ➤ Prolonged baseline QT intervals:
    - Correct electrolytes.
    - Other therapies:
    - Magnesium
    - Overdrive pacing
    - Isoproterenol
    - Phenytoin
    - Lidocaine
■ Stable wide-complex tachycardia, unknown type
  ➤ O$_2$ by face mask; ensure airway, IV access
  ➤ Attempt to establish a specific diagnosis.
  ➤ 12-lead ECG
  ➤ Esophageal lead
  ➤ Clinical information
  ➤ If persistent wide-complex tachycardia of unknown type, then assess cardiac function.
    - If preserved cardiac function (choose one):
    - DC cardioversion
    - Procainamide
    - Amiodarone
    - If poor EF (<40%), choose one:
    - DC cardioversion
    - Amiodarone
■ Stable atrial fibrillation/flutter
  ➤ Assess cardiac function.
  ➤ If preserved cardiac function, choose one:
    - Calcium channel blockers
    - Beta blockers
  ➤ If poor cardiac function (EF <40%), choose one:

- Digoxin
- Diltiazem
- Amiodarone
➤ Rhythm conversion, either chemically or DC cardioversion is indicated only when pt is unstable. For nonemergent cases, make a careful evaluation for thromboembolic events first.
■ Stable Wolff-Parkinson-White (w/ or w/o CHF)
➤ Avoid adenosine, beta blockers, calcium channel blockers, digoxin.
➤ Rate control w/ amiodarone
➤ Rhythm conversion only in unstable cases. Evaluate for thromboembolic events prior to nonemergent cardioversion.
■ Stable narrow-complex tachycardias
➤ O_2 by face mask; ensure airway, IV access
➤ Vagal maneuvers to help slow rate & allow for identification of rhythm
➤ Adenosine 3 mg IVP via central line or 6 mg IVP via peripheral IV
➤ Adenosine 6 mg IVP via central line or 12 mg IVP via peripheral IV
■ If junctional tachycardia, then assess cardiac function.
➤ If preserved cardiac function, then:
- Beta blocker
- Calcium channel blocker
- Amiodarone
- DC cardioversion
➤ If poor cardiac function (EF <40%), then:
- Amiodarone
- DC cardioversion
■ If ectopic or multifocal atrial tachycardia
➤ Assess cardiac function.
➤ If preserved cardiac function, then
- Beta blocker
- Calcium channel blocker
- Amiodarone
- DC cardioversion usually not successful
➤ If poor cardiac function (EF <40%), then
- Amiodarone
- Diltiazem
- DC cardioversion usually not successful
■ If PSVT

➤ Assess cardiac function.
➤ If preserved cardiac function, then
  • AV nodal blockade w/
  • Beta blocker
  • Calcium channel blocker
  • Digoxin
  • DC cardioversion
  • Antiarrhythmics
  • Procainamide
  • Amiodarone
  • Sotalol
➤ If poor cardiac function (EF <40%), then
  • DC cardioversion
  • Digoxin
  • Amiodarone
  • Diltiazem

ACLS ALGORITHMS: VF (OR PULSELESS VT)

CHRISTINE A. WU, MD

DESCRIPTION
■ Definition: Fine or coarse, rapid, fibrillatory movements of the ventricles that replace normal contractions of the heart

DIAGNOSIS
■ ECG monitor, pulse check

MANAGEMENT
■ Perform ABCs.
■ Check pulse. If no pulse initiate CPR (± precordial thump for witnessed arrest).
■ Check rhythm. If VF or VT:
  ➤ Defibrillate
    • Defibrillate 200 J. Check pulse & rhythm.
    • Defibrillate 300 J & recheck.
    • Defibrillate 360 J & recheck.
    • CPR if still no pulse, establish IV access, intubate.
  ➤ Epinephrine or vasopressin
    • Epinephrine 1 mg IV, repeat q3–5min
    • Vasopressin 40 U IV, single dose 1 time only
    • After each drug dose, defibrillate again w/ 360 J & recheck.

- ➤ Amiodarone 300 mg IV push
  - Can be redosed at 150 mg IV if VF/VT recurs
  - Max dose 2.2 g over 24 h
- ➤ Lidocaine
  - 1–1.5 mg/kg IV push
  - Can then give 0.5-mg/kg boluses q3–5min up to 3 mg/kg total
  - After each drug dose defibrillate w/ 360 J & recheck.
- ➤ Consider:
  - Magnesium 1–2 g IV for polymorphic VT or suspected hypo-magnesemic state
  - Procainamide 30 mg/min, max 17 mg/kg
  - Sodium bicarbonate 1 mEq/kg IV only if metabolic acidosis is suspected

---

AIRWAY BURN

MARC SCHROEDER, MD
JULIN TANG, MD, MS

DESCRIPTION
- ■ Burn injury to upper & lower airway due to fire, steam, electricity, or chemicals.
- ■ Inhalational burns increase mortality by 30–40%.
- ■ May be assoc w/ massive pulmonary edema.

DIAGNOSIS
- ■ Exam
  - ➤ Look for
    - Singed nasal hair or eyebrows
    - Soot in oropharynx
    - Burn to nose or mouth
  - ➤ Listen for
    - Stridor
    - Cough
    - Hoarseness
  - ➤ Examine for other signs of respiratory distress.
- ■ History: Increased risk of airway burn if
  - ➤ Fire in enclosed space
  - ➤ Longer time of exposure
  - ➤ Presence of toxic fumes

- Labs
  - CXR
  - ABG
  - Carbon monoxide level
    - Carbon monoxide has 200 times the affinity of oxygen for hemoglobin (shifts the oxygen/hemoglobin dissociation curve to the left).
    - If carbon monoxide is present, oxygen content can be low even though arterial oxygen partial pressure is normal.

MANAGEMENT

- Airway mgt
- Anticipate difficulty securing airway due to trauma & generalized body edema.
  - Avoid succinylcholine: it may increase K+ due to tissue damage.
- Ventilation
  - Increased alveolar ventilation needed due to increased metabolism from burn leading to increased CO_2 production
    - If carbon monoxide poisoning is suspected, administer 100% oxygen. This decreases the half-life of carboxyhemoglobin from 4 h to <1 h.
- Evaluate extent of injury by bronchoscopy & laryngoscopy once airway is secured.
- Anticipate prolonged intubation if there are large fluid losses/shifts or suspected airway edema.
- Extubation
  - Anticipate high risk of pulmonary edema & respiratory distress.
  - Be ready to reintubate.
- Chemical burns: anticipate difficult airway mgt & ARDS. Also worry about:
  - Oropharyngeal injury
  - Esophageal/gastric perforation
  - Aspiration
- Monitor clinical course w/
  - CXR
  - ABGs
  - Pulse oximetry
  - Co-oximetry for carboxyhemoglobin
- Prophylactic steroids & antibiotics are contraindicated.

AIRWAY FIRE

MARK ROLLINS, MD

DESCRIPTION

- Fire in the airway
- A fuel, oxidizer, & ignition source must be present to start a fire. Risk of fire increases w/:
  - Presence of an ET tube (fuel)
  - High FiO_2 or N_2O (both oxidizers)
  - Use of laser or electrocautery (ignition sources)
- High-risk surgeries involve use of laser or electrocautery near the trachea or esophagus. To reduce risk of fire:
  - Reduce FiO_2 to lowest possible (<30).
  - Avoid nitrous oxide (supports combustion).
  - Use intermittent apnea or jet ventilation rather than an ET tube if possible.
  - Use a fire-resistant tube or consider wrapping w/ metallic tape (no current tube or method of protection is completely laser- or fireproof).
  - Fill cuff w/ methylene blue-tinted saline; can help absorb heat & signal a rupture.
  - Place wet pledgets above cuff.
  - Place cuff as far distally as possible in the trachea.
  - Have a source of water (60-mL syringe) immediately available.

DIAGNOSIS

- Smoke, flame, or audible "pop" can signal an airway fire.

MANAGEMENT

- Stop ventilation & gas flow through ET tube.
- Remove ET tube.
- Inspect airway w/ DL.
- Mask ventilate w/ 100% oxygen & reintubate.
  - Important: Make sure fire is out before administering oxygen!
- Obtain consult immediately to assess lower airway damage w/ bronchoscopy.
- Follow blood gases to further assess gas exchange abnormalities.
- Head-up postop positioning to decrease edema
- Administration of postop humidified oxygen

- Long-term intubation & ventilation, bronchial lavage, and/or steroids may be required.

AIRWAY OBSTRUCTION

J. W. BEARD, MD
RICHARD PAULSEN, MD

DESCRIPTION
- Definition
  - Anatomic obstruction of gas movement leading to hypoventilation
  - Obstruction can primarily involve the upper (extrathoracic) or lower airways.
  - Obstruction can be total or partial.
  - Obstruction can be acute or chronic.
  - This chapter primarily deals w/ acute upper airway obstruction. Lower airway obstruction from bronchospasm is covered elsewhere.
- Cardiovascular manifestations: HTN, tachycardia, myocardial ischemia & bradycardia followed by cardiac arrest (if hypoxia present)
- Pulmonary manifestations: hypercarbia, hypoxia, negative pressure pulmonary edema
- Pts at high risk include
  - Those undergoing procedures resulting in dependent airway edema (eg, performed in prone or Trendelenburg position), esp if surgery was prolonged & fluid/blood requirements were significant
  - Procedures leading directly to airway compromise through edema/hematoma formation (usually involve the neck or airway structures directly)
  - Excessive sedation, leading to tongue sagging on posterior pharynx
  - Those at risk for laryngospasm
  - Those w/ a mediastinal mass
  - Obese pts
  - Pts w/ foreign body aspiration
  - Pts w/ a history of bronchospasm
  - Pts undergoing anaphylactic reaction

- Pts w/ recurrent laryngeal nerve palsy (obstruction usually occurs w/ bilateral palsies)
- Problems w/ the ETT can also cause obstruction, including
  - Kinked ETT
  - Cuff herniation
  - Obstruction from secretions or blood
- Pt may present in a variety of clinical settings, including the ER, preop, or postop.
  - Mild chronic obstruction may worsen in the postop setting.
  - Some causes of obstruction are more likely to present after extubation:
    - Laryngospasm
    - Oversedation (w/ tongue causing posterior pharyngeal obstruction)
    - Residual neuromuscular blockade
    - Bilateral vocal cord paralysis
    - Foreign body

DIAGNOSIS
- During spontaneous ventilation
  - Pts often use accessory muscles of respiration & display labored breathing pattern.
  - Other signs include
    - Paradoxical abdominal movement w/ respiration
    - "Rocking boat" ventilation
    - Stridor
    - Wheezing
    - Anxiety
- During mechanical ventilation
  - Increased peak airway pressure (usually w/ normal plateau pressure)
  - Decreased chest wall movement
  - CO_2 capnogram shows obstructed pattern.
  - Wheezing
- Decreased oxygen saturation, hypercarbia & altered mental status may occur quickly.
- Some specific causes of airway obstruction
  - Laryngospasm
    - Occurs usually after extubation; caused by irritative stimulus during light anesthesia
  - Residual neuromuscular blockade

- Evidence of insufficient reversal (<4/4 TOF, fade, no sustained head lift, rapid-shallow respirations)
➤ Airway edema
  - Obstruction usually after extubation in pt w/ other evidence of tissue edema (scleral, tongue, facial)
➤ Aspiration/foreign body
  - Obstruction caused by larger particles
  - Stridor and/or wheezing can be present.
➤ Mediastinal mass
  - Obstruction may present after switch from spontaneous to positive-pressure ventilation.
➤ Vocal cord paralysis (bilateral)
  - Can occur after thyroid, parathyroid, thoracic, tracheal surgery or traumatic tracheal intubation
  - Stridor w/o ability to phonate

MANAGEMENT
- First intervention is application of 100% oxygen & airway positioning (eg, backward tilt of head, anterior displacement of mandible).
  ➤ When obstruction is not immediately reversible, an oral or nasal airway may be used.
  ➤ Nasal airways are often better tolerated: oral may induce gagging, vomiting, laryngospasm.
- If airway continues to be obstructed, attempt positive-pressure mask ventilation.
- If cause of obstruction is determined or suspected, consider specific treatment.
  ➤ Laryngospasm
    - If occurs during induction, deepen anesthetic & reduce level of stimulation.
    - Provide continuous positive pressure.
    - If not successful, give small dose of succinylcholine (10–20 mg in an adult).
    - Use caution as succinylcholine may cause respiratory depression.
    - Intubate the trachea if obstruction continues.
  ➤ Mediastinal mass
    - Return to spontaneous ventilation if possible.
    - Intubate trachea & advance ETT distal to lesion if possible.
    - Consider CPB if readily available.

➤ Bilateral vocal cord paralysis
  - Intubate the trachea to relieve obstruction & protect airway.
➤ Airway edema/hematoma
  - Sit pt upright.
  - If partial obstruction, consider emergent evacuation of hematoma.
  - If total obstruction, intubate trachea.
  - Note leak pressure around ETT.
➤ Residual neuromuscular blockade
  - Administer acetylcholinesterase inhibitor if not already given.
  - Reduce work of breathing by sitting pt up & assisting w/ mask ventilation.
  - Reintubate trachea if pt fails to improve.
➤ Aspiration/foreign body
  - Clear upper airway.
  - Suction oropharynx.
  - Consider administering bronchodilators.
➤ Kinked ETT
  - Correct kink if possible.
  - If armored tube w/ severe kink or obstruction, remove tube & reintubate w/ new ETT.
➤ ETT secretions
  - Suction ETT w/ or w/o saline irrigation.
➤ ETT cuff herniation
  - Deflate cuff.
  - Gradually reinflate once airway patent.
  - If obstruction occurs again, consider reintubation w/ new ETT.
➤ For excessive sedation contributing to airway obstruction
  - Consider appropriate reversal agents (eg, naloxone, flumazenil).
■ If maneuvers described above fail to open airway, consider tracheal intubation.
  ➤ If obstruction occurs postop, look at anesthesia record for ease of intubation.
  ➤ Evaluate airway for potential difficulty (see also Technique chapter "Airway Assessment").
  ➤ If difficult airway suspected, recruit additional help (see also Critical Event chapter "Difficult Airway Management").
  ➤ Degree of obstruction & decreased oxygen saturation determine the available time for intervention.

➤ Consider whether surgical airway (eg, cricothyrotomy) may be urgently needed; obtain experienced personnel for this.

■ After successful intubation, consider evaluation by ENT surgeon to evaluate cause of obstruction.

➤ If obstruction is mild, ENT surgeon may perform flexible fiberoptic pharyngoscopy/laryngoscopy to evaluate cause of obstruction prior to intubation attempts.

■ If obstruction responds to initial therapy, consider whether additional measures may help improve obstruction.

➤ Steroid therapy

➤ Elevate head of bed.

➤ Suction airway secretions.

➤ Racemic epinephrine nebulizer treatment (may temporarily decrease airway mucosal edema; beware of rebound increase in edema)

➤ Helium-oxygen inhalation to decrease viscosity of inspired gas & decrease work of breathing

■ Depending on cause of obstruction & pt's response to therapy, consider whether pt should remain in a closely monitored setting (eg, PACU, ICU).

ALKALOSIS

MANUEL PARDO, JR., MD

DESCRIPTION

■ Definitions

➤ Alkalemia: pH >7.45

➤ Alkalosis: process that raises the pH

➤ Metabolic alkalosis: elevation in plasma bicarb concentration produced by bicarb administration or by H^+ loss. Respiratory compensation occurs by hypoventilation & increased pCO_2.

➤ Respiratory alkalosis: decreased pCO_2 caused by hyperventilation. Renal compensation occurs through bicarb loss in urine, w/ decreased plasma bicarb. For every 10-mmHg decrease in pCO_2, plasma bicarb level drops by 2 mEq acutely or 5 mEq chronically.

■ Metabolic alkalosis

➤ Common causes: diuretics, NG suction, vomiting, administration of sodium bicarbonate, metabolism of organic acids (eg, citrate in blood products, lactate, ketoacids)

➤ Excess mineralocorticoid activity is uncommon cause in periop setting.
➤ Volume depletion tends to maintain metabolic alkalosis by preventing excess bicarb excretion in urine.

■ Respiratory alkalosis
  ➤ Common causes
    • Central respiratory stimulation: pain, anxiety, head trauma, brain tumor, stroke, pregnancy
    • Peripheral respiratory stimulation: hypoxemia, pulmonary emboli, CHF, pneumonia, interstitial lung disease, asthma
    • Multiple or other mechanisms: liver failure, sepsis, mechanical ventilation

DIAGNOSIS

■ Clinical history may suggest underlying cause of alkalosis.
■ ABGs: for measurement of pH, pO_2, pCO_2. Calculated values include base excess, bicarbonate.
■ Electrolytes: measure to evaluate anion gap & electrolyte abnormalities
■ BUN/Cr: if elevated, supports volume depletion as contributing factor
■ Signs & symptoms of metabolic alkalosis
  ➤ Usually asymptomatic, but pt may have signs of volume depletion or hypokalemia
■ Signs & symptoms of respiratory alkalosis
  ➤ Important physiologic effect: decreased cerebral blood flow, CNS vasoconstriction
  ➤ CNS symptoms: irritability, light-headedness, paresthesias, carpopedal spasm, circumoral numbness
  ➤ Cardiac symptoms: arrhythmias
  ➤ Other: decreased potassium, decreased ionized calcium, left shift of oxyhemoglobin dissociation curve

MANAGEMENT

■ Review clinical history for clues to underlying processes.
■ Obtain ABGs, electrolytes, BUN, Cr.
■ Diagnose primary acid-base disorder. Primary disorder causes pH to shift in that direction.
■ Determine if compensation is appropriate & consider additional primary disorder.
■ Treat underlying disease process discovered. Other considerations:

➤ Metabolic alkalosis: consider volume administration if pt is hypovolemic
➤ Respiratory alkalosis: if pt on mechanical ventilation, determine if pt is breathing above set ventilator rate. If not, reduce tidal volume or respiratory rate. If pt is breathing above ventilator rate, can try narcotic administration but may not be effective in reducing minute ventilation.

ALTERED MENTAL STATUS POSTOP

MADELEINE BIBAT, MD

DESCRIPTION

■ Definition: Postop change in:
  ➤ Level of consciousness
  ➤ Cognitive function
  ➤ Attention
  ➤ Behavior
■ Etiologies (differential diagnosis)
  ➤ Cardiovascular
    • Hypotension
    • Severe HTN
    • Tachycardia/bradycardia
    • Cardiac arrhythmias
  ➤ Pulmonary manifestations
    • Hypoxemia
    • Hypercarbia
  ➤ Drug-related: sensorium of pts w/ preexisting neuro abnormalities may be particularly sensitive to the effects of depressant drugs:
    • Benzodiazepines
    • Volatile anesthetics
    • IV anesthetics (barbiturates, propofol, ketamine)
    • Opioids
    • Anticholinergics
    • Steroids
    • Local anesthetic toxicity
    • Antidopaminergic drugs (phenothiazines & butyrophenones [eg, Haldol, droperidol])
    • Total spinal

- Retrobulbar block w/ inadvertent subarachnoid injection of local anesthetic & subsequent brain stem anesthesia
- CNS
  - Stroke
  - CNS infection
  - Cerebral ischemia
  - Seizure or postictal state
  - Coma
  - Increased ICP
  - Anxiety
  - Underlying psychiatric disease
  - Pain
  - Blindness
- Metabolic/toxic
  - Acidosis/alkalosis
  - Hyponatremia (eg, TURP syndrome)
  - Hypernatremia
  - Hypoglycemia
  - Uremia
  - Hepatic encephalopathy
  - Hypothermia
  - Hyperthermia
  - Hypo- or hyperthyroidism
  - Adrenal crisis
  - Other electrolyte abnormalities (ie, $K+$, $Ca++$, $Mg++$)
  - Drug withdrawal (eg, alcohol withdrawal)
- Infectious
  - Sepsis
  - CNS infections: meningitis, encephalitis, abscess, AIDS
- Procedures w/ increased risk: cerebrovascular, neuro, cardiac surgeries
- Severity: ranges from reversible anesthetic drug effects to permanent CNS impairment
- Postop delirium can be of unclear etiology.
- Sedation or anesthesia can lead to a recrudescence of prior focal neuro deficits (eg, in pts w/ a history of stroke that has resolved or TIA).
  - These symptoms are limited in duration.

DIAGNOSIS
- While evaluating pt, consider differential diagnosis (above) in light of

- Pt age, history
- Type of anesthetic
- Drugs administered
- Intraop events, mgt
- Assess ventilation, oxygenation, circulation.
- Evaluate vital signs; perform neuro exam.
- Try to discern whether mental status change is due to lingering anesthetic effects or permanent neuro damage (eg, focal deficit).
- Rule out metabolic etiology. Check:
  - Electrolytes
  - Glucose
  - ABGs
  - Consider blood or urine toxic screen.
- Obtain EKG.
- Consider reversal agents as diagnostic/therapeutic maneuver.
  - Narcotics: use naloxone in 40-mcg doses.
  - Benzodiazepines: use flumazenil in 0.2-mg doses.
- If focal neuro findings are present, consider a neurology consult.
- For a nonfocal neuro exam of unclear etiology, consider pain issues, residual drug effects, or possible postictal state.
  - If symptoms do not improve, consider a neurology consult.
- Emergence delirium usually occurs in the immediate waking period & is more common in those w/:
  - Preexisting cognitive impairment
  - History of alcohol or drug abuse
  - Elderly pts

MANAGEMENT
- Make sure pt is well oxygenated & ventilating well.
  - Provide supplemental oxygen as needed.
  - Manage airway as required.
- Consider reversal agents:
  - Naloxone for suspected narcotic overdose
  - Flumazenil for residual sedation from benzodiazepines
  - Physostigmine for possible continued anticholinergic effects
- Correct metabolic & acid/base derangements.
- Avoid hypothermia, which can increase the effects of CNS depressants.
- Treat suspected alcohol withdrawal.
- Provide adequate pain medicine to pts who are conscious, have a normal neuro exam, & are agitated.

- Inform surgeon of the problem.
- Obtain neurology consult as needed.

AMNIOTIC FLUID EMBOLUS

TESSA COLLINS, MD

DESCRIPTION

- Definition: Embolization of amniotic fluid into the maternal circulation, antepartum, intrapartum, or in the early postpartum period
- Cardiovascular manifestations
  - ➤ Hypotension
  - ➤ Dysrhythmias (EMD, V-tach or V-fib)
  - ➤ Hemodynamic collapse (cardiac arrest)
- Pulmonary manifestations
  - ➤ Hypoxia
  - ➤ Dyspnea
  - ➤ Bronchospasm
  - ➤ Pulmonary edema; ARDS
- Other manifestations
  - ➤ Seizures
  - ➤ Fetal distress
  - ➤ Coagulopathy
  - ➤ Uterine atony
  - ➤ Postpartum hemorrhage
- Risk factors
  - ➤ Abortion
  - ➤ Amniocentesis
  - ➤ Multiparity
  - ➤ "Tumultuous labor"; can also occur spontaneously during third trimester
  - ➤ Cesarean section
  - ➤ Abdominal trauma
- Severity: significant maternal mortality (26–61%); a large percentage of survivors are neurologically impaired. Fetuses also are at high risk of mortality & neuro damage.

DIAGNOSIS

- Most specific signs: a diagnosis of exclusion
  - ➤ Amniotic fluid material in the maternal pulmonary circulation can be found but not usually useful in acute setting.

■ Most sensitive signs: classic triad of acute hypoxia, hypotension, coagulopathy

MANAGEMENT
■ Notify obstetrician; get help.
■ Secure airway w/ ETT; ventilate w/ 100% FIO_2.
■ Initiate CPR as needed.
■ Monitor fetus; deliver fetus & placenta ASAP.
■ Supportive care
  ➤ IV access
  ➤ Fluid & vasopressors/inotropes as needed
  ➤ Central access
  ➤ Consider pulmonary artery catheter for monitoring
■ Assess & treat coagulopathy.
  ➤ Follow labs (PT, PTT, fibrinogen, fibrinogen split products, plt, Hct/Hb).
  ➤ Give FFP, cryoprecipitate, platelets, blood as needed.

ANAPHYLAXIS/ANAPHYLACTOID REACTION

GRETE H. PORTEOUS, MD

DESCRIPTION
■ Definition
  ➤ Anaphylaxis: severe allergic (type I hypersensitivity) reaction caused by IgE-mediated release of histamine, leukotrienes, prostaglandins, & other humoral agents
  ➤ Anaphylactoid reaction is clinically similar but is not IgE-mediated.
■ Cardiovascular manifestations
  ➤ Decreased SVR, increased capillary permeability, & direct myocardial depression can cause:
    • Hypotension
    • Tachycardia
    • Dysrhythmias
    • Cardiac arrest
■ Pulmonary manifestations
  ➤ Bronchospasm
  ➤ Laryngeal edema
  ➤ Pulmonary edema
  ➤ Cough

- Dyspnea
- Hypoxemia
- Skin findings
  - Urticaria (hives)
  - Flushing
  - Peripheral edema
  - Pruritus
- Other manifestations
  - Nausea, abdominal pain
  - DIC
- Risk & predisposing factors
  - Incidence is 1:2,000–1:20,000 anesthetics.
  - Prior allergic history
    - Hay fever
    - Drug allergy
    - Food allergy
    - Pts w/ hx of atopy or severe allergy are at highest risk.
  - Muscle relaxants & antibiotics (esp cephalosporins) are most common drugs implicated in anaphylaxis during anesthesia.
  - Other agents to consider:
    - Latex (esp w/ multiple prior exposure to latex products)
    - Colloid volume expanders (eg, dextran)
    - Thiopental
    - Blood products
    - Protamine (esp if pt has fish allergies or is taking NPH insulin)
    - IV contrast is a relatively common cause of anaphylactoid reaction.
- Severity: Onset to parenteral antigen ranges from 2–15 min to several hours (rarely). Incidence of death or severe neuro injury can be as high as 10% in the OR.

DIAGNOSIS
- Most specific signs: In the anesthetized pt, look for triad of cardiovascular changes (eg, hypotension, tachycardia), pulmonary changes (eg, bronchospasm/increased airway pressures), & skin findings (urticaria, flushing).
- Most sensitive signs: hypotension, tachycardia, wheezing, urticaria
- There is no common laboratory test to confirm diagnosis.
  - Elevated serum tryptase levels suggest mast cell degranulation & an allergic reaction, but test usually takes several days.

MANAGEMENT

■ Treatment

➤ Stop any potential antigen.

• Higher-risk agents listed above

• If etiology of anaphylaxis is unclear, consider latex allergy.

➤ Administer IV fluids. Adults typically need at least 1–2 L crystalloid.

• Administer epinephrine.

• 10 mcg IV for mild hypotension

• 100–500 mcg IV for moderate to severe hypotension

• Can also give IM or SC, but IV preferable

➤ Administer 100% O_2 & consider tracheal intubation for signs of laryngeal edema or airway swelling.

➤ Consider other drug treatments.

• H1 blocker: diphenhydramine 50 mg IV

• Glucocorticoid (eg, methylprednisolone 50–125 mg IV)

• H2 blocker

• Glucagon 1 mg IV (when epinephrine contraindicated)

■ Prevention in high-risk pt

➤ Avoid administration of known or related allergen.

➤ Premedicate w/ H1-antagonist diphenhydramine & corticosteroids.

➤ Watch for signs of anaphylaxis; treat promptly.

AUTONOMIC HYPERREFLEXIA

ROBERT M. DONATIELLO, MD

DESCRIPTION

■ Definition

➤ Occurs following spinal injury, when descending inhibition is interrupted

• Most common w/ transections at T5 or above

• Rare w/ lesions below T10

➤ Assoc w/ chronic spinal cord injury (ie, occurs after acute symptoms of spinal shock have resolved)

➤ Inciting stimulus is usually below the level of the lesion. Common etiologies include

• Bladder distention

- Foley catheter placement
- Surgery w/ light anesthesia, or during recovery from anesthesia
- Procedures on bowel or bladder (eg, endoscopy, cystoscopy)
- ➤ "Mass reflex" refers to the intense autonomic reflexes, including sympathetic discharge & baroreceptor abnormalities, that are brought on by visceral or cutaneous stimulation.
- Cardiovascular manifestations
  - ➤ Sympathetic discharge = HTN & vasoconstriction below the lesion
  - ➤ Baroreceptor-mediated = reflex bradycardia & vasodilation/flushing above the lesion
  - ➤ Cardiac dysrhythmias commonly occur.
  - ➤ Myocardial ischemia, as a result of severe hypertension, can occur.
- Pulmonary manifestations
  - ➤ Severe HTN can cause pulmonary edema.
- Other manifestations
  - ➤ Severe HTN can lead to cerebral hemorrhage.
  - ➤ Sweating occurs above the lesion.
  - ➤ There is a speculated increase in the sensitivity of adrenoreceptors, explaining the exquisite sensitivity to exogenously administered pressors.
  - ➤ Cutaneous vasodilation, coupled with the pt's inherent inability to shiver, may lead to hypothermia.
- Procedures w/ increased risk
  - ➤ Any procedure, such as cystoscopy or TURP, or colonoscopy/laparoscopy, that distends the viscera or body cavities below the lesion
  - ➤ Cutaneous stimulation, theoretically even mild forms, may elicit this reflex.
- Severity: this reflex may lead to mortality & morbidity through myocardial ischemia, CNS hemorrhage, hypothermia or pulmonary edema, as noted above

DIAGNOSIS

- Can be best diagnosed w/ the following combination of signs in an at-risk pt w/ a mid-to-high thoracic transection
  - ➤ Dramatic rise in BP
  - ➤ Flushing & sweating of the face
  - ➤ Reflex (potentially dramatic) bradycardia

■ Other signs may include dysrhythmias, hypothermia.

MANAGEMENT
■ Preop
  ➤ Identify & note the level of the transaction.
  ➤ Assume that a susceptible pt will manifest this reflex; be prepared.
  ➤ Obtain history of triggering events.
■ Selection of anesthetic
  ➤ Although the pt may not have sensation in the surgical area, a "normal" anesthetic is necessary to prevent this reflex.
  ➤ GA or spinal anesthesia is effective in preventing the mass reflex in these pts.
  ➤ Have a vasodilator, such as nitroprusside, & an alpha antagonist (phentolamine) available.
  ➤ A clonidine patch may be useful in the periop period.
■ Monitoring
  ➤ Due to the potential rapidity of this critical event, frequent cuff pressures or an arterial line should be used.
  ➤ Temp should be carefully monitored.
  ➤ Maintain awareness of the subtle cues of sweating & flushing throughout the procedure.
■ Treatment
  ➤ Ensure adequate depth of anesthesia.
  ➤ Treat severe HTN w/
    • Phentolamine
    • Sodium nitroprusside
  ➤ Tachycardia can be treated w/ beta-blockers after vasodilators have been administered.

BRONCHOSPASM

IVAN ZEITZ, MD

DESCRIPTION
■ Definition: Contraction of smooth muscle in the walls of bronchi & bronchioles, causing severe airflow obstruction
■ Incidence: approx 0.2% of anesthetics
■ Risk factors
  ➤ History of asthma or COPD
  ➤ Irritation of airway
  ➤ Instrumentation of airway (eg, laryngoscopy, intubation)

- Smoking
- Inhalation of dust, smoke, noxious fumes
- Drug-related
  - Beta blockers
  - Histamine release
  - Cholinergic stimulation
- Highest-risk pts
  - Previous intubation for asthma exacerbation
  - Repeated hospitalization for asthma
  - Requirement for chronic systemic steroid therapy

DIAGNOSIS
- Increased peak inspiratory pressures, w/ unchanged plateau pressure
- Wheezing
  - Usually expiratory
  - May be absent in severe bronchospasm as airflow decreases
- Upsloping expiratory tracing on CO_2 capnograph
- Consider other diagnoses, including:
  - Mechanical obstruction in anesthetic circuit or ETT
  - Aspiration
  - Endobronchial intubation
  - Pneumothorax
  - Pulmonary embolism
  - Pulmonary edema
- Airway secretions & mucous plugging in pts w/ bronchospasm can worsen air flow obstruction.

MANAGEMENT
- Increase inhaled O_2 to 100%.
- Confirm diagnosis.
  - Ventilate by hand to assess pulmonary compliance.
  - Auscultate chest.
  - Suction airway to rule out kinked tube, mucous plug, aspiration.
  - Compare peak & plateau inspiratory pressures: high resistance from bronchospasm will cause peak > plateau.
- Increase depth of anesthesia.
  - Inhalational agents may be best choice, as they cause bronchodilation at high concentration (>1 MAC).
  - IV propofol may also have mild bronchodilating properties.
  - Consider temporarily stopping surgical stimulation.

- Administer inhaled beta agonist (eg, metaproterenol or albuterol).
  - Use spacers or nebulizers to optimize delivery.
  - Synchronize administration w/ inspiration.
  - Titrate several (5–10) puffs & assess effect.
  - Repeat as needed.
- Adjust ventilator settings.
  - Use a slow respiratory rate to allow adequate expiratory time.
  - If exhalation is incomplete, air trapping will occur, potentially leading to barotrauma or circulatory depression.
  - Allow hypercarbia if necessary to minimize air trapping.
- Administer IV steroids.
  - Consider methylprednisolone IV up to 2 mg/kg initial dose.
  - Consider early administration, as time to peak effect is unclear.
  - Most studies on deaths in asthmatics suggest that steroids were underutilized or underdosed.
- Consider infusion of IV sympathomimetics (epinephrine or isoproterenol).
  - Start at 1 mcg/min.
  - Titrate to bronchodilator effect.
  - Tachycardia & BP response will limit the dose that can be given.
- Postop care: consider ICU care for pt w/ severe or persistent bronchospasm.
- Prevention
  - Ketamine has sympathomimetic properties & may be useful for induction.
  - Be sure anesthetic depth is adequate prior to intubation.
  - IV lidocaine 1–2 mg/kg prior to intubation may be helpful.
  - Consider regional anesthesia to avoid instrumentation of airway.
  - Consider periop IV or PO steroid therapy, esp in high-risk pt.

CARDIAC TAMPONADE

DWAIN SKINNER, MD

DESCRIPTION
- Definition: Accumulation of fluid or blood in the pericardial space, resulting in a fall in cardiac output due to limitation of ventricular diastolic filling & reduction in stroke volume
- Amount of fluid necessary to cause pericardial tamponade is variable, depending on the rapidity of accumulation.

- Most common causes of cardiac tamponade
  - Cardiac surgery
  - Trauma
  - TB
  - Tumor
- Other etiologies
  - Acute viral or idiopathic pericarditis
  - Postradiation pericarditis
  - Renal failure

DIAGNOSIS
- Clinical manifestations
  - Dyspnea
  - Orthopnea
  - Jugular venous distention
  - Low arterial BP
  - Distant heart sounds
  - Kussmaul's sign (distention of the jugular veins on inspiration) may also be seen.
  - Pulsus paradoxus: BP decrease >10 torr during inspiration
- ECG: Electrical alternans may be seen.
- PA line. May see equalization of
  - Pulmonary artery wedge pressure
  - R atrial pressure
  - R ventricular pressure
  - Pulmonary artery diastolic pressures
- Echocardiography may demonstrate presence of
  - Pericardial fluid
  - R atrial & ventricular diastolic collapse
- CXR: serial chest films typically show progressive mediastinal widening
- Urine output usually diminished

MANAGEMENT
- Choice of anesthetics
  - Agents must be chosen to meet hemodynamic goals.
    - Maintain adequate preload.
    - Preserve afterload.
    - Do not depress HR.
  - Ketamine may be the induction drug of choice.
    - Even ketamine may induce hypotension in pts under maximal sympathetic stress.

- ➤ Doses of other anesthetics should be titrated to effect.
- ■ Maintain spontaneous ventilation until pericardial fluid is drained.
  - ➤ Positive-pressure ventilation may worsen cardiac tamponade by further restricting venous return to the heart.
- ■ Do not induce anesthesia until pt is prepped & draped & the surgeon is ready to cut.
- ■ Evacuation of pericardial fluid is achieved via
  - ➤ Pericardiocentesis: a small catheter advanced over a needle inserted in the pericardial space allows drainage of pericardial fluid
  - ➤ Pericardiotomy via subxiphoid window, often under local anesthesia
  - ➤ Pericardiectomy

DIABETIC KETOACIDOSIS (DKA)

JIENY M. HAN, MD

DESCRIPTION
- ■ Definition: Acute complication of diabetes mellitus characterized by hyperglycemia, ketonemia, & anion-gap metabolic acidosis.
  - ➤ The acidosis results from accumulation of organic acids from the catabolism of free fatty acids into ketone bodies.
  - ➤ Sustained hyperglycemia leading to osmotic diuresis & volume depletion is also a feature of DKA.
  - ➤ DKA occurs almost exclusively in type 1 diabetics. It is the result of either:
    - • Inadequate insulin therapy (eg, NPO pt who doesn't take insulin; pt who is vasoconstricted & doesn't absorb SC insulin well)
    - • Increased insulin requirement due to significant physical stress (infection, surgery, trauma) or emotional stress
- ■ Cardiovascular manifestations
  - ➤ Consequences of hypovolemia
    - • Tachycardia
    - • Hypotension
    - • Cardiovascular collapse secondary to severe dehydration
  - ➤ Depressed myocardial contractility
  - ➤ Decreased SVR
- ■ Pulmonary manifestations

➤ Increased respiratory rate & minute ventilation (Kussmaul's respiration).
  • This is respiratory compensation for the metabolic acidosis.
■ Other manifestations
  ➤ Anion-gap metabolic acidosis
  ➤ Osmotic diuresis
    • Polyuria if volume status is good
    • Oliguria if pt is hypovolemic
  ➤ Obtundation
  ➤ Coma
  ➤ Lowered serum sodium
    • This is an artifact of hyperglycemia; sodium is lowered 1.6 mEq/L for every 100 mg/dL of glucose in the blood.
  ➤ Hyperkalemia despite total body potassium deficit
■ Diabetics may have chronic neuropathy & nephropathy superimposed on DKA.
■ Procedures w/ increased risk: Diabetics w/ local or systemic infectious process requiring surgery (eg, appendicitis, gangrene, abscess) may develop DKA as a result of the infection.
■ Severity: Depends on degree of hypovolemia, metabolic acidosis, & coexisting disease. Children may be more susceptible to cerebral edema.

DIAGNOSIS
■ Most specific signs:
  ➤ Combination of hyperglycemia, positive serum ketones, metabolic acidosis
■ Most sensitive signs:
  ➤ Hyperglycemia
  ➤ Positive urine test for ketones
■ Other signs:
  ➤ Signs of dehydration
    • Orthostatic hypotension
    • Decreased skin turgor
    • Dry mucous membranes
    • Thirst
  ➤ Nausea or vomiting
  ➤ Anorexia
  ➤ Abdominal pain, which can mimic acute abdomen
  ➤ Depressed sensorium
  ➤ Increased urinary frequency

MANAGEMENT

■ Determine factors that precipitated DKA.
■ Decide whether to perform surgery in pt w/ DKA:
  ➤ Correct ketoacidosis before elective surgery.
  ➤ However, surgery may be required to treat the underlying cause of DKA in some pts (eg, pt w/ an abscess).
  ➤ Consider 1–4 h of medical stabilization prior to surgery.
■ Monitor following labs until DKA resolves. Initially, consider lab frequency of 1–2 h.
  ➤ ABG
  ➤ Glucose
  ➤ Electrolytes, BUN, Cr
■ Aggressively rehydrate w/ NaCl.
  ➤ Typical fluid deficit: 4–6 L
  ➤ Switch fluids to 5% dextrose-containing solution when serum glucose falls to <250 mg/dL.
  ➤ Fluid administration is the most important step in initial mgt & should be started before IV insulin bolus
■ Replace potassium.
  ➤ Watch ECG for signs of hyperkalemia.
  ➤ Administer potassium when K <5.5 as long as pt is not in acute renal failure.
■ Give regular insulin bolus (10 units IV or 0.1 U/kg), then continuous insulin infusion (5–10 U/h or 0.1 U/kg/h), titrated to glucose of 150–250.
■ Sodium bicarbonate therapy is not usually necessary.
  ➤ May worsen intracellular acidosis
  ➤ Consider bicarbonate therapy only if pH <7.0, & administer in small doses (eg, 50–100 mEq in 1 h).
  ➤ Acidosis will improve as perfusion & hydration improve.
■ If pt w/ DKA requires surgery, consider the following implications:
  ➤ Monitors
    • Serum glucose
    • Serial electrolytes (see above)
    • Urine output
    • CVP catheter in severe hypovolemia
    • Consider PA catheter if pt has myocardial dysfunction.
  ➤ Airway
    • If stiff joint syndrome related to diabetes is present, intubation may be difficult.

- Consider aspiration risk from diabetic gastroparesis.
➤ Induction
  - Severe hypotension may occur on induction of anesthesia in a hypovolemic pt, or from sympathectomy if a spinal or epidural is used.
  - Consider use of etomidate to induce GA.
  - Be prepared to give pressors & continue repletion of intravascular volume.
➤ Maintenance
  - Treat hemodynamic instability due to volume deficiency, acidosis, & pre-existing disease (eg, neuropathy).
➤ Postop period
  - Be prepared to continue to monitor labs & treat pt for DKA in the PACU or ICU.
  - Hypoglycemia may ensue if surgery corrected the cause of the DKA.

DIFFCULT AIRWAY MANAGEMENT

WYNDA W. CHUNG, MD
GERALD DUBOWITZ, MB CHB

DESCRIPTION
■ The ASA has published guidelines for the mgt of the difficult airway. The recommendations in this chapter are consistent with those guidelines.
■ Definitions (according to the ASA)
  ➤ Difficult airway mgt: clinical situation in which conventionally trained anesthesiologist has difficulty w/ mask ventilation, tracheal intubation, or both
  ➤ Difficult tracheal intubation
    - >3 attempts at conventional laryngoscopy required
    - >10 min of laryngoscopy required
■ Failed airway mgt can lead to cerebral hypoxia, myocardial ischemia, cardiac arrest, death.
  ➤ The greatest risk of complications occurs in the pt who cannot be ventilated or intubated.

DIAGNOSIS
■ Evaluation of the airway

➤ See also Technique chapter "Airway Assessment."
➤ Overall goal is to detect factors that may lead to problems w/ airway mgt. This may lead to a change in the approach to securing the airway.
  • Consider whether difficulty may arise w/ mask ventilation, tracheal intubation, or both.
➤ Approach includes history & physical & possibly other diagnostic tests.
➤ Direct laryngoscopy requires four anatomic features. History & physical should address conditions that affect these anatomic features:
  • Mouth opening
  • Pharyngeal space
  • Atlanto-occipital neck extension
  • Submandibular compliance
➤ The type of surgery may affect plans for airway mgt.
  • Surgery that can be done safely w/ local anesthesia w/o sedation offers a different risk profile than surgery that requires a major nerve block or neuraxial anesthesia.
  • If regional block fails, the pt may require urgent tracheal intubation, which increases the difficulty of airway mgt.
■ Inform the pt of the risks & possible procedures related to mgt of the difficult airway.
■ Assess the pt's ability to cooperate with attempts at awake tracheal intubation.

MANAGEMENT
■ Overall recommendations
  ➤ Perform careful airway assessment preop.
  ➤ If difficult airway anticipated, prepare specialized equipment & personnel.
  ➤ Develop a strategy to airway mgt in the pt based on the pt's medical problems, proposed surgery & planned anesthetic.
  ➤ Use more than one confirmatory test for intubation, including a reliable method such as CO_2 capnography.
  ➤ Develop a strategy for extubation that includes the possibility of urgent need for reintubation.
■ Prepare specialized equipment.
  ➤ Maintain a mobile "difficult airway cart" containing routine & specialized equipment for difficult airway mgt.
  ➤ Contents of the cart should include

- Standard equipment for mask ventilation, in a variety of sizes: face masks, oral airways, nasal airways
- Standard laryngoscopy equipment: handles, blades of varying lengths & shapes, Magill forceps
- ETTs: a variety of sizes, including small sizes & small diameter-longer than normal ETT (eg, "microlaryngeal")
- Fiberoptic airway mgt equipment: fiber, light source, swivel adaptor, intubating oral airways, face mask allowing fiberoptic access
- Blind intubation equipment such as tracheal tube introducers ("intubating stylets," light wand)
- Retrograde intubation equipment
- Surgical airway device (eg, cricothyrotomy kit)
- Other equipment to facilitate ventilation: consider LMA (now includes LMA designed to facilitate blind intubation), transtracheal catheter, jet ventilation equipment, ventilating (hollow) tracheal tube introducer, esophageal-tracheal Combitube
- Portable CO_2 detector
- Specialized laryngoscopy equipment: consider short or swiveling handle, tubular blade (eg, Bainton), other "nonconventional" blades, Bullard or Wu laryngoscope

➤ Most important: familiarize yourself w/ the equipment in your particular difficult intubation cart. In an emergency, this familiarity may translate into more expedient mgt.

■ Optimize pt factors.

➤ Provide supplemental oxygen. This may include
- Mask preoxygenation prior to induction of anesthesia
- Oxygen delivery by face mask, nonrebreather mask or nasal cannula
- Transtracheal insufflation or jet ventilation prior to intubation attempts
- The uncooperative pt who cannot be safely sedated may limit the amount of supplemental oxygen, so consider whether sedation would be beneficial or detrimental.

➤ For pt w/ full stomach (eg, trauma, pregnant)
- Administer nonparticulate antacid (eg, 30 mL PO Bicitra).
- Maintain cricoid pressure as long as possible unless it is clearly hindering intubation.
- For fasting pt, regurgitation still possible as insufflation of stomach may inadvertently occur during difficult airway mgt

➤ Carefully position pt to optimize laryngoscopy attempts. Consider building a "ramp" w/ blankets to support shoulders, neck, head. This is most important in the obese pt.

■ Develop strategy for intubation.

➤ Most important concept is to have a strategy for both difficult intubation & difficult mask ventilation.

➤ Basic mgt options include

• Awake intubation (eg, fiberoptic). This approach may be the safest, since both consciousness & respiratory drive can be maintained.

• Intubation after GA induction. Also consider risk of muscle relaxant & opiate administration, which will interfere w/ respiratory muscles or respiratory drive.

• Primary surgical airway

➤ As discussed above, regional anesthesia may be risky in the pt w/ a known difficult airway, because an inadequate or failed block may necessitate urgent airway mgt.

■ For unanticipated difficult intubation, w/ pt anesthetized, mgt includes

➤ Call for help early.

➤ Increase FiO_2 to 1.

➤ Ensure adequate mask ventilation.

➤ Ensure that an optimal laryngoscopy attempt was made. This may include

• Use external laryngeal manipulation.

• Change type of blade.

• Change length of blade.

• Optimize or change pt head position.

• Allow more experienced practitioner to attempt laryngoscopy.

• Ensure adequate depth of anesthesia or muscle relaxation (if used).

➤ Continue mask ventilation & allow the pt to awaken.

• This is influenced by anesthetic agents given.

• Pt receiving so-called "fixed agents" (eg, opiates, muscle relaxants) may not awaken promptly or may have persistent muscle relaxation or respiratory depression.

• Inhaled anesthetics require adequate ventilation for elimination.

• Once pt is awake, can pursue awake tracheal intubation.

➤ Place LMA.

➤ Attempt fiberoptic intubation.

➤ Use a difficult airway laryngoscope or blade.

➤ Attempt other method of difficult airway mgt (depends on skills of practitioner); may include blind intubation, tracheal tube introducer ("intubating stylet"), retrograde intubation.

➤ Place surgical airway.

■ For pt w/ difficult mask ventilation & difficult intubation ("can't intubate, can't ventilate")

➤ Consider steps to improve mask ventilation.

- Place oral airway or nasal airway.
- Reposition head & neck.
- Release cricoid pressure.
- Use 2-person mask ventilation: one person with two hands on face mask, the other performing manual ventilation.

➤ Institute emergency surgical or nonsurgical airway, because hypoxemia can develop rapidly & lead to cardiac arrest.

➤ The particular method will depend on the skills & experience of the practitioner but may include

- LMA
- Esophageal-tracheal Combitube
- Transtracheal jet ventilation or insufflation
- Cricothyrotomy

■ Strategy for extubation of pt who required difficult airway mgt

➤ As w/ intubation attempts, decide on a systematic approach to extubation.

➤ Consider whether the pt is at risk of postop respiratory failure or airway obstruction. This will depend on the pt & the surgery performed.

➤ Pts at high risk of respiratory failure may benefit from postop mechanical ventilation in the ICU until the risk decreases.

➤ Consider whether extubation w/ a ventilating tracheal tube introducer may be beneficial. This can be used to facilitate reintubation, although the introducer itself may interfere with ventilation & replacement of the ETT may not be straightforward.

➤ Consider the setting of extubation attempt. If airway obstruction is anticipated & emergent surgical airway may be needed, this may be more safely accomplished in the OR, w/ an ENT surgeon present.

■ Provide pt follow-up care.

➤ Clearly document the type & nature of airway mgt problems in the pt's chart.

- Describe whether difficulty was w/ mask ventilation, tracheal intubation, or both.
- Describe the airway mgt techniques that were used & the reasons for success or lack of success.
➢ Inform the pt about the difficulty w/ airway mgt. Stress that this is important for any future procedure requiring anesthesia.
➢ Evaluate the pt for complications of difficult airway mgt. These vary w/ the clinical situation but may include
  - Airway trauma (tracheal or esophageal perforation, possibly w/ pneumothorax)
  - Airway edema or bleeding
  - Pulmonary aspiration
  - Myocardial ischemia or infarction
  - CNS injury from cerebral hypoxia
- Clinical mgt pearls
  ➢ Always expect the unexpected. Preop assessment does not guarantee there will be no difficulty at intubation.
  ➢ Carefully position pts, especially when preop assessment suggests difficulty.
  ➢ Always consider preoxygenation.
  ➢ Consider viability of mask ventilation before committing to long-acting anesthetic, opiate, or muscle relaxant drugs.
  ➢ When using cricoid pressure, remember that this may interfere w/ intubation; consider releasing it if the alternatives are worse than maintaining it.
  ➢ Know where your emergency airway equipment is kept.
  ➢ Maintain regular practice w/ emergency airway techniques to optimize your performance in a real airway crisis.
  ➢ Cerebral hypoxic injury may occur with as little as 3–4 min of severe hypoxemia. Consider this when planning mgt strategy.

ELECTRICAL SAFETY

ART WALLACE, PHD, MD

DESCRIPTION
- Definition: Proper mgt & control of electric currents & voltages to avoid burns, shocks, dysrhythmias, & associated morbidity & mortality.

➤ Electrical ground: Point in an electrical circuit where the voltage is defined as zero. Instantaneously capable of supplying or receiving arbitrarily large amounts of electrical charge.

➤ Electrical isolation: Power is isolated from electrical ground.

➤ Line isolation monitor: Verifies that power output lines from isolation transformer are isolated from ground.

➤ Resistive coupling: Direct connection of two circuits by a wire or resistor. $V = I*R$

➤ Capacitive coupling: Electrical connection that occurs because of alternating current. More prevalent the higher the frequencies involved. Impedance (ohms) $= 1/(2pF*C)$

➤ Macroshock: Application of large currents or voltages to skin or tissue. Injury or death results from burn or arrhythmias. Range >0.1 Amps.

➤ Microshock: Application of very small voltages or currents directly to the heart or IV. May cause death from arrhythmias. Range >0.1 milliamps (mA).

➤ Leakage current: Smallest current allowed in electrodes or catheters that contact the heart. Fibrillation requires 50 microamps (uA), so 10 microamps (uA) is the limit.

➤ Electrosurgery: Electrosurgical units (ESU) (Bovie) operate at frequencies between 300,000 and 2 million cycles per second (300 kHz to 2 MHz) to avoid ventricular fibrillation. They deliver a large current that burns tissue, heats collagen to contract it, stops bleeding, & disrupts tissue.

➤ Unipolar: Source & ground of electrical circuit are in separate locations. For ESU ground pad is on pt's buttocks or leg. Hand-held device is source.

➤ Bipolar: Source & ground provided in hand-held device. Used in neurosurgery to avoid neuronal injury; also used in ovarian surgery, bowel surgery, & w/ implanted devices.

■ Current (milliamps): 1
➤ Effect: Threshold of perception

■ Current (milliamps): 5
➤ Effect: Accepted maximum harmless current

■ Current (milliamps): 10–20
➤ Effect: Sustained muscle contraction

■ Current (milliamps): 50–100
➤ Effect: Pain, possible fainting, exhaustion, mechanical injury,

■ Current (milliamps): 100–2,500
➤ Effect: Ventricular fibrillation

- Current (milliamps): 6,000 or more
  - ➤ Effect: Sustained myocardial contraction, respiratory paralysis, burns
- Cardiovascular manifestations: ventricular tachycardia or fibrillation
- Pulmonary manifestations: respiratory arrest
- Other manifestations: W/ macroshock: burns, electrical dysrhythmias, & permanent neuro injury are possible.
- Procedures w/ increased risk: neurosurgery
- Severity: death

DIAGNOSIS
- Most specific signs: arrhythmias
- Most sensitive signs: arrhythmias
- Other signs: line isolation monitor alarms

MANAGEMENT
- All electrical equipment used in the OR should be grounded.
- All electrical equipment used in the OR should be routinely inspected by biomedical engineering for leakage currents.
- Do not connect pts to the OR ground.
- When electrosurgical cautery is used, connect pt to the ESU ground pad.
- Do not place ESU ground pad near pacemakers or defibrillators.
- If increasing current levels are needed for ESU, check ground pad.
- If the line isolation monitor goes off, unplug the offending piece of equipment & send to biomedical engineering for testing.
- Use a bipolar ESU in neurosurgery, pts w/ pacemakers & defibrillators.

ELEVATED INTRACRANIAL PRESSURE (ICP)

ALEX KAO, MD
DHANESH K. GUPTA, MD

DESCRIPTION
- Definition: Although normal ICP is <10 mmHg, elevated ICP is usually defined as >20 mmHg
- Cardiovascular manifestations
  - ➤ Cushing's triad (HTN, bradycardia, respiratory irregularities)

- W/ an increased ICP, a higher MAP is needed to maintain cerebral perfusion pressure (CPP), resulting in decreased HR due to baroreflex.
- Neuro manifestations
  - Mental status changes ranging from confusion to drowsiness to obtundation
  - Cranial nerve palsy (eg, pupillary dilation)
  - Irreversible neuro injury may result from
    - Inadequate CPP leading to cerebral ischemia
    - Herniation
- Conditions w/ increased risk
  - Any intracranial procedure
  - Blunt trauma (eg, motor vehicle accident)
  - Head trauma
  - Recent stroke
- Severity
  - Variable, depending on degree of ICP elevation
  - At mild ICP elevations, mental status changes can be subtle.
  - As ICP increases further, herniation is a risk.
- The pt w/ elevated ICP may present for a variety of procedures, ranging from diagnostic tests (CT scan) to therapeutic intervention (bur hole, craniotomy). Pt may also require non-neurologic intervention (eg, multiple trauma).

DIAGNOSIS
- Clinical evaluation
  - Evaluate carefully if pt at risk for intracranial process.
  - In addition to altered mental status, pt may have nausea/vomiting.
  - Neuro exam may reveal decreased level of consciousness, cranial nerve deficit, motor or sensory deficit.
- ICP monitors
  - Epidural or subdural fiberoptic monitor (eg, Camino bolt): no CSF drainage possible
  - Ventriculostomy (aka external ventricular drain [EVD]): CSF drainage possible

MANAGEMENT
- Depends on where & when pt presents w/ elevated ICP. Some special populations:

➤ Intraop craniotomy (discussed in craniotomy chapters)
➤ Postop craniotomy pt in general will require urgent craniotomy w/ or w/o head CT.
➤ Epidural or subdural hematoma related to head trauma
  • Head trauma pt may develop increased ICP in ICU, or while undergoing diagnostic test or therapeutic intervention for another indication.
➤ Pt w/ acute stroke may present in ER or ICU w/ worsening mental status. Anesthesia provider may be called for tracheal intubation.

Approach to Anesthetic Management
■ Avoid premed, which may depress respiration.
  ➤ Hypercarbia can further increase ICP.
■ Induction
  ➤ If pt is conscious, ask pt to hyperventilate prior to induction.
  ➤ Provide adequate depth of anesthesia for laryngoscopy.
  ➤ Sympathetic activation from laryngoscopy can lead to increases in ICP.
  ➤ Coughing on induction or emergence can increase ICP.
■ Maintenance of anesthesia
  ➤ Facilitate cerebral venous drainage.
    • Keep head & neck position neutral.
    • Consider elevating head of bed.
    • Minimize elevations in intrathoracic pressure: use adequate neuromuscular blockade or opiates to prevent coughing or breathing.
  ➤ Keep inhaled agent & N_2O levels low (<0.5 MAC) to reduce effects of cerebral vasodilation on ICP.
  ➤ To avoid cerebral vasodilation from inhalation agent, administer IV propofol & oxygen.
  ➤ Propofol, STP, & hypothermia decrease ICP by decreasing $CMRO_2$.
  ➤ Narcotics are neutral w/ respect to $CMRO_2$, but must keep CO_2 controlled.
■ Mild hyperventilation to $PaCO_2$ 30–35 mmHg
  ➤ Decreased CO_2 leads to decreased CBF.
■ Diuresis w/ mannitol or furosemide if necessary
■ Steroids useful in some circumstances (eg, edema from tumors)
■ Definitive treatment depends on reason for elevated ICP.

ELEVATED PEAK AIRWAY PRESSURE

EMILY REINYS, MD
WILLIAM A. SHAPIRO, MD

DESCRIPTION

- A variety of anesthesia equipment problems as well as bronchospasm, pneumothorax, bronchial intubation, or increased airway secretions may lead to elevated peak airway pressure.
- Increased airway pressure can occur whenever an equipment malfunction creates:
  - ➤ **High-pressure delivery** (due to a faulty pressure regulator or open oxygen flush valve)
  - ➤ **Obstructed gas flow** (due to kinks or foreign bodies in the breathing circuit/endotracheal tube, insertion of the PEEP valve in the inspiratory limb, expiratory valve malfunction, or cuff overinflation)
  - ➤ **Inadequate pressure release** (due to closed pop-off valve or a pressure relief valve stuck in the closed position)
- Cardiovascular manifestations: hypotension, decreased cardiac output
- Pulmonary manifestations: barotrauma, hypoxemia/hypercapnia (w/ pneumothorax or airway occlusion)
- Procedures w/ increased risk of elevated peak airway pressure: any surgery requiring a small-diameter ETT (eg, direct laryngoscopy procedures); any procedure in which a pneumothorax is more common, such as interscalene or supraclavicular nerve blocks, subclavian or internal jugular central line placement, positive-pressure ventilation
- Severity: depends on underlying cause; equipment problems should be easily correctable, whereas etiology such as tension pneumothorax could be rapidly lethal if undetected

DIAGNOSIS

- The easiest way to confirm or exclude equipment-related causes is to turn off ventilator & manually control ventilation using reservoir bag on the anesthesia machine, or from a separate oxygen source such as an E-cylinder. If the problem resolves, the anesthesia system is the underlying cause; if not, the problem lies elsewhere.

- Check for bilateral breath sounds to confirm ETT placement or rule out pneumothorax (absent breath sounds on affected side); assess for presence of wheezing.
- Assess depth of ETT to rule out migration into R mainstem bronchus.
- Deflate & reinflate cuff to rule out overinflation.
- Pass suction catheter through endotracheal tube.

MANAGEMENT
- Intervention must be specific to the underlying problem:
  - Relief of circuit or ETT obstruction
  - Suctioning of copious airway secretions or administration of glycopyrrolate to decrease secretions
  - Correction of ETT positioning (R mainstem bronchus)
  - Chest tube placement for pneumothorax
  - Administer aerosolized bronchodilators for pts w/ underlying COPD/asthma.
  - Ensure ventilator I:E ratio of 1:2 or less to prevent air trapping in pts w/ obstructive pulmonary disease.
- Adequate preop assessment of anesthesia machine/breathing circuit to detect misconnections or obstructions
- Preop assessment & possible administration of aerosolized beta-agonist (eg, albuterol) for pts w/ COPD/asthma

---

ENDOBRONCHIAL INTUBATION

JONATHAN CHOW, MD

DESCRIPTION
- Definition: Placement of ETT into the R or L mainstem bronchus
  - R mainstem intubation more common than L due to anatomy of tracheobronchial tree
- Pulmonary manifestations
  - Decreased oxygen saturation (depending on FiO_2)
  - Typically results in atelectasis of contralateral lung
  - Unilateral or asymmetric breath sounds & chest rise
  - Increased A-a gradient on ABG
  - Increased peak inspiratory pressure
  - End-tidal CO_2 tracing usually normal
- Procedures w/ increased risk
  - Pt position involving Trendelenburg position
  - Head flexion during surgical procedure

- ETT can advance 2–3 cm w/ head flexion from neutral position

DIAGNOSIS

- Initial diagnosis made on physical exam
  - Bilateral chest movement & breath sounds
- Most sensitive & specific test: flexible fiberoptic bronchoscopy
  - Must differentiate carina from more distal bronchial bifurcations
- Other specific tests
  - CXR
    - May show ETT in mainstem
    - With R endobronchial intubation, may show atelectasis of L lung & R upper lobe
    - Optimal position is w/ ETT tip 2–4 cm above carina
  - Fluoroscopy
  - Palpation of ETT cuff in suprasternal notch rules out endobronchial location.
- Look for other pulmonary manifestations described above.

MANAGEMENT

- Check position of ETT after intubation.
  - Auscultate chest for symmetric breath sounds.
  - Observe symmetry of chest rise w/ ventilation.
  - Palpate ETT cuff at sternal notch.
  - Check depth of ETT insertion.
    - Adult man typically 23 cm at teeth
    - Adult woman typically 21 cm at teeth
- If endobronchial location confirmed, reposition ETT as necessary & recheck position.
- Use caution when withdrawing ETT: excess withdrawal may lead to accidental extubation.

HEMOPTYSIS

MANUEL PARDO, JR., MD

DESCRIPTION

- Definition: massive hemoptysis: 500 cc or more expectorated blood in 24 h
- Pulmonary manifestations: hemoptysis, hypoxemia, tachypnea, respiratory failure

- Other manifestations: pt may have signs of volume depletion
- Severity: Exsanguination is rare. Morbidity is related to hypoxemia & asphyxiation from coagulated blood in airways of tracheobronchial tree.
- Factors contributing to pt outcome: amount & rate of bleeding, concurrent pulmonary disease, effectiveness of cough, anticoagulation
- Bronchial artery is source of bleeding in 95% of pts. Inflammatory lung disease (eg, TB, bronchiectasis) most common cause.
- Pulmonary circulation bleeding less common, but can be related to PA catheter, AV fistulas, pulmonary embolism w/ infarction.
- Non-bronchial systemic artery bleeding least common. Possible causes: vascular trauma, aneurysm erosion, post-tracheotomy tracheoinnominate fistula.

DIAGNOSIS

- Hemoptysis. Have pt quantitate amount of bleeding. Ask pt if side of bleeding is already known.
- Exclude upper GI tract as source of bleeding.

MANAGEMENT

Periop Hemoptysis

- Postpone elective surgery in any pt w/ massive hemoptysis.
- Consider avoidance of tracheal intubation if pt w/ hemoptysis requires surgery.
- Avoid arterial hypertension.

Approach to Initial Mgt

- Transfer pt to monitored setting (eg, ICU or PACU).
  - ➤ Administer supplemental humidified oxygen.
  - ➤ Consider antitussive rx (eg, narcotics) as excess coughing may increase hemoptysis.
  - ➤ Oral intubation w/ 8.0 ETT for pt w/ overwhelming hemoptysis (hypoxemia, respiratory failure)
  - ➤ Consider consult by pulmonologist and/or thoracic surgeon. Flexible bronchoscopy may be useful in identifying side & location of bleeding. Rigid bronchoscopy may be needed to better evacuate blood & can provide a patent airway & route for ventilation.
  - ➤ CXR not reliable in detecting side of bleeding
  - ➤ If side of bleeding known, consider keeping that lung dependent to minimize bleeding into normal lung. Other options: advance

single-lumen ETT into non-bleeding side w/ fiberoptic guidance.
Double-lumen ETT may not provide adequate lung separation,
& narrow lumens not favorable for suctioning.

Definitive Therapy

■ May include bronchial or pulmonary artery embolization by interventional radiologist, balloon tamponade, or thoracotomy & lung
resection.

HEMORRHAGE

RICHARD PAULSEN, MD

DESCRIPTION

■ Definition: This chapter deals w/ acute blood loss.
■ Cardiovascular manifestations
  ➤ Decreased preload
  ➤ Tachycardia
  ➤ Hypotension
  ➤ Myocardial ischemia or infarction
  ➤ Metabolic acidosis
  ➤ Hemorrhagic shock
  ➤ Cardiac arrest
■ Pulmonary manifestations: decrease in end-tidal CO_2 from elevated
physiologic dead space
■ Other manifestations (mostly signs of end-organ ischemia)
  ➤ Stroke
  ➤ Oliguria
  ➤ Acute renal failure
  ➤ Peripheral vasoconstriction
  ➤ Anemia
■ Procedures w/ increased risk
  ➤ Trauma surgery
  ➤ Cardiac surgery
  ➤ Major vascular surgery
  ➤ Spine surgery, including fusion
  ➤ Liver resection, liver transplant
  ➤ Splenectomy
  ➤ Other surgery involving highly perfused organs/tissue

DIAGNOSIS
- Acute blood loss is commonly underestimated.
- Estimated blood volume (EBV) in adults = 70 mL/kg
- EBV in infants = 80–100 mL/kg
- Estimated allowable blood loss = (Starting Hct – Allowable Hct) × (EBV) divided by (Mean of Starting Hct & Allowable Hct)
- Classification of hemorrhage
  - ➤ It is important to understand the typical graded response to acute hemorrhage. Keep in mind these signs may be masked by anesthetic drugs, cardiovascular meds, or pt disease.
  - ➤ Class I: <15% blood volume loss (500 mL EBL in 70-kg pt)
    - Mild tachycardia
  - ➤ Class II: 15–30% blood loss (750–1,500 mL EBL in 70-kg pt)
    - Tachycardia
    - Slight hypotension possible
    - Decreased pulse pressure
    - Anxiety, restlessness
  - ➤ Class III: 30–40% blood loss (1,500–2,000 mL EBL in 70-kg pt)
    - Marked tachycardia
    - Hypotension
    - Tachypnea
    - Oliguria
    - Altered mental status
  - ➤ Class IV: >40% blood loss (EBL >2,000 mL in 70-kg pt)
    - Life-threatening level of bleeding
    - Extreme tachycardia
    - Hypotension, tachypnea
    - Oliguria
    - Markedly decreased mental status
    - Cool, clammy, pale extremities

MANAGEMENT
- Goal is to achieve adequate circulating blood volume, then adequate hemoglobin while surgeons identify & correct source of hemorrhage. Other goals include prevention of end-organ ischemia.
  - ➤ To manage hemorrhage, two main priorities are obtaining adequate IV access & obtaining blood products.
  - ➤ Definitive mgt of bleeding may also require intervention outside the OR (eg, interventional radiology suite for embolization).
- Call for help early.

➤ Among other tasks, additional personnel may be needed to place peripheral IVs, central line & arterial line & obtain, check & transfuse blood products.

■ Management of ABCs
  ➤ 100% oxygen
  ➤ Tracheal intubation & mechanical ventilation if necessary
    • Prepare for decrease in preload from positive-pressure ventilation.

■ IV access
  ➤ Two large-bore peripheral IVs usually provide better flow than one central line because of shorter length of catheter.
  ➤ Consider rapid infusion catheters, which use Seldinger technique to place short (6-cm), large-bore (up to 8.5 Fr) peripheral access.

■ Monitoring issues
  ➤ Place arterial line to facilitate close monitoring of BP & lab values.
  ➤ Central line may be useful in assessing volume status.
  ➤ Monitor hemoglobin, hematocrit, platelet count, electrolytes & coag parameters closely.
  ➤ It is important to diagnose coagulopathy early because it takes at least 45 min to obtain FFP.

■ Take measures to avoid hypothermia.
  ➤ Warm all fluids.
  ➤ Consider forced air warmer.

■ Consider what transfusion threshold to maintain.
  ➤ Important: interpret hemoglobin level w/ regard to pt's volume status. Pt who is still severely hypovolemic despite fluid therapy may require blood transfusion despite "acceptable" hemoglobin.
  ➤ W/ severe acute hemorrhage, consider whether a higher transfusion threshold should be maintained compared to the stable pt.
    • For healthy pt, hemoglobin of 8
    • For pt w/ systemic disease affecting vital organs (eg, coronary artery disease, cerebrovascular disease), hemoglobin of 10 may be more appropriate.

■ Fluid & blood replacement issues
  ➤ Replace volume w/ crystalloid (3 cc/1 cc blood lost) or colloid (1 cc/1 cc) & lost blood cells w/ PRBCs (1 unit increases Hgb by ~1).
  ➤ Estimated volume of blood to transfuse = (Desired Hct – Current Hct) × (EBV/transfused blood Hct)

➤ If cross-matched blood not available
  • Can give O-negative blood (immediately available) while ordering cross-matched blood
  • Cross-matched blood typically ready in 30–45 min
  • Can consider O-positive blood unless pt is woman in child-bearing years, since Rh-incompatible blood does not lead to hemolysis
  • Type-specific blood usually available in 10–15 min
  • If >2 units O-neg whole blood transfused, continue w/ O-neg to avoid hemolysis. O-neg blood may contain anti-A & anti-B antibodies. Can recheck blood type to confirm.
➤ Correction of coagulopathy is crucial, since bleeding may be uncontrollable until coag status returns to normal.
■ Considerations for massive transfusion (>1 blood volume transfused within several hours)
➤ Watch for the following & treat accordingly.
  • Coagulopathy (dilutional thrombocytopenia, DIC, lack of coagulation factors)
  • Metabolic problems (hyperkalemia, citrate toxicity & hypocalcemia, hypothermia, metabolic acidosis, impaired oxygen-carrying capacity)
  • Pts are at increased risk for transfusion-related acute lung injury, w/ development of pulmonary edema.
■ Follow-up care
➤ Pt may benefit from ICU care, especially if resuscitation is inadequate, bleeding is ongoing, or complications have developed.
➤ Before considering tracheal extubation, consider whether bleeding has been controlled & resuscitation is adequate.
➤ Evaluate pt postop for complications of hemorrhagic shock, including myocardial infarction, acute renal failure, acute stroke.

HYPERCARBIA

JAMES HSU, MD

DESCRIPTION
■ Definition: pCO_2 >45
■ Cardiovascular manifestations
  ➤ HTN
  ➤ Tachycardia

- ➤ PVCs
- ➤ Hypotension (w/ very high CO_2)
- ■ Pulmonary manifestations
  - ➤ Tachypnea
    - CO_2 <90 mmHg is a respiratory stimulant.
    - CO_2 >90 mmHg is a respiratory depressant.
  - ➤ Pulmonary vasoconstriction
  - ➤ Bronchodilation w/ increasing CO_2
- ■ Other manifestations
  - ➤ Obtundation
  - ➤ Increased ICP
  - ➤ Compensatory metabolic alkalosis from chronic hypercarbia
  - ➤ Hyperkalemia
- ■ Causes: hypercarbia results from decreased CO_2 elimination, increased CO_2 production, or CO_2 rebreathing
  - ➤ Decreased CO_2 elimination
    - Hypoventilation (eg, inadequate minute ventilation in ventilated pt, leak in breathing circuit, ventilator malfunction, obstructed airway, low tidal volumes after upper abdominal surgery, residual neuromuscular blockade)
    - Respiratory depression (eg, drug-related, such as from opioids or anesthetics)
    - Lung pathology leading to high dead space fraction (COPD, ARDS, PE)
  - ➤ Increased CO_2 production
    - Malignant hyperthermia
    - Thyrotoxicosis
    - Fever, sepsis
    - Shivering
    - Overfeeding from parenteral nutrition
    - Bicarbonate administration
    - CO_2 insufflation (laparoscopy)
  - ➤ CO_2 rebreathing (eg, stuck expiratory valve, inadequate oxygen flow rate, depleted CO_2 absorber)

DIAGNOSIS
- ■ Most specific signs: increased pCO_2 on ABG
- ■ Most sensitive signs
  - ➤ Increased pCO_2 on ABG
  - ➤ HTN
  - ➤ Tachycardia

- ➤ Respiratory distress
- ➤ Increased end-tidal CO_2
  - Assumes normal relationship between end-tidal & arterial CO_2
  - If pt develops increased physiologic dead space, pCO_2 may increase while end-tidal CO_2 remains same or decreases.
- ➤ Other signs: obtundation, signs of increased ICP (in susceptible pt)
- ■ Rebreathing of CO_2 indicates an equipment malfunction & is diagnosed using capnography by the presence of CO_2 on inspiration.

MANAGEMENT
- ■ Make sure pt has adequate oxygenation.
- ■ Establish an open airway & adequate ventilation.
  - ➤ This may require airway mgt including intubation & mechanical ventilation if other maneuvers fail.
- ■ Monitor vital signs, EKG, ABG.
- ■ Identify & treat underlying etiology of increased CO_2 production.
  - ➤ Hypercarbia from insufflation of CO_2 during laparoscopy may respond to decreasing the insufflation pressure.
  - ➤ Equipment malfunctions must be identified & fixed:
    - Leaks in circuit
    - Malfunctioning valves
    - Exhausted CO_2 absorbent
    - Ventilator failure
- ■ Manage sympathetic stimulation to ensure hemodynamic stability.

HYPERKALEMIA

KALEB JENSON, MD

DESCRIPTION
- ■ Plasma potassium (K+) concentration >5.5 mEq/L
- ■ Causes
  - ➤ Increased K+ intake
    - Blood transfusion
    - IV infusion
    - PO supplements
    - Ingestion of K+-rich foods in the face of renal insufficiency
  - ➤ Decreased K+ excretion
    - Renal failure (acute or chronic)
    - Drugs: potassium-sparing diuretics, ACE inhibitors

- Adrenal insufficiency/Addison's disease
- Intracellular to extracellular shift in K+
  - Acidosis
  - Succinylcholine
  - Cell death: burns, rhabdomyolysis, muscle trauma, hemolysis
  - Release of tourniquet on extremity
  - Release of vascular cross-clamp
  - Malignant hyperthermia
- Pseudohyperkalemia
  - Hemolysis of blood sample
  - Increased white cell or platelet count

DIAGNOSIS
- Plasma K levels
- ECG
  - Peaked T waves
  - Widened QRS complex
  - PVCs
  - Ventricular arrhythmias (wide complex "sine-wave" appearance)
  - Cardiac arrest
- Weakness or paralysis in awake pts

MANAGEMENT
- If a high K+ is suspected:
  - Measure stat serum K+.
  - Stop giving any IV containing K+ (eg, lactated Ringer's).
- Important: If there are ECG changes, treat aggressively since hyperkalemia can cause cardiac arrest.
  - Stabilize cardiac membranes.
    - 1 ampule of IV Ca++ gluconate (10 mL of a 10% solution)
    - May repeat in 5 min if no change in ECG
  - Facilitate intracellular shift of potassium.
    - 10 units of regular insulin IV
    - 25–50 g glucose IV
    - Treat acidosis: hyperventilation, sodium bicarbonate 50–100 mEq IV, treat underlying metabolic acidosis.
    - Consider inhaled beta-agonist (eg, albuterol).
  - Remove potassium from body.
    - Facilitate urine output: administer IV fluid & diuretics (eg, furosemide 10–20 mg).

- Consider urgent hemodialysis. Will need to call nephrologist & place hemodialysis catheter.
■ Mild hyperkalemia
  ➤ 50 g sodium polystyrene sulfonate in 70% sorbitol (Kayexalate) PO, or 50–100 g as retention enema
  ➤ Repeat q2h as needed.

HYPERTENSION (HTN)

RICHARD PAULSEN, MD

DESCRIPTION
■ Definition
  ➤ This chapter primarily discusses intraop or postop HTN. The Coexisting Disease chapter "Essential Hypertension" covers the preop presentation of HTN.
  ➤ BP >180/110 or >40–50% increase in baseline value. Relative changes in BP may be important clues to light anesthesia or postop pain.
■ Cardiovascular manifestations may include myocardial ischemia or infarction, arrhythmias, CHF, valve dysfunction, aortic dissection.
■ Pulmonary manifestations may include pulmonary edema.
■ Other manifestations can include stroke, elevated ICP, encephalopathy, platelet activation, renal injury, hemorrhage, wound hematoma in postop pts.
■ Severity: Consider carefully the clinical situation & pt's history. Remember that chronic HTN leads to right shift of the organ perfusion autoregulation curve.

DIAGNOSIS
■ Primary causes
  ➤ Noxious or painful stimulus
    - For instance, inadequate anesthesia during surgery, pain during emergence, postop pain
    - May be more common in pts w/ chronic HTN
  ➤ Metabolic problem
    - Most important to exclude hypoxemia & hypercarbia as causes
  ➤ Other causes
    - Hypothermia & shivering
    - Meds
    - Increased ICP

- Spinal cord injury
- Bladder distention

■ Secondary causes: Consider undiagnosed pheochromocytoma, thyroid storm

MANAGEMENT
■ Goal is to control HTN w/o compromising organ perfusion.
■ Important: Identify underlying causes of HTN, such as inadequate anesthesia or analgesia, hypoxemia, hypercarbia, & treat appropriately.
  ➤ Depending on cause, specific therapy may include increasing oxygen delivery, tracheal intubation, positive-pressure ventilation, increased dose of anesthetic agent, opiate or other analgesic therapy, regional nerve blockade.
■ Exclude artifactual reading.
■ Look for systemic manifestations of HTN, especially myocardial ischemia or stroke.
■ Continue outpt antihypertensive meds throughout periop period, especially beta blockers.
■ After attempts to correct underlying causes, consider additional pharmacologic therapy. Specific agent will depend on clinical setting & desired onset time for lowering BP.
  ➤ In general, BP is lowered until symptoms abate or BP is within 20–30% of baseline.
  ➤ Drug therapy may address specific clinical issue, for instance:
    - Fast speed of onset: nitroprusside is fastest & most reliable, but many other agents can be used
    - HTN w/ myocardial ischemia: consider beta-blocker therapy as well as nitroglycerin
    - HTN w/ tachycardia: consider beta blocker or calcium blocker
    - Vasoconstricted state: vasodilators (nitroglycerin, nitroprusside, hydralazine, fenoldopam)
  ➤ Refer to individual drug chapters for agent profiles & dosing recommendations.

HYPOGLYCEMIA

LISA SWOR-YIM, MD

DESCRIPTION
■ Glucose <70 mg/dL

DIAGNOSIS
- Serum glucose levels (venous or finger stick)
- Signs & symptoms
  - Irritability
  - Altered mental status
  - Seizures
  - Coma
  - Tachycardia
  - HTN
  - Sweating

MANAGEMENT
- Place IV catheter if not already in place.
- Consider IM or SC glucagon therapy if no IV access.
- If pt is awake, consider PO carbohydrate administration.
- Bolus D50 (50% dextrose solution)
  - 25–50 g IV in adults
  - 1 mL/kg IV in children
- Then start D5 (5% glucose) infusion at 1–2 mL/kg/min.
- Stop or reduce insulin dose.
- Check glucose frequently to guide therapy.
- Search for etiology of hypoglycemia:
  - Drug-related (insulin, oral hypoglycemic)
  - Discontinuation of TPN
  - Insulinoma
  - Newborn w/ diabetic mother
  - Starvation or fasting

HYPOKALEMIA

ANDREW CHUNG, MD

DESCRIPTION
- Plasma potassium <3.0 mEq/L
- Causes
  - GI losses
    - Vomiting
    - Diarrhea (eg, bowel prep)
    - NG suction
  - Renal losses

- K+-wasting diuretics
- Excess mineralocorticoid or glucocorticoid
- Renal tubular acidosis
➢ Extracellular to intracellular shift in K+
  - Alkalosis
  - Insulin use
  - Beta-adrenergic agonists
  - Alpha-adrenergic antagonists
  - Hyperaldosteronism
■ Cardiovascular manifestations
  ➢ Arrhythmias
  ➢ Decreased cardiac contractility
■ Neuromuscular manifestations
  ➢ Skeletal muscle weakness
  ➢ May be difficult to reverse muscle relaxants
  ➢ Tetany
  ➢ Ileus
  ➢ Rhabdomyolysis (rare)

DIAGNOSIS
■ Serum K+ measurement
■ EKG findings
  ➢ Flattened T waves
  ➢ Prominent U waves
  ➢ Prolonged PR interval
  ➢ ST-segment depression
  ➢ Atrial & ventricular arrhythmias

MANAGEMENT
■ Mild, asymptomatic hypokalemia (K+ >2.5)
  ➢ No treatment necessary
  ➢ Do not postpone surgery.
■ Symptomatic hypokalemia or K+ <2.5
  ➢ Replace K+ either PO or IV.
  ➢ IV rate: 0.2–0.5 mEq/kg/h
  ➢ Follow serum potassium level & ECG during treatment.
  ➢ If potassium is slow to increase, look for hypomagnesemia.
    - May need to increase magnesium level before potassium will rise appropriately
■ In pts on digitalis, digitalis toxicity is worsened by hypokalemia.

HYPOTENSION

JOHN R. FEINER, MD

DESCRIPTION

- Definition: Low arterial BP. The exact level varies between pts; however, a critical level of BP implies inadequate tissue perfusion pressure.
- Severity of hypotension is considered relative to a pt's baseline BP, although mean arterial pressure <50 mmHg would be considered significant in most cases.
- Cardiovascular manifestations: tachycardia is an appropriate cardiovascular response to hypotension; in severe hypotension, myocardial ischemia & arrhythmias may develop.
- Pulmonary manifestations: potential apnea in a spontaneously breathing pt or even increased ventilation in response to development of metabolic acidosis; increased alveolar dead space due to poor lung perfusion
- Other manifestations: most organs are affected by inadequate perfusion; neuro: changes in consciousness; renal: low urine output, w/ acute tubular necrosis in prolonged hypotension; liver: metabolic acidosis, w/ "shock" liver in severe cases
- Procedures w/ increased risk
  - ➤ Risk depends on both the procedure & the pt's coexisting disease.
  - ➤ Procedures w/ considerable risk include trauma cases, cardiac cases, major vascular surgery, liver transplantation.

DIAGNOSIS

- Diagnosis is made by noninvasive or invasive BP measurement. Should be confirmed by palpating a pulse.
- In an awake pt, symptomatic hypotension usually presents w/ dizziness, nausea, sympathetic responses such as sweating, & possibly loss of consciousness if severe enough.
- Other organ-specific signs related to hypotension stem from inadequate perfusion.
  - ➤ Kidney: low urine output
  - ➤ Brain: altered mental status, loss of consciousness
  - ➤ Heart: tachycardia, myocardial ischemia
- The essential diagnostic issue in hypotension is to determine the cause to help decide on the best treatment.
- Physiologic diagnosis

➤ The most rapid diagnostic technique for managing hypotension is to consider its physiologic cause.

➤ MAP = cardiac output (CO) × systemic vascular resistance (SVR)

➤ CO = heart rate (HR) × stroke volume (SV)

➤ SV determinants are
  • Preload
  • Contractility
  • Afterload (or SVR)

➤ This narrows the physiologic cause of hypotension to
  • HR
  • Preload (hypovolemia)
  • Contractility (pump dysfunction)
  • Afterload (low SVR)

➤ HR
  • Bradycardia may be a cause of hypotension. Treatment follows ACLS algorithms. Even if not the complete cause of hypotension, inadequate HR response may be contributory.
  • Tachycardia may also be a cause; treatment again follows ACLS algorithms.

➤ Preload
  • Often a source of physiologic confusion in ACLS algorithms
  • While we often consider low filling pressures (CVP, PA pressures) as diagnostic of low preload & high filling pressures excluding the diagnosis, several important causes of hypotension are assoc w/ high cardiac filling pressures & represent inadequate preload: cardiac tamponade & tension pneumothorax.
  • Furthermore, hypotension assoc w/ pulmonary embolism is caused by inadequate preload of the L heart, as is R ventricular dysfunction (eg, R ventricular MI). These events may be overlooked as causes of hypotension because they are physiologically confusing.

➤ Contractility
  • Contractility problems can cause hypotension. Examples include MI, drug effects, prior poor cardiac function.
  • Valvular dysfunction is usually considered within this category.

➤ Afterload/SVR
  • Low afterload (or SVR) may cause hypotension in cases such as anaphylactic/anaphylactoid reaction, drug effects, sepsis, liver failure, reperfusion syndrome, spinal shock.

■ Diagnostic workup

➤ The actual workup depends very much on the type of monitors already in place. We will consider a "graded" diagnostic approach, beginning w/ basic monitors, expanding to the most advanced monitors available. Clues from almost every monitor may be important in the ultimate diagnosis.

➤ Physical exam
  • Physical exam should never be neglected. Listening to the chest will confirm ventilation, equality of breath sounds (to exclude pneumothorax, gas trapping). Listening to the heart may suggest valvular problems & occasionally detects venous air embolism & the distant heart sound assoc w/ pericardial tamponade. Distention of neck veins (EJ) can usually be seen in cases of tension pneumothorax & tamponade. Skin warmth & appearance may suggest anaphylactic/oid reactions or other drug reactions.

➤ Basic monitors: ECG
  • Critical for examining heart rate, rhythm, presence of ST-segment depression

➤ Basic monitors: pulse oximeter
  • Some causes of hypotension are assoc w/ hypoxemia, such as tension pneumothorax.
  • Pulse oximeter signal is sensitive to perfusion pressure. A low BP reading occurring w/ loss of a pulse oximeter signal is usually severe hypotension.
  • Severe hypotension can occur w/ continued pulse oximeter signal, esp w/ newer models.
  • Continued pulse oximeter signal during hypotension may be a hint that the cause of hypotension is more likely low SVR than low CO.

➤ Basic monitors: airway pressure
  • Causes of hypotension assoc w/ high peak airway pressure include tension pneumothorax, hemothorax, gas trapping assoc w/ bronchospasm.

➤ Basic monitors: capnograph
  • Pulmonary embolism is assoc w/ a significant drop in end-tidal PCO_2 due to increased alveolar dead space.
  • Hypotension from many causes can be assoc w/ an increased dead space due to poor perfusion of zones of the lung, & therefore a drop in end-tidal PCO_2.

➤ Invasive monitors: arterial line
  • Waveform gives significant clues to the cause of hypotension.

- Systolic pressure variation is the changes in systolic pressure w/ ventilation. Changes in systolic pressure are exaggerated in conditions of inadequate preload, whether from hypovolemia or from other causes such as cardiac tamponade & tension pneumothorax.
- A characteristic waveform pattern may also occur in low SVR states.

➤ Invasive monitors: CVP
- Low CVP is helpful in distinguishing hypovolemia from other causes of hypotension.
- High CVP may occur in R heart failure, biventricular failure, tension pneumothorax, tamponade, PE.

➤ Invasive monitors: PA catheter
- Usually more useful than CVP alone (a PA catheter measures CVP too)
- Wedge pressure & pulmonary artery diastolic pressure reflect left ventricular filling pressure.
- PA catheter is also useful for diagnosis in pulmonary HTN assoc w/ elevated pulmonary vascular resistance.
- A thermodilution cardiac output will most clearly indicate whether hypotension is from low SVR or low cardiac output.

➤ Invasive monitors: transesophageal echo
- While not always available, placement of TEE can often be done rapidly & may help identify causes of hypotension that haven't been clearly identified.
- The physiologic cause of the hypotension can usually be identified quickly, & the specific cause such as valvular dysfunction, pericardial tamponade & occasionally emboli can be identified quickly.

■ Conclusions
➤ More than one cause of hypotension is frequently operating. The greatest confusion occurs in such cases.
➤ Interaction between preload & SVR is important to consider: profound vasodilatation will always drop preload, & the good therapeutic response to volume administration is usually misinterpreted as a sign that hypovolemia was the primary cause.
➤ In anaphylaxis, a common cause of profound vasodilatation, extravasation of fluid also occurs & hypovolemia is always an associated feature.

MANAGEMENT
- Preop
  - ➤ Pt w/ significant hypotension could require surgery in an emergent situation.
  - ➤ Mgt requires a rapid workup of contributing cause, invasive monitoring & setting up appropriate drug infusions.
- Intraop
  - ➤ Diagnostic workup
  - ➤ Establish more invasive monitors.
  - ➤ Consider getting assistance in extremely critical situation.
  - ➤ Fluid bolus & IV administration of a pressor/inotrope is first empiric measurement.
  - ➤ Continued treatment includes
    - Fluid/blood product administration as needed
    - Inotrope
    - Pressor
    - Chronotrope
    - Specific therapeutic maneuvers for identified causes
  - ➤ The balance between use of inotropes vs pressors depends on suspected causes.

HYPOTHERMIA

ALISON G. CAMERON, MD

DESCRIPTION
- Definition: Core body temp <35 degrees C
- Causes
  - ➤ Anesthetic-induced
    - Redistribution of heat
    - Decreased metabolic rate
    - Depression of central thermoregulatory threshold
      - ○ Thermoregulatory defenses (shivering, vasoconstriction) won't occur until the new, lower thermoregulatory threshold is reached.
  - ➤ Loss to environment
    - Conduction: due to direct skin contact w/ cold object or solution
      - ○ Convection: secondary to airflow over/on skin
      - ○ Radiation
      - ○ Evaporative loss (usually a minor effect)

- Pts most at risk
  - Elderly
  - Infants
  - Burn pts
  - Trauma victims
- Procedures most assoc w/ hypothermia
  - Massive blood transfusions if blood is not warmed
  - Large open abdominal/thoracic surgery
  - Long cases
  - Procedures using irrigation solutions below body temp (eg, TURP)
  - CPB & neurosurgery, where it is intentional

DIAGNOSIS

- Diagnosis is by measurement of temp.
  - Nasopharyngeal probe accurately reflects core temp if properly placed.
  - Esophageal temp probe placed in lower third of esophagus behind heart will also give accurate core temp.
    - Presence of heart tones helps confirm proper placement.
  - Rectal temp is slow to equilibrate but will eventually give accurate core temp.
- Signs & symptoms of hypothermia to 33 degrees C
  - Cardiovascular
    - HTN
    - Tachycardia
    - Increased cardiac output (stress response)
  - Pulmonary
    - Hyperventilation
    - Increase in V/Q mismatch
    - Decrease in hypoxic pulm. vasoconstriction
  - Other manifestations
    - Increased oxygen consumption
    - Hyperglycemia due to fall in plasma insulin levels
    - ADH suppression leading to "cold diuresis" w/ possible hypovolemia
    - Decreased metabolism: 50% reduction at 30 degrees C, 60% reduction at 25 degrees C
    - MAC decreases 5–7% with each degree centigrade drop in body temp.
    - Increased ACTH, adrenal cortical steroid excretion, epinephrine

- Viscosity increases 3% per degree centigrade decrease.
- Brain protected during focal & global ischemia
- $CMRO_2$ decreases 10% per degree centigrade.
- EEG suppression
- Increased PVR
- Altered mental status
- Poor wound healing
- Prolongs NM blockade

■ Signs & symptoms when hypothermia is to 28 degrees C
➤ Cardiovascular
- Hypotension
- Bradycardia
- ECG

■ Prolonged PR, QT interval
■ Widened QRS
■ J wave ("Osborne" wave) present
➤ Immediately follows QRS complex
- V-fib may occur.

■ Defibrillation is not effective <30 degrees C.
➤ Other manifestations
- Oxy-Hb dissociation curve shifted to left, impairing delivery of oxygen to tissues.
- Decreased O_2 consumption (if no longer shivering)
- Hypovolemia
- Thrombocytopenia due to platelet sequestering in portal circulation
- Increased hematocrit
- Metabolic acidosis
- Decreased drug metabolism

MANAGEMENT
■ Raise ambient temp.
➤ OR should be warmed to prevent significant heat loss.
- Pediatric pts require room temp of 28–30 degrees C.
➤ Consider infrared heating lamps.
➤ Use radiant warmer for neonate.
■ Warm IV fluids, blood.
■ Monitor & treat arrhythmias.
➤ Maintain normothermia to prevent hypothermia-induced v-fib.
■ Keep pt covered.

- Heat & humidify inspired gases or use low flow.
- Use a warming mattress.
- Use a forced air warming blanket.
- In extreme situations
  - Consider warm peritoneal, and/or pleural, and/or gastric lavage.
  - Consider CPB.
- Be alert to possible complications of rewarming:
  - Myocardial ischemia
  - Arrhythmias
  - Hypotension ("after drop")

HYPOXEMIA

ALICIA GRUBER, MD
JAMES HSU, MD

DESCRIPTION
- Definitions
  - Hypoxia: inadequate tissue oxygenation
  - Hypoxemia: decreased arterial oxygen tension
  - The importance of the degree of hypoxemia depends on coexisting illness: pts w/ coronary & cerebrovascular disease are at greatest risk.
- Age-related changes
  - In the elderly, a lower PaO_2 is expected as closing capacity increases w/ advancing age, eventually exceeding FRC.
  - Typical PO_2 based on age
    - May be calculated by mean $PaO_2 = 102 - (0.33 \times age\ in\ years)$
    - 60 years >80 mmHg
    - 70 years >70 mmHg
    - 80 years >60 mmHg
    - 90 years >50 mmHg
- Cardiovascular manifestations
  - Early: tachycardia, hypertension, cardiac arrhythmias
  - Late: bradycardia, hypotension, cardiac arrest
- Pulmonary manifestations
  - Increased respiratory rate (w/ PaO_2 <50 mmHg)
  - Increased PA pressure from hypoxic vasoconstriction
- CNS manifestations

- Confusion
- Restlessness
- Combativeness
- Obtundation
- Increased ICP
- Other manifestations
  - Metabolic lactic acidosis (anion gap) as cells undergo anaerobic metabolism
  - Increased hematocrit (w/ chronic hypoxemia)
- Situations w/ increased risk
  - Pts w/ pulmonary disease
  - Pts w/ cardiac disease
    - Pulmonary edema
  - Administration of respiratory depressant drugs
    - Opioids
    - Sedative-hypnotics
    - IV anesthetics
    - Muscle relaxants
  - Surgery involving or in close proximity to thorax
    - Upper abdominal or thoracic surgery
    - Placement of IJ or subclavian central line (risk of pneumothorax)

DIAGNOSIS
- Usually diagnosed by pulse oximetry or ABGs
  - Cyanosis is a late clinical finding.
  - Pulse oximetry susceptible to motion artifact
    - Will be late sign if pt is receiving high FiO_2
- Suspect hypoxemia in all pts w/ unexplained HTN, tachycardia, or AMS.
  - Confirm w/ pulse oximeter or ABGs.
- Differential diagnosis is large but can be broken down into four major categories:
  - Low FiO_2
  - Alveolar hypoventilation
    - Airway obstruction
    - Respiratory depressant effect of anesthetic or opioids
    - Residual effect of NM blockade
    - Splinting secondary to incisional pain or abdominal distention
  - Increased A:a gradient (V/Q mismatch or shunt)

- Bronchospasm
- Atelectasis
- Endobronchial intubation
- Aspiration
- Pulmonary edema
- Pneumothorax
- Pulmonary embolus (blood, fat or air)
➤ Decreased mixed-venous oxygen partial content
  - Related to decreased cardiac output or increased tissue oxygen extraction (eg, shivering/hyperthermia)
  - Anemia

MANAGEMENT
■ General principles for all pts
➤ Increase inspired oxygen delivery.
➤ Examine pt.
➤ Check pulse oximeter.
➤ Consider ABG measurement.
➤ Consider hematocrit to evaluate oxygen carrying capacity.
➤ Ensure hemodynamic stability & provide support if necessary.
  - Consider further cardiac testing (echo, left or right heart cath) if suspicious for cardiac lesion.
➤ Treatment depends on cause of hypoxemia. May include
  - Tracheal intubation & mechanical ventilation
  - PEEP
  - Noninvasive ventilation
  - Reversal of drug effect (eg, naloxone, flumazenil)
■ Considerations for intubated pt
➤ Increase FiO_2 to 1.
➤ Examine pt & oxygen delivery system.
➤ Hand-ventilate w/ large tidal volumes & auscultate lungs bilaterally.
➤ Check capnograph tracing for clues to etiology.
  - For instance, inadvertent extubation, bronchospasm
➤ If airway pressures are elevated, determine if secondary to elevated resistance (eg, obstructed tracheal tube, blood or mucous plug, bronchospasm). This is identified by peak-to-plateau pressure gradient.
  - Reduced lung/chest wall compliance (eg, pulmonary edema, pneumothorax, head-down position, abdominal CO_2 insufflation)

➤ If cause not obvious after initial evaluation, obtain ABG & consider stat portable CXR.

■ Considerations for pt w/o ETT

➤ Administer supplemental O_2 via non-rebreather face mask or high-flow face mask.

➤ Examine pt & oxygen delivery system.

➤ Physical exam may reveal clues to etiology.

  • For instance, upper airway obstruction, hypoventilation, pulmonary edema, aspiration

➤ If reversible cause not immediately identified & hypoxemia persists, consider tracheal intubation while evaluating underlying cause.

➤ Order stat CXR, ABG (w/ Hb), 12-lead EKG.

INFILTRATION/EXTRAVASATION INJURY

MANUEL PARDO, JR., MD

DESCRIPTION

■ IV solutions that end up extravascular can damage soft tissue.

■ This can result from backflow out of the catheter's entry site in the vein due to increased pressure or upstream obstruction, the catheter eroding out of the vein, the damage to the vein during IV placement, "back-walling," etc.

■ Risk factors for infiltration injuries include:

➤ Pts who can't communicate (GA)

➤ Debilitated or chronically ill pts

➤ Abnormal circulation in the limb being used (proximal tourniquets)

➤ Multiple punctures of the same vein

➤ IVs on dorsum of hand, foot, or ankle

➤ IVs older than 20 h

➤ IVs placed w/ difficulty

➤ Use of IV needles instead of catheters

■ Substances known to cause damage when infiltrated

➤ Thiopental (pH 10.5) can cause skin sloughing & nerve, muscle & tendon damage. Intra-arterial injections can cause gangrene & distal limb loss. Lower concentrations (2.5%) have reduced but not prevented these adverse effects.

- ➤ Vasopressors: Epinephrine, norepinephrine, dopamine can cause ischemic necrosis.
- ➤ Red blood cells, albumin & other colloids, & mannitol may cause compartment syndrome.
- ➤ Calcium, potassium, 10% dextrose, & $NaHCO_3$ can cause necrosis secondary to their hyperosmolality.
- ➤ Phenytoin (Dilantin) may cause necrosis due to cytotoxicity secondary to crystallization.
- ➤ Antibiotics (eg, nafcillin, penicillin) have been reported to cause skin necrosis; may be due to cytotoxicity related to the delivery vehicle.
- ➤ Parenteral nutrition & lipid agents can cause necrosis secondary to their hyperosmolality.
- ➤ Chemotherapeutic agents (eg, doxorubicin) can cause necrosis because of their cytotoxicity.
- ■ Agents that may be safer to use in questionable IVs (inject slowly!)
  - ➤ Propofol
  - ➤ Rocuronium
  - ➤ Succinylcholine
  - ➤ Fentanyl
  - ➤ MSO_4
  - ➤ Versed
  - ➤ Local anesthetics
  - ➤ Isotonic crystalloids
  - ➤ Other substances that one can normally give SC and/or IM

DIAGNOSIS
- ■ Slowed infusion rate
- ■ Swelling around IV site
- ■ Cooling & blanching of skin (no cooling if fluids are being warmed)
- ■ Confirm infiltration:
  - ➤ Palpate suspected site while flushing w/ an isotonic crystalloid (eg, normal saline, lactated Ringer's, or Plasmalyte).
  - ➤ Beware of what may already be in IV line: don't inject more of a potentially damaging substance.

MANAGEMENT
Precautions
- ■ When possible, administer dangerous substances in peripheral IVs that can be observed, or else via central lines.

- Check that IV is flowing appropriately before & after administering dangerous substances.
- Extravasation can occur at upstream venous puncture sites, esp if an infusion is pressurized.
- Beware of pressurized infusions.
- Beware of upstream constrictions (arms that are secured by folded sheets & tucked may swell & become constricted; leave room for swelling).
- Beware of the antecubital fossa. It is difficult to monitor as extravasations can occur in deeper fascial planes. Plus, the proximity of the median nerve puts it at increased risk for damage from extravasation.
- Watch for signs of infiltration/extravasation.

Treatment
- Hyaluronidase
  - 150–300 units diluted to 10 cc in NS. Give via infiltrated IV catheter & SQ surrounding the site of extravasation. Most effective if used early (<1 h).
  - Effective in animal models & humans
  - Excellent safety profile; only adverse effect reported is urticaria
- Specific antidote for vasopressors
  - Phentolamine 5 mg in 10–20 cc NS; give via the infiltrated IV & SQ in multiple injections around the site of extravasation
- Call plastic surgery consult early for extravasation of potentially dangerous substance.
  - Consider saline flushing (for details see Gault DT. Extravasation injuries. Br J Plast Surg 1993).
  - Fasciotomy, local excision, and/or skin grafting may eventually be required.
- Elevation
  - Decreases hydrostatic pressure in the capillaries, promoting absorption & decreasing edema
  - No studies of effectiveness but no deleterious effects (assuming arterial inflow & venous drainage are not compromised), so it is generally recommended
- Cold or heat
  - Cold has been shown to decrease necrosis due to chemotherapeutic agents, probably by decreasing local metabolic rate.
  - Heat has been shown to improve absorption of hyperosmolar drugs.

MONITORING

- For compartment syndrome
  - Tissue perfusion
  - Compartment pressures
  - Nerve conduction
- For tissue necrosis
  - Blistering
  - Pain beyond 2–4 h

LOCAL ANESTHETIC SYSTEMIC TOXICITY

MICHELLE PARAISO, MD

DESCRIPTION

- Definition: Excessive levels of local anesthetic in the blood, leading to systemic symptoms
- Can occur from:
  - Systemic absorption of anesthetic during & after nerve blocks
  - Inadvertent intravascular injection of local anesthetic
- Exacerbating factors: Local anesthetic toxicity is worsened by
  - Hypoxia
  - Hypercarbia
  - Acidosis
- Cardiovascular manifestations
  - Depressed myocardial contractility
  - Vasodilation, except for cocaine, which causes vasoconstriction
  - Arrhythmias
    - Bupivacaine is specifically assoc w/ ventricular arrhythmias refractory to resuscitation; pregnant patients seem to have a higher risk of cardiotoxicity.
- Pulmonary manifestations
  - Loss of airway reflexes/possible airway obstruction
  - Respiratory depression
  - Apnea
- CNS manifestations
  - Initially excitatory effects
    - Agitation
    - Confusion
    - Muscle twitching
    - Seizure

- ➤ Progresses to CNS depressive effects
    - Unconsciousness
    - Coma
- ➤ Other CNS manifestations
    - Tinnitus
    - Metallic taste
    - Circumoral numbness
    - Nystagmus
- ■ Procedures w/ increased risk: nerve blocks at sites w/ generous blood supply. Highest to lowest risk:
    - ➤ Intercostal
    - ➤ Caudal
    - ➤ Paracervical
    - ➤ Epidural
    - ➤ Brachial plexus
    - ➤ Sciatic
    - ➤ Subcutaneous
- ■ Can also occur w/ topical or IV administration (including Bier block)

DIAGNOSIS
- ■ Most specific signs: negative HR or BP response to local anesthetic containing epinephrine
- ■ Most sensitive signs: response to vasoconstrictors (eg, increase in HR & BP in the presence of epinephrine)

MANAGEMENT
- ■ Prevention
    - ➤ Limit total dose of local anesthetic during nerve block or local infiltration, including dose administered by surgeon.
    - ➤ Aspirate before injecting local anesthetic.
    - ➤ Use incremental injection of local anesthetic.
    - ➤ Consider benzodiazepine (eg, midazolam) premed to raise seizure threshold.
    - ➤ Monitor for signs & symptoms of systemic absorption (eg, pt report of perioral numbness; increase in HR w/ epinephrine-containing solutions of local anesthetic).
    - ➤ Stop injecting local anesthetic if there are signs or symptoms of toxicity.
- ■ Treatment
    - ➤ Establish patent airway, including intubation if necessary.
    - ➤ Administer 100% oxygen to avoid hypoxia.

➤ Prevent hypercarbia by maintaining ventilation.
➤ Support circulation w/ vasopressors.
➤ Stop seizures w/ 50–100 mg thiopental or w/ midazolam 0.5–1 mg repeated as needed, although seizures are usually brief.
➤ Treat arrhythmias pharmacologically or by cardioversion.
➤ For cardiovascular collapse from bupivacaine, consider CPB.

MALIGNANT HYPERTHERMIA (MH)

ALISON G. CAMERON, MD

DESCRIPTION

■ A disorder of muscle metabolism triggered by volatile anesthetics or succinylcholine, which leads to a life-threatening hypermetabolic state
■ Epidemiology
  ➤ Incidence: 1:4,500–1:60,000 general anesthetics
  ➤ Men more commonly affected than women
  ➤ Less frequent in infants & in adults >50 y
■ Etiology
  ➤ Abnormal excitation-contraction coupling in muscle produced by triggering agents, w/ prolonged actin-myosin interaction leading to muscle contracture
  ➤ MH shows autosomal dominant inheritance w/ partial penetrance.
  ➤ Mutation in ryanodine receptor is implicated as one cause of MH.
  ➤ Not all causes of MH have been elucidated.
■ Cardiovascular manifestations
  ➤ Tachycardia
  ➤ Arrhythmias
  ➤ HTN
■ Pulmonary manifestations
  ➤ Tachypnea
■ Other manifestations
  ➤ Metabolic/respiratory acidosis
  ➤ Increased sympathetic activity
  ➤ Hyperthermia
  ➤ Sweating
  ➤ Rigidity (75%)

- ➤ Rhabdomyolysis
- ➤ Cyanosis
- ➤ Mottling of the skin
- ■ Risk factors: pts w/
  - ➤ Duchenne's muscular dystrophy
  - ➤ Myotonia
  - ➤ Osteogenesis imperfecta
  - ➤ Strabismus
  - ➤ Masseter muscle spasm in response to succinylcholine
  - ➤ Family history of MH
- ■ Safe anesthetics/anesthetic adjuncts ("non-triggering agents")
  - ➤ Narcotics
  - ➤ Local anesthetics
  - ➤ IV anesthetics (thiopental, propofol, etomidate, ketamine)
  - ➤ Nondepolarizing muscle relaxants

DIAGNOSIS

- ■ Early signs
  - ➤ Elevated end-tidal CO_2
  - ➤ Overbreathing of ventilator, or increase in minute ventilation to maintain end-tidal CO_2, in ventilated pt
  - ➤ Tachycardia
  - ➤ Tachypnea in unventilated pt
- ■ Late signs
  - ➤ Fever
  - ➤ Metabolic acidosis
  - ➤ Coagulopathy, DIC
- ■ Other signs
  - ➤ Skeletal muscle rigidity
  - ➤ Elevated serum CK
  - ➤ Myoglobin in serum & urine
  - ➤ Increased serum K+, Ca++, lactate
  - ➤ Cardiac arrhythmias
  - ➤ Hemodynamic instability
- ■ Differential diagnosis
  - ➤ Pheochromocytoma
  - ➤ Infection, sepsis
  - ➤ Iatrogenic hyperthermia (eg, forced air warming)
  - ➤ Thyroid storm
  - ➤ Drugs: amphetamines, cocaine, neuroleptic malignant syndrome, centrally acting anticholinergics

MANAGEMENT

■ Treatment
- ➤ Confirm diagnosis (above)
  - When in doubt, treat for MH.
- ➤ Turn off volatile anesthetics & succinylcholine.
- ➤ Hyperventilate w/ 100% oxygen.
  - Use high flows of >10 L/min w/ anesthesia circuit.
  - It is not necessary to change the breathing circuit or anesthesia machine.
- ➤ Give dantrolene 2.5 mg/kg IV. This is the most important step in MH treatment.
  - Dantrolene is the treatment for MH & must be given ASAP!
  - Dedicate someone to mixing dantrolene. Mix 60 cc sterile water w/ each 20-mg vial of dantrolene.
  - May repeat dantrolene doses q5–10min to treat persistent physiologic/metabolic abnormalities of MH, up to a total dose of 10 mg/kg
  - After crisis, continue dantrolene (1 mg/kg q6h) for 24–48 h postop.
- ➤ Abort or complete surgery ASAP.
- ➤ Monitor & correct metabolic/physiologic abnormalities. ABG, electrolytes, coag status most useful.
  - Metabolic acidosis: administer sodium bicarbonate as guided by ABG analysis. In the absence of ABG, empirically give 1–2 mEq/kg IV.
  - Hyperkalemia is common. Usual mgt includes hyperventilation, calcium, sodium bicarbonate, insulin/glucose.
- ➤ Cardiac arrhythmias usually respond to treatment of acidosis. If necessary, administer standard antiarrhythmic agents, except calcium channel blockers.
- ➤ Maintain urine output at least 1–2 mg/kg/h.
  - Place urinary catheter.
  - Give IV saline.
  - Diurese if necessary, w/ furosemide 10–20 mg IV or mannitol 0.5–1 g/kg.
- ➤ Cool patient if hyperthermia is present. Consider the following cooling options & monitor temp closely to avoid inducing hypothermia:
  - Surface cooling blanket
  - Gastric lavage
  - Wound irrigation (eg, open peritoneal cavity)

- Arrange for postop care in ICU.
- Prevention
  - Pt suspected to be MH-susceptible should undergo testing prior to surgery. This includes muscle biopsy contracture testing & serum CK level (elevated in 70% of patients). If this is not possible (eg, emergency surgery), avoid triggering agents.
  - Prepare OR:
    - Remove vaporizers from machine.
    - Replace CO_2 absorber w/ fresh absorbent.
    - Flush machine w/ high-flow oxygen or air for at least 10 min.
    - Ensure availability of MH treatment cart.
  - Avoid triggering agents (volatile anesthetics, succinylcholine).
  - Monitor closely intraop & postop for signs of MH. For uneventful surgery, consider 3–5-h PACU stay prior to discharge.
- The MH Association of the U.S. sponsors a 24-hour hotline for questions or help treating acute episodes: 1–800-MHHYPER (1–800–644–9737).

METHEMOGLOBINEMIA

RICHARD PAULSEN, MD

DESCRIPTION

- Mostly acquired
- Methgb is oxidized Hgb (Fe^{3+} Hgb).
- Methgb cannot carry oxygen; hence, methemoglobinemia is pathophysiologically like anemia.
- Methgb is reduced mostly by NADH-dependent cytochrome B5 reductase: pts w/ NADH-dependant cytochrome B5 reductase deficiency are therefore more susceptible to methemoglobinemia.
- Causes: Agents that promote oxidation of Hgb or inhibit reduction of Methgb, such as
  - Amyl nitrite
  - NTG
  - NTP
  - Prilocaine
  - Benzocaine
  - Lidocaine
  - Mafenide acetate
  - Silver nitrate

➤ Aniline dyes
➤ Phenacetin

■ As w/ anemia, decreased delivery of oxygen may exacerbate/ promote ischemia.

DIAGNOSIS

■ Symptoms: weakness, fatigue, headache, dizziness, tachycardia.
■ Signs: cyanosis unresponsive to oxygen therapy; $SpO_2 = 85\%$.
■ Wide-range spectrophotometry can detect exact levels of Methgb (502 & 632 nm).
■ Blood appears chocolate-colored.

MANAGEMENT

■ Discontinue offending agent.
■ As w/ anemia, decision to treat is based on the oxygen-carrying capacity (ie, amount of normal, unoxidized hemoglobin the pt has, which equals Hb × [100 -%methgb]), symptoms, & pt factors (eg, presence of ischemic heart disease).
■ Treatment is methylene blue (1 mg/kg) infused over 5 min (to avoid toxic symptoms: restlessness, apprehension, tremor, & precordial pain).
■ Severe methgb is treated w/ exchange transfusion.
■ Do not give methylene blue to pts w/ glucose-6-phosphate deficiency (acute hemolysis will occur).

MYOCARDIAL ISCHEMIA/INFARCTION

CHRISTOPHER G. HATCH, MD

DESCRIPTION

■ Definition
➤ Myocardial ischemia results from an imbalance between oxygen supply & demand to the heart.
➤ If untreated, ischemia may lead to infarction (death of cardiac tissue).
■ Cardiovascular manifestations
➤ Hemodynamic instability
➤ EKG changes (ST segment elevation or depression)
➤ Changes in central filling pressures (generally increases) or cardiac output (generally decreases)

- ➤ Regional wall motion abnormalities (as visualized by TEE)
- ➤ Dysrhythmias (generally ventricular)
- ■ Pulmonary manifestations
  - ➤ Pts may develop pulmonary edema.
  - ➤ In the awake pt, this may manifest as increased shortness of breath or dyspnea.
  - ➤ In the anesthetized pt, this may manifest as worsening oxygenation.
- ■ Other manifestations
  - ➤ Awake pts may complain of chest pain, pressure, or discomfort.
  - ➤ Certain pts, especially those w/ diabetes, may have silent ischemic episodes.
- ■ Procedures w/ increased risk
  - ➤ Major vascular surgery (eg, requiring aortic cross-clamping)
  - ➤ Peripheral vascular surgery
  - ➤ Cardiac surgery (especially valvular or coronary artery procedures)
  - ➤ Major surgery (eg, prolonged surgery, large blood loss & fluid shifts), esp if case is an emergency
  - ➤ Intraperitoneal surgery
  - ➤ Intrathoracic surgery
- ■ Procedures w/ lowest risk
  - ➤ GI endoscopy (diagnostic)
  - ➤ Superficial surgery
  - ➤ Cataract surgery

DIAGNOSIS

- ■ Perform history & physical.
  - ➤ Ask the awake pt for symptoms of myocardial ischemia.
    - • Postop MIs are usually silent.
  - ➤ Compare vital signs to baseline values.
- ■ Multiple monitors can be used to help detect myocardial ischemia intraop:
  - ➤ ECG
  - ➤ ST segment analysis in multiple leads (usually leads II & V5) is the mainstay of periop detection of myocardial ischemia.
  - ➤ The most sensitive lead for detecting myocardial ischemia is V5.
  - ➤ ST segment elevation is highly specific for acute MI.
  - ➤ The sensitivity of ST segment monitors for TEE-diagnosed myocardial ischemia has been documented as 40%.

➤ The sensitivity of ST segment monitors for EKG-diagnosed myocardial ischemia has been documented as 75%.

■ PA catheter

➤ Sudden elevations in PA or PCW pressures are not sensitive or reliable indicators of ischemia.

■ TEE

➤ TEE is a sensitive detector of myocardial ischemia.

➤ Continuous real-time evaluation of ventricular function allows identification of new regional wall motion abnormalities, which may indicate ischemia.

➤ In animal studies & models, mechanical dysfunction (as visualized by TEE) precedes surface EKG changes when myocardial ischemia is produced.

➤ Studies have found that in pts w/ CAD undergoing major vascular or coronary surgery, regional wall motion abnormalities were more sensitive than ST segment changes on EKG in detecting myocardial ischemia.

➤ However, other studies have shown that TEE monitoring in pts undergoing noncardiac surgery has no benefit in predicting periop ischemic outcomes over EKG monitoring.

MANAGEMENT

■ Prevention

➤ Periop beta blockade of pts at known risk for myocardial ischemia has been shown to reduce the incidence of periop ischemia & infarction.

➤ During & after surgery, hemodynamics should be maintained as close to normal as possible. This is esp important during induction & emergence from anesthesia.

➤ In high-risk pts, PTCA, coronary stenting, or CABG may be indicated prior to elective surgery to reduce the risk of postop infarction. This should involve a discussion between pt, surgeon, anesthesia provider & cardiologist.

➤ Pain should be controlled postop to prevent HTN/tachycardia in response to pain.

■ Myocardial ischemia is managed by increasing oxygen supply to the myocardium and/or decreasing oxygen demand. The clinical scenario will dictate the best way to achieve this goal. Options include

➤ Correct hypoxemia & anemia to optimize myocardial oxygen delivery.

➤ Consider maintaining a hematocrit >30 in pts at risk for ischemia.

➤ Beta blockers are useful in the prevention or treatment of tachycardia, decreasing both HR & contractility.
  • IV preparations include propranolol, labetalol, esmolol, metoprolol.
➤ Nitrates: Nitroglycerin is most commonly used. This is predominantly a venodilator. It reduces venous return, thereby decreasing wall tension & myocardial oxygen demand. It may improve oxygen delivery by dilating coronary arteries.
  • Intraop it is infused starting at 0.5 ug/kg/min & titrating upwards as systemic BP allows.
➤ Vasoconstrictors: Phenylephrine is commonly used to help treat myocardial ischemia in the setting of hypotension as well as hypotension encountered w/ nitroglycerin infusions.
  • This alpha-adrenergic agonist improves coronary perfusion pressure but at the expense of increasing afterload & myocardial oxygen demand.
  • In the setting of hypotension, the increased coronary perfusion usually offsets the increased demand, making it a useful agent.
➤ Inotropes: Agents such as dopamine, dobutamine, or norepinephrine may be indicated when myocardial ischemia results in a significant reduction in cardiac output (ie, cardiogenic shock). If cardiogenic shock is present, a PA catheter and/or echocardiography may be useful in guiding therapy.
➤ Intra-aortic balloon counterpulsation (IABP) may ultimately be required to augment cardiac output if cardiogenic shock develops or persists despite these pharmacologic interventions.
➤ Heparinization & thrombolytic therapies are generally avoided intraop due to risks of excessive surgical bleeding, but they may be indicated & useful in certain circumstances.
■ Communicate w/ a cardiology consultant early if therapy such as IABP, cardiac catheterization, or thrombolysis is considered.

OLIGURIA

EDWIN CHENG, MD

DESCRIPTION
■ This chapter deals w/ acute oliguria unrelated to chronic renal failure.
■ Definitions

➤ Oliguria: urine output <0.5 mL/kg/h
➤ Acute renal failure (ARF): numerous definitions, including
  • 50% increase in baseline creatinine
  • 0.5-mg/dL increase in baseline creatinine
  • 50% decrease in creatinine clearance
➤ Important: Oliguria is often the first clinical manifestation of ARF. However, oliguria occurs in only 50% of ARF cases. In nonoliguric renal failure, elevated creatinine may be the only manifestation.
■ Differential diagnosis: Etiology of renal failure is divided into three categories.
  ➤ Prerenal: reversible renal hypoperfusion
    • Most common cause of ARF
  ➤ Renal: intrinsic renal injury that can occur at level of renal vessels, glomeruli, tubules (eg, acute tubular necrosis [ATN]), or tubulo-interstitium
  ➤ Postrenal: renal failure due to urinary tract obstruction
    • Can occur at different levels, including ureter, bladder, urethra, urinary catheter, etc
    • Least common cause overall

DIAGNOSIS
■ Most important part of evaluation is to look for likely causes of renal failure in the three main categories: prerenal, renal, postrenal.
■ Useful lab tests to supplement history & physical
  ➤ BUN, creatinine (including baseline level)
  ➤ Hct
  ➤ Electrolytes, esp potassium
  ➤ Fractional excretion of sodium (FENa): 100 × urine sodium/plasma sodium divided by urine creatinine/plasma creatinine
  ➤ Urinalysis to look for casts or other evidence of tubular damage

Prerenal Causes
■ Causes: look for disorders or conditions assoc w/ renal hypoperfusion.
  ➤ Hypovolemia
    • Look for pre-existing hypovolemia (eg, pt presenting w/ hemorrhage, vomiting, diarrhea, diuresis, fever, burns, sepsis).
    • Look for disorders w/ effective reduction in circulating blood volume: liver failure, heart failure, NSAID therapy, ACE inhibitor therapy.
    • Nature of surgical procedure will influence blood loss & fluid shifts.

- ➤ Hypotension
- ➤ Decreased cardiac output
- ➤ Surgical manipulation of renal arteries
- ➤ Aortic cross-clamp (either above or below renal arteries)
- ■ Diagnosis
  - ➤ Concentrated urine (urine osmolality >500 mosm)
  - ➤ Urine sodium <20
  - ➤ FENa <1
  - ➤ Improved urine output w/ fluid bolus

Renal Causes

- ■ Ischemic & nephrotoxin-induced ATN account for vast majority of renal causes.
- ■ Causes
  - ➤ Nephrotoxic drugs (aminoglycosides, contrast dye, chemotherapeutics)
  - ➤ Rhabdomyolysis
  - ➤ Hemoglobinuria
  - ➤ Prolonged renal hypoperfusion leading to ATN
- ■ Diagnosis
  - ➤ Identify potential causative agents.
  - ➤ FENa >1
  - ➤ Urine sodium usually >40
  - ➤ Urinalysis reveals granular casts.

Postrenal causes

- ■ Causes
  - ➤ Calculi
  - ➤ Clot retention
  - ➤ Surgical ligation or laceration of ureters
  - ➤ Kinking or obstruction of Foley catheter
  - ➤ Urine collection system disconnected (eg, pt who underwent bladder diversion procedure)
- ■ Diagnosis
  - ➤ Search for mechanical causes of obstruction or diversion of urine flow.
  - ➤ Irrigate Foley catheter to ensure patency.
  - ➤ Consider ultrasound to look for evidence of obstruction (eg, dilated collecting system).

MANAGEMENT

Prerenal oliguria

- ■ Mgt

> If hypovolemic, give crystalloid fluid bolus 5–10 cc/kg.
> In setting of poor cardiac output, diagnosis & treatment of the etiology for low cardiac output will improve prerenal oliguria.
> "Renal dose" dopamine (3–5 mcg/kg/min) will improve renal blood flow but has not been shown to reduce risk or improve outcome of renal failure. May cause tachyarrhythmias, peripheral vasoconstriction.
> Consider monitoring cardiac filling pressures w/ a central line to help guide fluid replacement.

Renal Oliguria
■ Mgt
> Discontinue causative agents or potential nephrotoxins.
> Diuretics (mannitol, furosemide) will promote urine output & may help w/ fluid mgt but do not change outcome of renal failure.
> Administer IV crystalloid to ensure that pt is euvolemic.
> Monitor electrolytes for hyperkalemia, which could cause life-threatening arrhythmias.
> For fluid overload w/ pulmonary edema, severe acidosis, or life-threatening hyperkalemia, may need to consult nephrologist to arrange urgent dialysis

Postrenal oliguria
■ Mgt
> Remove source of obstruction, if possible.
> Confirm proper placement of the Foley within the bladder & irrigate catheter.
  • Check for kinks or disconnections in the urine collecting system or catheter.
> If ultrasound reveals source of obstruction, may need to consult nephrologist or urologist for further mgt

---

OR FIRE

BETTY LEE-HOANG, MD

DESCRIPTION
■ A fuel, oxidizer, & ignition source must be present to start a fire.
■ Sources of ignition include static electricity, lasers, electrosurgical units.

- Flammable agents in the OR include surgical drapes, alcohol (including skin preps), petroleum-based products.
- O_2 & N_2O support combustion.
- Particularly dangerous: high levels of blow-by or insufflation of O_2 under surgical drapes
- Bowel gas, which consists of methane, hydrogen, & hydrogen sulfide, is highly flammable & may combust w/ the use of diathermy.

DIAGNOSIS
- Fire
- Smoke or burned odor
- Explosion or popping sound
- Heat

MANAGEMENT
- Smother fire on surgical field.
- Get help, activate fire alarms, call fire department.
- Extinguish fire if it is possible & safe to do so.
- Evacuate pt & OR personnel if fire cannot be controlled rapidly.
- Notify other ORs.
- Close door to OR & shut off gas supplies to affected OR.
- Treat pt & injured personnel.

PERIPHERAL NERVE INJURY

JASON LICHTENSTEIN, MD

DESCRIPTION
- Definition: Injury to a peripheral nerve that occurs during or as a consequence of an anesthesia-requiring procedure
- 15% of all legal claims assoc w/ anesthesia relate to peripheral nerve injuries. Can occur in assoc w/ general & regional anesthesia.
- Risk factors & predispositions
  - Male sex, extremes of body habitus, lengthy surgeries, poor positioning, prolonged positioning for surgery, prolonged tourniquet time (>2 h), pre-existing nerve entrapment, coexisting diseases (DM, ETOH abuse, rheumatoid arthritis, tobacco abuse, malnutrition, hypotension, PVD, cancer), meds (HIV meds), congenital anomalies (cervical rib)
- Possible causes: position-related nerve ischemia, stretch-related nerve ischemia, direct mechanical damage

- Some neuropathies may develop or become evident in the recovery room or ward. Can present as late as 7 days postop.
- Nerve injury can occur despite appropriate anesthesia care & proper padding.

Manifestations by nerve

- Ulnar: most common anesthesia-related neuropathy. Usually in males. Often from external compression by OR table or BP cuff. Common sites of injury: elbow at epicondylar groove (nerve is between skin and bone) or cubital tunnel. Manifests as inability to abduct all fingers or oppose fifth finger, decreased sensation in fourth and fifth digits, & later "ulnar claw."
- Brachial plexus: frequent site of stretch injuries due to long superficial course in axilla. Risk factors: arm abduction >90 degrees, contralateral head rotation, sternal retraction. Compression injury may result from poorly positioned axillary rolls. Manifests as motor deficits in median & radial nerve distributions, or sensory deficit in ulnar distribution (cardiac procedures).
- Radial: can be a result of pressure applied to lower humerus or arm falling off table, humeral fractures, & use of crutches. Manifests as inability to extend fingers or wrist; w/ proximal injury can find weakness of triceps. Decreased sensation may or may not be present in dorsum of 1 & 2 digits.
- Median: usually result of damage to nerve from injecting needle or extravasating drug in antecubital fossa. Results in wrist & 1–3 digits flexor weakness & inability to oppose first & fifth digits. Sensory loss in lateral palm.
- Common peroneal: most frequently injured lower extremity nerve, usually due to compression between head of fibula below the knee & operating table (metal frame used in lithotomy position to hold leg). It can occur while in the sitting position (neurosurgery). Manifests as "foot drop," inability to extend toes cephalad (dorsiflexion), & inability to evert foot. Sensory loss on dorsum of foot.
- Sciatic: most likely to occur as a result of stretch while in lithotomy position, esp when leg is externally rotated or extended at hip & knee. May appear as "foot drop," weakness in all lower leg muscle groups, including foot extensor or flexors. Decreased sensation in dorsum or sole of foot.
- Femoral: injured by compression at pelvic brim or extreme hip angulation. Manifests as diminished patellar reflex, weakness on

knee extension (quadriceps), hip flexion. Diminished sensation over anteromedial aspect of thigh.

DIAGNOSIS

- On initial evaluation, perform focused clinical neuro exam of involved area, including motor, sensory, & reflex exam. Gently palpate the areas of suspected nerve involvement. Skin exam may give clues to the etiology & anatomic location of the problem.
- Review records for risk factors for nerve injury, such as
  - ➤ Procedure performed
  - ➤ Duration & position during procedure
  - ➤ Pressure point padding descriptions
  - ➤ Distribution of regional anesthesia (nerve block)
  - ➤ History of prior neuropathies
  - ➤ Body weight
  - ➤ Site of compressive procedures, such as BP cuff or tourniquet
- Obtain neurology consult if symptoms & signs are moderate to severe, or if mild symptoms do not improve over few hours or few days, or if symptoms or signs increase. The neurology consultant can help decide when to perform further testing, such as electrophysiology or imaging.

MANAGEMENT

Prevention of Nerve Injury

- Assess positioning while pt is awake, if possible. Position pts in the most anatomic position allowed for the procedure.
- Rule of thumb: imitate position of your pt—if uncomfortable for you, then likely risky for pt.
- Pay close attention to the most frequently affected nerves: ulnar, peroneal, brachial plexus.
- Pad all pressure points to avoid compression between table & pt. Pay particular attention to elbow & lateral knees.
- Keep tourniquet times as short as possible. If >2 h, then deflate for 15 min q2h.
- Lithotomy: keep to <4 h if possible. Avoid compression of frame against lateral aspect of knee; keep hips & knees flexed w/ minimized external hip rotation.
- Supine: limit arm abduction to 90 degrees or less, elbow flexion to <110 degrees, & keep arms/forearms & wrist in mid-supination. Keep hips & knees flexed & minimize external rotation of hips.
- Lateral decubitus position: ensure that axillary roll is caudal to axilla.
- Important documentation issues

- Always document proper padding & positioning.
- Always document pre-existing neuro deficits.

Prognosis
- Most anesthesia-related peripheral nerve injuries will at least partially resolve in 6–12 wks. Avoid further trauma to affected nerve. In extreme cases there may be complete loss of function, & mgt may involve surgery to the affected nerve.
- Some pts require physical & occupational therapy.

PNEUMOTHORAX

JAMES BRANDES, MD

DESCRIPTION
- Definition: A simple pneumothorax is a collection of air within the intrapleural space. A tension pneumothorax results from continued collection of air via a one-way valve. An open pneumothorax is an open communication of the intrapleural space w/ the atmosphere.
- Incidence
  - W/ central line placement, 0.5–1%
  - In the mechanically ventilated ICU pt, 5–15%
  - In the ventilated ARDS pt, up to 60%
- Cardiovascular manifestations
  - Hypotension
  - Tachycardia
  - Cardiovascular collapse
  - Pulseless electrical activity
- Pulmonary manifestations
  - Absent breath sounds on affected side
  - Lung collapse leads to intrapulmonary shunt w/ resultant hypoxemia.
  - Progressively increasing peak inspiratory pressures
- Other manifestations
  - Hyperresonant to chest wall percussion
  - Tracheal shift
  - Distended neck veins
  - Subcutaneous emphysema
  - Wheezing
  - Chest pain, dyspnea, cough, & tachypnea manifest in the awake pt

- Procedures w/ increased risk
  - Central line placement
  - Positive-pressure ventilation
  - Intercostal nerve blocks
  - Perivascular subclavian nerve block
  - Paravertebral thoracic block
  - Tracheal intubation
  - Bronchoscopy
  - Mediastinal operations
  - Thyroidectomy
  - Neck explorations
  - Upper abdominal operations around the diaphragm (adrenalectomy/nephrectomy)
  - Laparoscopic surgery
  - Breast surgery (needle localization)
  - Thoracic spine operations
  - Lung biopsy
  - Pleurocentesis
- Pts w/ bullous emphysema & neonates are particularly at risk for barotrauma-induced pneumothorax.
- Severity: the entire spectrum from being an incidental finding on CXR to circulatory collapse resulting from mediastinal shift impeding return of blood to R side of heart
- Important: A clinically silent simple pneumothorax may result in a tension pneumothorax in the mechanically ventilated pt.

DIAGNOSIS
- Most signs are nonspecific.
- Subcutaneous emphysema is fairly specific except in laparoscopic surgical pts, who may have this finding commonly.
- Pneumothorax is often clinically silent or w/ minimal symptoms, w/ the diagnosis made only by CXR.
- Presentation of pneumothorax may be delayed 24–48 h after a procedure such as line placement.
- Films taken at end of expiration will be most sensitive, as at end of expiration the ratio of the volume of air in the pneumothorax to lung air is highest.
  - Films should be taken with pt upright to demonstrate presence of air in apical pleural space.
  - If films are taken in the supine pt (eg, ICU pt), air will collect in the basilar & subpulmonic areas & may be difficult to pick up.

- Clinical signs depend on severity of pneumothorax.
- Important: Never make the diagnosis of tension pneumothorax by CXR in the unstable pt! If you think of it & the pt is crashing, assume the diagnosis & treat accordingly.

MANAGEMENT

- Traditional therapy for pneumothorax is a chest tube placed to water seal.
- Specific therapy should be tailored to the etiology, pt status, & clinical setting.
- In the postop pt, a small (<20%) pneumothorax w/ minimal symptoms may be closely observed.
  - Give 100% oxygen to increase the gradient of nitrogen between the air in the pneumothorax & the venous circulation, theoretically decreasing the volume of the pneumothorax.
  - Repeat CXR in 6 h.
  - If pneumothorax is decreased in size, pt may be discharged w/ appropriate instructions.
  - If pneumothorax is same size or larger, it must be evacuated.
- A medium-sized (20–40%) or large (>40%) pneumothorax in the stable pt or any symptomatic pt may be treated w/ an 8F catheter placed over a guide wire in the fourth intercostal space along the anterior axillary line.
  - Air is aspirated, & the catheter may be left capped off with a 3-way stopcock.
  - Obtain repeat film in 6 h.
  - If the pneumothorax has resolved, the catheter may be pulled & the pt discharged.
  - Some clinicians advocate this therapy for all pneumothoraces, as if the pt is observed for 6 h first & then needs evacuation, the pt will remain in the hospital an extra 6 h.
- Pt in severe distress should immediately have a long 14g angiocath placed in the second intercostal space along the midclavicular line, followed by a chest tube for definitive treatment.
  - This is easy to do & is a lifesaving measure.
  - If the operative field is near the thorax, the surgeon may be able to evacuate the pneumothorax also.
  - Attaching the angiocath to a syringe w/ saline to aspirate for air bubbles may aid in placement. Listen for a rush of air. If the side of the pneumothorax is not apparent, the opposite side should be treated if symptoms don't improve quickly.

POSTOP NAUSEA & VOMITING (PONV)

BETTY LEE-HOANG, MD

DESCRIPTION
- Definition: Nausea & vomiting following surgery. PONV is one of the most common postop complaints. Risk for PONV depends on pt, surgical, & anesthetic factors.
- Pts at increased risk: young pts, females
- Surgeries that increase risk: intraperitoneal surgery (esp laparoscopy), GYN surgery, strabismus surgery
- Anesthetics & adjuncts that increase risk: volatile anesthetics, nitrous oxide, opioids, anticholinesterases
- Spinal or epidural anesthesia may produce hypotension, which may be accompanied by PONV.

DIAGNOSIS
- Subjective report of nausea, vomiting

MANAGEMENT
- Usual Rx: Common antiemetics include selective 5-hydroxytryptamine (serotonin) antagonists such as ondansetron & dolasetron, Compazine, metoclopramide, scopolamine. Due to risk of QT interval prolongation, do not use droperidol as an antiemetic.
- Prophylactically: treat high-risk pts w/ antiemetics before emerging from anesthesia, & avoid emetogenic anesthetics & adjuncts intraop. Propofol decreases the incidence if used as a continuous infusion.
- Postop, treat w/ antiemetics.

PULMONARY ASPIRATION

LEI WANG, MD

DESCRIPTION
- Aspiration of gastric contents into trachea/bronchi/alveoli
- Risk factors
  - Altered mental status
  - Full stomach
  - GERD
  - Bowel obstruction

➤ Obesity
➤ Pregnancy
➤ Diabetes
➤ Ascites
➤ Abnormal GI motility

Types of Aspirates
■ Particulate matter
➤ Large particles can cause significant obstruction of large airway, causing asphyxia.
➤ Small particles cause distal airway obstruction, resulting in V/Q mismatch & hypoxia.
■ Liquid gastric content: Severe pulmonary injury expected if
➤ pH <2.5
➤ Volume >25 cc (0.4 cc/kg)
■ Fecal material
➤ Prognosis is poor.
■ Blood
➤ Aspiration of blood does not cause pneumonitis.
➤ However, aspiration of large volume of blood may fill the alveoli, causing hypoxemia.

DIAGNOSIS
■ Significant pulmonary aspiration is usually witnessed in OR.
■ For unwitnessed pulmonary aspiration, pt usually presents w/ hypoxia & sometimes a mixed metabolic & respiratory acidosis. CXR findings are variable & delayed.

MANAGEMENT
■ For large pulmonary aspiration
➤ Place pt in Trendelenburg position.
➤ Suction mouth & pharynx quickly.
➤ Secure airway w/ ETT.
➤ Suction trachea through ETT before applying positive-pressure ventilation.
➤ Place pt on mechanical ventilation w/ 100% oxygen & PEEP.
➤ Supportive care
■ Bronchoscopy & lavage if pt aspirates large particulate mass to clear large airway obstruction.
■ Avoid corticosteroids.

- Prophylactic antibiotics recommended only if aspirates are grossly infected or feculent.
- Small aspirations may require only supplemental oxygen.

Prevention
- Pt scheduled for elective surgery should follow proper preop fasting guidelines.
- Nonparticulate antacids to raise stomach pH >2.5 should be given to pts at high risk for pulmonary aspiration.
- Consider IV meds in at-risk pts:
  - H2 blockers such as cimetidine, ranitidine
  - Metoclopramide stimulates gastric emptying & increases lower esophageal sphincter tone.
- Cricoid pressure should be applied during induction of anesthesia in at-risk pts.
- Extubate at-risk pts awake, when protective laryngeal reflexes have returned.

PULMONARY EDEMA

LINDA LIU, MD

DESCRIPTION
- Definition: Pulmonary edema can be from increased pulmonary capillary pressure (congestive heart failure, neurogenic pulmonary edema), increased pulmonary capillary endothelial permeability (ARDS, infection, shock, drug toxicity, massive transfusion, anaphylaxis, trauma, aspiration), or sustained reductions in the interstitial hydrostatic pressure (negative pressure pulmonary edema)
- Cardiovascular manifestations
  - Depends on etiology of pulmonary edema; S3 or JVP elevation if poor CO
  - Nonspecific manifestations; often just tachycardia
  - ECG changes are nonspecific: other than tachycardia, sometimes may reflect underlying cardiac disease (MI, LVH, rhythm disturbances)
- Pulmonary manifestations: desaturations, rales, low lung compliance
  - If pt is intubated, may have increased peak inspiratory pressures & copious secretion (pink-tinged)

- CXR signs depend on severity & chronicity; often just diffuse infiltrates.
- If from pulmonary venous hypertension, may see Kerley B lines, redistribution of pulmonary flow from bases to apices, infiltrates, pleural effusion

■ Other manifestations: if cardiac output is poor, will have poor peripheral perfusion & renal insufficiency

■ Procedures w/ increased risk
  ➤ Increased pulmonary capillary pressure can occur in any procedure w/ large volume shifts & overly aggressive volume resuscitation (intra-abdominal vascular surgery, major abdominal procedures, liver surgery, major spine surgery).
  ➤ It can be more likely in pts w/ poor underlying cardiac function.
  ➤ Neurogenic pulmonary edema is often seen in neurologic catastrophes (aneurysm surgery, neurologic hematoma evacuations).
  ➤ Negative-pressure pulmonary edema is often seen after airway obstruction or laryngospasm.

■ Severity: depends on baseline cardiovascular function & etiology of pulmonary edema

DIAGNOSIS
■ Most specific signs: interstitial infiltrates on CXR
■ Most sensitive signs: widened A-a gradient on ABG or decreasing pulse ox
■ Other signs: may have elevated PCWP if etiology is due to increased pulmonary capillary pressure, but will be normal if etiology due to increased capillary permeability

MANAGEMENT
■ Mgt including preop preparation
  ➤ Reschedule nonemergent cases.
  ➤ Diuresis to lower hydrostatic pressure in the lungs to lowest possible level while maintaining adequate organ perfusion
  ➤ Remove offending agent (ie, stop transfusion, start antibiotics, treat anaphylaxis).
  ➤ Intubation & mechanical ventilation may be required to maintain oxygenation & decrease work of breathing.
  ➤ Consider placing invasive monitors to follow cardiac filling pressures.
  ➤ Supportive care

PULMONARY EMBOLISM (PE)

ANNEMARIE THOMPSON, MD

DESCRIPTION

- PE is due to the entry of foreign material (eg, clot, air, fat, neoplastic cells, talc, septic emboli, amniotic fluid) into the pulmonary circulation, specifically the pulmonary arteries.
- Obstruction of the pulmonary arteries can
  - Increase dead space
  - Result in hypoxia
  - Increase pulmonary vascular resistance
  - Produce reflex bronchoconstriction
  - PE can also cause RV dysfunction & cardiac arrhythmias.
- Thrombus is the most common cause; therefore, this section will focus on pulmonary *thromboembolism*.
- Risk factors
  - Genetic predisposition: activated protein C resistance (aka factor V Leiden) is the most common
  - Hyperhomocysteinemia: caused by folate, B6, or B12 deficiency
  - Antiphospholipid antibodies or lupus anticoagulant
  - Pregnancy
  - Oral contraceptives or hormone replacement therapy
  - Neoplasm
  - Surgery, as late as 1 mo postop
- Anticoagulation w/ heparin & subsequently warfarin for at least 6 mo remains the mainstay of treatment for most cases.

DIAGNOSIS

- Most frequent symptom: dyspnea
- Most frequent sign: tachypnea
- Other signs may include findings of RV dysfunction
  - Neck vein distention
  - L parasternal lift
  - Loud second heart sound
  - T-wave inversion V1-V4 on ECG
  - R bundle branch block
  - Atrial fibrillation
- Other symptoms include pleuritic chest pain, cough.
- Intraop PE is rare & requires a high index of suspicion for diagnosis. Usually presents as

- Unexplained hypotension
- Hypoxemia
- Bronchospasm
- Decrease in end-tidal CO_2

■ TEE sometimes used intraop
  - About 40% of patients w/ PE have RV dysfunction that is characterized by free wall hypokinesis w/apical sparing.
  - Also a large thrombus may be seen in proximal pulmonary arteries w/ TEE.

■ PA catheters may reveal
  - Increased CVP (due to RV dysfunction)
  - Increased PA pressures w/ a normal PCWP

■ ABG/CXR
  - Profound hypoxia w/ a normal CXR strongly suggests PE, but ABG & A-a gradient are not diagnostic (according to PIOPED data).
  - CXR normal in only 12% of pts w/ PE in PIOPED study
  - Abnormal CXR does not exclude PE diagnosis.

■ D-dimer plasma levels
  - Elevated in 97% of pts w/ PE
  - Also elevated in many hospitalized pts w/o PE

■ Venous ultrasonography commonly used to identify source of thrombus
  - About 70% of pts w/ PE have evidence of lower extremity DVT.
  - Impedance plethysmography & venography are also used to look for DVT.

■ Ventilation-perfusion scans & spiral CT are used to identify PE.
  - Both are most sensitive for proximal pulmonary arteries.

■ Pulmonary angiography is gold standard.

MANAGEMENT

■ Heparin is the mainstay of therapy for most pts.
  - Usually a bolus of 5,000–10,000 units followed by continuous infusion starting at 18 units/kg/h (max 1,600 units/h)
  - Target PTT is 60–80 sec.

■ Oral anticoagulation w/ warfarin is started once therapeutic PTT is reached w/ heparin.
  - Continue warfarin for at least 6 mo, w/ a target INR of 2–3.

■ For pts w/ contraindications to anticoagulation (eg, hemorrhage) or failure of adequate anticoagulation, an inferior vena cava filter is an option.

> ➤ IVC filters should be strongly considered in postop pts where bleeding due to anticoagulation may be catastrophic (eg, postcraniotomy pt or pt w/ subarachnoid hemorrhage).
> ➤ Multidisciplinary consultation w/ the attending surgeon & an internist/hematologist should be initiated in such cases.
- Thrombolysis is indicated for pts w/ massive PE, cardiogenic shock, or hemodynamic instability. Thrombectomy/embolectomy is available at some centers when thrombolysis is contraindicated.
- Intraop treatment is supportive, w/ inotropes & IV fluids as well as oxygen.

SEIZURE

J. W. BEARD, MD

DESCRIPTION
- A seizure is an abnormal, excessive, synchronous discharge of neurons.
  - ➤ Etiologies include
    - Hyper/hypoglycemia
    - Hyponatremia
    - Uremia
    - Hypoxia
    - Local anesthetic toxicity
    - Substance withdrawal
    - Fever
    - CNS infection
    - Inadequate anticonvulsant therapy
- Epilepsy is a condition characterized by recurrent seizures.
  - ➤ Common etiologies include
    - Space-occupying lesion (eg, tumor)
    - Cortical irritation (eg, subarachnoid hemorrhage)
    - Head trauma
    - Hereditary disorders
    - Anatomic malformation
- Seizures can be classified as partial (focal) or generalized.
  - ➤ Partial seizures are believed to localize to discrete regions of the brain. Symptoms may be motor, sensory, or psychological.
    - If consciousness is preserved during the seizure, the seizure is termed a "simple-partial seizure."

- If consciousness is impaired, the seizure is termed a "complex-partial seizure."
- Generalized seizures are believed to involve synchronous, bilateral, diffuse regions of the brain, leading to loss of consciousness.
  - "Absence seizures" (petit mal) are lapses of consciousness w/o loss of postural control, usually lasting for a few seconds.
  - Generalized tonic-clonic seizures (grand mal) are assoc w/ tonic-clonic muscle activity that may last several minutes. Variants include tonic, atonic & myoclonic generalized seizures.
- Status epilepticus is defined as repeated or continuous seizure activity for at least 30 min.
  - Seizure may be convulsive or nonconvulsive.
  - Unabated status epilepticus may result in permanent neuronal injury.
- Cardiovascular manifestations of seizures may include tachycardia & hypertension.
- Pulmonary manifestations may include aspiration & hypoventilation (possibly accompanied by hypercarbia & hypoxia).
- Seizures are usually followed by a postictal state characterized by altered mental status, gradual wakening & headache that may last for hours.
- Severity depends on the occurrence of cardiopulmonary complications, as listed above.

DIAGNOSIS
- Made by clinical observation and/or EEG monitoring

MANAGEMENT
- Maintain control of airway, oxygenation & ventilation.
  - Intubate trachea if ventilation is impaired by continued seizure activity.
- Stop seizure w/ one of the following agents:
  - Diazepam 0.1–0.3 mg/kg IV
  - Lorazepam (Ativan) 0.1 mg/kg IV
  - Thiopental 25–100 mg IV
  - Midazolam 2–4 mg IV
  - Methohexital 30 mg IV
  - Phenobarbital 20 mg/kg IV, rate not to exceed 50 mg/min
- Propofol can produce anticonvulsive & epileptogenic activity. No current dose recommendations exist for acute treatment of seizure.

- Avoid ketamine & etomidate secondary to possible lowering of seizure threshold.
- Identify reversible causes (eg, electrolytes, glucose, hypoxia) & treat accordingly.
- Consider prophylactic Dilantin therapy w/ loading dose 15 mg/kg IV at 50 mg/min followed by oral maintenance doses (300 mg qHS) to prevent further seizures.
- If pt takes chronic anticonvulsant therapy, consider checking anticonvulsant level.

SPINAL & EPIDURAL COMPLICATIONS

STEVEN YOUNGER, MD
KEN DRASNER, MD

DESCRIPTION
- Complications of spinal & epidural anesthesia can manifest immediately or after the block has resolved. These delayed complications include:
  - Postdural puncture headache
  - Infection (epidural abscess or meningitis)
  - Epidural hematoma
  - Traumatic injury
  - Local anesthetic neurotoxicity
  - Transient neuro symptoms
- Acute complications are described in the epidural & spinal technique chapters.

Postdural Puncture Headache (PDPH)
- Postural headache assoc w/ CSF leak through previous dural puncture
- Dural puncture w/ an epidural needle has a high risk of PDPH.
- For spinal blocks:
  - Highest incidence in young women
  - Higher risk w/ cutting-tip needles (Quincke)
  - Lower risk w/ conical-tipped needles (Whitacre, Sprotte)

Epidural Abscess
- Although rare, can cause neuro injury & paralysis

Epidural Hematoma
- Can be devastating & result in permanent paralysis
- Uncommon in healthy pts not receiving anticoagulants
- Time from symptoms until surgical decompression correlates w/ neuro outcome.

Persistent Neuronal Injury
- Highly variable incidence dependent upon technique & pt-related factors. Major sensory & motor deficits relatively rare, likely one occurrence per several thousand.

Meningitis
- Infection of CSF/meninges
- Uncommon w/ meticulous sterile technique
- Possible higher risk following LP in presence of bacteremia

Local Anesthetic Neurotoxicity
- Seen in several settings:
  - Continuous spinal anesthesia: most recent cases involved small-bore catheters used to administer lidocaine. These catheters are no longer available. Risk remains w/ large-bore (epidural) catheters if high dose of anesthetic is administered.
  - Repeat injection after failed spinal block
  - Single-shot spinal

Transient Neurologic Symptoms
- Formerly referred to as transient radicular irritation (TRI), but name changed because mechanism is unknown
- Symptoms include pain or dysesthesia in buttocks and/or lower extremities.
- Most commonly seen in
  - Pts receiving lidocaine
  - Outpatient procedures
  - Lithotomy position, knee arthroscopy or other procedures that stretch the lumbar & sacral nerve roots

DIAGNOSIS

Postdural Puncture Headache
- Symptoms include
  - Postural headache relieved by supine position
  - Usually 6–24-h delay after dural puncture
  - Nausea/vomiting

➤ Absence of frank meningeal signs (meningismus, photophobia, fever)

Epidural Abscess

- Symptoms include
    - ➤ Fever
    - ➤ Chills
    - ➤ Meningeal signs
    - ➤ Pain at catheter site
    - ➤ Loss of sensory or motor function below catheter site
- Close postop monitoring for persistent motor or sensory block or new neuro symptoms helps in early diagnosis.
- Infusions should be turned off temporarily if necessary to evaluate pts for persistent abnormal neuro symptoms.
- Imaging (MRI) confirms the diagnosis.

Meningitis

- Signs/symptoms include
    - ➤ Fever/chills
    - ➤ Headache
    - ➤ Photophobia
    - ➤ Meningismus
    - ➤ Leukocytosis
- Diagnosis confirmed w/ LP

Epidural Hematoma

- Symptoms include
    - ➤ Back pain
    - ➤ Neuro deficits below the catheter or injection site
- Close monitoring of high-risk pts (see below) is indicated.
- Infusions may be turned off temporarily to evaluate pts for persistent abnormal neuro symptoms.
- Diagnosis confirmed w/ CT or MRI imaging

Traumatic Injury

- Persistent neuronal injury due to trauma usually occurs in distribution that corresponds to paresthesia during block placement.

Local Anesthetic Neurotoxicity

- Symptoms may include
    - ➤ Bowel & bladder dysfunction
    - ➤ Sensory loss or motor impairment

Transient Neurologic Symptoms
- Diagnosis by typical symptoms & time course
  - Pain or paresthesia in buttocks or lower extremities
  - Onset after resolution of spinal block
  - Resolution generally within 3 days, almost always within 1 wk

MANAGEMENT

Postdural Puncture Headache
- Many cases resolve spontaneously by 24 h.
- If headache persists, treatment w/ epidural blood patch is indicated (see Technique chapter "Epidural Blood Patch").
- Conservative strategies may alleviate symptoms, but high frequency of recurrence. These therapies include
  - Caffeine 300–800 mg PO
  - Aggressive hydration, IV or PO
  - Supine position as much as possible
  - Stool softeners
  - Abdominal binders
  - PO analgesics

Epidural Abscess
- Treatment
  - Requires immediate surgical intervention
- Prevention
  - Meticulous sterile technique
  - Avoid blocks when evidence of skin infection exists at proposed puncture site.
  - Controversial: blocks in the setting of bacteremia. If bacteremia suspected, antibiotics prior to the procedure may reduce infection risk.

Meningitis
- Treat w/ antibiotics ASAP. Do not delay antibiotics until after LP in cases w/ high clinical suspicion.

Epidural Hematoma
- Treatment includes immediate surgical consultation. Time from symptoms until surgical decompression correlates with neuro outcome. Stop anticoagulants & consider reversal.
- Prevention: Decide whether to do neuraxial block in pt receiving anticoagulants. Also, decide when to remove epidural catheter in pts receiving anticoagulants. Consider following American

Society of Regional Anesthesia guidelines for recommendations for specific drugs (detailed recommendations and updates available at www.asra.com).

➤ Low-dose subcutaneous unfractionated heparin: no contraindication to neuraxial block, including catheter placement. Consider delaying block (or catheter removal) until 3–4 h after last dose of heparin & starting SC heparin 1–2 h after block. Since heparin-induced thrombocytopenia may occur during heparin administration, pts receiving heparin for >4 d should have platelet count prior to neuraxial block.

➤ Intraop "full" anticoagulation w/ unfractionated heparin: take following precautions:

- Delay first dose of heparin at least 1 h after block.
- Check PTT prior to catheter removal. Remove catheter 1 h prior to subsequent heparin doses or 2–4 h after last dose.
- Monitor closely for postop neuro changes (eg, inappropriate motor or sensory blockade).
- Risk after bloody or traumatic block placement not defined & not an absolute contraindication to proceeding with case; communication w/ surgeon & aggressive postop monitoring essential.
- Avoid neuraxial block in pts on prolonged therapeutic heparinization.
- Avoid neuraxial block in pts taking meds that affect other clotting mechanisms (NSAIDs).
- Uncertain: risk of hematoma during cardiac surgery

➤ Low-molecular-weight heparin (LMWH)

- If pt on preop LMWH prophylaxis, single-shot spinal probably safest. Delay block for 10–12 h after last dose of LMWH. Delay for 24–36 h if pt on "full" LMWH anticoagulation (eg, enoxaparin 1 mg/kg q12 or 1.5mg/kg/d).
- If pt scheduled for postop LMWH, recommendations based on dosing pattern:
- Twice-daily dosing. Remove indwelling catheters prior to initiation of LMWH thromboprophylaxis. Delay first postop dose at least 24 h after block. Remove catheters 12–24 h after the last dose of LMWH & 2–4 h prior to starting LMWH. Some centers remove epidural catheter routinely on POD 1.
- Single daily dosing. Give first postop LMWH dose 6–8 h postop. Give the second postop dose no sooner than 24 h after the first dose. Indwelling neuraxial catheters may be safely

maintained. However, the catheter should be removed at least 10–12 h after the last dose of LMWH. Subsequent LMWH dosing should occur at least 2 h after catheter removal.

➤ Antiplatelet drugs
- NSAIDs alone do not increase risk of hematoma formation, but risk increased in combination w/ other drugs (eg, heparin, LMWH).
- IIb/IIIa inhibitors (ticlopidine, clopidogrel): uncertain risk

➤ Fibrinolytic/thrombolytic drugs
- Widely regarded as contraindication to neuraxial block
- For pts w/ unexpected fibrinolytic/thrombolytic therapy, unclear when safe to remove catheters. Continue vigilant neuro monitoring. Consider following fibrinogen levels. Limit local anesthetic dose in epidural infusion to minimize motor & sensory block.

➤ Oral anticoagulants
- Stop 4–5 days prior to neuraxial blockade, & check PT/INR.
- Caution: Soon after cessation of warfarin, PT & INR may be normal as factor VII levels normalize. However, factor II & X levels may not yet be adequate for normal hemostasis.
- Monitor postop neuro status closely. See ASRA guidelines for more detailed mgt algorithms regarding oral anticoagulants.

Traumatic Injury
■ Paresthesia requires removal or replacement of needle or catheter to avoid neuronal injury.
■ Pain on injection through needle or catheter may indicate nerve root compression or intraneural injection & requires immediate removal of needle or catheter.
■ Avoid injection or needle/catheter advancement if pt has paresthesia.

Local Anesthetic Neurotoxicity
■ Repeat injection after failed spinal block
   ➤ To avoid toxicity, total combined dose should be less than the max dose a clinician would consider prudent to administer as a single injection.
   ➤ Recommended max doses for spinal
   - Lidocaine 60 mg
   - Bupivacaine 15–20 mg
   - Tetracaine 15–20 mg

- Single-shot spinal
  - ➤ Toxicity may be greatest risk w/ lidocaine.
  - ➤ Avoid exceeding 60 mg lidocaine max dose.
  - ➤ Do not use epinephrine w/ lidocaine spinals.

Transient Neurologic Symptoms
- Symptoms usually self-limiting

TRANSFUSION REACTION/ACUTE INTRAVASCULAR HEMOLYSIS

DONAL RYAN, MD

DESCRIPTION
- Acute intravascular hemolysis usually due to ABO blood incompatibility
  - ➤ Reported frequency of 1 in 33,000 units
- Cardiovascular manifestations
  - ➤ Hypotension
  - ➤ Tachycardia
  - ➤ Shock
- Other manifestations
  - ➤ Acute renal failure
  - ➤ Hemoglobinuria
  - ➤ Coagulopathy (DIC)
- Severity proportional to amount of incompatible blood infused, type of incompatibility, time to treatment
  - ➤ If volume of incompatible blood is <5% of total blood volume, reaction is usually not severe.
  - ➤ Can be fatal (1 in 300,000 to 1 in 700,000 RBC transfusions)

DIAGNOSIS
- Most specific sign: hemoglobinuria
- Other signs under anesthesia
  - ➤ Unexplained hypotension
  - ➤ Tachycardia
  - ➤ Diffuse oozing in surgical field
- Symptoms in an awake pt include
  - ➤ Chills
  - ➤ Fever
  - ➤ Chest & flank pain
  - ➤ Nausea

■ Unexplained increase in temp of >1 degree C in the setting of a transfusion should arouse suspicion of a hemolytic reaction.

MANAGEMENT
■ Stop the transfusion as soon as a hemolytic reaction is suspected.
■ Notify transfusion service/blood bank immediately. All cross-matched units should be rechecked.
■ Maintain urine output at a minimum of 1 to 2 mL/kg/h by
  ➢ IV fluids
  ➢ Mannitol 12.5–50 g
  ➢ Furosemide 20–40 mg
■ Maintain BP.
■ Insert urinary catheter if not in place.
■ Low-dose dopamine may help preserve renal blood flow & support pressure.
■ Alkalinize urine w/ IV bicarbonate (start w/ 0.5–1 mEq/kg) to target urine pH of 8.
■ Recheck unit & blood slip & pt ID.
■ Verify hemolysis:
  ➢ Plasma-free hemoglobin & urine hemoglobin
  ➢ Direct antiglobulin test
  ➢ Bilirubin
  ➢ Haptoglobin
■ Send baseline coagulation studies:
  ➢ Platelet count
  ➢ PT, PTT
  ➢ Fibrinogen
■ Send pt's blood & transfused blood for repeat compatibility tests.
■ Platelets & FFP may be indicated in the presence of rapid blood loss.

TRANSFUSION REACTION, OTHER

DONAL RYAN, MD

DESCRIPTION
■ Allergic reactions
  ➢ Occur in 1–3% of all transfusions
  ➢ Allergen is usually a protein in the plasma of transfused blood to which the pt has been previously sensitized.
  ➢ Less likely to occur w/ packed cells than whole blood

- Anaphylactoid & anaphylactic reactions
  - Likely due to a transfused plasma protein, but exact cause is difficult to determine in most cases
  - Small percentage of cases related to anti-IgA deficiency (IgA-deficient pts w/ anti-IgA antibodies can have anaphylaxis to transfused IgA)
- Febrile nonhemolytic reactions
  - Febrile reactions occur in 1–3% of RBC transfusions, 20–30% of platelets.
  - Typically due to white cell or platelet sensitization
  - Fever may be the first sign of an acute hemolytic reaction or bacterial contamination.
- Bacterial contamination
  - Bacteria present in stored blood can multiply & produce toxins.
  - Likely due to contamination at the phlebotomy site or to transient donor bacteremia
  - Most common in platelet transfusions (1/12,000) as they are stored at room temp
- Transfusion-related acute lung injury (TRALI)
  - Noncardiogenic pulmonary edema occurring 1–6 h after transfusion of plasma containing blood components
  - Antibody (in donor plasma)/antigen (recipient) mechanism involving human leukocyte antigen & granulocyte antigens that stimulates complement activation
  - Mortality much lower than ARDS (<10%)
- Delayed hemolytic transfusion reaction (immune extravascular reaction)
  - Usually due to Rh & Kidd system antibodies. Occurs 2–21 days following transfusion.
  - Anamnestic response, so may not be predictable by cross-matching
- Graft-versus-host disease (GVHD)
  - Donor lymphocytes attack immunocompromised recipient.

DIAGNOSIS
- Allergic reactions
  - Severity ranges from mild urticaria to bronchospasm, laryngeal edema, severe hypotension, death.
  - The faster the onset, the more severe the symptoms.
- Anaphylactoid & anaphylactic reactions

- Severe hypotension, tachycardia, bronchospasm, and/or rash assoc w/ a transfusion
- See chapter on "Anaphylaxis."
■ Febrile nonhemolytic reactions
- Signs & symptoms include chills, fever, headache, myalgia, nausea, vomiting, nonproductive cough, hypotension, chest pain, dyspnea.
- Fever may be first sign of an acute hemolytic reaction or bacterial contamination.
■ Bacterial contamination
- Signs & symptoms include high fever, tachycardia, hypotension, chills, vomiting, diarrhea.
- Can also produce septic shock, oliguria, DIC
■ TRALI
- Noncardiogenic pulmonary edema, hypoxemia, tachycardia, fever, & hypotension occurring 1–6 h after transfusion of plasma containing components
■ Delayed hemolytic transfusion reaction (immune extravascular reaction)
- Often manifested only by decrease in hematocrit
- Presents 2–21 days after transfusion
- Can mimic postop bleeding; therefore consider checking bilirubin
- Jaundice & hemoglobinuria may occur.
■ GVHD
- Clinically evident 8–10 days after transfusion: fever, rash, diarrhea, leukopenia, thrombocytopenia

MANAGEMENT
■ Allergic reactions
- Stop transfusion for moderate to severe reactions (debatable whether it is necessary to stop a transfusion for mild urticaria only)
- Treat w/ antihistamines (H1 & H2).
- Consider giving antihistamines for future transfusions.
■ Anaphylactoid & anaphylactic reactions
- Stop transfusion.
- Treat w/ epinephrine, diphenhydramine, corticosteroids, supportive therapy.
- See "Anaphylaxis" chapter for further details.

➤ Any pt w/ an anaphylactic transfusion reaction must be worked up for IgA deficiency.
- Febrile nonhemolytic reactions
  ➤ Pts w/ history of febrile reactions should receive white cell-poor packed cells.
  ➤ Generally not dangerous, but symptoms can be unpleasant
  ➤ Look for developing signs of an acute hemolytic reaction or bacterial contamination.
  ➤ Conscious pts may benefit from acetaminophen for fever & meperidine for chills.
- Bacterial contamination
  ➤ Stop transfusion.
  ➤ Send transfusion blood for Gram stain & cultures.
  ➤ Supportive therapy
  ➤ See "Septic Shock" chapter for more details.
- TRALI
  ➤ Treat like ARDS (see "ARDS" chapter).
- Delayed hemolytic transfusion reaction (immune extravascular reaction)
  ➤ Look for signs of hemorrhage as alternate cause of falling Hct.
  ➤ Transfuse as needed.
- GVHD
  ➤ In susceptible pt use only irradiated blood products, as this virtually eliminates any risk.

VENOUS AIR EMBOLISM (VAE)

JULIN TANG, MD, MS
MANUEL PARDO, JR., MD

DESCRIPTION
- VAE occurs when air enters the venous system due to
  ➤ Subatmospheric venous pressure or
  ➤ Iatrogenic injection of gas
- Cardiovascular manifestations
  ➤ Hypotension
  ➤ PA HTN
  ➤ RV failure
  ➤ Cardiac arrest

- Pulmonary manifestations
  - Elevated physiologic dead space
  - Hypoxemia
  - ARDS
- VAE can occur in any procedure w/ operative site above the heart.
- Procedures w/ increased risk of VAE
  - Neurosurgery (esp sitting craniotomy)
  - Cardiac surgery
  - Liver surgery
  - Laparoscopic surgery
  - Major spine surgery
  - Central line placement & removal
  - Arthroscopy
- Severity depends on
  - Volume & rate of gas entrained
  - Presence of patent foramen ovale
  - Nitrous oxide
  - Baseline cardiovascular function

DIAGNOSIS
- Most specific signs
  - Increased end-tidal nitrogen
  - TEE (look for intracardiac air, RV dilation, TR)
  - Increased sounds from precordial Doppler monitor
  - "Mill-wheel" murmur on auscultation
- Most sensitive signs
  - TEE
  - Precordial Doppler
  - End-tidal nitrogen
  - Decreased end-tidal CO_2
- Other signs
  - Increased arterial pCO_2
  - Hypotension
  - Increased CVP
  - Hypotension
  - Hypoxemia

MANAGEMENT
- In highest-risk procedures such as sitting craniotomy, place central line & precordial Doppler.

➤ Confirm position of central line near junction of SVC/RA before starting case w/
  • CXR
  • Fluoroscopy or
  • Intravascular ECG
■ When VAE suspected:
➤ Inform surgeon.
➤ Flood surgical field w/ saline.
➤ Lower surgical field below heart.
➤ Increase FIO_2 to 1.0.
➤ Attempt aspiration of air from a central line.
■ VAE w/ hypotension & hypoxemia
➤ Trendelenburg w/ L lateral position
➤ IV crystalloid administration
➤ For cardiac arrest, CPR & ACLS resuscitation
■ If procedure must continue:
➤ Keep surgical field below heart.
➤ Discontinue nitrous oxide.
➤ Carefully monitor for signs of ongoing embolism.

PART FOUR

Techniques

AIRWAY ASSESSMENT

RICHARD PAULSEN, MD
MANUEL PARDO, JR., MD

INDICATIONS

- Difficult airway mgt is the cause of significant morbidity & mortality in anesthesia care.
- Airway assessment is designed to predict difficulty w/ mask ventilation or tracheal intubation.
- A pt w/ predicted difficult intubation may be a candidate for awake intubation prior to induction of general anesthesia.

PREPARATION

- Airway assessment involves history, physical, review of previous anesthesia records.
- The urgency of the surgery or the need for tracheal intubation will determine available time for preparation.

ANATOMY

- Direct laryngoscopy requires four anatomic features:
  - Mouth opening
    - Mouth opening must be adequate for laryngoscope to fit.
  - Pharyngeal space
    - Excess tissue (eg, from edema) can block the view of the larynx.
  - Atlanto-occipital neck extension
    - Necessary for proper alignment of the axes of the mouth, pharynx, & larynx.
  - Adequate submandibular compliance
    - W/ laryngoscopy, the submandibular tissue is displaced anteriorly to expose the larynx. If submandibular compliance is low (eg, from prior neck irradiation or submandibular abscess), it may be difficult to apply enough force to expose the larynx.

TECHNIQUE

- History
  - Check previous anesthesia records if available. Look for:
    - Method of intubation (eg, direct laryngoscopy, blind nasal, fiberoptic).
    - Ease of intubation.
    - Number of attempts.

- Grade of laryngoscopic view.
- Laryngoscope blade used.
➤ Congenital syndromes associated w/ difficult airway include:
  - Pierre Robin.
  - Goldenhar.
  - Down.
  - Treacher Collins.
  - Turner.
  - lippel-Feil.
➤ There are many pathologic states associated w/ difficult airway mgt. In general, they affect the required anatomy for laryngoscopy. These states include:
  - Obesity.
  - Ankylosing spondylitis.
  - Radiation therapy.
  - Acromegaly.
  - Cervical spine injury.
  - Basilar skull fracture.
  - Upper airway tumors.
  - Epiglottitis.
  - Abscess in neck or pharynx.
  - Papillomatosis.
  - Croup.
  - Tetanus.
  - Traumatic foreign body.
  - Maxillary/mandibular injury.
  - Laryngeal fracture.
  - Laryngeal edema.
  - Soft tissue/neck injury.
  - Rheumatoid arthritis.
  - TMJ syndrome.
  - Scleroderma.
  - Sarcoidosis.
  - Angioedema.
  - Diabetes.
  - Hypothyroidism.
  - Thyromegaly.
■ On physical exam, evaluate the anatomic features necessary for laryngoscopy. This includes:
  ➤ Mouth opening
    - >2 fingerbreadths is optimal in adults.

➤ Neck extension
  • At least 30 degrees from neutral is desirable.
➤ Thyromental distance
  • >3 fingerbreadths is normal in adults; less may indicate an "anterior" larynx.
➤ Mallampati classification should be determined. It is based on structures observed when pt opens mouth. For greatest accuracy, pt should be sitting & should not phonate or arch tongue during evaluation.
  • Smaller numbers indicate reduced chance for difficult intubation.
  • 1 = soft palate, fauces, entire uvula & pillars seen.
  • 2 = soft palate, fauces & uvula visualized.
  • 3 = soft palate & base of uvula observed.
  • 4 = only hard palate visible.
➤ Note loose teeth, dentures, caps, braces, damaged teeth, partials, crowns, trauma, masses.
➤ Check for patent nostrils, especially if nasal intubation is planned.
➤ Identify cricothyroid membrane.
➤ Auscultate neck for stridor.
➤ Note voice characteristics.
■ The following findings may predispose to difficulty w/ intubation:
➤ High arched palate.
➤ Large tongue.
➤ Long/narrow mouth.
➤ Short neck.
➤ Beard (may hide a receding mandible & cause difficulty w/ mask ventilation).
➤ Large upper incisors.
➤ Small/receding mandible.
■ Note any conditions that could interfere w/ pt cooperation. This is especially important if awake intubation is considered.

COMPLICATIONS
■ Unrecognized difficult intubation may result in hypoxemia during attempts at airway mgt. This may ultimately lead to cerebral hypoxia, myocardial ischemia & cardiac arrest.
■ Airway trauma may result from attempts at difficult airway mgt.

PEARLS
- Prepare additional equipment & personnel for suspected difficult airway mgt.
  - If possible, intubate trachea w/ pt awake.
  - If this is not possible (eg, due to lack of pt cooperation), consider attempts to maintain spontaneous ventilation.
- Recent anesthesia record indicating easy direct laryngoscopy is reassuring, but consider whether pt's airway anatomy has changed since then (eg, due to airway edema, c-spine disease, or other causes).
- Combining different physical exam tests may improve the ability to predict a difficult intubation, but no combination is infallible.

ANESTHESIA MACHINE CHECK

PATRICIA ROTH, MD

INDICATIONS
- In 1993, the U.S. FDA developed the latest guidelines for anesthesia machine checkout.

PREPARATION
- Before starting case, ensure familiarity w/ all equipment.
- Perform a complete anesthesia apparatus checkout at the beginning of each day.
- Perform an abbreviated checkout before each subsequent use that day.

ANATOMY
- Not applicable

TECHNIQUE
- Summary of FDA recommendations
  - Conduct checkout before administration of anesthesia.
  - Anesthesia system should conform to current & relevant standards, including ascending bellows ventilator, capnograph, pulse oximeter, oxygen analyzer, respiratory volume monitor (spirometer), & breathing system pressure monitor w/ high- & low-pressure alarms.

➤ Modify guidelines to accommodate current equipment design & variations in local clinical practice. Local modifications should have appropriate peer review.

➤ Refer to the operator's manual for the manufacturer's specific procedures & precautions, especially the low-pressure leak test (step #5).

➤ If anesthesia provider uses same machine in successive cases on the same day, steps marked with an asterisk (*) may be abbreviated or skipped after initial checkout.

■ Emergency Ventilation Equipment
➤ *1. Verify backup ventilation equipment is available & functioning.

■ High-Pressure System
➤ *2. Check oxygen cylinder supply.
• Open O_2 cylinder & verify at least half full (about 1,000 psi).
• Close cylinder.
➤ *3. Check central pipeline supplies.
• Check that hoses are connected & pipeline gauges read about 50 psi.

■ Low-Pressure Systems
➤ *4. Check initial status of low-pressure system.
• Close flow control valves & turn vaporizers off.
• Check fill level & tighten vaporizers' filler caps.
➤ *5. Perform leak check of machine low-pressure system.
• Verify that the machine master switch & flow control valves are OFF.
• Attach "suction bulb" to common fresh gas outlet.
• Squeeze bulb repeatedly until fully collapsed.
• Verify bulb stays fully collapsed for at least 10 sec.
• Open one vaporizer at a time & repeat previous two steps.
• Remove suction bulb & reconnect fresh gas hose.
➤ *6. Turn on machine master switch & all other necessary electrical equipment.
➤ *7. Test flowmeters
• Adjust flow of all gases through their full range, checking for smooth operation of floats & undamaged flowtubes.
• Attempt to create a hypoxic O_2/N_2O mixture & verify correct changes in flow and/or alarm.

■ Scavenging System
➤ *8. Adjust and check scavenging system.

- Ensure proper connections between the scavenging system & both APL (pop-off) valve & ventilator relief valve.
- Adjust waste gas vacuum (if possible).
- Fully open APL valve & occlude Y-piece.
- With minimum O_2 flow, allow scavenger reservoir bag to collapse completely & verify that absorber pressure gauge reads about zero.
- With the O_2 flush activated, allow the scavenger reservoir bag to distend fully, & then verify that absorber pressure gauge reads <10 cm H_2O.

■ Breathing System
➤ *9. Calibrate O_2 monitor.
- Ensure monitor reads 21% in room air.
- Verify low O_2 alarm is enabled & functioning.
- Reinstall sensor in circuit & flush breathing system w/ O_2.
- Verify that monitor now reads 90%.
➤ 10. Check initial status of breathing system.
- Set selector switch to "Bag" mode.
- Check that breathing circuit is complete, undamaged, unobstructed.
- Verify that CO_2 absorbent is adequate.
- Install breathing circuit accessory equipment (eg, humidifier, PEEP valve) to be used during the case.
➤ 11. Perform leak check of the breathing system.
- Set all gas flows to zero (or minimum).
- Close APL (pop-off) valve & occlude Y-piece.
- Pressurize breathing system to about 30 cm H_2O with O_2 flush.
- Ensure that pressure remains fixed for at least 10 sec.
- Open APL (pop-off) valve & ensure that pressure decreases.

■ Manual and Automatic Ventilation Systems
➤ 12. Test ventilation systems & unidirectional valves.
- Place a second breathing bag on Y-piece.
- Set appropriate ventilator parameters for next pt.
- Switch to automatic ventilation (ventilator) mode.
- Fill bellows & breathing bag with O_2 flush & then turn ventilator ON.
- Set O_2 flow to minimum, other gas flows to zero.
- Verify that during inspiration bellows delivers appropriate tidal volume & that during expiration bellows fills completely.
- Set fresh gas flow to about 5 L/min.

- Verify that the ventilator bellows & simulated lungs fill & empty appropriately w/o sustained pressure at end expiration.
- Check for proper action of unidirectional valves.
- Exercise breathing circuit accessories to ensure proper function.
- Turn ventilator OFF & switch to manual ventilation (Bag/APL) mode.
- Ventilate manually & ensure inflation & deflation of artificial lungs & appropriate feel of system resistance & compliance.
- Remove second breathing bag from Y-piece.

■ Monitors

■ 13. Check, calibrate and/or set alarm limits of all monitors: capnometer, pulse oximeter, oxygen analyzer, respiratory volume monitor (spirometer), pressure monitor w/ high & low airway alarms.

■ Final Position
➤ 14. Check final status of machine.
- Vaporizers off.
- AFL valve open.
- Selector switch to "Bag".
- All flowmeters to zero.
- Pt suction level adequate.
- Breathing system ready to use.

COMPLICATIONS

■ Machine malfunction is a significant cause of anesthesia accidents. Catastrophic events can include failure to ventilate, oxygenate, or deliver anesthetics.

■ It is wise to have a backup source of oxygenation & ventilation readily available at all times (eg, an oxygen cylinder w/ a transport delivery system attached).

PEARLS

■ The four most important checks are
➤ Oxygen analyzer calibration
- The oxygen analyzer is the only machine safety device that detects a malfunction (breakage & low-pressure leaks) downstream from the flowmeters.
➤ Low-pressure leak test
- This test checks the integrity of the anesthesia machine from the flowmeters to the common gas outlet.

➤ Circle system test
  • This test verifies the absence of low-pressure leaks in the system & proper function of the inspiratory & expiratory valves.
➤ Positive-pressure leak test
  • This quick test will detect one of the most common causes of machine leaks; that is, when the CO_2 absorbent is changed & not reseated properly.

ANKLE BLOCK

ROBERT M. DONATIELLO, MD

INDICATIONS
■ Common indication: surgical procedures of the foot not requiring a tourniquet above the ankle
■ Ideal for pts undergoing brief procedures, or those unable to withstand the potential hemodynamic changes assoc w/ general or neuraxial anesthesia, or the potential toxicity assoc w/ more proximal lower extremity blocks

PREPARATION
■ Equipment: Sterile gloves, Betadine, 3 x 10-mL syringes, 1 x 22g 1.5-inch needle, 2 x 25g 1.5-inch needles, local anesthetic of choice (see the Local Anesthetics topic for specific drug information).
■ Pt preparation: Supine position. An assistant may be necessary to position the lower extremity if pt is unable to do so.

ANATOMY
■ Posterior tibial nerve: Sensory to heel, medial sole, & portion of lateral sole of foot. Location: Behind posterior tibial artery at level of medial malleolus.
■ Sural nerve: Sensation to lateral foot. Location: Superficial between lateral malleolus & Achilles tendon.
■ Superficial peroneal nerve: Cutaneous sensation to dorsum of foot and all 5 toes. Location: Superficial, lateral to extensor digitorum longus at level of lateral malleolus.
■ Deep peroneal nerve: Sensory to medial half of the dorsal foot, esp the first & second toes, & motor to the toe extensors. Location: Lateral to flexor hallucis longus at the level of the medial malleolus (ant. tibial artery lies between nerve & tendon).

- Saphenous nerve: Superficial sensation to anteromedial foot. Location: Anterior to medial malleolus. It is the only nerve of foot not derived from the sciatic nerve.

TECHNIQUE

- Prep skin of ankle thoroughly w/ Betadine solution.
- Posterior tibial nerve: Palpate posterior tibial artery posterior to medial malleolus. Direct 22g needle adjacent to pulse w/ continuous aspiration, until bone contact is made or paresthesia is elicited. Inject 5 mL of local anesthetic.
- Sural nerve: Place 25g needle laterally between lateral malleolus & Achilles tendon & perform a deep subcutaneous fan infiltration of 3–5 mL local anesthetic.
- Superficial & deep peroneal & saphenous nerves: Envision a line on the dorsal surface of the foot between medial & lateral malleoli. Identify extensor hallucis longus tendon by having pt dorsiflex big toe. Palpate anterior tibial artery between this tendon & extensor digitorum longus tendon. Place a skin wheal of local anesthetic w/ the 25g needle just lateral to the arterial pulsation along the above line. The needle is directed directly perpendicular to the entry site, & 3–5 mL local anesthetic is injected after passing through the extensor retinaculum (a "pop" is felt). The same needle can be withdrawn to the subcutaneous level & directed medially, then laterally, to create a subcutaneous "ring" of 8–10 mL of local anesthetic bounded by the malleoli that anesthetizes the saphenous & superficial peroneal nerves, respectively.

COMPLICATIONS

- Pt discomfort: Best remedied w/ preemptive explanation of the block to pt & light sedation.
- Failed block: Allow adequate time for local anesthetic to set in.
- Intravascular injection: Avoid by aspirating at each block site prior to injecting.

PEARLS

- Avoid injecting excessive volumes of anesthetic, as the excess hydrostatic pressure may damage smaller nerves traveling within already tight fascial sheaths.
- DO NOT use epinephrine to prolong the block, as multiple end arteries are found in the foot.
- Consider the use of an assistant to manipulate the lower extremity.

■ Always query the surgeon as to whether a tourniquet will be used.

AXILLARY BLOCK

ARUL DORAISWAMY, MD

INDICATIONS
■ Common indications: Surgical procedures involving hand and/or forearm

PREPARATION
■ Equipment: Sterile gloves, sterile prep, 30–50 cc local anesthetic in a syringe connected to sterile extension tubing
  ➢ Nerve stimulator, EKG electrode, 22g 50-mm insulated b-beveled needle
  ➢ W/o nerve stimulator, a 22–23g b-beveled needle will suffice
■ Pt preparation: Supine w/ arm abducted 90 degrees at shoulder & flexed 90 degrees at elbow

ANATOMY
■ At the level of the axilla, the nerves of the brachial plexus are separated by fibrous septa & travel alongside the axillary artery.
■ The relative positions of the peripheral nerves are variable, but most commonly the median nerve is above, the radial nerve is behind, & the ulnar nerve is below the axillary artery.
■ The axillary & musculocutaneous nerves have already left the brachial plexus sheath, the latter passing through the coracobrachialis muscle before becoming subcutaneous distal to the elbow.

TECHNIQUE
■ Palpate & stabilize the axillary artery w/ the middle 3 fingers of your nondominant hand, as high in the axilla as possible. Fingers should point up the axilla, parallel to the artery.
■ Nerve stimulator technique: Starting just beyond your fingertips, advance needle inferior to the axillary artery at a 45-degree angle to the skin, directed toward the apex of the axilla. When muscle stimulation is elicited in the hand or forearm at <0.6 mAmps, instruct assistant to inject 15–20 cc local anesthetic, after aspirating to avoid intravascular injection. Repeat procedure w/ another 15–20 cc above

the axillary artery. Continue to advance needle into the body of the coracobrachialis muscle; when elbow flexion is elicited at <0.6 mAmps, inject ~10 cc local anesthetic to block the musculocutaneous nerve.

■ Transarterial technique: Advance needle cephalad at a 45-degree angle to the skin, toward the axillary artery, while assistant aspirates. When blood is aspirated, continue advancing until blood stops, then inject 30–40 cc local anesthetic, while aspirating for blood every 5–10 cc.

■ Field block technique: Using a "moving needle" technique, inject local anesthetic above & below the axillary artery & into the coracobrachialis. After ~1/2 of the local anesthetic is used, test the peripheral nerves. If needed, inject more local anesthetic using the same technique, focusing on the known location of the inadequately blocked nerves relative to the axillary artery.

COMPLICATIONS

■ Intravascular injection.
■ Intraneural injection.
■ Hematoma: More likely after transarterial technique. If extensive enough, it can potentially compress the brachial plexus & cause nerve damage.

PEARLS

■ If artery is difficult to palpate, reduce the degree of arm abduction.
■ Attempting to block the musculocutaneous nerve by injecting into the coracobrachialis muscle is often unreliable, unless a nerve stimulator is used. An alternative method is to block the cutaneous branches of this nerve by performing a subcutaneous ring block along the crease of the elbow, beginning at the biceps tendon & ending near the lateral epicondyle.
■ When injecting local anesthetic, apply digital pressure to the axillary artery distally to facilitate proximal spread of the solution.
■ After the first injection w/ the nerve stimulator, find the next nerve quickly before the local anesthetic diffuses into that area.
■ Success rate w/ the transarterial technique may be increased if half of the local anesthetic solution is deposited anterior to the artery, while the other half is deposited posterior.
■ If a paresthesia in the hand or forearm is elicited with any of these techniques, some would advocate injecting 15–20 cc local anesthetic right there after withdrawing the needle slightly. Confirm

that pain does not worsen, because that could indicate intraneural injection.

BIER BLOCK (INTRAVENOUS REGIONAL BLOCK)

JONATHAN CHOW, MD

INDICATIONS
- IV regional anesthesia (Bier block) is a suitable technique for short surgical procedures of the arm (duration <60 min). It is reliable & pt satisfaction is usually excellent.

PREPARATION
- Peripheral IV: 20g or 22g is adequate
- Esmarch bandage (for exsanguinating arm)
- Tourniquet
  - ➣ Consider double-cuffed tourniquet
- Local anesthetic: 50 cc plain lidocaine 0.5%

ANATOMY
- Block is produced from dilute local anesthetic injected into peripheral vein. Tourniquet prevents local anesthetic from leaving arm.

TECHNIQUE
- Place a small peripheral IV in the distal hand of the operative extremity. Attach a short IV extension tubing.
- Place a double-cuffed tourniquet on the upper arm.
- Elevate the arm & exsanguinate by wrapping it with an Esmarch bandage.
- Inflate the proximal tourniquet (the cuff closer to the shoulder) to a pressure at least 50 mm Hg greater than pt's systolic blood pressure.
- Remove the Esmarch bandage.
- Slowly inject 40–50 mL of 0.5% lidocaine through the IV.
- Anesthesia usually results in 5 minutes & will last for the duration of tourniquet inflation.
- Pt may begin to complain of tourniquet pain as early as 30 min.
  - ➣ When this occurs, inflate the distal cuff (the one closer to the hand). Then deflate the proximal cuff. Tourniquet pain should decrease in a few minutes.
- At the end of the procedure, ensure that at least 20 min have passed to prevent rapid IV bolus of local anesthetic when the cuff is deflated.

■ Deflate the cuff & observe pt for signs of local anesthetic toxicity.
   ➤ Some believe in deflating & reinflating the cuff to prevent a local anesthetic bolus from being delivered.

COMPLICATIONS
■ Seizure or arrhythmia from local anesthetic toxicity

PEARLS
■ Proper function of tourniquet is key to this block. Tourniquet failure can result in both lack of block & systemic toxicity from local anesthetic. Ensure that you understand how to use the double-cuffed tourniquet system. Once tourniquet is deflated, the block dissipates rapidly. Make sure the surgeon understands that tourniquet cannot be deflated during surgery. Tourniquet pain is usually the limiting factor for surgery longer than 60 min.

BLIND NASAL INTUBATION

ALISON G. CAMERON, MD

INDICATIONS
■ Blind nasal intubation is useful for urgent intubation in pts w/ limited mouth opening or limited neck movement, or outside the OR when paralysis is risky or not an option.
■ Done w/ pt awake or well sedated w/ good spontaneous ventilation

PREPARATION
■ Prepare ETT (7.0–7.5) & coat w/ lidocaine ointment or jelly.
   ➤ Also prepare slightly smaller ETT in case initial ETT too large for nasal passages.
■ Consider antisialogogue such as glycopyrrolate (0.2 mg IV) to help decrease secretions. This will improve effectiveness of topically applied anesthetics & vasoconstrictors.
■ Apply topical vasoconstrictor & local anesthetic to nose.
   ➤ 1% phenylephrine in 4% lidocaine (1:3 dilution).
   ➤ 4% cocaine on cotton-tipped applicators inserted deep into nasopharynx.
   ➤ Additional solution can be applied to nasal passages via a syringe w/ long IV catheter attached.
   ➤ This helps prevent epistaxis as well as reducing pt discomfort.
■ Can also perform superior laryngeal nerve block or apply local anesthetic spray ("Hurricaine spray" = Benzocaine 2-sec spray).

■ Nose may be predilated by inserting lubricated nasal airways in increasing sizes until size of ETT is reached. However, this may increase risk of nosebleed.

ANATOMY
■ Basic pharyngeal/hypopharynx anatomy
■ If superior laryngeal nerve block is chosen, it is approached externally between the greater cornu of the hyoid bone & thyroid cartilage. Use a 23g needle & inject 2–3 cc 1% lidocaine. (See also chapter on Superior Laryngeal Nerve Block.)

TECHNIQUE
■ Place oxygen in pt's mouth or nose via nasal cannula or nasal airway w/ adapter to ventilator circuit. This ensures adequate oxygenation while performing intubation.
■ Either nares may be used (depending on nasal patency); however, placing the ETT into the right nares will align the longer flat side of the ETT along the nasal septum & may help to prevent irritation/trauma of the turbinates.
  ➤ Advance well-lubricated ETT perpendicularly into nose until at laryngeal inlet; when pt inspires, advance ETT into trachea.
  ➤ To best hear breath sounds, place ear above ETT opening. If breath sounds disappear, the ETT has advanced into esophagus or pyriform sinus & must be withdrawn to above the level of the glottis & reinserted.
    • Can also use capnography to identify tracheal entry.
  ➤ Once tube is past glottic opening, swiftly pass it through the cords (ideally immediately before inspiration to minimize VC trauma).
  ➤ Manipulate the head, thyroid cartilage, or ETT as necessary to successfully place tube.

COMPLICATIONS
■ Aspiration
■ Epistaxis
■ Pharyngeal soft tissue trauma
■ Damage to nasal turbinates
■ Hypertension/tachycardia
■ Esophageal intubation

PEARLS
■ Soften the ETT in warm (not hot) bottle of irrigation fluid prior to use to facilitate placement.

- Consider use of Endotrol ETT, which has a ring & plastic cable mechanism that allows manipulation of ETT tip.
- To minimize chance of epistaxis w/ ETT insertion, place an esophageal stethoscope through ETT until soft rounded end protrudes from ETT. This reduces the chance of the ETT bevel injuring the nasopharynx or nasal turbinates.
- Attach Jackson-Reese circuit to ETT & when bag begins to inflate & deflate, tube tip will be above/through glottic opening.
  - Ask pt to "pant" to increase opening of glottis.
  - Use direct laryngoscopy & Magill forceps to guide tube. Mouth must open >2 cm for Mac 3 blade to help with use of Magills.
  - Attach earpiece to L-shaped elbow connector to ETT to listen w/o risk of secretions contacting face/skin as tube is inserted.
    - Alternately, attach capnograph tubing to ETT & use CO_2 tracing to guide ETT insertion.

BLOOD COMPONENT THERAPY

ELIZABETH DONEGAN, MD

INDICATIONS
- Annual blood use in the U.S.
  - Donations: 13.2 million
  - Transfusions: 12 million
- Safety
  - Blood transfusion has become increasingly safe w/ improved donor screening & testing procedures.
  - Nevertheless, transfuse only when necessary & obtain consent prior to transfusion whenever possible.

PREPARATION
- Likely transfusion:
  - Order a "type & screen": pt's blood will be tested for
    - Blood type (ABO, Rh)
    - Presence of common red cell antibodies (pt's serum + red cells w/ known antigens)
- Planned transfusion
  - Order "type & cross-match":
    - Pt's blood tested for blood type (ABO, Rh)
    - Red cells to be transfused are tested w/ pt's serum
- Emergency transfusion:

➤ Obtain a blood sample for blood type
➤ Transfuse O red cells
➤ Then accept "type-specific" blood

ANATOMY
■ Each whole blood donation (450 mL + 50 mL for testing) can be fractionated into:
➤ 1 unit of packed red cells (pRBCs) +
➤ 1 unit of fresh-frozen plasma (FFP) or 1 cryoprecipitate (cryo) +
➤ 1 platelet concentrate
■ At collection, blood is anticoagulated w/ citrate (binds calcium) & preserved for:
➤ 35 days: CPDA1, citrate-phosphate-dextrose-adenine solution
➤ 42 days: Adsol (AS-1), Nutrice (AS-3) additional adenine & dextrose
■ Apheresis is in-line donor centrifugation collection for platelets, FFP, or cryoprecipitate.
■ Plateletpheresis is equivalent of 6 platelet concentrates.
■ Whole blood donations may be "leuko-reduced" ($10^9 > 10^6$ WBC) to reduce alloimmunization & viral transmission.

TECHNIQUE
■ Important: Transfuse all blood components through a blood filter (170–260 microns).
➤ This removes small clots & tissue fragments.
➤ Use only IV saline as carrier.
■ Whole blood transfusion
➤ This is discouraged because valuable components are lost.
➤ Whole blood has no advantage over component therapy.
■ Irradiated red cells/platelets
➤ Used to prevent graft vs. host disease (GVHD) in severely immunosuppressed pts (ie, nonreconstituted bone marrow transplant recipients, premature infants weighing <=1,500 g)
■ CMV antibody-negative red cells/platelets. Use for:
➤ Premature infants <=1,500 g
➤ CMV-negative pts who are severely immunosuppressed to prevent fatal CMV infection
■ Designated donor blood from first-degree relatives requires pre-transfusion irradiation to prevent transfusion-associated GVHD.
■ Red cells:
➤ pRBCs are transfused for their oxygen-carrying capacity only.
➤ Precede the decision to transfuse w/ measurement of the hematocrit (or hemoglobin) whenever possible.

➤ Adults: The "transfusion trigger" depends on a number of factors.
  • Hemoglobin >=10: Transfusion rarely indicated
  • Hemoglobin <=7: Transfusion often indicated
  • Hemoglobin level 7–10: Transfusion is largely dependent on pt's cardiovascular status & the rapidity of blood loss.
  • In a 70-kg pt, 1 unit increases hematocrit by 3%.
  • Allowable blood loss (ABL) is calculated: ABL = estimated blood volume times (difference in initial & final Hct)
➤ Pediatric guidelines for older infants & children are similar to those for adults but:
  • Infants <24 h w/ Hbg <13 g/dL generally need pRBCs.
  • Infants <4 mo w/ cyanotic heart disease or failure, or severe respiratory disease, & infants >4 mo w/ respiratory failure on ventilatory support, transfuse for Hbg <13 g/dL.
  • Neonates w/ acute blood loss or phlebotomy >=5–10% blood volume may need pRBCs.
  • Stable newborns w/ signs/symptoms of anemia may benefit from pRBCs if Hbg <8 g/dL.
  • Transfusion may be indicated in children w/ certain hemoglobinopathies to suppress production of endogenous Hbg.

■ FFP
➤ Plasma (separated & frozen within 6 h of collection), maintains donor coagulation factors at 100%.
➤ FFP is most often transfused for single or multiple coagulation factor deficits, as documented by PT or PTT >=1.5 times midpoint of normal range.
➤ Bleeding due to a factor deficiency occurs when the blood level is <=30% of normal & replacement therapy requires 10–15 mL/kg body weight.
➤ FFP is also transfused for clinically significant factor XI deficiency and/or other congenital deficiencies for which no suitable clotting factor concentrate is available.
➤ Massive blood transfusion (>1 blood volume in several hours) may require use of FFP but should be guided by PT/PTT measurement when possible.
➤ Vitamin K deficiency (needed to activate FII, VII, IX, X, protein C & S) causes an elevated PT +/- elevated PTT & should be treated w/ vitamin K if time allows (several hours).
➤ FFP is also transfused to treat antithrombin III deficiency & thrombotic thrombocytopenic purpura.
➤ FFP is not indicated for volume replacement.

- Cryoprecipitate
  - Cryoprecipitate is licensed only for its factor VIII content but also contains fibrinogen, fibronectin, FXIII, von Willebrand's factor.
  - Used in the OR as a source of concentrated fibrinogen.
  - Each unit consists of ~15–30 mL & contains ~250 mg (minimum 150 mg) of fibrinogen.
  - Generally, 1 unit per every 10 kg body weight is transfused to pts w/ fibrinogen levels <=125 mg/dL.
  - Bleeding due to low fibrinogen occurs when the level is <=80 mg/dL.
- Platelets
  - Platelet transfusion is indicated w/ surgical bleeding & platelet counts between <=50,000 & 80,000 (<=100,000 in closed, vulnerable spaces such as orbit or brain).
  - Spontaneous bleeding occurs when the platelet count falls below 10,000.
  - Platelet count cannot be predicted by the volume of blood loss due to individual variations, initial platelet counts, bone marrow & splenic sequestration & release.
  - A platelet count should precede platelet transfusion.
  - Platelets are transfused as 1 concentrate per 10 kg body weight or 1 pheresis.

COMPLICATIONS
- Risks of transfusion
  - Transfusion reactions (see also "Transfusion Reactions" in Critical Events section):
    - Allergic 1–3% (if hives only, stop transfusion, treat w/ Benadryl 25–50 mg IV, then restart)
    - Febrile 1% (can be a sign of hemolytic transfusion reaction)
    - Transfusion-related acute lung injury: nonfatal 1:600, fatal 1:11,000
    - Hemolytic, immediate (intravascular, usually ABO incompatibility due to clerical error): nonfatal 1:20,000, fatal 1:600,000
    - Hemolytic, delayed (extravascular, usually other red cell antibodies): nonfatal 1:4,000–12,000, fatal 1:1.1 million
  - Infections transmitted by transfusion:
    - HIV 1:1.9 million
    - HCV 1:1.6 million
    - HTLV I/II 1:3 million
    - HBV 1:180,000

PEARLS
- Alternatives to transfusion
  - Blood salvage/reinfusion (red cells w/o coagulation factors, not used w/ bacterial contamination or cancer in the field)
  - Normovolemic hemodilution (lower the hematocrit to 21–25% preop, then reinfuse stored blood at the end of surgery)
- Autologous donations
  - Safest blood but is often not needed
  - Advisable if transfusion is likely
  - Replace iron if not transfused.
  - May donate every 3 days if Hct $>=34\%$
- Massive transfusion
  - Serum calcium, preferably ionized calcium, should be measured following multiple transfusions & replaced as needed. Citrate, the anticoagulant in blood components, works by binding calcium (factor IV in the coagulation cascade) & is in excess in blood components.
- Rh-negative transfusion recipients
  - When possible, Rh-negative pts should be transfused w/ Rh-negative red cells & platelets.
  - At times of limited availability, Rh-negative blood components should be reserved for females who may possibly become pregnant in the future.
  - If Rh-positive blood is transfused to females w/ child-bearing potential, Rh immune globulin (RhoGAM) should be considered immediately post-transfusion to prevent alloimmunization.
- Sickle cell disease/thalassemia: Pts requiring a lifetime of transfusion w/ a high potential for alloimmunization to red cell antigens may be transfused w/ red cells matched for major red cell antigens.

CAUDAL BLOCK, ADULT

MERLIN D. LARSON, MD
ALEX KAO, MD

INDICATIONS
- Adult caudal is a good technique for perineal procedures.

PREPARATION
- Place pt prone over hip bolsters.
- Use epidural kit w/ Crawford needle.
- Mild sedation.

ANATOMY

■ Sacral hiatus is located by placing the index finger on the coccyx. Hiatus is then usually below the proximal interphalangeal joint. Confirm by rocking finger sideways above the hiatus to feel the sacral cornu.

■ Beneath the sacrococcygeal ligament is the sacral canal. Injection should occur in the sacral canal, not the dural sac, which usually ends at S2.

TECHNIQUE

■ Place sponge between buttocks after positioning prone.

■ Sterilize sacral area (Betadine or alcohol).

■ Identify sacral hiatus w/ nondominant hand.

■ Anesthetize dermis, SQ, w/ 1.5% lidocaine & 25g needle. Insert 25g needle into caudal canal & inject 1–2 cc lidocaine.

■ Hold Crawford needle like a dart & firmly press it through the ligament. A pop will be felt as it enters the sacral canal.

■ Redirect needle cephalad & insert needle about 3 cm.

■ Inject small amount of air or saline into canal while pressing over the injection site. Failure to feel a bulge during injection confirms placement within sacral canal.

■ Thread catheter through needle & secure w/ Mastisol & Tegaderm.

■ Test dose similar to lumbar epidural.

■ 20 cc of 2% lidocaine is sufficient for operations on the perineum.

COMPLICATIONS

■ Inadvertent subarachnoid, intraosseus, or IV injection

■ Injection into soft tissue, leading to ineffective block

■ Patchy block

PEARLS

■ Sacral hiatus is absent in 5–10% of pts.

CAUDAL BLOCK, PEDIATRIC

ALEX KAO, MD

INDICATIONS

■ Suitable for procedures involving lower extremities, perineum, lower abdomen. Use as supplement to general anesthesia, or for postop pain control.

PREPARATION

■ 1.5–2-inch 22g short-bevel needle or 22g Angiocath

ANATOMY

- Sacral hiatus is the midline space between the sacrum & the coccyx, bounded laterally by 2 sacral cornu, & is covered by sacrococcygeal ligament.
- Beneath the sacrococcygeal ligament is the sacral canal, which contains the dural sac (usually ends at about S2).
- Injection should occur in the sacral canal, not the dural sac.

TECHNIQUE

- Position lateral decubitus, w/ knees & shoulders flexed, pt facing anesthetist.
- Sterilize sacral area (Betadine or alcohol).
- Identify sacral hiatus w/ nondominant hand.
- Insert needle at 45-degree angle, advance through sacrococcygeal ligament.
- After loss of resistance, lower needle angle to parallel to skin, advance 0.5–1 cm.
- If using Angiocath, pull needle out, leaving only the catheter in place.
- Inject 1–2 mL local anesthetic per spinal segment to be anesthetized.
- There should be little resistance to injection if the needle/catheter is in the correct location. About 15 mL total will fill the sacral canal.
- If, upon injection, a skin wheal appears, then injection is into soft tissue.

COMPLICATIONS

- Inadvertent subarachnoid or intraosseous injection
- Injection into soft tissue, leading to ineffective block
- Patchy block

PEARLS

- Convenient dosing: 0.25% bupivacaine, 1 cc/kg, max 15 cc.
- If using Angiocath, after injection, remove catheter & look for kink. Kink represents where the catheter passed through the sacrococcygeal ligament.
- Sacral hiatus is absent in 5–10% of pts.

CENTRAL LINE PLACEMENT

MANUEL PARDO, JR., MD

INDICATIONS

- Common indications

> Assess fluid status
> Administer vasopressor infusions
> High-flow venous access
- Other uses
  > Pt w/ poor peripheral IV access
  > Mgt of air embolism

PREPARATION
- Equipment
  > Central line kit
  > Gown
  > Sterile gloves
  > Skin prep solution
  > Saline flush
- Optional equipment
  > Ultrasound is extremely useful for vein localization
  > Skin marker to mark vein location
- Pt position: supine, in Trendelenburg position for subclavian (SCV), internal jugular (IJ), or external jugular (EJ) catheterization

ANATOMY
- IJ: IJ vein lies parallel & lateral to carotid artery within carotid sheath. Vein is typically located 1.5 cm beneath skin.
- EJ: typically runs near lateral border of sternocleidomastoid; if vein is not visible w/ pt in Trendelenburg position, select a different site.
- SCV: vein is located deep to clavicle. Typically, the pleura is only 0.5 cm deep to vein.

TECHNIQUE
- Use local anesthesia for awake pts. After positioning & skin prep, technique varies by site.
- IJ
  > Rotate head <30 degrees to opposite side.
  > Locate vein w/ finder needle/syringe. Puncture skin about 5 cm above clavicle to minimize risk of pneumothorax.
  > Switch to larger needle or IV catheter & enter vein.
  > Determine whether blood is arterial or venous based on color, pulsatility, transduction of pressure, or blood gas analysis.
  > Continue w/ Seldinger technique (place guidewire, remove needle or IV catheter, nick skin w/ scalpel, dilate catheter tract, place catheter, remove guidewire).

➤ Sew catheter to skin. From right IJ, catheter depth is typically 14 cm. From left IJ, 16 cm. Catheter position is checked postop by CXR.

■ EJ
  ➤ Use IV catheter to cannulate vessel.
  ➤ Continue w/ Seldinger technique as above.
  ➤ Sew catheter to skin at 16 cm.

■ SCV
  ➤ Use needle at least 2.5 inches long.
  ➤ Puncture skin at halfway point of clavicle, about 2–3 cm inferior to clavicle.
  ➤ Keep needle parallel to floor to avoid pneumothorax.
  ➤ Initially, aim needle towards inferior border of clavicular head.
  ➤ Hit clavicle w/ needle, then withdraw needle slightly & advance needle just beneath clavicle.
  ➤ If blood is not aspirated, fan needle towards superior border of clavicular head.
  ➤ When vessel is entered & venous blood confirmed, continue w/ Seldinger technique.
  ➤ Sew catheter at 16 cm depth.

COMPLICATIONS
■ Hematoma
  ➤ Worse w/ coagulopathy.
  ➤ Can obscure landmarks & even cause airway obstruction if vein is in neck.
  ➤ With SCV, pt may develop hemothorax w/ no visible hematoma. New CXR infiltrate & falling hematocrit may be signs of this.
■ Arterial puncture
  ➤ Can cause hematoma or arterial damage.
  ➤ If carotid is damaged, pt may develop stroke or require vascular surgery for repair.
■ Air embolism
  ➤ Risk is higher if pt is hypovolemic or spontaneously breathing, or not in Trendelenburg position.
■ Pneumothorax
  ➤ Highest risk w/ SCV (1–2%)
  ➤ Obtain CXR after all central line attempts.
■ Guidewire embolism
  ➤ Always keep wire visible & verify that full length of wire is present after procedure.

PEARLS

- Use 33-inch IV tubing filled w/ saline as a pressure manometer. Attach this to the needle or IV catheter to confirm venous location prior to dilating blood vessel. Injury from accidental arterial puncture is worse w/ vessel dilation.
- To minimize risk of vessel injury, dilate only subcutaneous tissue & 1–2 cm into vessel.
- IJ, SCV: when puncturing blood vessel, withdraw needle slowly because blood commonly enters syringe on withdrawal.
- IJ: aim needle slightly away from carotid to minimize risk of arterial puncture.
- IJ: don't palpate carotid artery while inserting needle into vein; this compresses the IJ & makes access more difficult.
- EJ: if wire meets resistance at level of clavicle, withdraw wire by 10 cm, place traction on IJ vein, pass wire again.
- SCV: consider placing rolled towel underneath thoracic spine to allow clavicle to angle down towards bed. This facilitates needle entry parallel to floor.
- SCV: if difficult cannulation, consider manipulating pt's shoulder & arm to reposition the anatomy more favorably.

CERVICAL PLEXUS BLOCKS (SUPERFCIAL & DEEP)

PERRY LEE, MD

INDICATIONS

- Anesthesia of the cervical plexus can be used for operations on the lateral or anterior neck, such as thyroidectomy, carotid endarterectomy, or as a supplement to brachial plexus blocks for shoulder surgery.

PREPARATION

- Equipment: Sterile gloves, Betadine, local anesthetic, syringes & needles.
- Pt preparation: For both the deep & superficial block, pt is placed supine w/ head turned slightly to the side opposite that being blocked.

ANATOMY

- Deep cervical plexus block

➤ The cervical plexus is formed by the ventral rami of C2–4, which run anteriorly along the transverse process of the cervical vertebrae. These serve as the targets for the deep cervical plexus block.

■ Superficial cervical plexus block
➤ The superficial branches of the cervical plexus merge behind the midpoint of the posterior aspect of the sternocleidomastoid, usually at the level of C4 & at the point where the external jugular vein crosses the sternocleidomastoid.

TECHNIQUE
■ Deep cervical plexus block
➤ A line between the mastoid process & the clavicular insertion of the sternocleidomastoid muscle is drawn. A second line, drawn approx 0.5 cm below this line, approximates the line along which the transverse process of the C2–4 vertebrae lie. The transverse process of the C2 vertebra can be found approximately 1.5 cm below the mastoid process, along the posterior line, w/ the transverse processes of the C3–4 vertebrae lying 1.5 cm caudad along this line.
➤ Skin wheals are raised over the approximate locations of the transverse processes.
➤ A 1.5-inch needle is then inserted perpendicular to the skin & directed slightly posteriorly & caudad until the transverse processes are contacted.
➤ Paresthesias are not sought; rather, 5 mL of local anesthetic is injected after the transverse process is contacted & negative aspiration is confirmed.
➤ This is repeated along the other two cervical vertebrae.
■ Superficial cervical plexus block
➤ A skin wheal is raised at the midpoint point of the posterior edge of the sternocleidomastoid, followed by the insertion of a 2-inch needle along the plane of the muscle.
➤ 10 mL of local anesthetic is infiltrated as the needle is advanced & withdrawn in both anterior & posterior directions along the posterior edge of the muscle.

COMPLICATIONS
■ Deep cervical plexus block
➤ Accidental injection into the vertebral artery, epidural space, or subarachnoid space is possible. Frequent aspiration as well as

maintaining a slightly caudad direction during needle insertion is important to minimize these complications.

➤ Phrenic nerve as well as recurrent laryngeal nerve blockade can also occur, which may compromise respiratory function in pts w/ pre-existing contralateral phrenic or recurrent laryngeal nerve paralysis.

■ Superficial cervical plexus block

➤ Complications include IV injection of local anesthetic into the external jugular vein.

PEARLS

■ Superficial block is technically easier to accomplish & has fewer complications.

CRICOTHYROTOMY

EDWIN CHENG, MD

INDICATIONS

■ A temporary, emergent surgical airway placed in the event of an upper airway obstruction or failed intubation w/ inadequate mask ventilation.

■ The airway can be a 14g IV catheter connected to a jet ventilator, or a larger cannula or tube that can be connected to the anesthesia circle system.

■ A definitive tracheostomy should follow the cricothyrotomy as soon as possible.

PREPARATION

■ Rapid sterile prep

■ Equipment: Either (1) A cricothyrotomy kit or (2) a 14g IV catheter (as long as possible) attached to a 5- or 10-cc syringe, low-compliance (stiff) tubing to attach to the catheter & jet ventilator, & the jet ventilator

■ Surgical personnel to perform a tracheostomy

ANATOMY

■ The cricothyroid membrane is between the thyroid cartilage & the cricoid cartilage.

■ If the thyroid cartilage is difficult to identify, the cricoid cartilage is the first solid ring cephalad to the suprasternal notch.

TECHNIQUE
- With pt supine, extend the neck (do not extend neck in the setting of c-spine precautions).
- Puncture the cricothyroid membrane in the midline w/ a 14g IV catheter attached to a syringe.
- Aspirate for air to confirm entry into the lumen of the trachea.
- Advance the catheter & remove the syringe & stylet.
- Connect the catheter to low-compliance tubing.
- Secure the catheter to the neck.
- Ventilate via jet ventilation, which may require up to 50 psi to generate adequate flow through the IV catheter.
- Alternative method: Use the Seldinger technique, in which a guidewire is threaded through the IV cannula after puncture of the cricothyroid membrane, & the puncture site is dilated. A large cannula is then introduced into the trachea & attached to the anesthesia circle system.

COMPLICATIONS
- Dislodgement can lead to pneumothorax, subcutaneous emphysema, & mediastinal emphysema.
- Other complications include bleeding into the airway, false passage, & esophageal puncture.
- Long-term complications include tracheal stenosis.

PEARLS
- The IV catheter used for jet ventilation must be securely held in position.
- Inadequate expiration time using the jet ventilator can lead to barotrauma.
- Avoid jet ventilation in cases of complete upper airway obstruction.

DIGIT BLOCK

GERALD DUBOWITZ, MB CHB

INDICATIONS
- Block used for surgery on the finger
  - ➤ Generally better for surgery to the distal parts of the digit

PREPARATION
- Standard monitors.

- As w/ all blocks, resuscitation equipment should be available.
- IV access is optional.
- Needle: 25g or smaller, 16 mm or longer.
- Syringe: 10 mL.
- Prep: iodine or alcohol prep to skin between digits.
- Local anesthetic: can use lidocaine 1–2% (w/ or w/o bicarbonate) or bupivacaine 0.25–0.5%. More concentrated solutions are favored because of relatively small volume of injection.
- Do not use epinephrine as this can make the digit ischemic.

ANATOMY
- Common digital nerves are derived from the median & ulnar nerves & divide distal to the palm to make up the volar digital nerves.
- The smaller dorsal collateral nerves supply the back of the fingers as far as the interphalangeal joint.
- The dorsal surface of the thumb is innervated by the superficial radial nerve, which can alternatively be blocked by injecting the flexor sheath of the thumb.
- The upper branch of the ulnar nerve innervates the dorsal side of the fifth finger & can be blocked 5 cm above the wrist.

TECHNIQUE
- Positioning
  - ➤ Perform sterile skin prep & use aseptic technique.
  - ➤ Lay hand on flat sterile surface or drapes w/ fingers spread.
- Injection
  - ➤ Both digital nerves can be blocked by injecting local anesthetic into the interdigital space at the metacarpal phalangeal joint.
  - ➤ This may be easier w/ the needle bent at 45 degrees to allow placement parallel to fingers.
  - ➤ Alternatively, the needle can be inserted vertically at the lateral aspects of the fingers at their base.
  - ➤ Inject 2–3 mL of local anesthetic into the interdigital space.
  - ➤ This can be supplemented by a ring block, by injecting about 1–2 mL of local anesthetic subcutaneously around the base of the digit to be blocked.

COMPLICATIONS
- IV injection: aspirating before injection will minimize this.
- Intraneural injection: prevent by checking for paresthesia.
- No block/inadequate block: supplement the block if needed.

PEARLS

- Use the smallest-gauge needle available, as the injection can initially be quite painful.
- Inject slowly at first.
- Don't use epinephrine.

DIRECT LARYNGOSCOPY AND TRACHEAL INTUBATION

HELGE EILERS, MD

INDICATIONS

- Direct visualization of larynx w/ epiglottis & vocal cords, insertion of tube into trachea through mouth or nose
- Indications
  - ➤ Facilitate positive-pressure ventilation (most common indication for use during general anesthesia)
  - ➤ Maintain patent airway
  - ➤ Airway protection from aspiration
  - ➤ Respiratory failure or insufficiency
  - ➤ Need for pulmonary toilet
- Most commonly performed under anesthesia & muscle relaxation; can also be done in conscious pt (w/ sedation & topical anesthesia of pharynx)

PREPARATION

- Pt evaluation: thorough airway exam important to determine appropriate technique for intubation & to anticipate difficulties
- Endotracheal tubes (ETT)
  - ➤ Most commonly polyvinylchloride w/ high-volume/low-pressure cuff
  - ➤ For pediatric pts often uncuffed tubes
  - ➤ Average tube sizes (internal diameter in mm)
    - Adult man: 7.5–8
    - Adult woman: 7–7.5
    - Preemie: 2.5
    - Newborn: 3.0
    - 1–6 mo: 3.5
    - 6–12 mo: 4.0
    - >1 year: uncuffed ETT size = $(16 + \text{age})/4$
- Laryngoscope

- Light handle w/ interchangeable blades
- Have different sizes & types available
  - Curved (Macintosh)
  - Straight (Miller, Jackson-Wisconsin)
- Other equipment
  - Gloves
  - Stylet
  - Magill forceps
  - Tooth guard
  - Stethoscope
  - Suction
  - Breathing circuit or anesthesia machine
  - Oxygen source
- Pt position: sniffing position (cervical flexion & atlanto-occipital extension) is used to align the axes of mouth, pharynx, & larynx; use a firm support for head (eg, folded towels)
- Anesthetics & muscle relaxants

ANATOMY
- Larynx: at the level of fourth to sixth cervical vertebrae, framework of cartilages, surface landmarks: thyroid & cricoid cartilages
- Laryngeal innervation
  - Superior laryngeal nerve, internal division—sensory above vocal cords, no motor; external division—sensory to anterior subglottic mucosa, motor to cricothyroid muscle
  - Recurrent laryngeal nerve—all other motor & rest of subglottic sensory innervation
- Glottic opening: triangular space between VC, apex of triangle anterior, joins base of epiglottis
- Vallecula: space between base of tongue & pharyngeal side of epiglottis
- Trachea: 10–15 cm from vocal cords to carina
- Pediatric airway anatomy compared to adult
  - Narrowest part is the subglottic cricoid ring
  - Larynx is more cephalad (level of C3)
  - Epiglottis omega-shaped, longer
  - Smaller pharynx
  - Larger tongue
  - Larger occiput
  - Narrow nares

TECHNIQUE
- Description for right-handed individual
- Open mouth w/ fingers of right hand, thumb on lower and first digit on upper incisors.
- Hold laryngoscope firmly in left hand.
- Insert laryngoscope blade on right side of mouth.
- Sweep tongue to left out of way & advance blade.
- Position tip of curved blade in vallecula.
  - Advance straight blade beneath laryngeal surface of epiglottis.
- Pull in the direction of axis of laryngoscope handle; this will lift epiglottis & expose glottic opening.
- Classification of quality of exposure (Cormack & Lehane)
  - Grade 1: glottic opening fully exposed
  - Grade 2: only arytenoids & posterior opening visible
  - Grade 3: only epiglottis visible
  - Grade 4: no laryngeal structures visible
- Pass ETT through glottic opening.
- Inflate cuff.
- Ensure proper position (auscultation, chest movement, condensation in ETT, capnography, fiberoptic bronchoscopy).
- Secure ETT w/ tape.
- Average depth of ETT at the lips
  - Adult man: 23 cm
  - Adult woman: 21 cm
  - Child: 1 kg: 7 cm
  - 2 kg: 8 cm
  - 3 kg: 9 cm
  - Other children: 12 cm + (age/2)
- Tips for nasal intubation
  - Use wider nares (ask pt through which side it is easier to breathe)
  - Anesthetize & vasoconstrict nasal mucosa (4% cocaine or 3:1 mix of 4% lidocaine & 1% phenylephrine)
  - Dilate passage w/ lubricated nasal airway
  - Pass ETT through nasal passage
  - Perform DL & advance ETT through glottic opening
    - May need Magill forceps
    - Rotating the ETT may also help

COMPLICATIONS
- Endobronchial intubation: after 1 year of age mostly to right side

- Esophageal intubation: sometimes difficult to recognize—if you think the ETT is in the esophagus, it probably is.
- Soft tissue injury (mostly lips or gums)
- Dental injury: use tooth guard, preintubation dental exam
- Tracheal injury; excess cuff pressure leads to mucosal ischemia
- Inadequate anesthesia may lead to hypertension & tachycardia, coughing, bronchospasm, laryngospasm; cough may increase intraocular & intracranial pressure
- Aspiration of gastric contents: use precautions for pt at risk
- Epistaxis or false submucosal passage can result from nasal intubation

PEARLS
- Prepare optimally for "best first attempt"; subsequent attempts likely more difficult (soft tissue injury, swelling, bleeding, secretions).
- External manipulation of larynx (most commonly to right & cephalad) may improve view of glottic opening.
- Obese pt: use blankets to build ramp under upper body to reduce impairment by excess tissue.
- Pediatric pt: use towel under shoulder instead of head.
- Be careful w/ head positioning after intubation: head extension withdraws, flexion advances ETT.
- Eschmann-type introducer can help if vocal cords cannot be visualized.
- Cuffed ETT can be used in children <8 y (keep leak pressure of 15–20 cm H_2O to avoid mucosal ischemia).
- "Awake look" (view of vocal cords under direct laryngoscopy w/ pt awake) does not guarantee successful intubation after induction of anesthesia.

DOPPLER CARDIAC OUTPUT MONITORING

GERALD DUBOWITZ, MB CHB

INDICATIONS
- Noninvasive method of measuring cardiac output (CO) using Doppler ultrasound

PREPARATION
- Pt is intubated for continuous monitoring.

ANATOMY

■ Doppler principle relies on the fact that moving objects reflect ultrasound waves at different frequencies. This is known as the Doppler shift.

■ w/ blood flow, the RBCs are moving; therefore, their velocity can be calculated. Pulsed-wave Doppler velocity vs time area under the curve is traced, yielding stroke distance (eg, the average red cell travels 20 cm in one beat). Diameter of descending aorta is measured by M-mode.

TECHNIQUE

■ Two approaches to Doppler cardiac output monitoring
  ➤ Pencil probe (transcutaneous) placed at sternal notch
    • Requires user training
    • Difficult to do in OR
  ➤ Esophageal Doppler
    • Can be performed w/ standard TEE machine & probe, though dedicated & smaller Doppler cardiac output devices now marketed
■ Esophageal Doppler
  ➤ Measured w/ probe in esophagus at approx 35 cm
    • Adjust probe to get max signal (sound) from aorta.
  ➤ Descending aorta flow measured
  ➤ For quantitative measurement, calibration is needed (eg, w/ suprasternal probe or nomogram)
    • Not reproducible for quantitative results
    • Very good for qualitative measurements
■ Advantages
  ➤ Minimally invasive, easy to use, good safety profile compared to PA catheter (PAC)
  ➤ Beat-to-beat measurement of CO
■ Limitations
  ➤ Only an estimate of CO
  ➤ Not reliable w/ aortic cross-clamp or bypass because of unknown variations in CO
  ➤ Should not use in pt w/ esophageal pathology
  ➤ Unreliable in pts w/ disease of aortic valve or thoracic aorta

COMPLICATIONS

■ Potential for esophageal perforation

PEARLS
- Not necessarily a replacement for the PAC, but may be a useful monitor of CO trends in high-risk pts who have relative contraindications to a PAC
- Can be used to direct pt resuscitation & assess volume status

---

DOUBLE-LUMEN ENDOBRONCHIAL TUBE PLACEMENT

MARC SCHROEDER, MD

INDICATIONS
- The double-lumen endobronchial tube (DLT) is the most reliable & widely used approach for endobronchial intubation to control the ventilation of each lung
- DLTs facilitate lung deflation & secretion removal
- Indications
  - ➤ Enhance surgical exposure
  - ➤ Avoid contamination or spillage from one lung to another (blood or purulent drainage)
  - ➤ Control the distribution of ventilation in cases of bronchopleural fistula or giant unilateral lung cysts
- Commonly used for the following surgical procedures
  - ➤ Thoracoscopy
  - ➤ Pneumonectomy
  - ➤ Lobectomy
  - ➤ Thoracic aortic surgery
  - ➤ Thoracic spine surgery
  - ➤ Esophageal resection

PREPARATION
- Review CXR, chest CT scan, results of bronchoscopy for abnormal findings.
  - ➤ Finding of a markedly distorted carina and/or proximal endobronchial tumor may contraindicate placement of DLT or require fiberoptic-guided endobronchial intubation of the contralateral bronchus.

ANATOMY
- Right mainstem bronchus is shorter (2 vs 5 cm) & wider (1.6 vs 1.3 cm) than the left mainstem bronchus.
- Tracheobronchial dimensions are 20% larger in men than women.

- Choosing right or left-sided DLT.
  - ➤ Left-sided DLT is preferred because uniform ventilation to all lobes will most likely be achieved.
  - ➤ Right-sided DLT is undesirable for most procedures requiring lung separation because of the short & variable length of the right mainstem bronchus.
  - ➤ Other aspects of right-sided DLT.
    - Right-sided DLT designs incorporate a separate opening in the bronchial lumen to permit ventilation of right upper lobe.
    - Nevertheless, inadequate lung separation and/or collapse of right upper lobe is likely unless tube is precisely positioned.
    - Malpositioning occurs in >90% of cases when using only physical examination.
    - Proper positioning must include fiberoptic assessment.
  - ➤ Indications for right-sided DLT.
    - Left mainstem bronchus mass (eg, tumor).
    - Left mainstem distortion (eg, thoracic aneurysm).
- Important characteristics of the DLT.
  - ➤ Clear disposable PVC tubes that resemble Robertshaw design.
  - ➤ Two separate lumens, one terminating in the left mainstem bronchus & the other in the distal trachea.
  - ➤ Cuffs are high volume, low pressure.
  - ➤ Bronchial cuff is blue, facilitating fiberoptic visualization.
  - ➤ Radiopaque markers identify tracheal & bronchial distal lumens.
- Selection of DLT size
  - ➤ In general 35–37 Fr can be used in most adult women, 39 Fr in most adult men.
  - ➤ More precise selection of tube size can be made by measurement of tracheal width (TW) from CXR.
  - ➤ Measured TW: recommended left-sided DLT
    - TW >=18 mm: 41 Fr
    - TW >=16 mm: 39 Fr
    - TW >=15.5 mm: 37 Fr
    - TW >=15 mm: 35 Fr
    - TW >=13 mm: 32 Fr
    - TW >=12 mm: 28 Fr

TECHNIQUE

- General anesthesia, neuromuscular blockade.
- Macintosh blade is preferred because of the bulky nature of the DLT & because the tracheal cuff tears easily on the teeth.

- The DLT is passed w/ the distal curvature concave anterior.
- Once the endobronchial lumen has passed through the larynx, the stylet is removed & the tube is rotated 90 degrees toward the left.
- Advance DLT until moderate resistance is felt. Average depth is 29 cm for a 170-cm-tall person.
- Confirming proper position of left-sided DLT.
  - ➤ A sequence of cuff inflation & positive-pressure ventilation is performed to determine tube position & functional isolation of the lungs. Nevertheless, proper positioning frequently requires fiberoptic bronchoscopy.
  - ➤ Physical examination
    - Inflate tracheal cuff. Ventilation through both lumens should produce bilateral breath sounds.
    - Inflate bronchial cuff slowly w/ 1–2 mL of air & clamp tracheal lumen. Ventilation through bronchial lumen should produce only left lung movement, indicating the bronchial lumen has entered the left mainstem bronchus.
    - Unclamp tracheal lumen & clamp bronchial lumen. Ventilation through tracheal lumen resulting in only right lung ventilation indicates tracheal lumen above the carina.
  - ➤ Fiberoptic visualization of a properly placed left-sided DLT
    - Pass fiberscope through tracheal lumen.
    - Confirm correct positioning of the tube by visualizing the carina, an unobstructed view of the right mainstem bronchus, & the blue bronchial cuff just distal to the carina.
    - Pass fiberscope through the bronchial lumen, observing the bronchial carina w/ unobstructed views of the left upper & lower lobes. Troubleshooting malpositioned left-sided DLT
- Bronchial lumen in too deep in left mainstem or bronchial cuff herniated over carina obstructing right mainstem bronchus.
  - ➤ Clinical signs: ventilation through bronchial lumen produces left lung ventilation, but ventilation through tracheal lumen met w/ increased resistance.
  - ➤ Corrective action: fiberoptic visualization through tracheal lumen & repositioning of DLT.
- Bronchial lumen in right mainstem bronchus.
  - ➤ Clinical signs: ventilation through bronchial lumen produces right lung ventilation.
  - ➤ Corrective action: manual reinsertion.

- Withdraw DLT (5 cm) above the carina.
- Abduct pt's head & neck to the right while readvancing the tube.
- Ventilate through bronchial lumen for left lung movement.
- If right lung ventilation persists, proceed to fiberoptic-guided approach.

➤ Corrective action: fiberoptic-guided reposition
  - Advance fiberscope through bronchial lumen.
  - Identify bronchus intermedius.
  - With both cuffs deflated, withdraw the DLT & fiberscope simultaneously above the carina.
  - Advance fiberscope into the left mainstem bronchus, stopping 1 cm above the bronchial carina.
  - Advance DLT over the fiberscope until the rim of the bronchial lumen comes into view.
  - Advance fiberscope through the tracheal lumen, confirming proper tube position.

■ Insertion technique for right-sided DLT.
  ➤ General anesthesia, neuromuscular blockade.
  ➤ Insert right-sided DLT into distal trachea using direct rigid laryngoscopy.
  ➤ Insert fiberscope through bronchial lumen & advance into right mainstem bronchus.
  ➤ Flex tip of fiberscope anteriorly, visualizing the center of the right upper lobe.
  ➤ Return fiberscope to neutral position, viewing the bronchus intermedius.
  ➤ Advance DLT until rim of bronchial lumen comes into view.
  ➤ Withdraw fiberscope & flex anteriorly, visualizing the right upper lobe through the ventilation slot.
  ➤ Advance fiberscope through the tracheal lumen for inspection of the bronchial cuff at the carina.

Contraindications to use of DLT
■ Difficult or impossible direct laryngoscopy.
■ Anatomic constraints within tracheobronchial tree.
■ Predicted difficulty w/ exchange of DLT to single-lumen tube when ventilatory support anticipated postop.
■ Full stomach.
■ When DLT is contraindicated, consider use of a bronchial blocker technique.

COMPLICATIONS
- Hypoxemia & hypoventilation due to malpositioning
- Tracheobronchial tree disruption
  - Potential manifestations include pneumothorax, subcutaneous emphysema.
- Traumatic laryngitis
- Inadvertent suturing of DLT to bronchus

PEARLS
- Use pediatric fiberscope (3.6–3.9 mm).
  - These sizes will fit through a 35–41 Fr DLT.
  - Lubricate well w/ silicone spray.
- Repeat fiberoptic bronchoscopy after positioning pt for surgery because DLT may move up to 2 cm.
  - This is especially important when using the right-sided DLT.
- When using a left-sided DLT for a left pneumonectomy, prevent stapling of DLT to bronchus.
  - Immediately prior to surgical stapling of the left mainstem bronchus, stop ventilation temporarily & withdraw DLT above the carina, guided by fiberoptic visualization.
  - Following bronchial stapling, resume ventilation through the bronchial lumen.
- To aid lung collapse, apply suction to the nondependent lung.

ENDOTRACHEAL TUBE (ET) EXCHANGE

LINDA LIU, MD

INDICATIONS
- Indications
  - Need for larger or smaller ET tube
  - Cuff leak in existing tube
  - Need to change from nasal to oral route or vice versa
  - Change from double-lumen ET tube to single-lumen or vice versa

PREPARATION
- Equipment: New ET tube, laryngoscope
- Optional equipment: Ventilating tube changer or fiberoptic scope if laryngoscopy may be difficult

■ Pt preparation: Place on FiO_2 1.0, ensure adequate sedation, consider paralysis if ET exchange will be facilitated

ANATOMY
■ Laryngeal inlet anatomy

TECHNIQUE
■ If larynx is easy to see by direct laryngoscopy (DL): Perform DL & withdraw old ET tube under direct visualization of laryngeal inlet, replace w/ new tube, confirm placement.
■ If pt has a difficult airway, options include:
  ➤ Place ventilating tube changer down old ET tube, slide off ET tube, & place new ET tube over tube changer & slide into place.
  ➤ Load new ET tube on fiberoptic scope, place scope down side of existing ET tube, confirm it is in trachea, then slide out old ET tube while sliding down new ET tube.
  ➤ Perform DL, place tube changer down side of old ET tube, confirm tracheal placement, slide down new ET tube on the tube changer while removing old ET tube.

COMPLICATIONS
■ Trauma to lip or oropharynx
■ Tube exchanger is placed too distally, causing bronchial tear
■ Peak inspiratory pressures too high w/ jet ventilation via tube exchanger, leading to pneumothorax
■ Dislodgement of old or new ET tube
■ Pt may become hypoxic or hypercarbic & have hemodynamic instability

PEARLS
■ Prepare for the worst-case scenario.
■ Be sure that the reason for the ET tube exchange is important, because there is always the risk of losing an already secured airway.

EPIDURAL BLOOD PATCH

GERALD DUBOWITZ, MB CHB

INDICATIONS
■ Indications: Postdural puncture headache

PREPARATION
- Equipment
  - Gown
  - Mask
  - Sterile gloves
  - For placement of the epidural: Epidural kit
    - Tuohy needle or similar loss of resistance syringe
    - Local anesthetic, syringe & needle for infiltration
    - Iodine or other skin prep solution
  - For the blood draw
    - Syringes to draw 30 mL blood
    - 20g needle
    - Alcohol skin wipe
    - Tourniquet
- Where possible use a trained assistant
- Optional equipment: Fluid column for confirmation of epidural space
- Pt position: sitting or lateral
- Bear in mind the dural puncture may have been a result of a difficult epidural placement previously; plan accordingly
- Sitting will be uncomfortable for a pt w/ a postural headache.
- Check coagulation status
  - Do not proceed if a coagulopathy is present

ANATOMY
- See "Epidural Neuraxial Blockade" chapter.

TECHNIQUE
- Blood draw
  - With assistance:
    - Ask assistant to prepare pt for a sterile blood draw of 30 mL blood.
    - Do not draw the blood until the epidural space is identified.
  - Without assistance:
    - Consider inserting a 14–20g IV into the antecubital vein before doing the epidural, to facilitate drawing blood for the blood patch. Using sterile technique, prep & drape the site prior to blood draw.
- Epidural
  - Position pt.
  - Find the space corresponding to the level of the dural puncture.

➤ Prep skin; infiltrate local anesthetic.
➤ Place the epidural needle.
➤ Instill up to 30 mL of autologous fresh blood into the epidural space, or until the pt feels significant pressure at the site of injection, whichever comes first.
➤ Withdraw the epidural needle.

COMPLICATIONS

■ Blood draw
  ➤ Failed cannulation
  ➤ Hematoma
  ➤ Infection
  ➤ Arterial puncture: can cause hematoma or arterial damage
■ Epidural
  ➤ Failed placement
  ➤ Dural puncture
  ➤ Neuropathy/spinal cord nerve root damage
  ➤ Epidural hematoma or abscess

PEARLS

■ Plan carefully & use an assistant.
■ Injection of blood must be reasonably close to the original site.
  ➤ Injecting within 2 levels should suffice.
■ If you get a wet tap, withdraw the epidural needle & try again.
■ If the original approach was reported as difficult, try another technique:
  ➤ Paramedian rather than midline.
  ➤ Lying rather than sitting.
■ Blood can be injected through the epidural catheter if it is still in place.
  ➤ Cutting the catheter will reduce its length & hence its resistance to injection.
  ➤ A smaller syringe will be easier to inject with (eg, 10 mL rather than 30 mL).
■ Most patients get relief a few seconds to minutes after the blood patch. If there is no relief, the patch has failed.
  ➤ Consider repeating or
  ➤ Reconsider the diagnosis.
■ Repeated patches mean repeated complication risk.
  ➤ Discuss benefits & risks carefully with pt.
  ➤ Consider obtaining expert assistance.

EPIDURAL NEURAXIAL BLOCKADE

STEVEN YOUNGER, MD

INDICATIONS
- Epidural blocks are used in a variety of clinical settings: outpatient surgery, inpatient surgery, postop pain, chronic pain, & obstetric anesthesia & analgesia
- Can consider epidural for any operation below the nipple line
- Contraindications
  - ➢ Absolute
    - Coagulopathy
    - Infection near site of puncture
    - Pt refusal
  - ➢ Relative
    - Hypovolemia
    - Sepsis
    - Severe back deformity

PREPARATION
- Epidural kit: Contents include epidural needle, catheter, saline, local anesthetic, syringe for loss of resistance. Verify that kit has not expired.
- Common epidural needle sizes: 17g or 18g Tuohy or Hustead
- Local anesthetic solution for epidural use
- If epidural local anesthetic will be immediately given, prepare standard equipment, monitoring, & drugs, including those required for induction of general anesthesia.
- Obtain baseline hemodynamic values prior to block. Correct hypovolemia–sympathectomy from epidural can cause sinus arrest in hypovolemic pts.
- Catheter can be placed in preop or block area & dosed in the OR.

ANATOMY
- The epidural space is 3–6 mm thick & is occupied by epidural fat, lymphatics, vascular tissue.
- The epidural space runs the length of the spinal column. Cephalic limit is the foramen magnum.
- Epidural space boundaries: Dura at deep margin, ligamentum flavum superficially .

- The spinous processes of the T6-T9 thoracic vertebrae angle down sharply, making midline approaches more difficult.
- Approaching the space from the midline, the layers encountered from superficial to deep are skin, subcutaneous tissue, supraspinous ligament, interspinous ligament, ligamentum flavum, epidural space, dura, arachnoid, CSF.
- Markings on epidural needle & epidural catheter allow measurement of depth of epidural space & depth of catheter insertion.

TECHNIQUE

Position

- Can choose lateral decubitus or sitting.
- Lateral decubitus: Greatest pt comfort & preferable for heavily sedated pt.
- Sitting: Encourages flexion & facilitates recognition of the midline, important in obese pts.

Midline approach

- Recommended for lumbar, low thoracic, & C7-T1 placement
- Identify interspace, consider marking w/ skin marker, & prep w/ Betadine solution.
- Administer local anesthetic w/ 25g needle. A long needle can help identify the space between spinous processes & other bony anatomy, esp in pt w/ abundant subcutaneous fat. In very thin pt, avoid entering the subarachnoid space w/ needle.
- Insert epidural needle into chosen interspace & advance until it is felt to "seat" in firm tissue. This is easiest to feel in lumber region, where the ligamentum flavum is thickest.
- Attach loss of resistance (LOR) syringe to epidural needle. Seek LOR to identify epidural space. Options include:
  - ➤ Saline-filled syringe
  - ➤ Saline-filled syringe w/ air bubble. Compression of air bubble can help to quantify amount of pressure on plunger.
  - ➤ Air-filled syringe
- Depress plunger of the syringe w/ thumb of the right hand while advancing needle w/ left hand. Brace left hand against pt's back to avoid uncontrolled advancement of needle.
- Slowly advance needle while applying pressure to syringe plunger. Two approaches: Intermittent "tap-tap" of plunger vs. "continuous pressure" on plunger. Should feel firm resistance to pressure on plunger if needle tip is in ligamentum flavum.

- Stop needle advancement when LOR encountered.
- Remove syringe from needle. Consider saline administration to facilitate catheter placement. Insert catheter 3–4 cm past tip of needle.
- A brief paresthesia may occur while threading catheter. For persistent paresthesia or for pain during injection, withdraw needle or catheter to minimize risk of neuronal injury.
- Attach connector to end of catheter. Aspirate for blood or CSF.
- Secure catheter w/ occlusive dressing (eg, Tegaderm).

Paramedian approach
- Recommended for midthoracic approach (T6-T9) & in pts w/ osteoarthritis, compression fractures, & poor spine flexion
- Administer local anesthetic approximately 1–1.5 cm lateral to the midline. Can use this as "finder" needle to identify the spinal lamina of the vertebra forming the lower border of the interspace.
- Insert epidural needle perpendicular to the skin, advance to lamina, then angle 45 degrees cephalad & 45 degrees toward the midline & "walk" over the edge of the lamina into the ligamentum flavum.
- Halt the needle at the first sign of paresthesia, as this approach can place the needle tip close to the spinal roots if the angle of the needle is too shallow or too acute.
- Seek LOR as above. Continue w/ remainder of procedure described for midline approach.

Test dose
- Main purpose of test dose is to identify inadvertent subarachnoid or IV placement of catheter.
- Administer test dose in monitored setting through the catheter.
- Note blood pressure, heart rate prior to test dose.
- Typical test dose: 3 cc 1.5% lidocaine w/ 1:200,000 (5 mcg/cc) epinephrine.
- IV detection: 1 min after injection—look for heart rate response to epinephrine. Typically increases > 15 bpm if intravascular. 3 min after injection—look for subarachnoid block (eg, lower extremity numbness, motor block).
- Test dose is less reliable in elderly, OB pts, & during general anesthesia.

COMPLICATIONS
- General

➤ Immediate complications include hypotension, bradycardia, total spinal block, seizure. Nausea/vomiting frequently accompanies significant hypotension.

➤ Delayed complications include urinary retention, backache, postdural puncture headache. Rare but severe complications include meningitis, epidural abscess, epidural hematoma w/ paralysis, neurologic injury from spinal cord or nerve root trauma. (See also chapter on delayed complications of neuraxial block.)

■ Hypotension
  ➤ Anticipate effects of sympathectomy in pts w/ significant aortic or mitral valve stenosis. Prepare medication to increase afterload (eg, phenylephrine)

■ Total spinal
  ➤ Can be seen w/ inadvertent placement of epidural catheter into subarachnoid space
  ➤ Signs/symptoms: High sensory level, loss of consciousness, respiratory arrest, cardiovascular collapse
  ➤ Treatment: Prompt airway mgt including intubation & hemodynamic support w/ vasopressors until block wears off

■ Local anesthetic toxicity
  ➤ Seizure: Control airway & oxygenate; sedate & paralyze if necessary
  ➤ Cardiovascular collapse: ACLS protocol

PEARLS

■ Guide to dose lumbar catheters w/ 2% lidocaine & epi = 2 cc/segment for pt 5 foot tall, add 0.1 cc/segment for every 2 inches over 5 feet. Decrease dose in pregnancy, elderly, & those w/ thoracic catheters.

■ Use broken stick, ice, or laryngoscope handle for sensory level testing instead of needle.

■ Sensory nerves not blocked by epidural: Vagus, glossopharyngeal, trigeminal

---

FEMORAL BLOCK

GERALD DUBOWITZ, MB CHB

INDICATIONS

■ Can be used for lower limb surgery, esp knee arthroscopy

■ For more extensive coverage, use 3 in 1 block (femoral, obturator & lateral femoral cutaneous) combined w/ sciatic nerve block

PREPARATION
■ Standard monitors, resuscitation equipment
■ IV access
■ Iodine or alcohol prep
■ Needles
    ➤ 20–24g, 25 mm or longer
    ➤ Consider insulated needle for use w/ nerve stimulator.
■ Two 20-mL syringes
■ Local anesthetic solution (eg, lidocaine 1% or bupivacaine 0.25%)

ANATOMY
■ Femoral nerve lies in the anteromedial aspect of the upper thigh.
■ Can be located 1–2 cm lateral to the femoral artery as it passes through the femoral sheath below the inguinal ligament.

TECHNIQUE
■ Place pt in supine position.
■ Prep the groin area & inguinal crease.
■ Palpate the femoral artery in the groin.
■ Insert the needle lateral to this at 90 degrees to the skin.
■ Nerve can be located using paresthesia, but this may be more accurately achieved using a nerve stimulator.
    ➤ With nerve stimulator, quadriceps muscles will twitch, moving the patella superiorly. The needle is advanced until minimally acceptable threshold is achieved that still produces a twitch (eg, <0.5 mA).
■ After aspirating to ensure no intravascular injection, infiltrate 20–30 mL of local anesthetic. Larger volume will block more nerves (see Techniques chapter "Lumbar Plexus Block").

COMPLICATIONS
■ IV injection: aspirate to be sure of needle placement before injection.
■ Intraneural injection: check for painful paresthesia on injection; redirect needle if this occurs.
■ No block/inadequate block: supplement the block if needed.

PEARLS
■ Rarely of use on its own. Better when combined w/ distal pressure & greater volume to achieve the 3 in 1 block.

FIBEROPTIC AIRWAY MANAGEMENT

ROBIN STACKHOUSE, MD

INDICATIONS

- Note: Preparation of pt & equipment for fiberoptic airway mgt takes time. Consider whether pt's condition allows this time. For instance, pt w/ severe hypoxemia or airway obstruction may need immediate emergency surgical or nonsurgical airway mgt.
- Indications
  - ➤ Intubation of pt w/ cervical spine instability.
    - Examination & intubation of pts w/ blunt or penetrating airway trauma.
  - ➤ Pt is predicted to be difficult to intubate.
- Four main anatomic problems predict difficult intubation:
  - ➤ Limited oropharyngeal space
    - Perform a Mallampati exam to assess.
  - ➤ Limited atlanto-occipital (A-O) extension
    - Normal A-O extension is 35.
    - A decrease of >1/3 is assoc w/ an increased risk of difficult airway mgt.
  - ➤ Limited pharyngeal space
    - Decreased thyromental distance.
    - Space-filling pharyngeal illnesses (infections, edema, hematoma, tumors).
    - Subtle signs of limited pharyngeal space include use of accessory muscles, difficulty managing secretions, sitting upright w/ airway held in the "sniffing" position, restriction of maximal inspiratory flow.
  - ➤ Decreased submandibular compliance
    - Limits ability to displace the soft tissues of the pharynx anterior to the line of view on direct laryngoscopy.
    - May be caused by infiltrating processes or scarring.
- Contraindications
  - ➤ Insufficient time: Pt must have adequate oxygenation & ventilation for the time it takes to perform the technique.
  - ➤ No pharyngeal space.
  - ➤ Excessive secretions or blood in the airway.

PREPARATION

- Monitors, oxygen, judicious sedation for pt

- Fiberoptic bronchoscope w/ compatible light source
- Endotracheal tube (ETT), medications for topicalization & blocks
- Suction equipment (Yankauer, ETT suction catheter)

ANATOMY

- Anesthesia to nose (for nasal intubation), pharynx, larynx, trachea must be provided.
- The nose is innervated by branches of the ophthalmic & maxillary divisions of the trigeminal nerve (anterior ethmoidal nerve, nasopalatine nerve, sphenopalatine ganglion).
- The oropharynx is innervated by the lingual & glossopharyngeal nerves.
- The larynx & trachea are innervated by the recurrent laryngeal nerve & the superior laryngeal nerve (both are branches of the vagus nerve).

TECHNIQUE

- Provide vasoconstriction & topical anesthesia to nasal mucosa for nasal intubation. Instill lidocaine 3% & phenylephrine 0.25% or cocaine 4% into nose w/ cotton swabs or pledgets.
- Provide topical anesthesia to oropharynx.
  - ➤ Lingual & glossopharyngeal nerves (oropharynx): Use aerosolized local anesthetic (preferably lidocaine) or bilateral glossopharyngeal nerve block.
  - ➤ Recurrent laryngeal nerve & superior laryngeal nerve: Topicalization of both distributions may be accomplished by local anesthetic aerosol. Alternatively, perform transtracheal & superior laryngeal nerve block.
  - ➤ Transtracheal block
    - Fill 5-cc syringe w/ 4 cc of 2–4% lidocaine & connect to a 20g IV catheter.
    - Identify the cricothyroid membrane & prep skin w/ alcohol or Betadine.
    - Insert IV at 90-degree angle through the cricothyroid membrane until air is aspirated.
    - Remove needle.
    - Reconfirm intratracheal location by air aspiration.
    - Inject the local anesthetic. Pt may cough, but this will facilitate spread of local.
  - ➤ Superior laryngeal nerve block
    - Prepare syringe w/ 22g needle & 2 cc local anesthetic (eg, lidocaine 1–2%).

- Prep skin overlying the cornua of hyoid bone w/ alcohol or Betadine.
- Insert needle over cornu & advance until bone is contacted.
- Direct needle caudally until contact w/ bone is lost, & inject local anesthetic.

■ Use a channel to assist in aiming the fiberoptic bronchoscope (FOB) toward the airway.
  ➤ ETT for nasal intubations
    - Nasal tubes cause less trauma if they are softened in warm water & lubricated prior to insertion.
    - Advance a nasal ETT to 14–16 cm in an adult.
  ➤ Oral intubating airway for oral intubations
■ Suction any secretions in the pharynx prior to inserting the FOB.
■ Advance the FOB through the ETT w/o manipulating it until it is past the end.
  ➤ Do not let the ETT exit through the Murphey eye.
■ Keep the FOB taut.
  ➤ Use flexion & rotation to identify airway structures.
■ Keep the view of the airway centered as the scope is advanced.
■ If difficulty is encountered w/ pharyngeal space, secretions, or aiming the FOB anterior enough to enter the airway, inflate cuff of the ETT w/ 10–20 mL air.
  ➤ Remember to withdraw the air prior to advancing the ETT through the vocal cords.
■ Advance the FOB through the vocal cords & thread the ETT over the FOB.

COMPLICATIONS

■ Laryngospasm, particularly w/ inadequate topicalization
■ Bleeding from nerve blocks or ETT in nose (vasoconstriction recommended)
■ Gagging or vomiting, aspiration

PEARLS

■ 11 essentials of fiberoptic intubation:
  ➤ Appropriate pt.
  ➤ Adequate time.
  ➤ Pharyngeal space.
  ➤ Minimal blood & secretions.
  ➤ Prepared FOB (cleaned, focused, defogged).

➤ Use an appropriate channel.
➤ Aim the channel.
➤ Supply supplemental oxygen.
➤ Sedate, but don't put the airway in jeopardy.
➤ Adequate topicalization/blocks.
➤ Develop your expertise.
➤ If the view through the FOB becomes obscured, try wiping the tip against the mucosa to clear.
➤ If unsuccessful, remove the scope & wipe the secretions off.

■ When localizing structures cannot be identified, withdraw the scope slightly to obtain a wider field of view.
■ If resistance is felt in advancing the ETT through the nose, use 90 degrees of counterclockwise rotation so that the bevel of the ETT will more easily make the caudad turn in the posterior nasopharynx.
■ If resistance is felt when advancing the ETT over the FOB into the airway, rotate the tube while gently advancing.
■ If pt does not have an identifiable thyroid cartilage, feel the contours of the trachea beginning at the sternal notch & moving cephalad. The cricoid cartilage is both wider & higher than the other cartilages.

GLOSSOPHARYNGEAL NERVE BLOCK

ROBIN STACKHOUSE, MD

INDICATIONS

■ Glossopharyngeal nerve (GPN) is also known as cranial nerve IX (CN IX).
■ GPN supplies sensation to the vallecula, anterior surface of the epiglottis, pharynx, soft palate, tonsillar pillars & posterior third of the tongue. It provides motor innervation to the stylopharyngeus muscle.
■ Bilateral GPN block attenuates the gag reflex & allows for oropharyngeal examination in the awake pt.

PREPARATION

■ Lidocaine 0.5–2%, 4–10 mL in syringe (preferably a control syringe to allow for easy aspiration during injection)
■ 22–25g 9-cm spinal needle

ANATOMY

- CN IX exits the skull through the jugular foramen, anterior to the vagus & spinal accessory nerves, the internal carotid artery, & the internal jugular vein.
- Traveling anterior, it passes behind the styloid process & between the internal jugular vein & carotid artery into the mucosa posterior to the palatopharyngeal arch, where it divides into peripheral branches.

TECHNIQUE

- Pt should be sitting w/ mouth open wide, tongue protruding.
- Stand facing the pt & use a tongue depressor or laryngoscope blade to retract the tongue to the contralateral side from where the block is to be done.
- Anterior approach
  - ➤ The spinal needle is inserted to a depth of 0.25–0.5 cm into the base of the palatoglossal arch at a 45-degree angle to both the transverse & sagittal planes.
  - ➤ An aspiration test must be performed to ensure that the needle has not passed through the tissue into the pharynx or into the internal jugular vein or carotid artery.
  - ➤ After negative aspiration, inject 2–5 mL of the local anesthetic.
  - ➤ The block is then repeated on the contralateral side.
- Posterior approach
  - ➤ Put a 45-degree bend at the distal 1 cm of the spinal needle.
  - ➤ Position pt & retract tongue as w/ anterior approach.
  - ➤ Insert needle to a maximum depth of 1 cm at the base of the palatopharyngeal arch.
  - ➤ Perform an aspiration test. If negative, inject 2–5 mL of local anesthetic.
  - ➤ Repeat on contralateral side.

COMPLICATIONS

- Intravascular injection may result in headache, seizure, dysrhythmias & hematoma. All are more common w/ the posterior approach.

PEARLS

- Posterior approach more reliably blocks the pharyngeal branches of CN IX. Anterior approach may get these branches through retrograde spread.
- External approach (between the mastoid & styloid processes) is not appropriate when being used for airway mgt because the

need for bilateral block also results in bilateral block of the vagus nerve.

ILIOINGUINAL-ILIOHYPOGASTRIC BLOCK

GERALD DUBOWITZ, MB CHB

INDICATIONS
■ Used for abdominal incisions around the inguinal region, including inguinal hernia repair

PREPARATION
■ Standard monitors, resuscitation equipment
■ IV access
■ Prep w/ iodine or alcohol
■ Needle 25g, 25 mm or longer, blunted or b-bevel
■ Two 20-mL syringes
■ Local anesthetic
  ➢ Can use lidocaine 1% (w/ or w/o bicarbonate) or bupivacaine 0.25% (plain)

ANATOMY
■ Ilioinguinal & iliohypogastric nerves lie between the internal oblique muscle & the aponeurosis of the external oblique muscle.

TECHNIQUE
■ Positioning
  ➢ Pt in supine position
  ➢ Sterile technique
  ➢ Iodine or alcohol prep
  ➢ Prep the abdomen lateral to the umbilicus & down to the inguinal crease.
  ➢ Use a short-bevel or pencil-point spinal needle. Alternatively, blunt the needle on the inside of a sterile glass vial.
■ Injection
  ➢ Place needle vertical to skin, 3 cm medial & inferior to anterior superior iliac spine.
  ➢ Insert through skin; feel click through external oblique aponeurosis.
  ➢ Fan out while injecting 15 mL local anesthetic here.

- ➤ Reinsert needle at medial end of inguinal ligament (1–2 cm lateral to symphysis pubis).
- ➤ Fan out while injecting 10 mL local anesthetic.
- ➤ Insert needle subcutaneously at the midline & inject 5 mL of anesthetic from umbilicus inferiorly to symphysis pubis.

COMPLICATIONS

- ■ IV injection: Aspirate to be sure of needle placement before injection.
- ■ Intraneural injection: Check for painful paresthesia during injection.
- ■ No block/inadequate block: Supplement the block if needed. Be aware of maximum (toxic) dose of local anesthetic.

PEARLS

- ■ Supplementary blocks may be useful
  - ➤ May block the ilioinguinal nerve at the internal ring (care w/ the ilioinguinal artery, which is nearby)
  - ➤ Subcutaneous injection at the site of incision
- ■ Blunting the needle allows much better appreciation of the fascial layers but makes skin penetration more difficult. Use sharp needle to make a hole in the skin

---

INFORMED CONSENT

MIMI C. LEE, MD, PHD

INDICATIONS

- ■ Informed consent involves the discussion of the planned anesthetic, alternatives, risks & benefits in language appropriate for the pt or proxy.
- ■ Early rapport can facilitate a constructive & open communication between pt & anesthesia provider.

PREPARATION

- ■ Interview pt in a relaxed but focused manner. Ensure privacy & minimize distractions & interruptions.
- ■ Reassure pt that you or another anesthesia provider will be there for the duration of surgery.
- ■ Use layperson's language when possible. Explain any concepts not immediately grasped by pt, & continue until pt expresses understanding.

- Obtain translators to facilitate communication as appropriate. Family members may not always perform this properly & may inappropriately filter the information.

ANATOMY
N/A

TECHNIQUE
- Discuss your anesthetic plan. Include alternatives or anticipated outcomes, pending intraop events
- Where appropriate, discuss the following, including explanations of risks & benefits of each:
  - Endotracheal intubation, w/ special attention to oral vs nasal & awake vs asleep
  - Mechanical ventilation intraop as well as prolonged mechanical ventilation postop
  - Invasive hemodynamic monitoring, including arterial lines, central lines, pulmonary arterial catheters
  - Regional, general, & monitored anesthesia care
  - Blood product transfusion
  - Postoperative PACU, ICU, or stepdown care
- Discuss risks pertinent to pt's medical problems (eg, risk of bronchospasm in pt w/ asthma, dental injury in pt w/ loose teeth, risk of worsening CHF in pt w/ cardiomyopathy).
- Describe actions or therapies that may modify these risks, & discuss w/ surgeon if appropriate (eg, continuing factor therapy intraop & postop in pt w/ hemophilia, beta blocker therapy in pt w/ significant CAD).
- Document all that was discussed, including risks & benefits. Document whether anyone else was present with pt. Note whether all questions were answered, if pt expressed understanding of everything discussed, & if pt agrees to proceed as planned. Also, document if certain issues were discussed w/ surgeon.

COMPLICATIONS
- Jehovah's Witnesses must be informed of the increased risks of excessive bleeding. Some hospitals have specific release forms to document this.

PEARLS
- Documentation of the consent is crucial. If a problem occurs, this can show that pt did express understanding of risks.

- Some patients ask for risk estimates for certain complications. This will clearly vary w/ anesthetic, surgical, & pt-specific factors. Some general risks include:
  - Risk of death related to anesthesia: 1 in 185,000
  - Risk of transfusion-related hepatitis C: 1 in 500,000
  - Risk of transfusion-related hepatitis B: 1 in 65,000
  - Risk of transfusion-related HIV: 1 in 1.5 million
  - Risk of fatal hemolytic (ABO) transfusion reaction: 1 in 500,000
  - Risk of major cardiac complications (MI, cardiac arrest, complete heart block, ventricular fibrillation, pulmonary edema) in elective, noncardiac surgery
    - Factors: high-risk surgery (intraperitoneal, intrathoracic, suprainguinal vascular), history of CHF, history of ischemic heart disease, history of cerebrovascular disease, insulin treatment, renal failure (creatinine >2 mg/dL)
    - No risk factors: 0.5% risk
    - 1 risk factor: 1% risk
    - 2 risk factors: 5% risk
    - 3 risk factors: 10% risk

INTERCOSTAL BLOCK

LEI WANG, MD

INDICATIONS

- Indications: Pain relief for upper abdominal & thoracic surgery; rib fracture; minor procedures on upper abdomen (gastrostomy tube placement) or chest (chest tube placement)

PREPARATION

- Equipment: 22g 38-mm short-bevel needle; 10-cc control syringe
- Agents: Bupivacaine 0.25%, ropivacaine 0.2%, lidocaine 1%, mepivacaine 1% for sensory block; bupivacaine 0.5%, ropivacaine 0.5%, lidocaine 1.5% for motor block
- Pt preparation: IV sedation w/ benzodiazepines, opioids, or ketamine, prone position

ANATOMY

- Intercostal nerve is located inferior to intercostal artery & vein at the inferior border of each rib. Each intercostal nerve gives out five major branches, including white rami communicantes, gray rami communicantes, dorsal rami, lateral cutaneous branch, anterior cutaneous branch.

TECHNIQUE
- Mark the midline & draw paramedian lines at the posterior angle of the ribs, just lateral to the paraspinous muscles. Mark each rib on the paramedian lines.
- Make skin wheals at each injection site using 1% lidocaine w/ 30g needle.
- Begin at the lowest rib. Use index & middle fingers of the left hand to retract wheal site up & over the rib. Needle is inserted between the tips of the two fingers & advanced until it contacts the rib. Keep the needle steady. Adjust the left hand so that the hub of the needle is held between the index & middle fingers, w/ the hypothenar eminence resting on the back. Walk the needle off the inferior border of the rib. Advance the needle 2–4 mm past the edge of the rib into the intercostals groove. Inject 3–5 cc of local anesthetic. Repeat for each nerve to be blocked.

COMPLICATIONS
- Pneumothorax: Incidence <1%
- Local toxicity: Intercostal space is highly vascularized. Pt needs to be monitored for 15–20 min after performing the block.

PEARLS
- Adequate sedation is important so that pt can tolerate the procedure.
- Control syringe allows better control during aspiration & injection.
- Avoid intravascular injection of local anesthetics w/ negative aspiration.

INTERSCALENE BRACHIAL PLEXUS BLOCK

CHRISTOPHER HATCH, MD

INDICATIONS
- Interscalene blockade is the most proximal approach to the brachial plexus.
- It is the most suitable block for proximal procedures on the arm or shoulder.
- The C8 & T1 nerve roots may prove difficult to block; therefore, this block is less suitable for surgery involving the distal arm or hand,

unless a supplementary peripheral ulnar nerve block is also performed.

■ Indications for this block include
  ➤ Surgery on the shoulder or upper arm.
  ➤ Surgery on the distal arm or hand (w/ appropriate supplemental blockade as mentioned above).
  ➤ Reduction of dislocated shoulder, arm, or wrist fractures.

■ In addition to applications for surgical anesthesia, other uses for interscalene block include
  ➤ Diagnostic tool in the evaluation of shoulder & upper extremity pain.
  ➤ Palliation for acute pain emergencies such as acute herpes zoster, brachial plexus neuritis, shoulder & upper extremity trauma, cancer pain.
  ➤ Alternative to stellate ganglion blockade for treatment of reflex sympathetic dystrophy of the shoulder & upper extremity.

PREPARATION

■ Place peripheral IV & standard monitors.
■ Prepare equipment for resuscitation & airway mgt.
■ Premedicate w/ anxiolytics and/or analgesics as needed.
■ Block equipment includes
  ➤ Antiseptic skin preparation solution
  ➤ Syringes (20-cc or 30-cc sizes)
  ➤ Needles
    • 25–27g for local anesthetic skin wheal
    • 23g 32 mm for block placement
    • Alternatively a 22g 40-mm insulated nerve stimulator needle (if using a nerve stimulator)
  ➤ IV extension tubing
  ➤ Nerve stimulator (if using this technique)
  ➤ Local anesthetic of choice

ANATOMY

■ The brachial plexus is made up of nerve roots from C5 to T1.
■ As they leave their vertebral foramina, they pass laterally in a deep groove or "gutter" along the superior surface of the cervical vertebrae transverse process.
■ This groove separates the transverse process into anterior & posterior tubercles, which are the origin of the anterior & middle scalene muscles, respectively.

- As these nerve roots leave the transverse processes, they pass into the space between the anterior & middle scalene muscles—the paravertebral or interscalene groove.
- At this point they merge to form the three trunks of the brachial plexus & are enclosed in fascial sheath.

TECHNIQUE
- Pt position
  - Pt is lying supine w/ head turned slightly to the side opposite of that being blocked, w/ the shoulder slightly depressed.
- Landmarks
  - Pt is asked to temporarily lift the head to facilitate palpation of the posterior border of the sternocleidomastoid muscle (SCM).
  - The interscalene groove is palpated by rolling the fingers laterally from the SCM & over the belly of the anterior scalene muscle.
  - A mark may be placed on the pt indicating this groove.
  - The cricoid cartilage is then palpated & a line is extended laterally to intersect the previous mark indicating the interscalene groove.
  - This intersection of these lines is used as the point of needle insertion; usually around the level of the sixth cervical vertebra.
- Needle insertion and injection
  - After antiseptic skin preparation & placement of a skin wheal w/ local anesthetic at the insertion point, a 22g or 23g short-beveled needle is inserted perpendicular to the skin w/ a 45-degree caudad & slightly posterior angle.
    - This angle is important to avoid accidental IV or intrathecal injection.
  - The needle is then advanced carefully while assessing its proximity to the brachial plexus.
    - If using a regular needle, it is necessary to elicit a paresthesia to indicate appropriate placement.
    - When using a nerve stimulator w/ a special insulated needle, correct placement is indicated by twitching of the arm below the level of the shoulder at <0.5 mA current. Note that stimulation of the diaphragm indicates too anterior an approach.
  - Once a paresthesia or appropriate stimulation is attained, the needle is stabilized & aspirated to ensure the needle is not intravascular or intrathecal (aspirate for blood or CSF).
  - Once correct placement is confirmed, slowly inject 20–30 cc of local anesthetic.

- Some advocate reaspiration once or twice during injection to ensure the needle has not migrated.

COMPLICATIONS

- Inadvertent epidural or intrathecal injection
- Vertebral artery injection w/ subsequent seizure & loss of consciousness
- Phrenic nerve blockade is frequently produced; therefore, do not perform bilateral blocks
- Recurrent laryngeal, vagus & cervical sympathetic blockade
- Pneumothorax is very rare but can happen w/ very deep needle placement
- Ecchymosis & hematoma formation at the block site

PEARLS

- The key to successful & safe use of this block is clear knowledge & identification of the anatomy surrounding the brachial plexus.
- Paresthesia or nerve stimulation should occur very superficially (rarely deeper than about 1 inch in most people).
- Supplemental peripheral nerve blocks are likely to be needed for surgery involving the distal arm or hand, as the C8 and T1 nerve fibers are inadequately blocked w/ this technique.

INTRAOSSEOUS (IO) LINE PLACEMENT

PATRICK ROSS, MD

INDICATIONS

- Common indications: vascular access for pediatric resuscitation, primarily in children <6 y
- Any fluid that can be given IV can be given via IO line
- Can be achieved much more quickly than venous cutdown
- Should be used for temporary access & removed when pt is resuscitated & secure venous access obtained

PREPARATION

- Equipment
  - ➤ Jamshidi-type bone marrow aspiration needles are preferred. Spinal needles have walls that are too thin to work; hypodermic needles will become clogged

➤ Betadine or other skin prep
➤ Gloves
■ Pt preparation: supine w/ towel roll under knee

ANATOMY

■ Preferred site is proximal tibia. Use the flat anteromedial surface of tibia 1–3 cm below the tibial tuberosity.
■ Distal femur can be used, but overlying tissue makes this more difficult.

TECHNIQUE

■ Palpate the tibial tuberosity. Plan insertion 1–2 fingerwidths below this.
■ Prep the skin.
■ Align the bevels of the stylet & needle.
■ Support the knee w/ a firm surface & stabilize the leg w/ the non-dominant hand.
■ DO NOT allow any portion of your hand to be behind the insertion site.
■ Insert needle through skin & direct into bone perpendicular to flat portion of tibia. Aim slightly caudad, away from growth plate.
■ Stop advancing when you feel sudden loss of resistance.
■ Unscrew cap & remove stylet.
■ Stabilize the needle & slowly inject 10 mL of saline.
■ Check for any sign of extravasation, (Image not available on the Palm) circumference of leg, or (Image not available on the Palm) resistance.
■ Secure w/ a bulky dressing & attach infusion set.
■ If the test injection results in infiltration, remove the needle & attempt on the other leg.

COMPLICATIONS

■ Complications occur in <1% of pts.
■ Reported complications include tibial fracture, compartment syndrome, skin necrosis, osteomyelitis.

PEARLS

■ Any drug can be given in IO line but should be followed w/ 5–10 mL of flush.
■ Fluid will need to be administered under pressure to overcome resistance.
■ Insertion likely successful if

- ➤ There was sudden loss of resistance
- ➤ The needle can remain upright without support
- ➤ There is no evidence of extravasation
- Marrow cannot always be aspirated into the syringe. This does not necessarily indicate a misplaced IO line.
- Higher flow rates will be achieved w/ an IO line vs small IV catheters.

LATERAL FEMORAL CUTANEOUS NERVE BLOCK

JAMES BRANDES, MD

INDICATIONS

- The lateral femoral cutaneous nerve provides purely sensory innervation to the lateral thigh.
- It is typically used in conjunction w/ other peripheral nerve blocks of the lower extremity (eg, femoral & sciatic nerve blocks) for operations on the lower extremity; especially helpful for tourniquet pain.
- It can be the sole anesthetic for skin grafting from the lateral thigh.
- It can be used diagnostically & therapeutically for pts w/ chronic pain of the lateral thigh (meralgia paresthetica).
- Since this is purely a sensory nerve, a more dilute concentration of local anesthetic may be used since a motor block is not needed. This will allow for use of a larger volume, which will increase the success of this block.

PREPARATION

- 20-cc syringe, alcohol prep, 3- to 4-cm small-gauge needle, 0.25% bupivacaine

ANATOMY

- This nerve is a branch of the lumbar plexus (L2 & L3 nerve roots) that travels lateral to the psoas muscle & courses through the fascia inferior & medial to the anterior superior iliac spine.
- It has an anterior branch that terminates at the knee & forms a part of the patellar plexus.
- The posterior branch covers the lateral buttock & thigh.

TECHNIQUE

- Stand on the side of the pt that corresponds to the dominant hand of the operator.

- Identify the anterior superior iliac spine. The injection point is 2 cm medial & 2 cm inferior to this landmark.
- Advance the needle in a perpendicular fashion to the skin & feel for a characteristic "pop" through the fascia lata.
- Aspirate & inject 10–15 cc of local anesthetic, fanning the needle in a medial to lateral direction, injecting above & below the fascia lata.

COMPLICATIONS
- This block is very safe, but nerve injury is possible.

PEARLS
- No paresthesias necessary. Stimulator won't work because there is no motor component.
- This is one of the easiest blocks to learn & have a high degree of success with.

LMA PLACEMENT

TESSA COLLINS, MD

INDICATIONS
- LMA is indicated for use for surgical procedures in which tracheal intubation is not necessary.
- LMA is contraindicated for:
  - Pt at risk for regurgitation or aspiration.
  - Pt w/ very poor pulmonary compliance (obese, pregnant, trauma pt, etc).
  - Generally pt should be spontaneously ventilating, although PPV at low pressures is possible.
  - In general, the contraindications for an LMA are the same as for a face mask.
- Other devices in the LMA family include
  - ProSeal: Has a different cuff design than LMA classic. Has a lumen that allows placement of nasogastric tube into stomach.
  - Fastrach: Facilitates blind intubation through a rigid LMA.
  - Unique: Disposable LMA.
  - Flexible: Useful for procedures about the face.

PREPARATION
- Choose appropriate size LMA according to the following guidelines:

> LMA size, pt size, weight range, cuff volume
> LMA size 1: infant, <5 kg, up to 4 mL
> LMA size 1.5: infant, 5–10 kg, up to 7 mL
> LMA size 2: child, 10–20 kg, up to 10 mL
> LMA size 2.5: child, 20–30 kg, up to 14 mL
> LMA size 3: child to small adult, 30–50 kg, up to 20 mL
> LMA size 4: adult, 50–70 kg, up to 30 mL
> LMA size 5: adult, 70–100 kg, up to 40 mL
> LMA size 6: adult, >100 kg, up to 50 mL

ANATOMY
N/A

TECHNIQUE
- Fully deflate cuff & lubricate back side w/ water-soluble lubricant.
- Induce anesthesia.
  > Propofol is the agent of choice for IV inductions.
  > Deep vapor induction provides adequate anesthesia for children.
- Place pt's head in sniff position.
- Hold LMA like a pen, guide LMA along the hard palate w/ index finger, push cranially, advance until an increased resistance is felt.
- Inflate cuff just enough to obtain a seal; do not overinflate.
- When cuff is properly positioned, longitudinal black line faces cephalad.
- When cuff is inflated, the LMA will pop up slightly.
- Attach breathing circuit & confirm proper positioning w/ gentle hand ventilation.
- Deflate & remove LMA at end of procedure.

COMPLICATIONS
- LMA is a supraglottic airway device, so does not protect pt from aspiration or laryngospasm.

PEARLS
- LMA may be used as an emergency nonsurgical airway for pt w/ difficult tracheal intubation & difficult mask ventilation (can't intubate, can't ventilate).
- LMA can act as a guide ("channel") for fiberoptic intubation.
- Do not overinflate cuff: 60 cm H_2O is max cuff pressure.
- To minimize trauma & sore throat, do not force LMA.
- Alternate insertion technique is to place LMA into mouth backwards & simultaneously advance & rotate the LMA 180 degrees.

LOWER EXTREMITY NEURAL BLOCKADE AT THE KNEE

SUNDEEP MALIK, MD

INDICATIONS

- Somatic blockade at the level of the knee is a primary anesthetic technique as well as an adjunct to general anesthesia.
- Knee blocks (popliteal block & saphenous nerve block) are useful for lower extremity surgery involving the ankle or foot.
- A popliteal block can be performed in three ways: posterior (anatomical), lithotomy, or lateral approach.
- A saphenous block is often used to supplement the popliteal block when the medial portion of the ankle may be involved or a tourniquet is used.
- The posterior & lateral approaches to the popliteal block & a field block for the saphenous nerve at the knee are described here.

PREPARATION

- Betadine prep for skin.
- Equipment: a nerve stimulator & a 22g 2-inch (5-cm) insulated needle for posterior approach & a 22g 4-inch (10-cm) insulated needle for the lateral approach to the popliteal block. For a saphenous block, a 10-cc control syringe w/ a 25g 1.5-inch needle is chosen.
- Local anesthetic solution
  - ➤ Popliteal block: 40 mL of any of the following: 0.5% bupivacaine, 0.5% ropivacaine, 0.5% levobupivacaine, 1.5% mepivacaine, 1% lidocaine.
  - ➤ Saphenous block: 10 mL of any of the above local anesthetic solutions.
  - ➤ Use of epinephrine in local anesthetic solution is not recommended.

ANATOMY

- Sciatic nerve: divides into the tibial & common peroneal nerve at the upper end of the popliteal fossa.
  - ➤ The tibial nerve is the larger of the two branches & provides sensory innervation to the majority of the plantar surfaces of the foot as well as the posterior ankle. Its motor innervation includes the gastrocnemius muscle.

➤ The common peroneal nerve provides sensory innervation from the lateral calf to the lateral malleolus as well as the dorsal surface of the foot. Motor innervation is to peroneal muscles
■ Femoral nerve: the saphenous nerve is the terminal end of the femoral nerve.
➤ This provides sensory innervation from the medial calf to the medial malleolus.

TECHNIQUE

Popliteal Block (Lateral Technique)
■ Identify the most prominent point of the lateral femoral epicondyle. Mark a point 7 cm cephalad, in the groove between the tendons of the vastus lateralis & the biceps femoris.
■ Prep skin w/ Betadine solution & make a skin wheal w/ local anesthetic.
■ Insert a 10-cm insulated needle attached to a nerve stimulator (initial current at 2 mA) perpendicularly to the skin surface until the femur is contacted.
■ Withdraw the needle to the skin & then redirect 30 degrees posteriorly to the lateral plane.
■ If the nerve is contacted, as demonstrated either by ankle flexion or extension, the nerve stimulator is turned down to 0.4 mA & the needle position is optimized to produce ankle flexion or extension.
■ After a negative aspiration confirms that the needle is not intravascular, the local anesthetic solution is injected.
■ If the nerve is not located, the needle should be reinserted 5–10 degrees anterior to the previous approach. If this is still unsuccessful, then the needle is reinserted 5–10 degrees posterior.
■ If these redirections still do not produce nerve stimulation, confirm that the correct anatomical location was marked. If the position is correct, then a new skin puncture should be made approximately 0.5 cm posterior to the initial insertion site.

Popliteal Block (Posterior Approach)
■ The pt is positioned prone.
■ With a marker, a triangle is drawn consisting of
➤ The medial edge of the biceps femoris muscle.
➤ The lateral edge of the semitendinosus muscle.
➤ The skin crease along the popliteal fossa.

- A line is drawn in the midline from the upper tip of the triangle to the middle of the skin crease.
- A point 7 cm superior to the skin crease & 1 cm lateral to the midline of the triangle is marked.
- After Betadine prep, a skin wheal is raised w/ local anesthetic at the marked point.
- A 2-inch 22g insulated needle attached to a nerve stimulator (set at 2 mA) is then advanced at an angle of 60 degrees to the skin in an anterior superior direction until the nerve is stimulated (plantar flexion or extension will be observed).
- Optimize the needle location w/ the stimulator set at 0.4 Hz (plantar flexion or extension should be observed again).
- Aspirate the needle to rule out intravascular placement of the needle.
- Inject local anesthetic solution.
- The needle insertion sites should be moved laterally in 5-mm increments if the nerve cannot be stimulated.
- Stimulation of the biceps femoris muscle indicates an insertion that is too lateral; medial movement of the puncture site should be attempted.

Saphenous Block
- An area 5 cm below the medial surface of the tibial condyle is identified. Alternatively, choose a point just distal to the posterior edge of the medial condyle of the femur.
- After skin prep with Betadine, a 25g needle on a control syringe is inserted deeply subcutaneously & a field block is performed using 5–10 cc of local anesthetic solution.

COMPLICATIONS
- Contraindications: local disease (eg, infection), pre-existing paresis or neuritis
- Specific complications may include local infection, nerve damage, or vascular lesions (ie, hematoma). The reported incidence of these is low.

PEARLS
- As always when conducting regional anesthesia, have resuscitation equipment available, including an anticonvulsant.
- In the popliteal fossa the nerves are superficial to the popliteal vessels.

■ For the popliteal blocks a paresthesia method can be attempted, although the nerve stimulation method may be more generally reliable for producing an adequate block.

■ Knee blocks can be supplemented w/ ankle blocks.

LUMBAR PLEXUS BLOCK

JASON WIDRICH, MD

INDICATIONS

■ Lumbar plexus is responsible for sensation to anterior leg, lower abdomen, thigh & medial aspect of lower leg.

■ Can be combined w/ sciatic nerve block or popliteal block for lower extremity procedures.

■ Can be used to provide postop analgesia for procedures to thigh & knee (eg, total knee arthroplasty).

■ For pts who are anticoagulated, this block carries a lower risk of complications than neuraxial regional anesthetics.

■ Nerves affected include ilioinguinal (L1), genitofemoral (L1–2), iliohypogastric (T12-L1), obturator (L2–4), lateral femoral cutaneous (L2–3), femoral (L2–4).

PREPARATION

■ Location for injection should be prepped w/ either an alcohol or Betadine solution. Sterile technique should be used as much as possible.

ANATOMY

■ The lumbar plexus is found lateral to the lumbar spine, anterior to the transverse process & quadratus lumborum, posterior to the psoas muscle.

■ The inferior aspect of this space is bordered by the psoas, iliacus & quadratus muscles.

TECHNIQUE

■ Posterior approach
  ➤ This procedure can be performed in the prone or lateral position.
  ➤ After sterile preparation, the location for skin entry is identified & anesthetized 4–5 cm lateral & 3 cm inferior to spinous process at L4.

➤ The goal is to pick a location that will allow the needle to contact the L5 transverse process (usually at 7–9 cm depth).
➤ The needle should then be directed slightly superior & deep to the process, in the direction of the lumbar plexus.
➤ Location of the nerve can be accomplished w/ a nerve stimulator, a paresthesia, or a loss of resistance technique (between the quadratus & psoas muscles, loss of resistance feels similar to an epidural).
  • The stimulator technique tends to be the most precise when a quadriceps "twitch" is noticed at <0.5 mA.
➤ At this point, local anesthetic may be injected through the needle, or a catheter for continuous infusions (5 cm past the needle tip) may be placed. 30–40 cc of local anesthetic is administered in divided doses & the needle is removed.
■ Inguinal approach
➤ This technique is an anterior approach to the nerves at a lower point in the leg.
➤ A quadriceps twitch (<0.5 mA) or a paresthesia is elicited by location of the femoral nerve (lateral to the femoral artery, 1 cm below the inguinal ligament, depth 3–5 cm).
➤ Pressure is placed inferior to the needle as the local anesthetic (30–40 mL) is injected.
➤ The idea is to "push" the anesthetic up the femoral sheath to block the lateral femoral cutaneous, obturator & femoral nerves (hence the name 3 in 1 block).

COMPLICATIONS
■ Epidural or intrathecal injection is possible w/ posterior technique.
■ Needle directed too far superiorly may pierce peritoneum in inguinal technique.
■ Intravascular injection is possible.
➤ Consider adding epinephrine 1:200,000 to local anesthetic solution (sudden HR increase >10 w/o other stimuli is suspicious for intravascular injection).
■ Local anesthetic toxicity, seizure, arrest possible w/ high doses or intravascular injections.

PEARLS
■ When used alone this procedure is better for postop analgesia than for surgical block. Consider supplementing with GETA or general + LMA.

OBTURATOR NERVE BLOCK

PHILIP BICKLER, MD

INDICATIONS

- This block is combined w/ sciatic, femoral & lateral cutaneous nerve blocks for surgical procedures on or above the knee & is used alone for localization of hip joint pain as a diagnostic procedure.
- Relieves hip joint pain and/or spasm of the adductor group of muscles in the leg.
- It is an uncommonly used block because alone it anesthetizes a restricted region of the body.

PREPARATION

- Pt lies supine w/ legs slightly abducted.
- An X is marked on the skin 1 cm below & 1 cm lateral to the pubic spine (pubic tubercle).
- The area from the pubic symphysis halfway to the anterior superior iliac spine is prepared w/ Betadine.
- Because no paresthesia is sought or is typical, usually no sedation is necessary. If used in combination w/ femoral or sciatic nerve blocks, sedation w/ small doses of fentanyl or midazolam may be advised.

ANATOMY

- The obturator nerve arises from the 2th lumbar nerves, leaving the pelvis via the obturator foramen.
- Divides into anterior & posterior branches on entering the thigh. The anterior innervates the hip joint & adductor longus, gracilis & adductor brevis. The posterior innervates other adductors & the knee joint.

TECHNIQUE

- At the marked site, make a skin wheal & infiltrate locally with a 25-g needle & carbonated 1% lidocaine.
- Using a 22-g 1.5-inch needle, infiltrate 3–5 cc of local anesthetic down to the inferior ramus of the pubic bone (about 3–4 cm deep). Keep the needle perpendicular to the skin surface.
- Use a 3-inch 22-g spinal needle for the block. Insert the block needle perpendicular to the skin & advance it until the inferior ramus of the pubic bone is contacted.

- Withdraw the needle 1 cm & direct laterally about 15 degrees & cephalad about 5 degrees so that it slides past the inferior pubic ramus toward the obturator foramen.
- Advance the needle 2–3 cm beyond where the pubic ramus was contacted & toward the obturator foramen.
- Slowly inject 15 cc of local anesthetic (eg, 0.25% bupivacaine, 0.5% ropivacaine, or 1.5% lidocaine w/ epinephrine 1:200,000) while moving the needle forward & backward 1 cm.
- Inject an additional 10 cc of local anesthetic as the needle is slowly withdrawn.

COMPLICATIONS
- Toxic reactions to local anesthetics

PEARLS
- A common error is directing the block needle too cephalad toward the abdominal cavity, not the obturator foramen.
- A paresthesia is rarely seen during the block.
- Do not exceed the safe dose of local anesthetic.
- The block is difficult in obese pts.

PA CATHETER PLACEMENT

MANUEL PARDO, JR., MD

INDICATIONS
- Pressures measured: PA systolic, diastolic, mean, wedge pressure (PCWP)
- Other information: temp, thermodilution cardiac output (CO), mixed venous PO_2. Morphology of PA tracing may suggest specific valvular lesions (eg, mitral regurg).
- Consider PA diastolic or PCWP as volume status monitor in pt w/ LV systolic dysfunction undergoing stressful surgery w/ large volume shifts.
- CO measurement may guide mgt in pt w/ severe hypotension not responding to initial rx. Mgt would differ if low BP from low CO vs. normal or high CO w/ very low SVR.
- TEE may provide similar information on cardiac status.
- Base decision to place PA cath on pt, surgery, & practice setting.

PREPARATION
- Equipment needed: PA catheter kit, pressure transducers & cables, introducer sheath kit, cables for thermistor & injectate temp, CO module for monitor, cath shield
- Place shield over cath, flush all ports of cath, test balloon, connect to transducer & zero.

ANATOMY
- Catheter will pass from insertion site to vena cava, right atrium, right ventricle, & pulmonary artery.
- Important: Must recognize morphology of RA, RV, PA, PCWP tracings.

TECHNIQUE
- Refer to "Central Line Placement" chapter for placement of introducer sheath.
- Advance cath to 20 cm; inflate balloon w/ 1.5-cc syringe volume. Advance only w/ balloon up; withdraw only w/ balloon down.
- Watch for tracing to change. Speed of advancing: 1–2 cm/sec until PA; 0.5–1 cm/sec until PCWP.
- After wedging catheter, deflate balloon & withdraw by 2 cm before securing. Cath will soften at body temp & move distally.
- CXR can confirm placement.

COMPLICATIONS
- Arrhythmias: Most commonly PVCs when traverses RV. Consider lidocaine if ventricular arrhythmias are persistent or assoc w/ hypotension.
- Heart block: Transient RBBB most common. If pt has LBBB, obtain transcutaneous pacer prior to procedure (risk of complete heart block).
- PA rupture: Can present w/ hemoptysis & massive hemorrhage. Risk factors: Anticoagulation, PA HTN, elderly pt, balloon inflation w/ distally placed cath. Prevention: keep cath as proximal as possible in PA; consider never wedging cath.
- Catheter knotting: Presents as difficulty removing cath. CXR confirms dx. May need IR to remove.

PEARLS
- Don't blow up balloon too often: PA rupture risk.

- If cath appears to be coiling in RA or RV, consider rotating cath (alters angle of cath curve), changing pt position (Trendelenburg, tilt left or right), guidewire PA cath, echo guidance, fluoro.
- Easiest insertion route is from right IJ: most direct path to RA.
- When inserting catheter, verify that pressure you are looking at is from distal port.
- Typical distances: from right IJ to RV, 25–40 cm; PA, 35–55 cm; PCWP, 45–65 cm.

PARACERVICAL BLOCK

DWAIN SKINNER, MD

INDICATIONS
- Common Indications: analgesia for procedures involving cervix & uterus such as cervical biopsies, conization, dilatation & curettage
- Other uses: analgesia for the first stage of labor for pts in whom epidural analgesia is contraindicated

PREPARATION
- Needles (see technique below for needle options), syringes, local anesthetic, prep solution, resuscitative equipment
- Pt position: supine in lithotomy (use care in positioning pregnant pt)
- Sedation is optional. Supplemental O_2 required if using sedation.
- Standard ASA monitors
- Fetal & uterine contraction monitoring if intrauterine pregnancy

ANATOMY
- Sensory innervation to uterus, cervix & upper vagina originates from T10-L1.
- All sensory visceral nerve fibers are located in Frankenhauser's ganglion.
  - Frankenhauser's ganglion is situated in the lateral fornix of the vaginal canal.
  - Blockade of this ganglion may be used for analgesia in the first stage of labor (the second stage being transmitted via pudendal nerve S2-S4).

TECHNIQUE

- Maternal vaginal exam to determine location of fetal presenting part & relation to fornix.
  - ➤ To avoid intravascular injection, a 12- to 14-cm, 22g needle is used w/ a guide (eg, Iowa Trumpet) so that the needle point extends only 5–7 mm beyond guide.
  - ➤ Following a sterile prep, the guide, w/ the needle tip protected, is directed into the lateral fornices using the index & middle fingers between 3 & 4 o'clock & between 8 & 9 o'clock so that the tip of the guide does not injure the fetal presenting part.
  - ➤ Five to 10 mL of chosen local anesthetic is injected into each lateral fornix after negative aspiration to rule out intravascular injection.
  - ➤ An alternative technique uses a short-beveled needle w/o the guide.
  - ➤ The addition of epinephrine to chosen local anesthetic may increase duration of action but may also inhibit uterine contractions.

COMPLICATIONS

- Paracervical hematoma or abscess
- Intravascular injection
- Fetal local anesthetic injection or absorption resulting in toxicity & fetal bradycardia (incidence 5–70%), depression, acidosis, or death
- Uterine arterial vasoconstriction

PEARLS

- For the pregnant pt, paracervical block should be avoided in the presence of prematurity, uteroplacental insufficiency, or fetal distress because the incidence of abnormal FHR changes is significantly higher in the presence of pre-existing FHR abnormalities.

PENILE BLOCK

ALISON G. CAMERON, MD

INDICATIONS

- Used in pediatric & adult anesthesia, either as adjunct to general anesthesia or as sole anesthetic for procedures on the penis such as circumcision, hypospadias repair, urethral dilatation, papilloma laser fulguration
- Provides anesthesia to the distal 2/3 of the penis only

PREPARATION
- Sterile prep of area
- 5-cc syringe w/ 25g or 27g needle
- Local anesthetic of choice (bupivacaine, levobupivacaine, ropivacaine excellent choices for longer duration of block). Do not use epinephrine.

ANATOMY
- The dorsal penile nerves are bilateral & midline, lateral to the dual midline dorsal arteries of the penis, & are covered by Buck's fascia.
- The penile nerves are terminal branches of the pudendal nerve (S2–4) & emerge under the pubis near the symphysis & provide sensation to the penis.
- At the base of the penis, the nerves spread out & encircle the entire penis before terminating at the glans.

TECHNIQUE
- Several techniques exist.
  - Most common: Dual injection of local anesthetic (1–5 mL depending on age of pt) at base of penis deep to Buck's fascia after negative aspiration for blood
  - Alternate technique: Subcutaneous ring block by circumferential injection at base of penis
  - Third technique: Palpate lower border of symphysis, insert needle until it contacts symphysis, withdraw & reinsert just below symphysis until "pop" felt; if negative aspiration for blood, inject local anesthetic.

COMPLICATIONS
- Hematoma
- Intravascular injection
- Accidental addition of epinephrine to solution, resulting in ischemia of the penis

PEARLS
- Avoid epinephrine (causes vasoconstriction & possible necrosis in isolated circulations).
- Holding pressure after injection helps avoid hematoma formation.
- Intermittent injection helps minimize risk of intravascular injection.

PERIPHERALLY INSERTED CENTRAL VENOUS CATHETER (PICC) LINE

WILLIAM RHOADS, MD

INDICATIONS
- Common indications
  - Long-term (1 wk to 3 mo) IV access
  - Central venous access for parenteral nutrition

PREPARATION
- Equipment: PICC line kit. Two major types:
  - Catheter insertion inside needle
    - Kit includes breakaway introducer needle (usually 16g), curved forceps, measuring tape, PICC catheter.
  - Seldinger technique
    - Kit includes IV for initial placement into vein, PICC catheter w/ guidewire, peel-away introducer sheath, guidewire for sheath, measuring tape.
- Pt preparation: supine, arm extended at a 90-degree angle. As w/ other central lines, need sterile gloves, Betadine prep, transparent dressing, lidocaine for local anesthesia.

ANATOMY
- Identify palpable cephalic or basilic vein in the antecubital fossa.

TECHNIQUE
- Apply tourniquet to upper arm.
- Use sterile prep, drape, & aseptic technique throughout.
- Use local anesthesia for awake pts.
- Flush catheter w/ saline.
- Measure distance from insertion site to desired catheter tip location in subclavian vein or SVC.
- Cut catheter to desired length.
- Next steps depend on PICC kit used.
  - Catheter-inside-needle kit.
    - Insert introducer needle into vein until brisk blood return occurs.
    - Using curved forceps, advance catheter through introducer needle to desired length.

- Holding the catheter in place, fully withdraw introducer needle, press wings of needle together until the needle snaps & peel the needle away from the catheter.
  - ➤ Seldinger-based kit
    - Insert IV into peripheral vein. Depending on guidewire size, can use IV as small as 20g.
    - Place guidewire into IV into vein, then remove IV.
    - Nick skin w/ scalpel, place peel-away introducer sheath over guidewire, then remove guidewire.
    - Insert PICC catheter w/ guidewire into introducer sheath.
    - When PICC catheter fully inserted, peel away introducer sheath.
    - Remove guidewire from PICC catheter.
- ■ After either method
  - ➤ Flush catheter w/ saline.
  - ➤ Secure catheter to skin w/ Steri-Strips, suture, or transparent dressing.
  - ➤ Obtain CXR to confirm line placement.

COMPLICATIONS
- ■ Inadvertent arterial puncture
- ■ Phlebitis
- ■ Clotting or breakage of catheter
- ■ Malposition of line into noncentral vein
- ■ For instance, inadvertent passage of catheter cephalad through the internal jugular vein

PEARLS
- ■ Seldinger technique offers more flexibility in PICC line insertion technique.
- ■ If the peripheral vein is small, consider using a Seldinger-based PICC kit.
- ■ Can use IV as small as 20g, vs 16g needle required for catheter-inside-needle kit
- ■ If difficult to advance catheter, consider flushing catheter while advancing, or repositioning pt's arm.
- ■ Never pull the catheter back w/ the introducer needle in place, as this may shear off the catheter.
- ■ In some institutions, the catheter tip is bevel-cut at 45 degrees before placement to mark the end of the catheter.
- ■ Fluoroscopy may be useful to identify location of line during insertion, or to reposition line after placement.

PUDENDAL BLOCK

ALISON G. CAMERON, MD

INDICATIONS
- The pudendal nerve supplies the pelvic floor & perineum w/ sensation. This block will also provide motor blockade to perineal muscles & external anal sphincter.
- Block of this nerve can provide pain relief for many OB/GYN procedures & act as an adjunct to IV sedation or general anesthesia.
- Indicated procedures include
  - Second stage of labor pain
  - Assistance w/ forceps/vacuum deliveries
  - Malignancies
- Block will not provide sufficient anesthesia for procedures such as manual removal of retained placenta or repair of lacerated upper vagina/uterus.

PREPARATION
- 22g 8.75-cm needle
- Iowa Trumpet (needle guide)
- 5–20 mL local anesthetic (lidocaine, bupivacaine, levobupivacaine, ropivacaine, 2-chlorprocaine)
- Sterile prep to area to be injected (perineal vs vaginal)

ANATOMY
- Pudendal nerve is formed from S2–4 nerve roots, passes through the greater sciatic foramen, goes around the ischial spine & then through the pudendal canal in the lesser sciatic foramen.
- Once the nerve passes through the pudendal canal, it branches to form 3 nerves: the inferior rectal nerve, the perineal nerve & the dorsal nerve of the clitoris/penis.
- Pudendal nerve blockade will anesthetize the posterior two thirds of the scrotum/labia & part of the buttocks.

TECHNIQUE
- Two different approaches: transperineal & transvaginal.
- Transperineal.
  - Place pt in lithotomy position.
  - Inject skin wheal of local anesthetic 2.5 cm posterior & medial to ischial tuberosity, continuing to move needle deeper, infiltrating local anesthetic.

> Change to long 8.75-cm needle & use index finger of free hand to locate the ischial spine & sacrospinal ligament.
> Aim needle posterior to these two structures, w/ assistance from the rectal finger. After aspirating to ensure no intravascular injection, inject 5–20 mL local anesthetic.

■ Transvaginal approach (more common)
> Place pt in lithotomy position.
> Use Iowa Trumpet to protect needle tip as it is advanced into vagina, guided by free finger within vagina to ischial spine.
> Needle tip will penetrate sacrospinal ligament w/ resistance.
> After negative aspiration for intravascular injection, local anesthetic is injected.

■ Block will need to be repeated on opposite side.

COMPLICATIONS
■ Local anesthetic toxicity
■ Unintended nerve blockade
■ Intravascular injection

PEARLS
■ Usually performed by obstetrician or gynecologist

RETROBULBAR BLOCK

GERALD DUBOWITZ, MB CHB

INDICATIONS
■ Block used for eye surgery.
■ Provides motor block of extraocular muscles as well as sensory anesthesia.
■ Facial nerve innervates orbicularis oculi muscle.
■ Commonly performed by ophthalmologists for cataract, cornea & anterior chamber procedures.
> For cataract surgery, some surgeons may prefer topical anesthesia.

PREPARATION
■ Resuscitation equipment, IV access
■ Local anesthetic eye drops
■ Needle: 25g, 25 mm long

- 10-mL syringe: 5 mL 2% lidocaine w/ 5 mL 0.75% bupivacaine & 150 units hyaluronidase for retrobulbar injection
- Contraindications (some relative)
  - Previous retinal detachment surgery in same eye
  - Large eye (>29 mm)
    - Theoretically, if there is no gap between the globe & the orbit (bone), the needle can puncture the globe more easily. Also, there may be decreased space for large-volume injection or hemorrhage
  - Other pathology in the orbit (affecting anatomy/landmarks)
  - Penetrating eye injury
  - Warfarin therapy

ANATOMY
- Sensation to eye occurs via ophthalmic nerve (long & short ciliary nerves)
- Innervation of orbicularis oculi muscle via facial nerve
- Ophthalmic artery lies just lateral to optic nerve

TECHNIQUE
- Apply local anesthetic drops to eye.
- Eye in neutral position.
- May ask pt to look slightly cephalad.
- Retrobulbar technique.
  - Insert needle at inferolateral border of orbit, aimed at apex of orbit.
  - Direct the needle tangential to the equator of the globe, w/ the bevel inward toward the globe, then direct to the superior orbital fissure.
  - May feel needle "pop" into the extraocular muscle cone.
  - Aspirate before injection.
  - Inject approx 2–4 mL local anesthetic into the muscle core.
  - After injection, apply pressure to the eye either w/ digit or weighted dressing.
- Peribulbar technique.
  - Insert needle in similar fashion to retrobulbar technique.
  - Direct needle lateral to the lateral rectus muscle so that needle does not enter extraocular muscle cone.
  - Aspirate before injection of 5–10 mL local anesthetic.
- Facial nerve block.

➤ May be necessary to block orbicularis oculi to minimize pt squinting during surgery.
➤ Can be performed at inferolateral orbital rim (Van Lint method).
➤ Can be performed at mastoid process (Nadbath method).

COMPLICATIONS
■ Retrobulbar hemorrhage
   ➤ Occurs in 1–3% of cases
   ➤ Can be venous or arterial in origin
   ➤ Minimize by avoiding injection in superomedial quadrant
■ Penetration of the eye
   ➤ Effects
     • Retinal detachment
     • Intraocular toxicity of local anesthetic
   ➤ Symptoms
     • Sudden loss of vision
     • Acute pain
     • Loss of ocular tone
     • Movement of eye w/ needle
■ Penetration of optic sheath & injection of local anesthetic
   ➤ Can lead to cardiorespiratory arrest
   ➤ May occur secondary to CNS spread via optic nerve or from intravascular injection
■ Extraocular muscle damage
■ Oculocardiac reflex (bradycardia & other arrhythmias)
■ Chemosis
■ Postop diplopia (self-limiting within 24 h)
■ Inadequate or incomplete block

PEARLS
■ Keep needle at a tangent to the eye to avoid ocular trauma.
■ Use Luer-Lok syringes.
■ Keep bevel of needle toward the eye; always know where it is.
■ Avoid long needles.
■ Avoid injection into the inferior & lateral rectus muscles (muscle damage).
■ Avoid injection into the superomedial quadrant (hemorrhage).
■ Watch closely for signs of hemorrhage, as this can lead to cancellation of surgery.
   ➤ Pressure on the eye after injection may minimize bleeding risk.

RETROGRADE TRACHEAL INTUBATION

HELGE EILERS, MD

INDICATIONS

- Indication: Emergency airway procedure can be used if endotracheal intubation w/ direct laryngoscopy has failed.
- Most commonly used in anesthetized pt; can also be done in conscious pt w/ anticipated difficult airway using sedation & topical anesthesia.

PREPARATION

- Pt position: Supine, neck slightly extended to facilitate palpation of landmarks
- Equipment: J-wire & needle large enough to pass the wire
- 20g IV catheter w/ 0.021-inch J-wire will work well
- Syringe
- Kits are commercially available
- Alternatively, an epidural catheter w/ matching needle can be used
- Optional: Endotracheal tube (ETT) changer
- ETT
- Local anesthetic (when performed in conscious pt)
- It is helpful to have a second person help to control & keep tension on the wire

ANATOMY

- Cricothyroid membrane: Soft membranous connection between thyroid & cricoid cartilages, only few centimeters below vocal cords

TECHNIQUE

- Position pt.
- Palpate cricothyroid membrane.
- In conscious pt use local anesthetic to infiltrate skin above cricothyroid membrane & topical anesthetic to anesthetize the pharyngeal mucosa.
- With syringe attached to needle, advance needle through cricothyroid membrane, bevel facing cephalad.
- Aspirate while you advance the needle.
- Once needle enters trachea, air will be freely aspirated.

- In conscious pt inject 1–2 mL of 4% lidocaine into the trachea to anesthetize the subglottic part of the airway. The pt will cough; be careful not to dislodge the needle.
- Pass the wire through the needle until it appears in the pharynx.
- Pull wire out of mouth.
- Securing both ends of the wire, remove the needle.
- Hold wire under mild tension while advancing ETT over wire into trachea.
- Tip of ETT will be only a short distance past the vocal cords when reaching entry point of wire into trachea.
- It can be difficult to determine if ETT is in the trachea or caught on the anterior commissure.
- Carefully remove wire & advance ETT further into trachea.

COMPLICATIONS
- Bleeding: Accidental puncture of blood vessels or thyroid gland
- Injury of thyroid gland: Insertion of needle too far caudad or into accessory lobe of thyroid gland
- Infection
- Inability to advance ETT
- Loss of control over distal end of wire

PEARLS
- If you have difficulty palpating the cricothyroid membrane, start at the most prominent part of the thyroid cartilage & slowly move caudad until you feel a softer membranous structure.
- If there is too much tension on the skin from excessive neck extension, it might be difficult to feel the membrane.
- If nasal intubation is desired, you can tie the end of the wire to a catheter passed through the nose into the mouth & then pull catheter & wire out the nose so you can pass an ETT over the wire through the nares.
- To increase control over the distal end of the wire, you can hold it with a clamp.
- If you have difficulty passing the ETT, it might be caught at the anterior commissure. Try to rotate the ETT while you carefully advance it.
- You can pass an ETT changer or the suction channel of a fiberoptic bronchoscope over the wire, carefully remove the wire & advance the tube changer or bronchoscope further into trachea, then pass

ETT over scope or tube changer. The advantage is that the tip of your introducer will be more distal than the entry point of the wire.

■ The use of a larger-diameter catheter, tube changer, or fiberoptic scope will make it easier to pass an ETT (the smaller the difference between outside diameter of the guiding catheter/wire & the inside diameter of the ETT, the easier it will be to pass the ETT into the trachea).

SCIATIC NERVE BLOCK

JAMES HSU, MD

INDICATIONS

■ Sciatic nerve supplies cutaneous innervation to the posterior thigh & to all of the leg & foot, except for a thin medial strip that is supplied by the saphenous nerve.

■ Even though it is the largest nerve in the body, very few surgical procedures can be performed with a sciatic block alone.
  ➤ To obtain surgical anesthesia below the knee, the sciatic block is combined w/ a femoral or saphenous nerve block.
    • However, this does not provide analgesia for a thigh tourniquet.
  ➤ For surgical anesthesia above the knee, the sciatic block can be combined w/ a femoral, lateral cutaneous femoral, and/or obturator nerve block.

■ The anterior sciatic block is useful for pts who cannot be positioned for the classic block because of pain or lack of cooperation.

■ Patient selection
  ➤ Informed consent & pt cooperation are required.
  ➤ The block is indicated for surgical procedures of the lower leg, ankle & foot when combined w/ the other blocks, as described above.
  ➤ These blocks are especially useful for pts who can't tolerate a sympathectomy associated w/ a neuraxial block (eg, pt w/ severe aortic stenosis).

PREPARATION

■ 20–25 cc of local anesthetic solution
  ➤ 22g 10- to 12-cm needle
  ➤ Nerve stimulator (optional)
  ➤ Sterile prep solution

■ Most importantly, need adequate TIME for the block to take effect

ANATOMY

- Classical approach: posterior superior iliac spine, sacral hiatus, greater trochanter
- Anterior approach: anterior superior iliac spine, pubic tubercle, greater trochanter
- The sciatic nerve is formed from the fusion of two nerve trunks.
  - ➤ One is the tibial nerve, "medial" sciatic nerve, which comprises the anterior branches of the L4-S3 ventral rami.
  - ➤ The other trunk is the peroneal nerve, which is made up of the posterior branches of the L4-S3 ventral rami.
  - ➤ The roots merge on the anterior surface of the piriformis muscle.
- The posterior cutaneous nerve of the thigh joins the sciatic nerve as it exits from the pelvis.
- At the inferior border of the piriformis, the sciatic nerve is equidistant between the ischial tuberosity & the greater trochanter.
- The nerve travels through the thigh along the posterior medial aspect of the femur & divides into the common peroneal & tibial nerves at the superior border of the popliteal fossa.

TECHNIQUE

- Classical approach
  - ➤ Pt is placed laterally w/ the side to be blocked in the nondependent position.
  - ➤ The nondependent leg is flexed w/ the heel braced against the knee of the dependent leg.
  - ➤ A line (line 1) is drawn from the posterior superior iliac spine to the greater trochanter.
  - ➤ Another line is then drawn from the sacral hiatus to the greater trochanter (line 2).
  - ➤ A perpendicular line is then drawn bisecting the first line in a caudomedial direction for 5 cm.
  - ➤ The needle insertion point is the intersection between the perpendicular line and line 2.
  - ➤ The needle is then inserted (usually pointing slightly caudally) until paresthesia, nerve stimulation, or bone is contacted.
  - ➤ If bone is contacted, then the needle needs to be directed in a systematic direction either medially or laterally until paresthesia or nerve stimulation, at which point the local anesthetic is injected.
- Anterior approach

➤ Pt lies in a supine position w/ the leg to be blocked in neutral position, not tilting laterally or medially.

➤ A line drawn between the anterior superior iliac spine & the pubic tubercle is trisected.

➤ A second line is drawn parallel to this first line from the greater trochanter.

➤ A third line is drawn perpendicularly from the medial-middle junction of the trisected first line in a caudolateral direction.

➤ The intersection of the second and third line is the needle insertion site, where contact with the medial aspect of the femur should occur.

➤ Once contact is made, the needle is directed slightly medially to slide off the femur.

➤ Nerve contact should occur about 5 cm past the contact point w/ the femur & the local anesthetic is then injected.

➤ Heavy sedation is sometimes required as this block is often very painful for the pt.

COMPLICATIONS
■ May be difficult to perform, especially the anterior approach
■ Hematomas
■ Infections
■ Nerve damage (persistent paresthesias are generally self-limited)

PEARLS
■ Positioning is the most important key to the success of the block.
■ Moderate to heavy sedation may be required for the anterior technique, as it can be quite painful.
■ With the anterior technique, it is extremely important to keep the leg in a neutral position & not to let it deviate medially or laterally.
■ Adequate time must be allowed for the block to take effect.

SPHENOPALATINE GANGLION BLOCK

CHRISTOPHER HATCH, MD

INDICATIONS
■ This block is used mostly for the treatment of facial pain syndromes, including
  ➤ Acute migraine headache
  ➤ Acute cluster headache
  ➤ Status migrainosus
  ➤ Chronic cluster headache

> Various facial neuralgia syndromes (eg, Sluder's, Vail's, Gardner's syndromes)

■ There are two approaches to this block: transnasal & via the greater palatine foramen

PREPARATION

■ Premed w/ anxiolytics and/or analgesics may be given as indicated.
■ The block should be performed in the OR or other procedure area after obtaining venous access & application of standard monitors.
■ Appropriate agents & equipment should be readily available for resuscitation & airway mgt should the need arise.
■ Block equipment includes
> For transnasal approach
   • 2% viscous lidocaine or 10% cocaine solution drawn up in a sterile 5-cc syringe
   • Cotton-tipped applicators (3.5 inch)
   • Local anesthetic
> For greater palatine foramen approach
   • Dental needle w/ 120-degree angle
   • Local anesthetic

ANATOMY

■ The sphenopalatine ganglion (also known as the pterygopalatine, nasal, or Meckel's ganglion) is located in the pterygopalatine fossa just posterior to the middle nasal turbinate.
■ A very thin layer (1–2 mm) of mucous membrane & connective tissue encloses it.
■ From this ganglion, branches are sent to multiple ganglia (including the gasserian & superior cervical), as well as to trigeminal & facial nerves & the carotid plexus.

TECHNIQUE

■ Transnasal approach
> Pt is placed in a supine position & the anatomy of the nares is inspected.
> The neck is slightly extended to draw the nose upward & about 0.5 cc of local anesthetic (2% viscous lidocaine or 10% cocaine, as stated above) is instilled into each naris for topicalization.
> Two of the 3.5-inch cotton-tipped applicators are soaked in a local anesthetic of choice & then one is placed into each naris.
> Each applicator is advanced along the superior aspect of the middle turbinate until the tip comes into contact w/ the nasal mucosa overlying the sphenopalatine ganglion.

➤ 1 cc of local anesthetic is then instilled over the applicators, which are allowed to remain in place for about 20 min & are then removed.

■ Greater palatine foramen approach
  ➤ Pt is placed in a supine position w/ slight cervical spine extension.
  ➤ The greater palatine foramen is located on the posterior portion of the hard palate, just medial to the gumline near the third molar.
  ➤ A dental needle w/ a 120-degree angle is inserted about 2–3 cm into the foramen at a superior & slightly posterior angle.
  ➤ If the needle is advanced too deeply, a maxillary nerve paresthesia may be elicited.
  ➤ The needle is aspirated gently & 2 cc of local anesthetic is injected slowly.

COMPLICATIONS

■ The region of this block is very vascular; therefore, significant systemic absorption of local anesthetic is possible, resulting in a risk of local anesthetic toxicity.

■ With the transnasal approach, epistaxis is the most common complication.

■ Significant orthostatic hypotension has been documented after this block; therefore, this should be monitored closely & pt should initially be allowed to ambulate only w/ assistance.

PEARLS

■ The transnasal approach is clearly a much simpler technique & may be done at the bedside, in the ER, as well as in the pain clinic

■ If anatomic abnormalities (eg, nasal polyps, tumors, previous trauma) preclude the use of the transnasal approach, then the greater palatine foramen provides an alternative.

■ Data suggest that up to 80% of cluster headaches can be aborted w/ this technique.

STELLATE GANGLION BLOCK

MICHELLE PARAISO, MD

INDICATIONS

■ Indicated for upper extremity autonomic dysfunction such as circulatory insufficiency or hyperhidrosis; pain from reflex sympathetic dystrophy, herpes zoster, neoplasm, or phantom limb pain

PREPARATION
- Sterile skin prep
- Needle: 1.5–3 inch, 22–25g
- Syringe w/ local anesthetic

ANATOMY
- In the cervical region, the sympathetic chain is located anterolateral to the vertebral bodies in a fascial plane bounded anteriorly by the carotid sheath & posteriorly by the prevertebral muscles.
- The nerve fibers in the sympathetic chain fuse to form ganglia.
- The first thoracic & inferior cervical ganglia often fuse to form the stellate ganglion.
- These fibers supply the head, neck & upper extremity.
- The stellate ganglion lies in proximity to the transverse process of C6 (Chassaignac's tubercle), which is located at the level of the cricoid cartilage.
- The ganglion can also be blocked at C7, but w/ greater risk of puncturing the vertebral artery or pleura.

TECHNIQUE
- Although other approaches have been described, the paratracheal approach described here is most frequently used.
- Pt should be supine w/ mild neck extension.
- The sternocleidomastoid muscle & the contents of the carotid sheath are moved laterally.
- After local skin infiltration with local anesthetic, a 1.5–3-inch, 22–25g bevel needle is inserted just lateral to the trachea at the level of C6.
- Once contact is made with the transverse process of C6, located approximately 1–2 cm deep in the average pt, withdraw the needle 2 mm & inject 10–15 cc of local anesthetic in increments between aspiration.
- A 0.5-cc test dose is recommended to rule out vertebral artery injection.

COMPLICATIONS
- More common complications
  - Horner's syndrome (ptosis, miosis, anhydrosis)
  - Nasal congestion
  - Vasodilation & increased skin temp
  - Hematoma
  - Recurrent laryngeal nerve block (hoarseness, dysphagia)

- Uncommon complications
  - Phrenic n. block
  - Cardioaccelerator n. block
  - Brachial plexus block
  - Epidural or subarachnoid block
  - Pneumothorax
  - Punctured esophagus
  - Punctured intervertebral disc
  - Osteitis of transverse process or vertebral body
- Most severe complications
  - Vertebral artery injection (loss of consciousness, seizure)
  - Intradural injection resulting in total spinal
  - Osteomyelitis of vertebral body or discitis

PEARLS
- Increased skin temp by at least 2 degrees C is the most conclusive sign of blocking the sympathetic nervous system at this level.

SUBARACHNOID BLOCK (SPINAL ANESTHESIA)

KENNETH DRASNER, MD

INDICATIONS
- Viewed by many as preferred technique for procedures involving lower abdomen, perineum, or lower extremities
- Particularly well suited for unstable pts having perineal or lower extremity procedures where limited block may be adequate
- Can use alone in select cases involving upper abdomen, but potential for discomfort & respiratory effects are significant drawbacks
- Some advocate use in combination w/ general anesthesia to decrease anesthetic requirement, blunt stress response, & optimize postoperative analgesia.
- Contraindications: Bleeding diathesis, significant anticoagulation, elevated intracranial pressure, infection at site of puncture, pt refusal
- Relative contraindications: Pre-existing neurologic disease, abnormal anatomy. May be wise to forego in cases where there might be a perceived relationship between procedure & exacerbation of an underlying condition (eg, back pain) even though no true medical contraindication exists.

PREPARATION

- Spinal kit. May choose different needle or local anesthetic than supplied. Verify that kit & anesthetic have not expired.
- Standard equipment, monitoring, & drugs, including those required for induction of general anesthesia
- Obtain baseline hemodynamic values & correct hypovolemia prior to block—sympathectomy from spinal can cause hypotension.

ANATOMY

- Spinal cord generally terminates at T12-L1 or L1–2 because of differential growth of spinal cord & vertebral column. Below this level, nerve roots run parallel to the longitudinal axis, resembling a horse's tail, or cauda equina.
- Spinal cord is surrounded by CSF & meninges.
- Dura (outermost meningeal layer) originates at the foramen magnum & terminates between S1 & S4.
- Arachnoid lies on inner surface of dura & forms the major barrier to drug diffusion from the epidural space.
- Pia (innermost meningeal layer) is a highly vascular structure closely applied to the cord.

TECHNIQUE

General

- Single-injection technique is most common.
- Repetitive injection through a catheter (continuous spinal anesthesia [CSA]) permits titration of block & greater control of duration.
- Combined spinal & epidural (CSE) is accomplished by passing spinal needle though epidural needle prior to epidural catheter placement.

Position

- Can use lateral decubitus, sitting, or prone.
- Lateral decubitus: Greatest pt comfort & is preferable for heavily sedated pt.
- Sitting: Encourages flexion & facilitates recognition of the midline, particularly important in the obese pt. Sitting also raises CSF pressure & distends the dural sac. This facilitates placement & aids in recognition of the subarachnoid space.
- Prone: Technically more demanding due to limited flexion, low CSF pressure, contracted dural sac. Rarely used except for perineal procedures performed in jack-knife position.

Interspace

- To avoid spinal cord trauma, do NOT perform lumbar puncture above L2 in adult (or L4 in infants). In 2% of pts, spinal cord terminates below L2. Unfortunately, there is a higher failure rate associated w/ more caudal injections. At L4–5 interspace, incidence of failed spinal block is >7%.
- For CSA w/ catheter: Choose a low interspace & do not advance catheter >4 cm beyond needle tip.

Technique

- Midline approach
  - ➤ Technically easier & produces less discomfort as the needle passes through less sensitive structures
  - ➤ Needle is inserted just rostral to the lower spinous process & advanced w/ a slight cephalad orientation through the supraspinous ligament, interspinous ligament, ligamentum flavum, & the epidural space to pierce the dura/arachnoid.
- Paramedian approach
  - ➤ Useful in challenging pts where there is narrowing of the interspinous space, calcification of the ligaments, or inability to flex
  - ➤ Needle is generally inserted 1–2 cm off the midline & slightly less cephalad
  - ➤ L5-S1 interspace cannot be generally accessed from the midline because of the orientation of the L5 spinous process. Use paramedian (Taylor) approach.
- Small-gauge needles (<=22g) are most often used w/ an introducer to prevent needle deflection.
- Although needles generally penetrate the dura & arachnoid, injection of drug into the subdural space can occur & result in failure of the technique (typically associated w/ an unusual or patchy sensory block). Failure may also be more likely w/ pencil-point needles due to the proximal extension of the side hole. To minimize this possibility, advance needle slightly after obtaining CSF.

COMPLICATIONS

General

- Immediate complications include hypotension, bradycardia, total spinal block. Nausea or vomiting, particularly if there is significant hypotension.
- Delayed complications include backache, postdural puncture headache. Rare but severe complications include meningitis,

epidural abscess, epidural hematoma w/ paralysis, neurologic injury, local anesthetic neurotoxicity. (See also chapter "Delayed Complications of Neuraxial Block.")

Hypotension
- Anticipate effects of sympathectomy in pts w/ significant aortic or mitral valve stenosis. Prepare medication to increase afterload (eg, phenylephrine).
  - ➤ Cardiac arrest after spinal. ASA closed-claims database documents cases of healthy patients developing profound bradycardia leading to cardiac arrest under spinal anesthesia for relatively minor surgical procedures. Usually presents 20 min after block & can be fatal despite proper resuscitation. Maintain heart rate & treat severe bradycardia or asystole immediately & aggressively w/ full resuscitation dose of epinephrine.

Total Spinal
- Lower risk w/ isobaric rather than hyperbaric solutions. Very high incidence w/ spinal performed after failed epidural.
- Signs/symptoms: High sensory level, altered mental status, respiratory arrest, hypotension, cardiovascular collapse.
- Treatment: Prompt airway management including intubation & hemodynamic support w/ vasopressors (eg, ephedrine, phenylephrine, epinephrine).

Local Anesthetic Neurotoxicity
- Recent occurrence of permanent neurologic injuries (eg, cauda equina syndrome) after spinal anesthesia has refocused attention on local anesthetic neurotoxicity & led to modifications in practice.
- Repeated spinal injection after failed spinal poses significant risk of toxicity as anesthetic may distribute in the same restricted fashion, resulting in neurotoxic concentrations. Safest approach is to assume any local anesthetic administered was actually injected into the subarachnoid space. Total local anesthetic from the two injections should not exceed the maximum reasonable dose for single-injection spinal anesthesia.
- Lidocaine: Neurotoxic injury may occur at the high end of the dose range previously recommended for lidocaine (100 mg). This risk might be increased by concurrent use of epinephrine. Consider limiting dose to 60 mg & avoiding vasoconstrictors.
- Bupivacaine & tetracaine doses customarily range from 5 to 15 mg but should never exceed 20 mg.

- To minimize risk of local anesthetic neurotoxicity w/ CSA:
  - ➤ Administer local anesthetic at the lowest effective concentration. For lidocaine, do not exceed 2% solution. If anticipate prolonged procedure, bupivacaine likely poses less risk.
  - ➤ Administer a test dose, followed by assessment of the extent of blockade.
  - ➤ Use maneuvers to increase the spread of local anesthetic should maldistribution occur (eg, alter the lumbosacral curvature, use a local anesthetic w/ a different baricity).
  - ➤ Limit the amount of local anesthetic used to establish a block to the maximum reasonable dose for single-injection spinal anesthesia.
  - ➤ Abandon the technique if well-distributed sensory anesthesia is not achieved before the dose limit is reached.

Transient Neurologic Symptoms
- Generally defined as pain/dysesthesia in the buttocks/lower extremities.
- Previously termed "transient radicular irritation" but abandoned because implies specific etiology that has not been established.
- Frequently follows lidocaine spinal anesthesia.
- Onset after resolution of spinal block & generally resolves by day 3.
- Higher incidence in outpts & increased risk for pts in lithotomy or those undergoing knee arthroscopy.
- Concentration of glucose, osmolarity of the anesthetic solution, & the injected concentration of lidocaine do not affect incidence.
- Risk may be reduced if lidocaine dose is limited to 25 mg & combined w/ fentanyl.
- Bupivacaine has a dramatically lower incidence of transient neurologic symptoms than lidocaine & should be used in cases where longer duration is acceptable.
- Prilocaine may have lower risk than lidocaine but adequate data are lacking.

PEARLS
- Stream trajectory
  - ➤ Needles having side ports should be positioned to take advantage of the directional flow of the local anesthetic stream. Bevel direction of a cutting needle has no effect on the stream.
- Needle bevel

➤ The path of a cutting needle tends to veer away from the bevel, particularly with smaller needles used w/o an introducer. This can be used to advantage.

➤ If a cutting needle (eg, Quincke) is used, orient the bevel parallel to the longitudinal axis to promote spreading of the dural fibers & reduce the risk of postdural puncture headache.

SUPERIOR LARYNGEAL NERVE BLOCK

ANNEMARIE THOMPSON, MD

INDICATIONS

■ Common indications: To provide adequate analgesia & blunt airway reflexes during awake airway mgt involving intubation or endoscopic procedures

■ The superior laryngeal nerve (SLN) can also be permanently blocked for pain relief due to diseases of the larynx.

■ SLN is a branch of the vagus nerve that divides just above the hyoid cartilage into an external & internal branch.

➤ External branch supplies motor innervation to the cricothyroid muscle.

➤ Internal branch supplies sensory innervation to inferior aspect of epiglottis & laryngeal inlet as far down as the vocal cords.

PREPARATION

■ Equipment
➤ Gloves
➤ Alcohol or Betadine
➤ 1% lidocaine (3 cc for each side)
➤ 2.5-cm 25g needle on a syringe

■ Pt preparation: Head extended, clinician standing on side to be blocked

ANATOMY

■ SLN is blocked inferiorly to the greater cornu (the most lateral prominences) of the hyoid bone.

TECHNIQUE

■ Consider premed to alleviate anxiety.

■ Apply pressure to contralateral greater cornu of the hyoid bone to aid in identification of landmarks on the side to be blocked.

- Insert 25g needle onto the greater cornu of the hyoid bone near the tip, then "walk off" the inferior border of the greater cornu.
- Penetrate the thyrohyoid membrane at the "walk off" point (about 1 cm deep); aspirate to ascertain that the pharynx has not been entered (signaled by air in the syringe) or that a vascular structure has not been entered (signaled by blood in the syringe).
- Inject 3 cc local anesthetic into space between thyrohyoid membrane & pharyngeal mucosa.
- Repeat SLN block on contralateral side.

COMPLICATIONS
- Intravascular injection
- Hematoma
- Infection
- Nerve damage

PEARLS
- Relatively easy block to perform

SUPRACLAVICULAR BLOCK

KURT DITTMAR, MD

INDICATIONS
- Provides anesthesia at the level of the brachial plexus trunks
- Effective for hand, forearm & elbow surgery
- Usually rapid-onset, dense block excellent for distal upper extremity surgery

PREPARATION
- Supine, head turned to contralateral side
- Sterile prep & drape
- 22g 1.5-inch short-bevel needle
- 20–30 cc local anesthetic
- Nerve stimulator (optional)

ANATOMY
- The brachial plexus trunks are located cephaloposterior to the subclavian artery in the interscalene groove.
- The neurovascular bundle passes between the first rib & midpoint of the clavicle.

TECHNIQUE
- Plumb-bob approach.
  - Needle is advanced perpendicular to the ground at the clavicular insertion of the lateral border of the SCM.
  - The plexus is identified w/ either a nerve stimulator or by paresthesia.
  - Slight caudad or cephalad correction along the first rib in the plane parallel to the head & neck can aid in locating the plexus.
- Traditional approach.
  - Advance the needle in a caudal direction after entering the interscalene groove one fingerbreadth above the clavicle.
  - The plexus is identified w/ either a nerve stimulator or by paresthesia.
  - If the first rib is encountered, anterior & posterior movements along the rib can assist in localization of the plexus.
- For both approaches, inject the appropriate volume of local anesthetic after negative aspiration for blood & air.

COMPLICATIONS
- Pneumothorax; most cases are subclinical
  - Incidence of 1–6%
- Intravascular injection
- Horner's syndrome
- Phrenic nerve blockade

PEARLS
- Direct needle laterally, since medial direction increases incidence of complications.
- Aspiration of air necessitates a CXR to rule out PTX.

TEE INSERTION & BASIC EXAMINATION (ADULT)

JASON WIDRICH, MD
ALEX KAO, MD
RENEE ROBERTS, MD
KIM SKIDMORE, MD

INDICATIONS
- Use of an ultrasonic probe in the esophagus provides excellent 2-D images of the structure & function of the heart, valves & major vessels.

- Contraindications to TEE placement include esophageal tear, stricture, or recent variceal bleed.
- Indications for the use of TEE include
  - Unexplained hypotension
  - Suspected pericardial effusion
  - Suspected aneurysm or aortic dissection
  - Evaluation of valvular function & pathology
  - Assessment for emboli (plaque, air)
  - Evaluation of cardiac anatomy after surgical repairs & for abnormal anatomy
  - LV preload, segmental wall motion abnormalities (SWMA) & global function assessment before & after cardiopulmonary bypass, or during other major hemodynamic perturbations
- Pulsed-wave (PW) Doppler measures the Doppler shift in ultrasonic frequency as objects move toward & away from a pinpoint location within the 2-D image, relative to the probe tip.
  - Color flow mapping, a subtype of PW, allows the diameter of regurgitant or shunt jets to be measured.
  - Velocity vs time curves can be "traced" to yield an area under the curve.
  - For example, PW in the left ventricular outflow tract (just proximal to the AV annulus) yields cm traveled by an average red cell in a cardiac beat.
  - Multiplication of this number by the heart rate & by the area of the LVOT = pi* (LVOT diameter/2)^2 yields the cardiac output. This is well validated compared to thermodilution.
  - Similarly, Qp:Qs can be calculated if the area under the curve is traced for both the RVOT & LVOT.
- Continuous-wave Doppler samples Doppler shift at a higher frame rate.
  - Therefore, it is more useful when velocities are >1 m/s (eg, peak gradient across a stenotic valve).
  - Maximum velocity can be "calipered" & thus pressure gradients inferred (DP = 4v^2).
- Contractility is evaluated best by the percent thickening of the myocardium during systole.
  - Normal to mild hypokinesis is 30–50%; severe hypokinesis is <30% thickening.
  - Endocardial excursion toward the center of the chamber is also useful, where >30% is normal, 10–30% mild hypokinesis, <10%

severe hypokinesis, 0% akinetic of a given segment of the LV (apical, basal, mid, septal, anteroseptal, anterior, posterior, inferior, lateral) during systole.

➣ SWMA may be an indicator of
  • Myocardial ischemia or infarction.
  • Artifact such as hypovolemia.
  • Open pericardium.
  • Left bundle branch block.
  • Pacemakers.
  • Translational motion of nearby WMA.

PREPARATION

■ Probe can be placed under conscious sedation or under general anesthesia w/ an intubated trachea. Some pts may not be able to tolerate the probe awake or may have reflux significant enough to warrant intubation.

■ If pt is not receiving deep sedation or neuromuscular relaxation, a bite block should be used to protect pt & probe.

■ The most common method of insertion in conscious pts:
  ➣ First, suction stomach to evacuate air & fluids.
  ➣ Place a bite block (for intubated pt, can place after probe insertion).
  ➣ A head tilt or jaw thrust will help improve alignment for insertion of the probe.
  ➣ Direct probe down the esophagus.
  ➣ Guide probe midline over the tongue, alongside a gloved finger in the left side of mouth reaching deep into the posterior pharynx. Flex the end of the probe to assist w/ placement into the esophagus.
  ➣ For difficult placement, use a laryngoscope to assist w/ visualization & insertion into the esophagus.

ANATOMY

■ Obtaining a particular view on TEE is described by the following nomenclature:
  ➣ Degrees of rotation of the ultrasonic plane to the axis of the probe
  ➣ Level or depth from upper incisors
    • Upper esophageal (UE): 25–30 cm
    • Midesophageal (ME): 30–35 cm
    • Transgastric (TG): 35–40 cm
    • Deep transgastric: 40–45 cm

➤ Rotation of the probe in reference to the esophagus
  • 0 degrees (leftward) or 180 degrees (rightward) clockwise to vertical axis of the body
➤ Anteflexion or retroflexion of the distal end of the probe
➤ Longitudinal (long axis [LAX], usually 90 degrees) or transverse (short axis [SAX], usually 0 degrees) view of the object of interest

TECHNIQUE

■ Basic assessment (** = the most important views in cardiac assessment)
■ **ME AV SAX (25–40 degree plane): for visualization of the aortic valve
  ➤ Visualize leaflets, area, coronary arteries, color flow.
  ➤ Aortic stenosis
■ ME AV LAX (90–140 degree plane): LA, upper LV, aortic root, LVOT
  ➤ Mitral valve function, left atrial masses
  ➤ Aortic insufficiency, pathology of aortic root
■ ME bicaval (rotate probe clockwise, 110–120 degree plane): SVC on right side of screen, IVC on left side of screen
  ➤ ASD, atrial tumor, air embolus
■ ME RV inflow-outflow (70 degree plane, turn probe counterclockwise): RV inflow & outflow along w/ aortic valve view
  ➤ Pulmonic valve disease/insufficiency, RVOT pathology
  ➤ Air embolus
  ➤ Identify PA catheter
  ➤ CVP+maximal TR velocity by CW = PA systolic pressure estimate
■ **ME four chamber (0–10 degree plane): four chambers, LVOT, MV, TV
  ➤ Used to assess hypotension
  ➤ Chamber enlargement/cardiomyopathy
  ➤ Can assess MV/TV function & pathology
  ➤ Comparison of RV vs LV size
  ➤ Can assess for masses, effusions, air embolus
■ ME two chamber (90 degree plane): LV, LA
  ➤ Used to assess pathology & contractility at LV apex (& basal, mid) of the anterior & inferior walls
  ➤ LA appendage, mass, or thrombus

- ME LAX (90–120 degree plane): LA, entire LV, aortic root
  - LV contractility at basal & mid (& apical) segments of the anteroseptal & posterior walls
  - Masses, effusions
- **TG midpapillary SAX (90 degree plane): LV midpapillary
  - To assess contractility of the segments of LV representing all three coronary arteries
  - Hypovolemia diagnosed by approximation or "kissing" of papillary muscles
  - To assess LV preload & function
  - LVH (In diastole, "caliper" the thickness of the myocardial wall. LVH is >11 mm.)
  - Masses, effusions
  - Fractional area change
    - "Trace" the endocardial area.
    - Fractional area of change (FAC) = (End-diastolic area [EDA] - End-systolic area [ESA])/EDA.
    - Normal FAC is 0.36 to 0.64; is nearly as accurate as EF in estimating global contractility.
    - The EDA itself yields an estimate of preload (assuming there is no LVH). Normal preload is 5.5–11.9 cm^2/m^2 body surface area.
- Views to evaluate aneurysmal or atheromatous disease of thoracic aorta
  - UE aortic arch LAX (0 degree plane): arch
  - UE aortic arch SAX (90 degree plane): arch, PA, PV
  - ME ascending aortic SAX (0–60 degree plane): cross-section of ascending aorta, SVC, PA
  - ME ascending aortic LAX (100–150 degree plane): ascending aorta, right PA
  - Descending aortic SAX (0 degree plane): aorta, left pleural space
  - Descending aortic LAX (90 degree plane): aorta, left pleural space
- Additional views described by the American Society of Echocardiography
  - TG two chamber (80–100 degree plane): RV, LV, MV, chordae, papillary muscles
  - TG basal SAX (0–20 degree plane): LV, RV, MV, TV
  - ME mitral commissural (60–70 degree plane): MV, LV, LA

> TG LAX (90–120 plane): longitudinal view of LV
  • Useful for CO measurement
> Deep TG LAX (0 degree plane w/ anteflexed probe): LV at apex
  • Useful for CO measurement
> TG RV inflow (100–120 degree plane): RV, RA, TV, chordae
  • Useful for TR CW for PAS estimate

COMPLICATIONS
■ Lip injury, hoarseness, dysphagia
■ Esophageal stricture, tear. Electrical leakage test should be performed frequently in each probe to prevent strictures.
■ Response to insertion could cause hypoventilation, HTN, tachycardia, and/or ischemia.

PEARLS
■ Moving through a basic standardized exam in a systematic fashion from upper esophageal to mid-esophageal to transgastric cardiac views will improve speed (4 minutes) & limit missed diagnoses.
■ Obtain the views of the descending aorta after the basic exam.
■ TEE measures the velocity of an object moving toward or away from the probe. The PW or CW Doppler interrogation line must be aligned parallel w/ direction of blood flow to get accurate velocity measurements.
■ Unexplained sudden hypotension intraop or in the ICU is an important indication for the use of TEE.
  > The TG SAX midpapillary view and the four-chamber ME views are most often employed. They can be used to distinguish between:
    • Hypovolemia: decreased end-diastolic area, increased ejection fraction
    • Myocardial depression: increased end-diastolic area, decreased ejection fraction
    • Mitral regurgitation: increased ejection fraction, regurgitant color jets
    • Tamponade: fluid surrounding left ventricle
    • Cardiac arrest: increased end-diastolic area, no ejection fraction
    • Valvular disease: turbulent (mosaic of colors) jets are seen when the "scale" is reasonably set (ie, always set color bar to >0.5 m/s)

TRACHEAL TUBE INTRODUCER PLACEMENT (INTUBATING STYLET PLACEMENT)

GERALD DUBOWITZ, MB CHB

INDICATIONS
■ Facilitates intubation in pts w/ difficult tracheal intubation

PREPARATION
■ Many different types of tracheal tube introducers. Known by different names, including tracheal tube introducer, intubating introducer, gum elastic bougie (GEB).
  ➤ Some introducers have a hollow core to allow oxygen insufflation or ventilation.
  ➤ Introducers vary in their rigidity & curvature.
■ Tracheal tube introducer is designed for placement into trachea, then ETT is passed over stylet into trachea.
  ➤ This is contrasted to the standard disposable intubating stylet placed within ETT.
■ Test the introducer for size in the ETT by inserting it AND removing it before use. If the ETT & introducer do not easily pass over each other before insertion, lubricate further or select a larger ETT.

ANATOMY
■ Tracheal tube introducers are used in combination w/ direct laryngoscopy.
■ Large epiglottis or other anatomic feature may make glottic visualization difficult.

TECHNIQUE
■ Standard intubating stylet
  ➤ The widely used disposable intubating stylet is metal, typically w/ soft plastic wrapping. This is designed to be placed within the ETT.
  ➤ The stylet is inserted into the ETT until it is flush w/ or slightly proximal to the end of the ETT.
    • A small amount of lubricant will make it easier to insert & remove the stylet.
  ➤ Fold the proximal end of the stylet to prevent it from migrating into the ETT.

➤ Make a bend in the ETT as needed to facilitate passage between the vocal cords.
  - The stylet increases rigidity & can impart the proper shape for passage into the glottic opening. It also allows the ETT to move past a floppy epiglottis.
➤ After passing the tube past the cords, hold the endotracheal tube VERY firmly & if possible get an assistant to withdraw the stylet.
➤ Once the stylet is removed, attach breathing circuit & confirm placement.
■ Tracheal tube introducer
  ➤ Lubricate the introducer well w/ viscous jelly or silicone spray.
  ➤ Pass the introducer through the vocal cords under direct laryngoscopy.
  ➤ If the cords are not visible or barely visible, pass the introducer as close to the epiglottis as possible (anteriorly & in the midline) & insert blindly.
    - The GEB has an anterior bend in the tip to facilitate this.
  ➤ Once the introducer is past the cords, pass it a further 3–5 cm.
  ➤ Stabilize it in this position & pass the ETT over the introducer, taking care not to let go of the introducer.
  ➤ Once the ETT is placed, remove the introducer & confirm placement.

COMPLICATIONS
■ Esophageal intubation
■ Failed intubation
■ Tracheal injury
■ Pneumothorax

PEARLS
■ Preoxygenation is crucial in increasing time for intubation.
■ Problems do not necessarily occur from a failure to intubate; they occur from failure to ventilate. If in doubt stop the procedure & ventilate the pt's lungs.
■ If the intubation is considered difficult, have a backup plan (eg, fiberoptic intubation). See also Critical Events chapter "Difficult Airway Management."
■ Problems such as failure of ETT to pass into trachea are more common if introducer is placed too shallow rather than too deep.
  ➤ However, problems such as tracheal injury are more common if introducer is placed too deep.

- If the ETT will not easily pass between the cords when using introducer, rotate the ETT while advancing, or use a smaller ETT.
  - ➤ Do not force ETT, as this may damage the cords.
- A flexible introducer (eg, GEB) can be used for nasal intubations.

TRANSTRACHEAL JET VENTILATION (TTJV)

ALISON G. CAMERON, MD

INDICATIONS
- Used emergently in the "can't ventilate, can't intubate" scenario, via an emergency needle or catheter cricothyrotomy
- Used electively via rigid bronchoscope, ventilating laryngoscope, or catheter passed between vocal cords

PREPARATION
- For placement through cricothyroid membrane
  - ➤ Long 14–16g cannula
  - ➤ Special reinforced catheter designed to minimize kinking
  - ➤ As an alternative, can use vessel dilator from 7–9g introducer sheath
- To attach jet ventilator to catheter, the correct Luer-Llok adapter must be available as part of the jet ventilator.
- Oxygen may be insufflated (but not jet ventilated) via
  - ➤ A 5-mm ETT adapter attached to the catheter
  - ➤ A 3-cc syringe barrel (plunger removed) attached to the catheter at one end & to a 7.0-mm ETT adapter at the other
    - The adapter is attached to an anesthesia circuit or directly to the oxygen flush valve of the anesthesia machine
- Jet injector powered by wall oxygen or regulated tank
  - ➤ Saunders injection system is one system allowing adjustable inspiratory pressure
  - ➤ Alternative: fresh gas outlet on anesthesia machine

ANATOMY
- Cricothyroid membrane is located between thyroid cartilage & cricoid cartilage on anterior surface of neck.
- Cricothyroid membrane is at level of transverse process of C6 (Chassaignac's tubercle).

TECHNIQUE
- If a cricothyrotomy is necessary
  - Perform transtracheal local anesthesia if time permits.
    - Pierce cricothyroid membrane, aspirate air & inject 2–3 mL 2% lidocaine via a plastic IV catheter (pt will cough on injection & risk tracheal injury if a metal needle is used).
  - Insert catheter through cricothyroid membrane at 45-degree angle directed caudally, aspirate air, then advance catheter.
    - Advance the catheter several inches into the trachea; if not advanced far enough, it may migrate out of the trachea.
    - Massive subcutaneous emphysema may result from ventilation through a misplaced catheter.
- Attach catheter, bronchoscope, or ventilating laryngoscope to jet ventilator.
- Keep inspiratory jet burst approximately 1–2 sec (watch chest rise to assess for adequate amount of ventilation).
  - Venturi effect will entrain room air into lungs in addition to 100% oxygen from jet ventilation.
- Watch for chest to deflate after inspiration is stopped.
- During jet ventilation, inhaled anesthetic is not possible, so IV or IM anesthesia must be used.
- After ventilation is ensured, consider placement of a definitive airway.

COMPLICATIONS
- Hyperinflation
- Barotrauma, including pneumothorax & tension pneumothorax
- Cardiac output compromise
- Cricothyrotomy complications
  - Tracheal injury
  - Subglottic stenosis
  - Hoarseness

PEARLS
- Insufflation of oxygen at low flows (1–3 L/min) can prevent hypoxemia & allow time for more definitive airway mgt.
- Call for surgical assistance early if a surgical airway is contemplated.
- In complete upper airway obstruction, there may be difficulty w/ expiration, which may lead to hyperinflation & tension pneumothorax.

➤ Cardiac output may become compromised, necessitating immediate chest tube or needle thoracostomy.

WRIST BLOCK

JAMES M. SONNER, MD

INDICATIONS

■ Hand surgery can be accomplished by blocking the median, ulnar, radial & lateral cutaneous nerve of the forearm at the wrist.

PREPARATION

■ Use sterile prep of the wrist & aseptic technique.
■ 21 cc of local anesthetic of choice (eg, 1.5% lidocaine).
■ In most pts a short needle (eg, 5/8 inch) is adequate.

ANATOMY

■ Ulnar nerve: Innervates the ulnar side of the hand, both palmar & dorsal surfaces, the fifth finger & the medial aspect of the fourth finger. Located dorsal & lateral to the tendon of the flexor carpi ulnaris.
■ Median nerve: Innervates most of the radial side of the palm, the second & third fingers & part of the thumb & fourth finger. On the dorsal surface, it innervates the tips of the thumb, second & third finger & the lateral aspect of the tip of the fourth finger. Located between the tendons of the flexor carpi radialis & palmaris longus.
■ Radial nerve & lateral cutaneous nerve of the forearm (a branch of the musculocutaneous nerve): The radial nerve innervates the radial side of the dorsum of the hand, excluding the tips of the thumb & second & third fingers. Laterally, it innervates part of the thenar eminence. The lateral cutaneous nerve of the forearm innervates the radial side of the forearm. These nerves run lateral to the radius, in the superficial fascia.

TECHNIQUE

■ Three injections are performed.
■ Ulnar nerve: Block is performed 1 inch from the crease of the wrist. Insert needle perpendicular to the ulnar side of the wrist. Inject 5 cc local anesthetic deep, **beneath the tendon of the flexor carpi ulnaris** & 2 cc superficially.

- Median nerve: Block is performed 1 inch from the crease of the wrist. Inject 5 cc local anesthetic deep, **between the tendons of the flexor carpi radialis & palmaris longus**, & 2 cc superficially.
- Radial nerve & lateral cutaneous nerve of the forearm: Block is performed 3 inches from the crease of the wrist. Inject 7 cc local anesthetic subcutaneously in a ring over the radius.

COMPLICATIONS

- Like an ankle block, this is a relatively safe block & can be performed in the preop area. Complications include
  - ➤ Local anesthetic toxicity: Lessen risk by minimizing total volume of local anesthetic.
  - ➤ Intravascular injection: Minimize by periodic aspiration of needle, or keeping needle in motion during injection.
  - ➤ Intraneural injection: Watch for extreme pain during local anesthetic injection; withdraw needle if this occurs.
  - ➤ Nerve injury: This will not be evident until after the local anesthetic effect dissipates.

PEARLS

- OK to use a forearm tourniquet w/ this block.
- Not all nerves need to be blocked for all hand procedures; nerves can be selectively blocked at the wrist according to the operation.

PART FIVE

Drugs

2-CHLOROPROCAINE (NESACAINE, NESACAINE-MPF)

GRETE H. PORTEOUS, MD

INDICATION
- Local anesthesia for infiltration, peripheral nerve block, epidural & caudal blocks
- Not for spinal anesthesia

DOSE
- Depends on route of administration
  - Brachial plexus block, 30–40 mL of 2% solution
  - Lumbar epidural anesthesia, 2–2.5 mL per segment of a 2% solution (usual total volume 15–25 mL) is given. Repeat dose 2–6 mL less than original dose at 40- to 50-min intervals to maintain block.
- Reduce dose if given w/ epinephrine, in the elderly, debilitated, acutely ill, children & those w/ severe hepatic impairment or cardiac disease.
- Max dose: 11 mg/kg alone (total 800 mg in adults) or 14 mg/kg w/ 1:200,000 epi (not to exceed 1 g)

ONSET
- Rapid, usually 6–12 min

KINETICS
- Duration: about 60 min
- In vitro plasma half-life in adults is about 20 sec, in neonates about 40 sec
- Rate of systemic absorption depends on dose, site of injection, use of vasoconstrictors.
- Metabolized in plasma by hydrolysis of ester linkage by pseudocholinesterase (ester local anesthetic)

PREPARATION
- 1%, 2% solutions w/ methylparaben & EDTA for peripheral nerve block & infiltration
- 2%, 3% solutions methylparaben-free (MPF) for epidural & caudal anesthesia, as well as peripheral nerve blocks & infiltration

MECHANISM
- Binds to open sodium channels in sensory & motor neurons & blocks propagation of nerve impulses

COMMENTS
- Methylparaben preservative can trigger allergic reactions.
- Metabolites impair the action of sulfonamide drugs.
- Major toxicity, like all local anesthetics, is neurologic (confusion, agitation, tremors, seizures) & cardiovascular (dysrhythmias, hypotension, cardiovascular collapse).
- Because of rapid onset & short duration, popular for blocks in ambulatory surgery.
- Epidural chloroprocaine may interfere w/ action of subsequent neuraxial opiates (mechanism unknown).
- Epidural chloroprocaine has been assoc w/ severe back pain.
- Inadvertent subarachnoid injection has resulted in neurotoxicity.

ACETAMINOPHEN

MARK BOMANN, MD

INDICATION
- Mild to moderate pain mgt
- Adjunct to other analgesics
- Antipyretic

DOSE
- Adults and children >12 y
  - ➤ 650–1,000 mg PO q4–6h. Limit 4 g/day for acute therapy in healthy pts, 3 g/day for chronic therapy in healthy pts, 2 g/day for pts w/ chronic illness, liver or kidney disease, or malnourishment
- Children 6–11 y
  - ➤ 10–15 mg/kg PO q4–6h, max 4–5 doses per day for short-term therapy
- Children <6 y
  - ➤ 10–15 mg/kg PO q4–6h, max 4–5 doses per day for short-term therapy. Doses of 20–25 mg/kg (or more) PR have been used immediately prior to surgery in children not already on chronic therapy.

ONSET
- 30–60 min PO; variable onset PR

KINETICS
- Duration: 4–6 h
- Elimination half-life: 1–4 h

- Hepatic metabolism
- Renal excretion

PREPARATION
- Chewable tabs 80, 120, 160 mg
- Tabs 120, 160, 325, 500, 650 mg
- Capsules 325, 500 mg
- Gelcaps 500 mg
- Extended-release caplets 650 mg
- Suppositories 80, 120, 125, 300, 325, 650 mg
- Liquid (multiple concentrations of solution & suspension)
- Oral powders 80, 160 mg
- No IV formulation currently available in U.S.

MECHANISM
- Analgesia from increased pain threshold (specific site of action is unclear).
- Antipyretic action appears to be from direct action on the hypothalamus to block the effect of endogenous pyrogen.

COMMENTS
- Along w/ NSAIDs, it is the first-line pain treatment per the World Health Organization pain treatment protocol.
  - ➤ Commonly found in combination w/ oral narcotic preparations
  - ➤ Commonly used in pediatric pts as adjunct/first-line therapy for pain
  - ➤ Does not cause platelet dysfunction
  - ➤ Overall minimal side effect profile
- Can cause severe or even fatal hepatic toxicity w/ overdosage, perhaps less commonly in young children. Symptoms of hepatotoxicity may be delayed for days. Consider check of acetaminophen levels if overdose suspected. Oral acetylcysteine is a specific antidote; most effective when administered early in the course.

ADENOSINE

MARK BOMANN, MD

INDICATION
- Treatment for PSVT; includes PSVT from accessory bypass tracts (eg, WPW syndrome)

DOSE

- Rapid IV bolus 6–12 mg, may repeat in 1–2 min. Lower doses may be effective if administered via central vein.
- Pediatric dose: 0.05–0.25 mg/kg

ONSET

- <20 sec

KINETICS

- Cellular uptake & metabolism

PREPARATION

- Injection, 3 mg/mL

MECHANISM

- Slows conduction through AV node & reentrant pathways
- Endogenous nucleoside w/ antiarrhythmic activity

COMMENTS

- Contraindicated in pts w/ second- or third-degree heart block or sick sinus syndrome unless pt has a pacemaker
- Not effective in atrial flutter, atrial fibrillation, or ventricular tachycardia
- Potentially harmful for rapid afib in pts w/ WPW
- ECG monitoring required for safety & rhythm interpretation
- Pts w/ asthma can have bronchoconstriction.
- Decreases peripheral resistance & arterial pressure; If given at a slow rate a reflex tachycardia can develop due to decreased SVR.

ALBUTEROL

IVAN ZEITZ, MD

INDICATION

- Bronchospasm (prophylaxis & treatment)

DOSE

- 2 inhalations q4–6h is typical maintenance regimen.
- For acute intraop bronchospasm in mechanically ventilated pt, may need 10 inhalations or more because of delivery through ETT or ventilator circuit.
- 2.5 mg diluted to 3 cc w/ sterile saline by nebulizer tid/qid.

ONSET
- Bronchodilation begins within 5–15 min of inhalation.

KINETICS
- Peak effect in 0.5–3 h
- Effect usually lasts 4 h but may last 6 h.
- Elimination half-life: 3.8 h
- Hepatic metabolism
- Renal excretion

PREPARATION
- Premixed aerosol metered-dose inhaler (MDI) 0.09 mg/inhalation
  - Nebulizer solution 2.5 mg in 3 cc NS

MECHANISM
- Synthetic sympathomimetic amine; beta-2 > beta-1 effects on smooth muscles from trachea to bronchial tree (muscle relaxation resulting in bronchodilation)

COMMENTS
- Dose-limiting toxicity is cardiac (arrhythmias, tachycardia).
- May redose more frequently than recommended to treat bronchospasm (limited by cardiac toxicity).
- Because of specificity, efficacy, & relatively low toxicity, it is a first-line agent to treat bronchospasm.
- For mechanically ventilated pt, use spacer system to improve delivery of MDI, or use nebulized drug.

ALFENTANIL

MARK BOMANN, MD

INDICATION
- Analgesia
- Anesthesia adjunct

DOSE
- All opioid doses should be titrated to effect depending on a variety of factors, including
  - Pt age
  - Body weight
  - Physical status of pt

➤ Coexisting disease
➤ Other CNS depressant drug administration
➤ Surgery or procedure performed

■ IV
➤ Alfentanil (high-dose): 130–245 mcg/kg, followed by infusion at 0.5–1.5 mcg/kg/min. Inadequate for use as a sole anesthetic. Anticipate need for postop mechanical ventilation.
➤ Periop sedation/analgesia: 12.5–100 mcg/dose, depending on pt response. Children >12 yo: 0.5–1 mcg/kg/dose.
➤ Adjunct to GA, surgery <30 min
  • Induction 8–20 mcg/kg
  • Maintenance 0.5–1 mcg/kg/min or intermittent dose of 3–5 mcg/kg
➤ Adjunct to GA, surgery <1 h
  • Induction 8–50 mcg/kg
  • Maintenance 0.5–1 mcg/kg/min or intermittent dose of 3–15 mcg/kg
➤ Adjunct to GA, surgery >1 h
  • Induction 50–75 mcg/kg
  • Maintenance 0.5–3 mcg/kg/min
➤ Analgesia: 250–500 mcg IV (5–10 mcg/kg)

■ IM: up to 30 mcg/kg

ONSET
■ 1–2 min IV
■ <5 min IM

KINETICS
■ Duration: 10–15 min IV, 10–60 min IM
■ Peak effect: 1–2 min IV, 15 min IM
■ Elimination half-life: 90–110 min
■ Hepatic metabolism, renal excretion of metabolites

PREPARATION
■ 500 mcg/mL

MECHANISM
■ Mu opioid receptor agonist

COMMENTS
■ Comparison to fentanyl
➤ Alfentanil is one-eighth to one-tenth as potent.
➤ Alfentanil has faster onset.

- Important respiratory effects
  - ➤ Like other opioids, will cause respiratory depression & hypoventilation, which can ultimately lead to apnea & respiratory arrest
  - ➤ Like other potent opioids, can cause significant chest wall rigidity & difficulty w/ ventilation, requiring muscle relaxant administration. This is very common w/ rapid IV administration of large dose.
- Important cardiac effects
  - ➤ In general, has minimal effects on hemodynamic status & has been widely used for cardiac surgery.
  - ➤ Like other potent opioids, can cause significant bradycardia & hypotension
  - ➤ When used in combination w/ other sedative medications (eg, benzodiazepines, barbiturates) hypotension can be more pronounced.
- Consider dose reduction in elderly or debilitated pt or pt w/ liver or renal failure.
- Opioids not considered suitable for use as a sole anesthetic because of breakthrough HTN, inadequate anesthesia, high incidence of recall, muscle rigidity & postop respiratory depression

AMINOCAPROIC ACID (AMICAR)

LUNDY CAMPBELL, MD

INDICATION
- Antifibrinolytic to reduce postop bleeding & transfusion requirements in pts undergoing CPB
- Also used to reduce bleeding in other high-risk surgeries (eg, liver transplant)
- May decrease postop bleeding in pts w/ certain bleeding disorders

DOSE
- General adult dosing regimen:
  - ➤ 4–5 gm loading dose followed by 1 gm/hr for 8 hr, or until cessation of bleeding
- Typical Cardiopulmonary bypass regimen:
  - ➤ Loading dose: 60–80 mg/kg (usually 5 gm) over 20–60 minutes
  - ➤ Maintenance infusion 30 mg/kg/hour
  - ➤ Terminate infusion approx 1–2 h after heparin neutralization

ONSET

■ Not applicable since delivered by infusion. Loading dose should begin prior to skin incision & should be completely infused before initiation of bypass.

KINETICS

■ Half-life: 4.9 h w/ normal renal function
■ Renal excretion/concentration
■ 50% excreted unchanged in urine within 12 h

PREPARATION

■ Each 20-mL vial contains 5 g aminocaproic acid (25% solution).

MECHANISM

■ Lysine analog: Binds to lysine binding sites on plasmin & plasminogen. Blocks conversion of plasminogen to plasmin & binding of plasmin to target fibrin.

COMMENTS

■ May rarely cause myopathy, muscle necrosis
■ Decreased dose required in renal failure
■ Contraindicated in DIC. Intravascular thrombus may result if administered during DIC.
■ Other hemostatic agents such as aprotinin may be more effective in reducing transfusion requirement during major surgery.

AMINOPHYLLINE (THEOPHYLLINE)

MARK BOMANN, MD

INDICATION

■ Chronic asthma
  ➤ Typically considered third-line agent
■ COPD
  ➤ Typically not useful for acute exacerbations

DOSE

■ Load 6 mg/kg (as aminophylline) IV over 20–30 min (dilute in 50 mL NS or D5W), drip 0.5–0.7 mg/kg/h (dilute 500 mg in 500 mL NS or D5W)
  ➤ Theophylline levels required for proper titration, 0.6-mg/kg increase will result in a 1-mcg/mL increase in serum theophylline

- Maintenance adjustments
  - ➤ 0.4 mg/kg/h for nonsmoking adults
  - ➤ 0.7 mg/kg/h for smoking adults
  - ➤ 0.3 mg/kg/h for age >60
  - ➤ 0.2 mg/kg/h w/ hepatic insufficiency
- Pediatric: 1 mg/kg/h IV
- Dose by ideal body weight (poor fat absorption)
- Oral dose not discussed, as anesthesia provider not likely to initiate PO therapy
- 100 mg of aminophylline is equal to 80 mg theophylline.

ONSET
- <2 min IV
- 30 min PO

KINETICS
- Peak effect: 1 h IV, 1–2 h PO
- Duration: PO 4–8 h
- Hepatic elimination via P450 (1A2) system

PREPARATION
- IV form: aminophylline
- PO form: theophylline
- IV: 1, 2, 25 mg/mL
- Tabs: 100, 200 mg
- Extended-release tab: 225 mg
- Oral solution: 105 mg/5 mL
- Rectal suppositories: 250, 500 mg

MECHANISM
- Aminophylline is a methylxanthine that is converted to theophylline.
- Exact mechanism is not known but is thought to involve inhibition of phosphodiesterase, thus increasing cAMP in bronchial smooth muscle.
- Also thought to involve blockade of adenosine receptors, antagonize prostaglandin E2 & directly affect mobilization of calcium.

COMMENTS
- Treatment for reversible bronchospasm in asthma & COPD (third-line)
- Adverse reactions include tachycardia, nausea, hypokalemia, hypoglycemia

- May be useful in treatment of bronchospasm secondary to anaphylactic/anaphylactoid reactions
- Serious ventricular dysrhythmias noted w/ concomitant use of halothane; recommend waiting three half-lives or 13 h
- Very low toxic/therapeutic ratio; toxicity increased at >20 mcg/mL but may be seen when therapeutic levels are achieved
- Reduce dose by 50% in cor pulmonale, sepsis, CHF, liver disease
- Increases gastric acid secretion, which can exacerbate peptic ulcer disease
- Decreased responsiveness to IV adenosine (increase dose by 50–100%)
- May be useful in medical mgt of postdural puncture headache (though not well studied)
  - Theophylline dose PO 225 mg q8h for 3–5 days

AMIODARONE (CORDARONE)

RENÉE J. ROBERTS, MD

INDICATION
- Pulseless VT/VF
- Resistant ventricular & supraventricular arrhythmias
- Atrial fibrillation

DOSE
- For pulseless VF or VT: 300 mg IV push
- For stable arrhythmia,150 mg over 10 min, followed by 360 mg over 6 h at 1 mg/min, followed by 540 mg over 18 h at 0.5 mg/min

ONSET
- Hours when given IV

KINETICS
- Complex pharmacokinetics due to avid binding to poorly perfused adipose tissue
- Duration 13–100 days
- Metabolism hepatic
- Elimination & excretion via bile

PREPARATION
- 150-mg (50-mg/mL) ampules (Cordarone IV)
- For infusion, use 1.5- to 1.8-mg/mL concentration

MECHANISM

- Considered mostly as a class III antiarrhythmic (ie, K+ channel blocker)
- But has weak electrophysiologic properties of other 3 classes of antiarrhythmics as well (ie, Na channel blocker, beta blocker, calcium channel blocker)
- Arteriolar vasodilation, prolongs atrial, AV nodal, & ventricular refractory period

COMMENTS

- Reduces clearance of digoxin, diltiazem, warfarin, theophylline, quinidine, procainamide, flecainide
- Hypotension most common adverse effect
- Can also cause bradycardia, AV block, prolonged QT, torsades
  - ➤ In pts w/ AV nodal disease, may produce bradycardia or heart block, requiring temporary pacemaker
- Other complications, usually w/ longer-term use:
  - ➤ Interstitial fibrosis from pneumonitis
  - ➤ Hypo/hyperthyroidism because preparation is iodinated
  - ➤ Blue-gray skin (usually nose)
  - ➤ After 9 wks, increased LFTs from hepatocellular necrosis
  - ➤ Corneal yellow-brown microcrystals (3 wks); microdeposits may cause peripheral visual halos & decreased acuity
  - ➤ Paresthesia, tremor, ataxia, headaches
- ACLS 2000 guidelines now include amiodarone as possible drug therapy for multiple arrhythmias, including shock-refractory VF or VT, SVT, & atrial fibrillation/atrial flutter.

AMPICILLIN

JEREMY NUSSBAUMER, MD

INDICATION

- Endocarditis prophylaxis
- Antibiotic for treatment of infection from susceptible gram-positive cocci & some gram-negative rods

DOSE

- Adults: 20 mg/kg IV q4–6h
- AHA-recommended bacterial endocarditis prophylaxis for dental, oral, esophageal procedures is 2 g IV 30 min before procedure; for GU procedures, gentamicin (1.5 mg/kg) is also given.
- Children: 100–200 mg/kg/day IV divided q6h

ONSET
- Rapid

KINETICS
- Duration: Peaks at 5 min
- Half life: 1–2 h
- Metabolism: Renal elimination

PREPARATION
- Powder for injection

MECHANISM
- Inhibits cell wall replication in non-beta-lactamase-producing bacteria

COMMENTS
- May need to adjust dosage in renal failure pts
  - Dose q6–12h for CrCl 10–30 & q12h for CrCl <10
- Low incidence of cross-reactivity w/ cephalosporins
- Presumed safe in pregnancy

ASPIRIN (ACETYLSALICYLIC ACID)

GERALD DUBOWITZ, MB CHB

INDICATION
- Treatment of pain, inflammation, fever
- Prophylaxis for CVA, MI
- Treatment of MI

DOSE
- Analgesic/anti-inflammatory/antipyretic: 325–650 mg PO q4–6h up to 2 g/day
- Antiplatelet: 81–325 mg PO qd

ONSET
- Rapid onset PO, absorbed from stomach & small intestine
- Absorption of suppositories incomplete & unreliable

KINETICS
- 50–80% protein bound
- Unbound form is active; bound serves as a reservoir.
- Metabolism: hepatic
  - Metabolic products inactive

- Urine excretion depends on urine pH.
  - ➤ Alkaline urine: 85% excreted unchanged
  - ➤ With normal pH, excretion is 25%.
- Cyclooxygenase is not regenerated within the life span of platelets, so one aspirin affects platelet function for a week.
- Mini-dose aspirin (<650 mg qd) appears to be cleared within 24 h; platelet function returns to acceptable levels within 48 h.

PREPARATION
- Tablets
- Suppository

MECHANISM
- Inhibits prostaglandin synthesis
- Irreversibly acetylates platelet cyclooxygenase, which converts arachidonic acid to prostaglandin endoperoxidases

COMMENTS
- Gastric irritation may be a problem; enteric coating helps but has slower onset.
- Interacts w/ significant number of drugs (esp warfarin)
- Not recommended in pts w/ preexisting GI complaints due to gastric irritation & ulceration. Enteric-coated aspirin helps overcome this.
- Stop aspirin 1 wk prior to elective surgery.
  - ➤ Platelet function restored after a week or w/ platelet infusion.

ATENOLOL (TENORMIN)

CHRISTINE A. WU, MD

INDICATION
- Tachycardia: Effective in prevention & mgt of sinus & supraventricular tachycardias. Reduces risk of atrial fibrillation after CABG.
- Hypertension: Especially efficacious in combination w/ a diuretic, in elderly pts w/ isolated systolic hypertension
- Angina: Reduces rate & subsequently oxygen consumption
- Acute MI: Has been shown to reduce risk of death
- Perioperative cardiac morbidity: Has been shown to reduce the risk of death in pts who have or who are at risk for coronary artery disease who are undergoing noncardiac surgery

■ Congestive heart failure: Beta blockade has been shown to improve function & prevent death. Dose needs to be started low & gradually increased.

DOSE
■ Periop cardiac risk
  ➣ All pts w/ known CAD, PVD, or 2 risk factors (HTN, DM, age >=65, smoking, cholesterol >=240 mg/dL) should be on a beta blocker for surgery.
  ➣ If heart rate >50 & systolic BP >100 mmHg, atenolol 10 mg IV over 10 min preop. Repeat dose postop.
  ➣ If not taking PO, atenolol 10 mg IV q12h. Switch to atenolol 100 mg PO QD or 50 mg PO BID postop when taking PO meds.
■ Acute MI
  ➣ Atenolol 5 mg IV over 5 min followed by 5 mg 10 min later
  ➣ Should be administered w/ monitoring of BP, HR, ECG
  ➣ If pt tolerated 10-mg dose, give 50 mg PO 10 min after last IV dose, 50 mg PO 12 h later.
  ➣ Subsequent dosing: 100 mg PO QD or 50 mg PO BID.
■ HTN
  ➣ Initial dose: 50 mg PO QD. Dosing may range from 25 to 200 mg PO QD.
■ Requires renal dosage adjustment for those w/ creatinine clearance <35 mL/min

ONSET
■ Oral: one hour
■ IV: 5 minutes

KINETICS
■ Very hydrophilic, w/ limited CNS penetration
■ 50% bioavailability w/ oral dosing
■ Elimination half-life 5–8 h
■ Elimination is in urine & feces
  ➣ Accumulates in pts w/ renal failure; dose must be adjust

PREPARATION
■ IV: 0.5 mg/mL
■ PO: 25-, 50-, 100-mg tablets

MECHANISM
■ B1-selective antagonist w/o any intrinsic sympathomimetic activity

COMMENTS
- Atenolol has been shown to improve cardiac outcome in at-risk pts undergoing noncardiac surgery.
- Beta blockade reduces mortality after MI & in pts w/ congestive failure.

ATRACURIUM (TRACRIUM)

RONNIE LU, MD

INDICATION
- Neuromuscular block

DOSE
- Intubation: 0.4–0.5 mg/kg
- Maintenance: 0.25 mg/kg then 0.1 mg/kg q15–30min
- Infusion: 5–10 mcg/kg/min

ONSET
- 3–5 min depending on dose

KINETICS
- Duration: 20–35 min
- Metabolism by nonspecific ester hydrolysis (unaffected by pseudo-cholinesterase)
- Metabolism by Hofmann elimination, independent of renal & hepatic function

PREPARATION
- 10-mg/mL solution

MECHANISM
- Nondepolarizing neuromuscular block
- Competes w/ acetylcholine at nicotinic receptor site on motor endplate

COMMENTS
- May cause histamine release & assoc hypotension, tachycardia, bronchospasm
- In pts w/ liver failure, may cause CNS excitation or seizure secondary to laudanosine, a byproduct of Hofmann elimination

ATROPINE

MADELEINE BIBAT, MD

INDICATION
- Bradycardia
- Antisialogogue
- Used in reversal of nondepolarizing muscle relaxants to reduce muscarinic side effects of anticholinesterases
- Antidote for anticholinesterases used in insecticides

DOSE
- Bradycardia
  - Adult 0.5–1 mg IV q3–5min; max 2 mg
  - Pediatric 0.01–0.03 mg/kg; max 0.4 mg
- Antisecretory
  - Adult 0.2–0.4 mg IV/IM/SC
  - Pediatric 0.1–0.4 mg IV/IM/SC
- As antimuscarinic in combination with cholinesterase inhibitor for reversal of neuromuscular blockade:
  - 7–10 mcg atropine per 1 mg edrophonium
  - 25 mcg atropine per 70 mcg neostigmine
- As antidote for organophosphate toxicity, 2–6 mg IV/IM q1h

ONSET
- Rapid IV
- 15 min IM/SC

KINETICS
- Duration variable
- Elimination half-life: 2–3 h
- Hepatic metabolism
- Renal excretion

PREPARATION
- Various concentrations for injection (eg, 0.4 mg/mL, 1 mg/mL)

MECHANISM
- Competitively antagonizes acetylcholine at muscarinic receptors

COMMENTS
- Use caution in pts w/ asthma, myasthenia gravis, glaucoma
- Can be administered via endotracheal tube

- Dilates pupils when applied topically or systemically
- May increase serum levels of digoxin
- MAOIs & phenothiazines potentiate anticholinergic effects.

BENZOCAINE

SAMIR DZANKIC, MD

INDICATION
- Topical anesthesia, pain relief

DOSE
- Max 250–300 mg
- Use spray for no more than 2 sec.

ONSET
- 30–60 sec

KINETICS
- Minimal absorption
- Clearance by plasma cholinesterase, to much lesser extent by hepatic cholinesterase
- Duration of action 15–20 min

PREPARATION
- 1–5% cream, 20% ointment, 20% aerosol, 20% solution

MECHANISM
- Reversible sodium channel blockage resulting in attenuation of neural action potential formation & propagation

COMMENTS
- Intended area of use: skin, tympanic membrane, mucous membranes (oral mucosa, pharynx, larynx, tracheobronchial tree, nasal cavity, urinary tract, vagina, rectum)
- Side effects
  - Methemoglobinemia is the main toxic effect.
    - May be more common in infants, young children
    - Usually occurs w/ administration of higher-than-recommended dose but can occur w/ normal dose
    - Draw arterial blood for co-oximetry to diagnose methemoglobinemia.
  - Contact dermatitis and/or angioedema

- Benzocaine is an ester local anesthetic & can have cross-sensitivity w/ other ester local anesthetics.
- Cholinesterase inhibitors inhibit metabolism of benzocaine.

BRETYLIUM

JEREMY NUSSBAUMER, MD

INDICATION
- Treatment of shock-resistant ventricular arrhythmias
- May be useful in treatment of ventricular arrhythmias due to bupivacaine toxicity
- Has been used for IV regional sympathetic block

DOSE
- IV 5 mg/kg bolus over 1 min, repeat 10 mg/kg q10min until rhythm converted or max dose 30–35 mg/kg reached
  - ➤ If successful, begin infusion 1–2 mg/min.
- Has been used for IV regional sympathetic block (Bier block) 5 mg/kg

ONSET
- IV 6–20 min

KINETICS
- Peak effect in 6–9 h
- Duration 6–24 h
- Half-life 7–17 h
- Excreted unchanged in urine
- Half-life 16–32 h in renal failure

PREPARATION
- 50 mg/mL.
- Use undiluted for bolus doses.
- For infusion, dilute to 10 mg/mL in D5W or NS.

MECHANISM
- Class III antiarrhythmic
- Causes initial release of norepinephrine from nerve terminals, then inhibits further release

COMMENTS
- Commonly causes hypotension in postresuscitation period
- Decrease dose in renal failure

■ Has been removed from current ACLS guidelines because of reduced availability but still considered an acceptable therapy for persistent or recurrent ventricular fibrillation or tachycardia

BUPIVACAINE (MARCAINE, SENSORCAINE)

MICHAEL H. FAHMY, MD

INDICATION
■ Local or regional anesthesia or analgesia

DOSE
■ Will vary depending on type of block; max recommended dose for local or nerve block: 175 mg, or 225 mg if epi added to solution
■ Spinal: 1–2 mL of 0.75% bupivacaine
■ Epidural: 10–20 mL of 0.25–0.5%
■ Caudal (children): 1 cc/kg of 0.25% bupivacaine, up to 20 cc

ONSET
■ 5–20 min depending on route

KINETICS
■ Local: 0.25% conc, 2–4 h duration
■ Peripheral nerve block: 0.25–0.5% conc, 4–12 h duration
■ OB epidural analgesia: 0.1–0.5%, 2–4 h duration
■ Surgical anesthesia: 0.5–0.75%, 2–5 h duration
■ Postop surgical analgesia: 0.1–0.25%, 2–4 h duration
■ Spinal: 12.5–15 mg, 2–4 h duration
■ Metabolism: hepatic

PREPARATION
■ 0.25–0.75% solutions

MECHANISM
■ Amide-linked local anesthetic, blocks generation & conduction of nerve impulses by increasing the threshold for electrical excitation at level of sodium channel

COMMENTS
■ Potential cardiac toxicity w/ excess intravascular absorption. Look for ventricular arrhythmias.

- 0.75% conc not recommended for OB use due to early reports of cardiovascular collapse from intravascular absorption
- Low concentrations (0.25% or less) block sensory more than motor nerves.

BUTORPHANOL TARTRATE

JASON WIDRICH, MD

INDICATION
- Analgesia

DOSE
- IM: 0.02–0.08 mg/kg q3–4h
- IV: 0.01–0.04 mg/kg q3–4h
  - ➤ Typical analgesic dose: 1 mg IV q3–4h
- IV/PCA: dose 4–6 mcg/kg, lockout 5–15 min
- Epidural dose: 1–2 mg diluted in 5–10 cc preservative-free saline

ONSET
- IV 1–5 min
- IM 10 min

KINETICS
- Hepatic & renal elimination
- Peak effect 5–10 min; IV duration 2–4 h, IM 30–60 min
- Epidural action 3–4 h

PREPARATION
- Mixed w/ normal saline for IV use & preservative-free solutions for epidural use

MECHANISM
- Synthetic opioid agonist-antagonist
- Opioid agonist effect at kappa receptor
- Partial agonist/antagonist effect at mu receptor
- Relative potency 5 times that of morphine, 35 times that of meperidine
- Causes analgesia & sedation

COMMENTS
- Ceiling effect on respiratory depression at 30–60 mcg/kg

- Excessive sedation or respiratory depression can be countered by naloxone.
- Decreases opioid agonist effectiveness
- Can precipitate withdrawal in the opioid-dependent pt
- Additive sedation w/ droperidol, barbiturates
- Can cause slight increase in BP, cardiac output
- Side effects: itching, nausea/vomiting, excessive sedation, respiratory depression, hypertension, palpations, euphoria
- Risk of biliary spasm present but less than morphine or fentanyl
- Decrease dose by 50% for GFR <10 mL/min, decrease by 25% for GFR 10–50 mL/min.
- Reduce dose in severe liver disease

CALCIUM CHLORIDE & CALCIUM GLUCONATE

SAMIR DZANKIC, MD

INDICATION
- Hypocalcemia
- Hyperkalemia
- Hypermagnesemia
- Need for inotrope (eg, hypotension)

DOSE
- 5–10 mL of 10% calcium chloride (500–1,000 mg) IV
- 5–20 mL of 10% calcium gluconate (500–2,000 mg) IV

ONSET
- Immediate

KINETICS
- Partially eliminated by GI tract & kidney. Taken up by many tissues, including bone.

PREPARATION
- Calcium chloride comes as 10% in 10 mL.
- Calcium gluconate comes as 10% in 10 or 50 mL.

MECHANISM
- Improved excitation–contraction coupling in cardiac muscle. Essential to the function of many enzymes.

COMMENTS
- Increases risk of dysrhythmias in digitalized pts
- Antagonizes calcium channel blockers
- Contraindicated for cardiac resuscitation in the presence of VF or in hypercalcemia
- Consider dose reduction in severe renal failure (creatinine clearance <25 mL/min).
- Rapid infusion of large bolus of calcium chloride may cause decreased blood pressure, cardiac arrhythmias, or sinus arrest.
- Risk of skin necrosis w/ extravasation
  - ➤ Do NOT administer IM.

CAPTOPRIL

SAMIR DZANKIC, MD

INDICATION
- HTN
- CHF
- Post-MI left ventricular dysfunction

DOSE
- Typical dose: 25–50 mg PO TID
- Max dose 450 mg/day in divided doses

ONSET
- 15 min

KINETICS
- Peak effect at 60–90 min
- Duration of effect dependent on dose
- Serum half-life <2 h
- Metabolized to disulfide in liver
- Renal clearance

PREPARATION
- Tablets: 12.5, 25, 50, 100 mg

MECHANISM
- By blocking conversion of angiotensin I to angiotensin II, ACE inhibitors prevent angiotensin II-mediated vasoconstriction. Renin secretion increases while aldosterone levels decrease.

COMMENTS

- ACE inhibitor therapy may predispose to hypotension during general anesthesia that may be less responsive to conventional therapy.
  - ➤ Consider whether to stop ACE inhibitor therapy prior to surgery.
- Drug interactions: potentiates hypotensive effect of anesthetics; elevates digoxin level; enhances hemodynamic effect of vasodilators, calcium channel blockers, beta blockers
- Side effects: cough, upper respiratory tract congestion, rhinorrhea, proteinuria, neutropenia, rash, angioneurotic edema, hyperkalemia, taste disturbance
- May cause acute renal failure in pts w/ severe bilateral renal artery stenosis or stenosis of artery to the solitary kidney

---

CEFAZOLIN (KEFZOL, ANCEF)

MARK ROLLINS, MD

INDICATION

- Broad-spectrum antimicrobial therapy, surgical wound infection prophylaxis, endocarditis prophylaxis
- First-generation cephalosporin
- Most active against gram-positive aerobic cocci (except enterococci)
- Moderately active against certain gram-negative rods: *Klebsiella, E. coli, Proteus, Shigella*

DOSE

- IV dose should be given over 3–5 min.
- Surgical prophylaxis: 1–2 g 30 min prior to incision. For long procedures an additional 0.5–1 g IM/IV may be given.
- Adult: usual dose 1 g IV/IM q8h to 1.5 g IV/IM q6h; max adult dose 12 g/day
- Renal impairment
  - ➤ Cr clearance 35–54 or Cr 1.6–3.0: full doses w/ 8 h minimum intervals
  - ➤ Cr clearance 11–34 or Cr 3.1–4.5: half usual dose q12h
  - ➤ Cr clearance <10 or Cr >4.6: half usual dose q18–24h
- Pediatric: usual dose 25–50 mg/kg daily divided into 3–4 equal IV/IM doses
- Typical pediatric dose for surgical prophylaxis is 25 mg/kg IV
- For severe infections 50–100 mg/kg daily divided into 3–4 equal IV/IM doses

ONSET
N/A

KINETICS
- Serum half-life: 1.8 h w/ normal renal function
- Peak serum levels after IM administration in 1–2 h
- Renal excretion of unchanged drug

PREPARATION
- For IV, 1 g powder; reconstitute w/ H_2O, D_5W, or NS
- For IM, reconstitute 500 mg or 1 g powder w/ 2 or 2.5 mL fluid, respectively

MECHANISM
- A bactericidal beta-lactam antibiotic that interferes w/ bacterial cell wall (peptidoglycan) synthesis

COMMENTS
- Thrombophlebitis in 1–2% of pts
- Allergic reaction 1–3%, usually rash; anaphylaxis rare (<0.02%)
- Consider avoiding in pts w/ Hx of penicillin sensitivity.
- One of the most commonly administered prophylactic antibiotics in surgery

CEFTAZIDIME

MARK ROLLINS, MD

INDICATION
- Third-generation cephalosporin
- Active against many gram-negative organisms, including *Pseudomonas aeruginosa*
- Decreased activity against gram-positive organisms compared to first-generation cephalosporins

DOSE
- Adult: usual dose 1 g IV/IM q8–12h
  - For meningitis, 2 g IV q8h
  - For pulmonary *Pseudomonas*, 30–50 mg/kg IV q8h
  - Max adult dose 6 g/day
- Adult dose in renal impairment
  - Cr clearance 31–50: 1 g q12h
  - Cr clearance 16–30: 1 g q24h
  - Cr clearance 6–15: 500 mg q12h
  - Cr clearance 5 or less: 500 mg q48h

- Pediatric: usual adult dose for children 12 & older
  - Usual dose for 1 mo to 12 y: 25–50 mg/kg IV q8h
  - For meningitis or *Pseudomonas*, 50 mg/kg IV q8h
  - Max dose 6 g/day

ONSET
N/A

KINETICS
- Serum half-life 1.8 h w/ normal renal function
- Peak serum levels after IM administration in 1 h
- No metabolism
- Primarily renal excretion of unchanged drug

PREPARATION
- For IV: 1 g reconstituted w/ 5–10 mL sterile water
- For IM: reconstitute 500 mg or 1 g w/ 1.5 or 3.0 mL sterile H_2O, respectively

MECHANISM
- A bactericidal beta-lactam drug that interferes w/ bacterial cell wall peptidoglycan synthesis

COMMENTS
- Thrombophlebitis in 1–2% of pts
- Allergic reaction 1–3%; usually rash; anaphylaxis rare (<0.02%)
- Caution in pts w/ history of penicillin sensitivity

CEFTRIAXONE (ROCEPHIN)

MARK ROLLINS, MD

INDICATION
- Third-generation cephalosporin
- Most active against gram-negative organisms
- Decreased activity against gram-positive organisms compared to first-generation cephalosporins

DOSE
- Surgical prophylaxis: 1 g IV 0.5–2 h prior to incision
- Adult: usual dose 1–2 g IV/IM once daily
  - For meningitis, 2 g IV q12h
  - Max adult dose 4 g/day
- Pediatric: usual adult dose for children 12 & older

> Usual dose for age 1 wk to 12 y is 50–75 mg/kg IV qd or divided q12h dosing, w/ 2 g/day max.
> For meningitis, 100 mg/kg IV qd or divided q12h dosing, 4 g/day max

ONSET
N/A

KINETICS
- Serum half-life: 8.5 h
- Peak serum levels after IM administration in 1.5–4 h
- Both renal & biliary excretion of unchanged drug

PREPARATION
- For IV, reconstitute powder (comes as 250 mg, 500 mg, 1 g, 2 g)
- For IM, reconstitute to concentration of 250 mg/mL w/ NS or H_2O

MECHANISM
- A bactericidal beta-lactam drug that interferes w/ bacterial cell wall peptidoglycan synthesis

COMMENTS
- Thrombophlebitis in 1–2% of pts
- Allergic reaction 1–3%, usually rash; anaphylaxis rare (<0.02%)
- Consider avoiding in pts w/ Hx of penicillin sensitivity
- Commonly used for prophylaxis prior to neurosurgical procedures

CEFUROXIME

MARK ROLLINS, MD

INDICATION
- Second-generation cephalosporin
- Activity against gram-positive organisms similar to first-generation cephalosporins w/ increased activity against gram-negative organisms, but narrower in spectrum than third-generation drugs
- Often used for prophylaxis in cardiac surgery pts
- Active against *E. coli, Enterobacter, Klebsiella, Neisseria*
- Inactive against enterococci, *Pseudomonas*

DOSE
- Surgical prophylaxis: 1.5 g IV, 0.5–1 h prior to incision; in lengthy operations an additional 750 mg IV q8h
- Adult: usual dose 750–1,500 mg IV/IM q8h
  > Max dose for meningitis: 3 g IV q8h

- Renal dosing
  - ➤ Cr clearance 10–20: 750 mg IV/IM q12h
  - ➤ Cr clearance <10: 750 mg IV/IM q24h
- Pediatric: usual adult dose for children 13 & older
  - ➤ Usual dose for 3 months to 13 years: 50–100 mg/kg/day IV/IM divided q6–8h dosing
  - ➤ For meningitis, 200–240 mg/kg/day IV divided q6–8h

ONSET

N/A

KINETICS

- Serum half-life: 1.3 h
- Peak serum levels after IM administration in 15–60 min
- No metabolism
- Excreted unchanged in urine

PREPARATION

- For IV: reconstituted as 100 mg/mL
- For IM: reconstitute 750 mg w/ 3.0–3.5 mL sterile H_2O

MECHANISM

- A bactericidal beta-lactam drug that interferes w/ bacterial cell wall peptidoglycan synthesis

COMMENTS

- Thrombophlebitis in 1–2% of pts
- Allergic reaction 1–3%; usually rash; anaphylaxis rare (<0.02%)
- Caution in pts w/ history of penicillin sensitivity

CHLORPROMAZINE (THORAZINE)

JEREMY NUSSBAUMER, MD

INDICATION

- Psychotic disorders
- Behavioral problems
- Nausea/vomiting
- Preop anxiety
- Treatment of intractable hiccups

DOSE

- Adult
  - ➤ 25–50 mg IV or 0.5–1.0 mg/kg IV QD-QID

- ➤ 10–25 mg PO q4–6h for nausea/vomiting
- ➤ 25–50 mg PO TID for intractable hiccups
- ➤ 12.5–25 mg IM or 25–50 mg PO 2–3 h prior to surgery as a premed for anxiety
- ■ Children
  - ➤ 0.55 mg/kg IV q6–8h
  - ➤ 0.25 mg/lb PO q4–6h
  - ➤ 0.25 mg/lb IM q6–8h

ONSET
- ■ IV 5 min, peak in 10 min
- ■ PO 30 min
- ■ IM 10 min

KINETICS
- ■ Duration: 4–8 h
- ■ Elimination half-life: 10–30 h
- ■ Hepatic metabolism
- ■ Renal excretion

PREPARATION
- ■ Dilute to 1 mg/mL w/ NS & give at rate <0.5 mg/min.

MECHANISM
- ■ Mechanism of antipsychotic action involves central dopaminergic receptor (DA-2, DA-1) blockade.
- ■ Also has strong alpha-adrenergic blockade & anticholinergic actions

COMMENTS
- ■ Adverse effects include
  - ➤ Orthostatic hypotension, tachycardia, drowsiness
  - ➤ Hepatotoxicity
  - ➤ Extrapyramidal symptoms, including acute dystonic reactions
    - • May require urgent treatment w/ diphenhydramine, benztropine or other anticholinergic
  - ➤ Can cause neuroleptic malignant syndrome
  - ➤ May precipitate narrow-angle glaucoma attack
  - ➤ Agranulocytosis, bone marrow depression, anemia (typically with longer-term PO therapy)
  - ➤ Lowering of seizure threshold
- ■ May have exaggerated CNS effects when combined w/ CNS depressants

- Use w/ caution in pts w/ hepatic disease.
- Consider decreasing dose by 1/2 to 1/3 in the elderly & pts w/ renal failure.

CIMETIDINE

JASON WIDRICH, MD
EMILY REINYS, MD

INDICATION
- Peptic ulcer
- Gastric acid hypersecretion
- Reduction of gastric pH & volume for prophylaxis against aspiration

DOSE
- 300 mg IV/IM/PO

ONSET
- IV: <45 min

KINETICS
- Metabolism: hepatic
- Elimination primarily renal, some biliary elimination
- Peak effect in 60–90 min
- Duration of action 4 h IV

PREPARATION
- 150 mg/mL for injection

MECHANISM
- Competitive inhibitor of H2 receptors, decreasing gastric acid secretion.
- Gastric acid that is secreted after administration of drug will have higher pH.

COMMENTS
- Cimetidine affects the cytochrome P450 sytem in the liver, which may inhibit the metabolism of many other drugs, such as benzodiazepines, caffeine, labetalol, lidocaine, calcium channel blockers, theophylline, sulfonylureas, Coumadin.
- Adverse effects: hypotension w/ rapid administration, confusion, somnolence, bronchospasm, thrombocytopenia.

CISATRACURIUM

RONNIE LU, MD

INDICATION
- Neuromuscular block

DOSE
- Intubation: 0.1–0.15 mg/kg
- Maintenance: 0.05 mg/kg then 0.01 mg/kg q15–20min
- Infusion: 1–2 mcg/kg/min

ONSET
- 3–5 min

KINETICS
- Duration 20–35 min
- Metabolism by Hofmann elimination, independent of renal & hepatic function

PREPARATION
- 2-mg/mL solution
- 10-mg/mL solution

MECHANISM
- Nondepolarizing neuromuscular block
- Competes w/ acetylcholine at nicotinic receptor site on motor endplate

COMMENTS
- Single isomer of atracurium
- Low risk of histamine release

CLINDAMYCIN (CLEOCIN)

JEREMY NUSSBAUMER, MD

INDICATION
- Treatment or prophylaxis of bacterial infection due to susceptible organisms including staphylococci & aerobic & anaerobic streptococci
  - ➢ Does not cover enterococci

➤ Limited gram-negative coverage
➤ Can be used for bacterial endocarditis prophylaxis in penicillin-allergic pts

DOSE
- Adults: 600–900 mg IV q6–8h
- Children: 20–40 mg/kg/d IV divided q6–8h

ONSET
- Rapid

KINETICS
- Duration: variable
- Elimination half-life: 2–3 h
- Metabolism: hepatic

PREPARATION
- 150 mg/mL for injection
- Recommended infusion rate <30 mg/min w/ concentration >18 mg/mL

MECHANISM
- Inhibits protein synthesis by binding bacterial ribosomal S50 sub-units

COMMENTS
- May potentiate neuromuscular blocking drugs
- Can lead to pseudomembranous colitis
- Presumed safe in pregnancy

CLONIDINE

MARK ROLLINS, MD

INDICATION
- HTN mgt
- Epidural infusion for cancer pain refractory to opiates
- Anesthetic adjunct (reduces anesthetic requirement)
- Mgt of opiate withdrawal
- Migraine prophylaxis
- Many unlabeled uses (eg, severe pain, dysmenorrhea)

DOSE
- HTN
  - PO
    - Initial adult dose: 0.05–0.1 mg PO bid
    - Increase by 0.1–0.2 mg daily until desired pressure achieved
    - Max dose 2.4 mg/day
    - Use 50–75% usual dose for Cr clearance <10 mL/min.
  - Transdermal
    - Initially, 0.1 mg/day patch applied each week
    - Weekly dosing adjustments up to 0.6 mg/day
- Cancer pain
  - Initial adult dose 30 mcg/h by continuous epidural infusion
  - Pediatric dose 0.5 mcg/kg/h by continuous epidural infusion

ONSET
- After PO administration, BP begins to decrease in 30–60 min w/ maximal effect after 2–4 h.
- Transdermal patch produces therapeutic plasma levels 2–3 days after initial placement.

KINETICS
- Serum half-life: 6–20 h
- Peak serum concentrations 3–5 h after oral dosing
- Peak serum concentration approx 20 min after an epidural bolus
- Excreted in urine
- Metabolized by the liver (50%)

PREPARATION
- Oral tablets: 0.1, 0.2, 0.3 mg
- Transdermal systems: 0.1, 0.2, 0.3 mg/day
- Parenteral: 100 mcg/mL preservative-free

MECHANISM
- Alpha-2 adrenergic agonist
- Acts centrally to inhibit peripheral vasomotor tone, decreasing peripheral & renovascular resistance
- Inhibits ascending pain pathways by stimulating alpha-2 adrenergic postsynaptic receptors in the dorsal horn of the spinal cord
- Stimulates acetylcholine release & inhibits substance P release

COMMENTS
- Side effects: sedation, dry mouth, respiratory depression, bradycardia, decreased GI motility.

- Epidural dosing can be accompanied by decreased HR & BP.
- Cessation of oral clonidine can result in rebound hypertension. Dosing should be tapered over 2–4 days to minimize this effect.
- Clonidine may decrease both anesthetic & analgesic requirements & potentiate action of other CNS depressants.
- Hypotensive effect inhibited by tolazoline & tricyclic antidepressants.
- Epidural clonidine may prolong blockade from other epidural local anesthetics.

COCAINE

JASON LICHTENSTEIN, MD

INDICATION
- Topical anesthesia of oral, laryngeal, or nasal mucosa

DOSE
- Varies; depends upon
  - Area to be anesthetized
  - Anesthetic technique used
- Usual dose is 4% solution topically, with maximum dose of 1–3 mg/kg

ONSET
- Rapid

KINETICS
- Plasma half-life approx 1 h
- Metabolism: hepatic
- Excretion: renal

PREPARATION
- 4%, 10% aqueous solutions

MECHANISM
- Has local anesthetic effect from blockade of sodium channels
- Blocks presynaptic uptake of norepinephrine. This leads to sympathetic nervous system stimulation, including vasoconstriction.

COMMENTS
- Provides both local anesthesia & localized vasoconstriction to reduce bleeding
- May be habit-forming
- Can cause HTN, coronary artery vasoconstriction, dysrhythmias

COX-2 INHIBITORS (ROFECOXIB, CELECOXIB, VALDECOXIB, VIOXX, CELEBREX, BEXTRA)

GERALD DUBOWITZ, MB CHB

INDICATION
- Pain relief
- Pain assoc w/ osteoarthritis, rheumatoid arthritis, headache, dysmenorrhea

DOSE
- Celecoxib (Celebrex)
  - 100–200 mg PO q24h
    - 100 mg, 200 mg reported to have similar effects, but 200 mg appears better for acute pain
- Rofecoxib (Vioxx)
  - 12.5–50 mg PO q24h
    - 50 mg equivalent to 500 mg naproxen or 400 mg ibuprofen
- Valdecoxib (Bextra)
  - 10–20 mg PO bid

ONSET
- In surgical pain, relief within 60 min

KINETICS
- Rofecoxib half-life approx 17 h
- Celecoxib half-life approx 11 h
- Metabolism mediated by cytochrome P450
- Inactive metabolites
- Excreted by hepatic metabolism
- <3% unchanged in urine & feces
- Crosses placenta & blood-brain barrier in animal models

PREPARATION
- Oral preparations
  - Celecoxib (Celebrex)
    - 100-, 200-mg tablets
  - Rofecoxib (Vioxx)
    - 12.5-, 25-, 50-mg tablets
    - Oral suspension 12.5 mg or 25 mg in 5 mL
  - Valdecoxib (Bextra)
    - 10-, 20-mg tablets

MECHANISM
- NSAID
- Anti-inflammatory, antipyretic activity
- Inhibition of prostaglandin synthesis via inhibition of cyclooxygenase-2 (COX-2)
- Does not inhibit cyclooxygenase-1

COMMENTS
- No effect on platelets or bleeding time.
  - Therefore, regional anesthesia not contraindicated.
- Typically the full analgesic effect does not last 24 h.
- Less gastric side effects (including bleeding), although they can still occur.
- IV preparation may become available in the future.
- May cause fluid retention, peripheral edema, hypertension.

CYCLOSPORINE

JEREMY NUSSBAUMER, MD

INDICATION
- Immunosuppressant for organ transplant
- Severe autoimmune disease, such as
  - Rheumatoid arthritis
  - Psoriasis
  - Aplastic anemia
  - Ulcerative colitis

DOSE
- Should be based on ideal body weight
- PO dose is about 3x IV dose.
- IV 5–6 mg/kg 4–12 h before organ transplant, then 2–10 mg/kg/day divided bid to tid
- Dose adjusted to therapeutic blood levels
- PO dose for organ rejection prophylaxis: 15 mg/kg/day
- Rheumatoid arthritis typical dose: 2.5 mg/kg/day divided bid

ONSET
- PO onset in 1–2 h

KINETICS
- Hepatic metabolism

- Eliminated in bile
- Elimination half-life 8 h

PREPARATION
- Oral caplets
- IV formulation
  - For IV administration, dilute in 20–100 mL NS or D5W & administer over 2–6 h.

MECHANISM
- Cyclic polypeptide immunosuppressant
- Inhibits production & release of IL-2 & IL-2 activation of lymphocytes

COMMENTS
- Different oral preparations have different bioavailability (Neoral vs Sandimmune).
- Associated w/ hyperkalemia in renal transplant pts
- Hepatic toxicity may occur.
  - Usually causes mild cholestasis
- HTN common side effect
- Nephrotoxicity common
- Neuro complications of therapy
  - Tremor (common)
  - Headache
  - Seizures
  - Paresthesias
  - Confusion, encephalopathy
- Increases susceptibility to infection
- Long-term use may predispose to lymphoma.
- Can cause hirsutism

DANTROLENE (DANTRIUM)

JOHN TAYLOR, MD

INDICATION
- Treatment of malignant hyperthermia (MH)
- Treatment of neuroleptic malignant syndrome (NMS) – unlabeled use
- Skeletal muscle relaxant used to treat spasticity assoc w/ neural injury (eg, spinal cord injury)

DOSE
- MH: 2.5 mg/kg IV; may repeat dose up to a total of 10 mg/kg
- Continue administration until symptoms subside.
- Repeat regimen if MH symptoms reappear.
- Prophylaxis: 2.5 mg/kg IV over 1 h prior to anesthesia
- Post-crisis: 4–8 mg/kg/day in 4 divided doses administered for 1–3 days
- NMS: same as MH dosing

ONSET
- IV: <5 min
- PO: 1–2 h

KINETICS
- Metabolism: hepatic
- Half-life: 7–9 h
- Elimination: urine 25%; bile 50%
- Absorption: PO absorption is slow

PREPARATION
- Powder for injection: 20-mg vial reconstituted in 60 mL sterile water for injection (do not use bacteriostatic water for injection, 5% dextrose or saline solution)
- 25-mg, 50-mg, 100-mg capsules for PO use

MECHANISM
- Relaxes skeletal muscle by inhibiting calcium release from the sarcoplasmic reticulum

COMMENTS
- No contraindications when MH is suspected
- Relative contraindication for other uses: active hepatic disease

---

DDAVP (DESMOPRESSIN)

ANNE NOONEY, MD

INDICATION
- Neurogenic diabetes insipidus (DI)
- Mild hemophilia A (factor VIII deficiency)
  - ➤ Pt w/ >5% factor VIII activity
- Mild to moderate von Willebrand's disease (vWD)

- Hemostatic agent
  - Uremic bleeding
  - Major surgery (eg, cardiac): controversial benefit

DOSE
- Intranasal
  - For DI: 10–40 mcg
  - For hemophilia or vWD: 300 mcg
- IV
  - For DI: 2–4 mcg/day, usually in 2 doses
  - For hemophilia or vWD: 0.3 mcg/kg over 15–30 min (can also be given SC)
  - Hemostatic agent: 0.3 mcg/kg

ONSET
- 30 min from start of infusion (hemostatic effects)
- 1 h for antidiuretic effects

KINETICS
- Duration of hemostatic effects: approx 200 min
- Elimination half-life: 75 min

PREPARATION
- IV: 4, 15 mcg/mL
  - For IV use, dilute w/ 10–50 mL NS.
  - Store at 2–8 degrees C.
- Nasal: 10 mcg per inhalation
- PO: tablets: 0.1, 0.2 mg
  - PO dose used for DI
  - Not likely to be used during anesthesia care

MECHANISM
- Synthetic vasopressin analog
- Increases factors VIII & XII & von Willebrand levels by releasing them from vascular endothelium

COMMENTS
- Tachyphylaxis has been observed w/ multiple doses.
- Not recommended w/ factor VIII levels <5%
- Has been assoc w/ hypotension or slight HTN
  - Hypotension may be more common in post-bypass period.
  - Do not administer by rapid IV bolus.
- Can cause hyponatremia, seizures

➤ Symptoms can include headache, nausea, vomiting, altered mental status.
➤ Follow electrolytes & fluid balance carefully, esp in children & elderly.
■ Compared to vasopressin, desmopressin has a longer duration of action & fewer side effects.

DESFLURANE

ANTHONY ROMO, MD
EDMOND I EGER II, MD

INDICATION
■ Maintenance of GA

DOSE
■ MAC (in O_2): 9% (infants & children), 6% (30–60 years), 4.5% (80 years)
■ MAC-awake: one third of MAC
■ MAC-BAR: 9% (opioids markedly decrease)

ONSET
■ Seconds-minutes

KINETICS
■ Metabolism: 0.02% of desflurane taken up
  ➤ Lowest of all potent inhaled anesthetics
■ Elimination: pulmonary
■ Uptake
  ➤ Small relative to alveolar concentration because of low blood/gas (0.45) & tissue/gas partition coefficients (smallest of all potent inhaled anesthetics). Thus, the alveolar (end-tidal) concentration closely follows the inspired concentration, permitting close control of the anesthetic state & rapid recovery (most rapid among potent inhaled anesthetics; may lead to earlier OR & PACU discharge).
  ➤ Low uptake facilitates use of low-flow/closed-circuit anesthesia.
  ➤ Induction marred by respiratory irritation at concentrations >6% (MAC in 30- to 60-year-old pts)

PREPARATION
■ Clear, colorless nonflammable liquid (243–245 mL) in amber-colored bottles
■ No preservative required

MECHANISM

- Unclear
- Plausible basis: In vitro, volatile inhaled anesthetics enhance inhibitory channel (GABA, glycine, potassium) responses & block excitatory channel (glutamate, acetylcholine, sodium) responses.
  - ➤ However, these effects do not necessarily translate into mechanistic effects (eg, blockade of acetylcholine receptors does not decrease MAC).

COMMENTS

- Degradation by carbon dioxide absorbents
  - ➤ None in normal (wet) absorbent, even at higher temps (eg, closed circuit)
  - ➤ Degraded by desiccated absorbents to carbon monoxide
- Causes profound, dose-related muscle relaxation & enhances the effect of muscle relaxants; elimination decreases the effect of residual relaxants
- Side effects
  - ➤ Airway irritation
    - This occurs w/ concentrations >6% w/ coughing, breath-holding, laryngospasm & salivation on induction of anesthesia.
    - Irritation markedly decreased by administration of small doses of opioid & is less or no problem during maintenance.
    - When administered via LMA, desflurane does not produce more evidence of respiratory irritation than other inhaled anesthetics.
    - Irritation can produce desaturation during induction of anesthesia in infants & young children.
  - ➤ Transient tachycardia & hypertension
    - Increases in concentration >6%, particularly on induction of anesthesia, can cause transient (4–6 min) increases in HR & BP, esp w/ rapid increases in concentration.
    - Effect minimized by staying below 6%, by administration of small doses of opioid (eg, 100 mcg fentanyl) & by slowly increasing the concentration >6%
  - ➤ Higher concentrations depress heart/breathing (decrease BP, cardiac output & contractility; sustain systemic vascular resistance; increase $PaCO_2$), but no ventricular ectopy.
  - ➤ In 1- to 5-year-old children, recovery assoc w/ agitation (minimized by use of opioids or ketorolac)
  - ➤ Hypothermia
    - As w/ other inhaled anesthetics, desflurane decreases the set point for response to decreases in body temp.

➤ Like other potent inhaled agents, desflurane can trigger malignant hyperthermia; less potent trigger than halothane.
➤ Causes nausea/vomiting
➤ Desflurane's boiling point of 22.8 degrees C mandates use of a special (heated) vaporizer (Ohmeda Tec 6 vaporizer or ADU vaporizer).

■ Comparisons w/ other inhaled anesthetics
  ➤ Advantages
    • Lowest solubility & most rapid recovery
    • Greatest control over anesthetic state
    • Potentially earlier OR/PACU discharge
    • Greatest resistance to biodegradation or degradation by normal absorbents
    • Can use at low/closed-circuit inflow rates (most economical)
    • No ventricular ectopy
    • Produces muscle relaxation
    • Greatest capacity to protect against transient myocardial ischemia
  ➤ Disadvantages
    • At concentrations >6% it is a respiratory irritant & transient cardiovascular stimulant.
    • Postop agitation in preschool children
    • High acquisition cost
    • Degraded by desiccated absorbents to carbon monoxide

DEXAMETHASONE (DECADRON)

J. W. BEARD, MD

INDICATION
■ Long-acting corticosteroid to treat
  ➤ Cerebral edema
  ➤ Nausea/vomiting
  ➤ Inflammation

DOSE
■ Cerebral edema: 10 mg IV initial, then 4 mg IV q6h
■ Antiemetic
  ➤ Prophylaxis: 2.5–10 mg IV
  ➤ Treatment: 2–4 mg IV

ONSET
- Minutes

KINETICS
- Duration: up to 72 h
- Elimination half-life: 1.8–3.5 h in pts w/ normal renal function
- Elimination: renal, biliary
- Metabolism: hepatic

PREPARATION
- Available as 4, 10, 20 mg/mL & other concentrations for injection

MECHANISM
- Decreases inflammation by decreasing leukocyte migration. Has immune suppressive effects.

COMMENTS
- Pts w/ long-term steroid use may require stress doses during surgery.
- Steroids may lead to changes in glucose & lipid levels.
- Abrupt withdrawal of steroids may result in adrenal insufficiency or addisonian crisis (refractory hypotension & hyperkalemia may be seen).

DEXMEDETOMIDINE

MIMI C. LEE, MD, PHD

INDICATION
- IV anesthetic adjunct

DOSE
- Adult: 1 mcg/kg IV over 10–15 min, then 0.2–0.7 mcg/kg/hr or to therapeutic plasma levels of 0.4–1.2 ng/mL

ONSET
- 20–30 min

KINETICS
- Duration: 4 h
- Elimination half-life: 2.0–2.5 h
- Metabolism: liver & B-lymphoblastoid microsomal enzymes
- Excreted in urine

PREPARATION
- 100 mcg/mL

MECHANISM
- Selective alpha-2 agonist
- Decreases sympathetic nervous system activity (reduces plasma norepinephrine concentration)
- Yields analgesia, anxiolysis, hemodynamic stability, anti-shivering effects, antiemetic effects
- Sedation mediated at locus ceruleus

COMMENTS
- May cause bradycardia, hypotension
- Decreases MAC for inhalational agents
- Reduces postop opioid requirements
- Decreases cerebral blood flow w/o significantly altering cerebral O_2 metabolic rate ($CMRO_2$)
- Decreases cerebral blood flow & cerebral perfusion pressure w/o significantly altering ICP
- Decreases intraocular pressure
- Decreases opioid-induced rigidity during anesthesia induction

DIAZEPAM

JEREMY NUSSBAUMER, MD

INDICATION
- Sedation
- Treatment of
  - Anxiety
  - ETOH withdrawal
  - Status epilepticus

DOSE
- PO dosing more reliable than IM
- Adult
  - IV/IM 2–10 mg q3–4h prn
  - PO 2–10 mg q3–4h prn
  - For status epilepticus 5–10 mg IV q10–20min up to 30 mg in 8 h
- Children
  - IV/IM 0.04–0.2 mg/kg/dose q2–4h prn up to 0.6 mg/kg q8h
  - PO conscious sedation 0.2–0.3 mg/kg approx 1 h before procedure

ONSET
- IV: rapid
- PO: 25–60 min

KINETICS
- 20–50 h half-life in adults.
- Hepatic metabolism produces an active compound (desmethyl-diazepam) w/ 50–100 h half-life.
  - ➤ Use w/ caution in pts w/ hepatic impairment.

PREPARATION
- IV: 5 mg/mL
- PO: 2-, 5-, 10-mg tablets

MECHANISM
- Enhances GABA-A activity in CNS

COMMENTS
- Use w/ caution secondary to long-acting metabolite.
- Watch for exaggerated effects when used w/ opioids or other CNS depressants.
- Half-life is prolonged in the elderly; avoid use if possible.
- Contraindicated in pregnancy.
- Abrupt withdrawal can lead to seizures.

DIGOXIN (LANOXIN)

ALICIA GRUBER, MD

INDICATION
- CHF
- Atrial fibrillation/flutter, SVT (rate control)

DOSE
- Loading: 0.5–1.5 mg/day in 3 divided doses
- Maintenance: 0.125–0.5 mg QD

ONSET
- 5–30 min

KINETICS
- Well absorbed orally; 10% of individuals harbor enteric bacteria that inactivate digoxin in the gut, greatly reducing bioavailability
- Not extensively metabolized, excreted unchanged by the kidneys

■ Clearance correlates closely w/ creatinine clearance.
■ Elimination half-life: 40 h

PREPARATION
■ PO: 0.125-, 0.25-, 0.5-mg tablets
■ Parenteral: 0.1, 0.25 mg/mL

MECHANISM
■ Mechanical effects: Inhibits Na/K ATPase indirectly leading to a reduction of calcium expulsion from the cell by the sodium-calcium exchanger. Net result: increased cardiac contractility.
■ Electrical effects: At lower portion of dose range, cardioselective parasympathomimetic (atropine-like effect w/ delayed conduction through the AV node, prolongation of the PR interval). At toxic levels, sympathetic outflow is increased.

COMMENTS
■ Serum concentrations of potassium, calcium, & magnesium have important effects on sensitivity to digitalis. Hypokalemia, hypercalcemia, & hypomagnesemia increase the risk of a digitalis-induced arrhythmia.
■ Digoxin affects all excitable tissue, including smooth muscle & the CNS.
■ GI tract most common site of digoxin toxicity outside of the heart (anorexia, nausea, vomiting, diarrhea).
■ Most common cardiac manifestations include junctional rhythm, PVCs, bigeminy, second-degree AV block; however, digoxin can cause every variety of arrhythmia.
■ If digoxin toxicity is suspected, draw & correct underlying electrolyte abnormalities & send a digoxin level. For occasional PVCs or brief runs of bigeminy, oral potassium & withdrawal of the digoxin may be sufficient. For severe digoxin intoxication, pts are best treated w/ "Fab fragments" of digitalis antibody (Digibind).

DILTIAZEM (CARDIZEM)

DAN WAJSMAN, MD

INDICATION
■ Atrial fibrillation or atrial flutter
■ Paroxysmal supraventricular tachycardias

- Hypertension
- Angina

DOSE
- 0.25 mg/kg IV (usual adult dose: 15–20 mg) over 2 min
- Maintenance infusion: 5–15 mg/h

ONSET
- Within 3 min

KINETICS
- Duration: 1–3 h
- Elimination half-life: 3–4 h
- Cytochrome P450 metabolism
- Renal, biliary excretion

PREPARATION
- 5 mg/mL for injection

MECHANISM
- Inhibits the influx of calcium across the cell membrane of arterial smooth muscle, conductile & contractile myocardial cells. This dilates arterioles, slows nodal conduction & decreases cardiac contractility.

COMMENTS
- Avoid in wide complex tachycardia unless known to be supraventricular.
- Avoid in second- & third-degree AV block unless paced.
- Avoid in severe congestive heart failure.
- Avoid in pts w/ accessory bypass tracts, WPW or Lown-Ganong-Levine.
- Contraindicated for ventricular tachycardias.

DIPHENHYDRAMINE (BENADRYL)

MADELEINE BIBAT, MD

INDICATION
- Allergic reaction
- Urticaria, angioedema
- Anaphylaxis
- Sedation

- Antiemetic
- Treatment of drug-induced extrapyramidal reactions (eg, dystonic reaction)

DOSE
- Adult: 10–50 mg IV q4–6h. For dystonic reactions, 50 mg IV & repeat in 20–30 min if needed.
- Pediatric: 5 mg/kg/day IV divided q6h, max 300 mg.

ONSET
- <30 min

KINETICS
- Peak: 2–4 h
- Duration: 4–6 h
- Elimination half-life: 2 h
- Hepatic metabolism
- Renal excretion

PREPARATION
- 10, 50 mg/mL for injection

MECHANISM
- Histamine antagonist at H1 receptor sites; also binds to cholinergic receptors

COMMENTS
- Additive effects w/ other CNS depressants.
- MAOIs prolong anticholinergic effects.
- Use w/ caution in pts w/ asthma & increased intraocular pressure.
- No analgesic properties.

DOBUTAMINE

ALISON G. CAMERON, MD

INDICATION
- Any low cardiac output state, such as
  - ➤ Cardiac decompensation post-cardiac surgery
  - ➤ CHF
  - ➤ Acute MI

DOSE
- 2–20 mcg/kg/min IV

ONSET
- 1–2 min IV

KINETICS
- Duration: <10 min
- Elimination half-life: 2.4 min
- Metabolized by liver
- Excreted in urine

PREPARATION
- 250 mg in 250 mL D5W for 1-mg/mL dilution

MECHANISM
- Selective beta-1 agonist, w/ minimal beta-2 or alpha agonist actions
- Causes increased inotropy, dose-dependent increase in cardiac output, decreased SVR & PVR, mild chronotropy

COMMENTS
- For short-term use (up to 72 h)
- Avoid in IHSS since increased inotropy & low SVR will worsen CO.
- Avoid in pregnancy since low SVR may affect placental blood flow.
- May cause hypotension from beta-2 receptor-mediated vasodilation
  - ➤ May need to be used in combination w/ a vasoconstrictor (eg, phenylephrine)

DOPAMINE

ALISON G. CAMERON, MD

INDICATION
- Hypotension
- Oliguria

DOSE
- 1–20 mcg/kg/min
  - ➤ Renal vasodilation occurs at 0.5–3.0 mcg/kg/min IV.
  - ➤ HR & contractility increase at 3.0–10.0 mcg/kg/min IV.
  - ➤ Vasoconstriction occurs in the range of 10.0–20.0 mcg/kg/min IV.

ONSET
- <5 min IV

KINETICS
- Duration: 10 min
- Elimination half-life: 2 min
- Metabolized in liver, kidney, plasma
- Excreted in urine

PREPARATION
- 40 mg/mL, 5-mL bottle. Mix 80 mg in 50 cc D5W for 1,600-mcg/cc dilution.

MECHANISM
- Endogenous catecholamine, dose dependently acts via dopamine, beta- & alpha-adrenergic receptors.
- Low doses affect primarily dopamine receptors: increased renal, splanchnic, cerebral, coronary blood flow.
- Higher doses affect dopamine & beta-1 receptors: increased chronotropy & inotropy in addition to vasodilatory effects.
- Highest doses affect alpha-adrenergic receptors & produce vasoconstriction.

COMMENTS
- Unknown safety in pregnancy. Not safe in lactation.
- Evokes release of endogenous norepinephrine stores (predisposes to arrhythmias).
- High doses inhibit the release of insulin & can lead to hyperglycemia.
- Predisposes to arrhythmias w/ halothane.
- Simultaneous use w/ phenytoin may cause seizures.
- Contraindicated w/ pheochromocytoma, tachyarrhythmias.
- IV extravasation may cause tissue necrosis.
- Administration interferes w/ ventilatory response to hypoxemia.
- While low-dose dopamine increases urine production, there is no evidence that it improves renal function or outcome.

DOXACURIUM

JAMES CALDWELL, MB CHB

INDICATION
- Neuromuscular block
- Facilitation of tracheal intubation
- Maintenance of surgical relaxation

DOSE
- 0.05–0.08 mg/kg IV for tracheal intubation
- 0.005–0.01 mg/kg IV to maintain surgical relaxation

ONSET
- 4–5 min

KINETICS
- Metabolism: Does not occur
- Renal excretion: >90%
- Hepatic elimination: <10%
- Elimination half-life: 99 min

Duration
- Intubation dose: 90–150 min
- Maintenance dose: 30–45 min

PREPARATION
- 1 mg/mL solution in 5-mL vial (Nuromax)

MECHANISM
- Competitive antagonist of acetylcholine at neuromuscular junction
- Benzylisoquinolinium compound (atracurium-like)

COMMENTS
- Absence of cardiovascular effects
- Low risk of histamine release
- Very potent relaxant
- Slow onset
- Little role in clinical practice because of slow onset, long duration

DOXAPRAM (DOPRAM)

JEREMY NUSSBAUMER, MD

INDICATION
- Respiratory stimulant
- Can be used for anesthetic-induced respiratory depression

DOSE
- Adult: 0.5–1 mg/kg IV q5min up to 2 mg/kg total dose

ONSET
- 20–40 sec

KINETICS
- Hepatic metabolism
- Peak effect in 1–2 min
- Duration: 5–12 min

PREPARATION
- 20 mg/mL for injection

MECHANISM
- Acts on respiratory centers in medulla or carotid chemoreceptors

COMMENTS
- May cause seizures in higher doses
- Assoc w/ release of catecholamines
- Not a specific antidote to drug-induced respiratory depression
- Does not antagonize neuromuscular blockade
- Not for use in newborns due to benzyl alcohol content

DROPERIDOL (INAPSINE)

ANNE NOONEY, MD
DHANESH K. GUPTA, MD

INDICATION
- Nausea/vomiting
- Sedation
- Because of risk of arrhythmias, use is discouraged.

DOSE
- IV: 10–70 mcg/kg
- Usual antiemetic dose: 0.625–2.5 mg
- Usual sedation dose: 2.5–20 mg

ONSET
- Minutes

KINETICS
- Duration: 3–24 h
- Elimination half-life: 100–130 min
- Metabolism: liver
- Excretion in urine

PREPARATION
- 2.5 mg/mL in NS

MECHANISM
- Antagonizes dopamine receptors

COMMENTS
- New evidence of increased risk of Q-T prolongation & torsades rhythm disturbance has changed the indication & protocol of administration, requiring EKGs before administration & close monitoring after administration.
- Prolonged emergence may be seen in doses >1.25–2.5 mg.
- Combined w/ fentanyl, droperidol produces a state of analgesia, immobilization, & variable amnesia referred to as neuroleptanalgesia.
- Pts may feel anxious/restless/dysphoric despite outwardly calm appearance due to a dissociative state if droperidol is used for sedation. Consider benzodiazepine or diphenhydramine as adjuvant when droperidol is used.
- Contraindicated in pts w/ Parkinson's disease.
- May cause extrapyramidal symptoms; Rx w/ diphenhydramine.
- Mild alpha-adrenergic blocking activity may produce mild hypotension, esp in hypovolemic pts.

---

d-TUBOCURARINE (dTc, CURARE)

DON TAYLOR, MD, PHD

INDICATION
- Neuromuscular block, defasciculation

DOSE
- 0.3–0.6 mg/kg IV initially (divided dosage or slow push recommended due to histamine release), maintenance 10–50% of initial dose, defasciculating dose 3 mg IV (10% of intubating dose), infusion 1–6 mcg/kg/min

ONSET
- 3–5 min IV

KINETICS
- Duration: long-acting relaxant, 80–100 min to 25% recovery
- Elimination: primarily renal, 15–20% biliary excretion (increased in renal failure)

PREPARATION
- Supplied as 3 mg/mL, does not require refrigeration

MECHANISM
- Nondepolarizing neuromuscular block
- Competes w/ acetylcholine at nicotinic receptor site on motor end-plate

COMMENTS
- Histamine release is dose- and rate-dependent & may cause hypotension & tachycardia unless administered slowly (flushing, hives, bronchospasm, urticaria, etc as well).
- Pretreatment for defasciculation may cause diplopia, weakness & decreased vital capacity.
- Ganglionic blockade may cause hypotension.
- Except for defasciculation, little role in clinical practice because of slow onset & long duration.

EDROPHONIUM (REVERSOL, ENLON, TENSILON)

RONNIE LU, MD

INDICATION
- Reversal of neuromuscular block

DOSE
- 0.5–1 mg/kg

ONSET
- 1–2 min

KINETICS
- Duration: <1 h (variable depending on dose)
- Hepatic metabolism
- Renal excretion

PREPARATION
- 10 mg/mL solution

MECHANISM
- Noncovalent (competitive) inhibition of acetylcholinesterase

COMMENTS
- Administer w/ atropine 0.014 mg per 1 mg edrophonium to block muscarinic cholinergic effects.
- Low doses (<0.5 mg/kg) may result in duration of action shorter than that of long-acting muscle relaxants.
- Efficacy limited w/ deep block.

EPHEDRINE

RICHARD PAULSEN, MD

INDICATION
- Hypotension

DOSE
- 5–20 mg IV q5–10min
- 25–50 mg SC/IM

ONSET
- <1 min IV; variable onset IM

KINETICS
- Duration: 10–60 min
- Elimination half-life: 3–6 h
- Hepatic metabolism
- Renal excretion

PREPARATION
- 5 mg/cc in NS (mix one 50-mg/cc ampule w/ 9 cc NS)

MECHANISM
- Indirect-acting sympathomimetic; stimulates endogenous norepinephrine release

COMMENTS
- Affects uterine blood flow minimally
- Preferred pressor for hypotension in OB pt
- May get arrhythmias, esp w/ halogenated anesthetics
- MAOIs potentiate pressor effects

EPINEPHRINE

DAN WAJSMAN, MD

INDICATION
- Refractory hypotension
- Anaphylaxis
- Severe bronchospasm
- Cardiac arrest
- Symptomatic bradycardia
- Add to local anesthetics to prolong duration of action by decreasing absorption.

DOSE
- Cardiac arrest: 1 mg q3–5min; higher doses may be used if this fails
  - Can give intratracheal: 1 mg in adults, 0.1 mg/kg in children
- Bradycardia or hypotension: 1–10 mcg bolus; may infuse 1–10 mcg/min
- Bronchoconstriction
  - Adults: 0.1–0.5 mg SQ (use 1-mg/mL conc)
  - Children: 10 mcg/kg SQ
  - Nebulized: 0.25–0.5 mL racemic epi in 3 cc saline

ONSET
- IV: Rapid
- SQ: 6–15 min
- Inhalation: 1 min

KINETICS
- Duration: <1–4 h
- Metabolism: hepatic
- Excretion: renal, of metabolites

PREPARATION
- 0.1 mg/mL (1:10,000)
- 1 mg/mL (1:1,000)

MECHANISM
- Stimulates alpha-1, beta-1, beta-2 receptors

COMMENTS
- Causes cardiac irritability, usually PVCs
- Can treat accidental administration w/ nitrites or sodium nitroprusside or alpha blockers

ESMOLOL (BREVIBLOC)

CHRISTINE A. WU, MD

INDICATION
- Rapid-onset beta blockade of short duration
  - ➤ Can be used to treat intraop & postop hypertension & tachycardia, or to blunt hemodynamic response to intubation
  - ➤ SVT
  - ➤ Rate control in atrial fibrillation & flutter

DOSE
- Bolus: 0.5–1 mg/kg IV
- Infusion: load w/ 0.5 mg/kg IV over 1 min, followed by an infusion at 50 mcg/kg/min. A repeat loading dose may be given followed by increasing infusion in increments of 50 mcg/kg/min up to 300 mcg/kg/min.

ONSET
- Rapid

KINETICS
- Half-life: 9 min
- Low-potency metabolite w/ half-life of 4 h is excreted in urine & can accumulate w/ long infusions.
- Duration: depends on cumulative dose, typically 10–20 min
- Hydrolyzed by esterases in RBCs

PREPARATION
- IV: 10, 250 mg/mL

MECHANISM
- Beta-1 selective antagonist w/ little sympathomimetic activity & very short duration of action
- Lacks membrane-stabilizing actions

COMMENTS
- If continuous use is likely, substitute beta-blocker w/ longer half-life such as metoprolol.
- Consider smaller initial dose in elderly pts or those w/ impaired cardiovascular function.

ETIDOCAINE (DURANEST)

JASON WIDRICH, MD

INDICATION
- Local anesthetic for regional anesthesia

DOSE
- SQ/peripheral nerve block
  - 5–40 mL of 1% solution (50–400 mg) w/ epi 1:200,000
- Epidural
  - 10–30 mL of 1% solution (100–300 mg) w/ epi 1:200,000 or
  - 10–20 mL of 1.5% solution (150–300 mg) w/ epi 1:200,000
- Max recommended single dose in adults: 300 mg, or 400 mg w/ 1:200,000 epi

ONSET
- Infiltration onset: 3–5 min
- Epidural onset: 15–30 min

KINETICS
- Infiltration duration: 4–10 h
- Epidural duration: 6–10 h
- Hepatic elimination (amide local anesthetic)

PREPARATION
- 1%, 1.5% solutions

MECHANISM
- Binds to open sodium channels in sensory & motor neurons & blocks propagation of nerve impulses

COMMENTS
- Like other local anesthetics, can cause CNS & cardiovascular toxicity
  - Etidocaine toxicity causes seizures & carries a higher risk of cardiac toxicity than lidocaine or mepivacaine.
  - Can cause respiratory depression at high levels
- Not recommended for spinal/intrathecal administration
- Reduce dose in liver failure & the elderly.
- Compared to bupivacaine, etidocaine has:
  - Similar onset time
  - Longer duration of action
  - Greater motor blockade
  - Less sensory blockade
  - Similar cardiac toxicity profile

ETOMIDATE (AMIDATE)

EMILY REINYS, MD

INDICATION
- GA induction

DOSE
- 0.2–0.5 mg/kg

ONSET
- Usually <30 sec

KINETICS
- Rapid hydrolysis by plasma esterases & hepatic microsomal enzymes
- Redistribution responsible for reducing plasma concentration to awakening levels
- Renal excretion

PREPARATION
- Premixed solution 2 mg/cc

MECHANISM
- Enhances inhibitory effects of GABA on GABA-A receptors

COMMENTS
- Pain on injection
- Minimal cardiovascular depression
- Decreases cerebral metabolic rate, cerebral blood flow, ICP
- Long-term infusions lead to adrenocortical suppression

FENOLDOPAM

JAMES BRANDES, MD

INDICATION
- Short-term treatment of severe HTN
- Controlled hypotension

DOSE
- 0.1–1.6 mcg/kg/min (average dose 0.4–0.8 mcg/kg/min)
- Titrate in increments of 0.1 mcg/kg/min

ONSET
- 50% maximal onset in 15 min

KINETICS
- Distribution not known
- Does not cross blood-brain barrier
- Half-life: 4–10 min
- 50% of effect lost 15 min after stopping infusion

PREPARATION
- Supplied in 10-mg/mL solution.
- Dilute into 250 or 500 cc NS or D5W for infusion.
  - ➤ Diluted solution stable for 24 h.
  - ➤ No special tubing or light protection needed.

MECHANISM
- Peripherally acting dopaminergic agonist at dopamine DA1 receptors
- No effect on DA2 receptors
- Some effect on alpha-2 > alpha-1 receptors
- Dilates renal & mesenteric vascular beds
- Promotes natriuresis, diuresis, kaliuresis
- Does not change GFR

COMMENTS
- May cause reflex tachycardia
- Asymptomatic ST segment flattening in anterior & lateral leads common; may cause inverted T waves
- Increases intraocular pressure
  - ➤ Use w/ caution in glaucoma pts.
- May increase ICP
- Natriuretic & diuretic effects may be potentiated by ACE inhibitor or angiotensin II receptor antagonists.
- May increase portal venous pressure
- May also cause bradycardia, headache, flushing, dizziness
- Bolus doses not recommended
- Sometimes used in major vascular surgery because of purported renal protective effect

---

FENTANYL

JEREMY NUSSBAUMER, MD

INDICATION
- Analgesia

- Anxiolysis (oral transmucosal route)
- Anesthesia adjunct

DOSE
- All fentanyl doses should be titrated to effect depending on a variety of factors, including
  - Pt age
  - Body weight
  - Physical status of pt
  - Coexisting disease
  - Other CNS depressant drug administration
  - Surgery or procedure performed
- Dose for adults & children >12 years
  - IV
    - Cardiac surgery: 50–150 mcg/kg. Inadequate for use as a sole anesthetic. Anticipate need for postop mechanical ventilation.
    - Periop sedation/analgesia: 12.5–100 mcg/dose, depending on pt response
    - Children >12 years: 0.5–1 mcg/kg/dose
    - Adjunct to GA, low dose: 2 mcg/kg
    - Adjunct to GA, moderate dose: 2–20 mcg/kg, plus maintenance dose of 25–100 mcg as necessary. Some attenuation of stress response to surgery.
    - Adjunct to GA, high dose: 20–50 mcg/kg plus additional maintenance dose as necessary. For stressful surgery such as cardiac surgery, major abdominal or orthopedic surgery. May require postop mechanical ventilation at this dose.
  - IM
    - Premed for analgesia: 50–100 mcg. May repeat q1–2h.
  - Transdermal
    - Use only for chronic pain, not for acute or postop pain.
    - 25–100 mcg/h
    - Start at 25 mcg/h unless pt is opioid-tolerant.
  - Oral transmucosal
    - Analgesic or anxiolytic premed: 5 mcg/kg (400 mcg maximum)
    - Chronic pain relief in opioid-tolerant pt: Actiq 200–1,600 mcg, start at 200 mcg
  - Epidural
    - Postop analgesia 25–50 mcg/h
    - Can also combine fentanyl 1–5 mcg/mL w/ dilute local anesthetic solution for postop analgesia infusion

- Pediatric doses (2–12 years)
  - Supplement to GA: 2–3 mcg/kg
  - Sedation 1–3 years old: 2–3 mcg/kg/dose, may repeat q30–60min
  - Sedation 3–12 years old: 1–2 mcg/kg/dose, may repeat q30–60min
  - Oral transmucosal route for anxiolysis or analgesia: 5–15 mcg/kg (400 mcg max)

ONSET
- IV: 1–3 min
- IM: 7–8 min
- Oral transmucosal: 5–15 min
- Transdermal: 12–24 h
- Epidural: 20–30 min

KINETICS
- IV duration: 0.5–1 h (at 100-mcg dose)
- Elimination half-life: approx 220 min after IV injection
  - Context-sensitive half-life increases w/ prolonged infusions.
- IM duration: 1–2 h
- Epidural duration: 2–3 h
- Transdermal patch generally requires replacement q72h.
- Hepatic metabolism. Eliminated primarily in urine as metabolites.

PREPARATION
- 50 mcg/mL in 2-, 5-, 10-, 20-mL vials
- Transdermal Duragesic 25-, 50-, 75-, 100-mcg/h patches
- Fentanyl Oralet: 100-, 200-, 300-, 400-mcg buccal lozenges

MECHANISM
- Mu opioid receptor agonist

COMMENTS
- Fentanyl is 50–100 times more potent than morphine.
- Causes minimal histamine release
- Important respiratory effects
  - Like other opioids, will cause respiratory depression & hypoventilation, which can ultimately lead to apnea & respiratory arrest
  - Like other potent opioids, can cause significant chest wall rigidity & difficulty w/ ventilation, requiring muscle relaxant administration. This is very common w/ rapid IV administration of large dose.
- Important cardiac effects

- In general, fentanyl has minimal effects on hemodynamic status & has been widely used for cardiac surgery.
- Like other potent opioids, can cause significant bradycardia & hypotension
- When used in combination w/ other sedative meds (eg, benzodiazepines, barbiturates), hypotension can be more pronounced.

- Consider dose reduction in elderly or debilitated pts or those w/ renal failure.
- Opioids not considered suitable for use as a sole anesthetic because of breakthrough hypertension, inadequate anesthesia, high incidence of recall, muscle rigidity, postop respiratory depression
- Transdermal patches
  - Do not use solvents or warmth to remove transdermal patches; this may increase blood levels of fentanyl by 30%.
  - Do not apply patch to irritated or irradiated skin.
  - Do not cut patches in half, as this may affect drug delivery rate.
  - When transdermal fentanyl patch is removed, may take up to 17 h for fentanyl concentration to decrease by half.

FLUMAZENIL (ROMAZICON)

J. W. BEARD, MD

INDICATION
- Reversal of benzodiazepine sedation or overdose

DOSE
- Pediatric: Initial dose of 0.01 mg/kg (max 0.2 mg). Repeat doses of 0.01 mg/kg (max 0.2 mg) q1min to max total dose of 1 mg.
- Adult: Initial dose of 0.2 mg. Repeat doses of 0.2 mg q1min until desired level of consciousness obtained.
  - If resedation occurs, repeat doses of up to a total of 1 mg q20min (max 3 mg/h) may be used.

ONSET
- 1–3 min IV. 80% of response within first 3 min.

KINETICS
- Peak effect: 6–10 min
- Duration: up to 1 h
- Elimination half-life: 45 min (may increase in hepatic disease)

- Hepatic metabolism
- Hepatic elimination

PREPARATION
- Available as 0.1 mg/mL injectable

MECHANISM
- Benzodiazapine-specific competitive antagonism at the benzodiazepine/GABA-A receptor

COMMENTS
- Does not antagonize CNS effects of other agents acting at GABA-A receptors
- May induce seizures in pts at high risk (long-term BDZ sedation, TCA overdose, concurrent sedative-hypnotic drug withdrawal, myoclonic jerking/seizure activity prior to flumazenil administration, recent repeated parenteral BDZ administration)
- Resedation possible depending on benzodiazepine half-life/dose

---

FUROSEMIDE (LASIX)

MADELEINE BIBAT, MD

INDICATION
- Edema
- Hypercalcemia
- Hyperkalemia
- CHF

DOSE
- Adult: 10–40 mg IV; may repeat/increase dose in 1–2 h depending on response
- Pediatric: 1 mg/kg/dose initially; may increase in increments up to 6 mg/kg/dose depending on response

ONSET
- 5 min IV

KINETICS
- Duration: 2 h IV
- Elimination half-life: 1 h
- Hepatic metabolism (minimal)
- Renal excretion (80% excreted in urine)

PREPARATION
- 10 mg/ml solution

MECHANISM
- Inhibits Na-K-Cl co-transport in the ascending loop of Henle

COMMENTS
- Hypokalemia can result from furosemide use, which may prolong neuromuscular blockade.
- Increased risk for QT prolongation from furosemide-induced hypokalemia in the presence of class III antiarrhythmics.
- Enhances ototoxicity & nephrotoxicity of aminoglycosides & amphotericin B.
- May increase insulin dose requirements.
- Potassium supplements are often given to pts taking furosemide chronically.

GABAPENTIN (NEURONTIN)

JOHN KELTNER, MD, PHD

INDICATION
- Neuropathic pain
- Seizures

DOSE
- 300–4,800 mg/day PO in 3 divided doses

ONSET
N/A

KINETICS
- Half-life: 5–9 h
- Well absorbed by GI & excreted unchanged mainly in urine

PREPARATION
- 300-, 400-mg capsules; 600-, 800-mg tablets

MECHANISM
- Unknown

COMMENTS
- Dosing typically starts at 300 mg/day & increases daily over 1 month.
- Max dose limited by side effects (ie, somnolence, dizziness, headache).

GENTAMICIN

JEREMY NUSSBAUMER, MD

INDICATION
- Antibiotic used for gram-negative antibiotic coverage, especially *Pseudomonas* infection

DOSE
- Adults: 3–5 mg/kg/d IV divided q8h
- Adults: once-daily dosing at 4–7 mg/kg IV q24h
- Children: 1–2.5 mg/kg IV q8h
- Neonates <1 wk: 2.5 mg/kg IM q12h

ONSET
- IV peak level at end of infusion
- IM onset 30–90 min

KINETICS
- Duration: 6–12 h after single dose
- Elimination half-life: 2–4 h
- Excreted unchanged in urine (70–100%)

PREPARATION
- Vial is typically 80 mg in 2 mL diluent.
- Infuse over 30–60 min in 100–250 mL normal saline.

MECHANISM
- Aminoglycoside antibiotic
- Inhibits protein synthesis by binding bacterial ribosomal subunits

COMMENTS
- Considered unsafe in pregnancy
- Adverse effects include
  - Ototoxicity
  - Nephrotoxicity
  - Endotoxin reaction (sweating, fever, chills) has been reported w/ once-daily dosing w/ certain gentamicin preparations.
  - Can increase duration of neuromuscular blocking drugs & can itself cause neuromuscular blockade
    - A single dose of gentamicin in a pt w/ normal neuromuscular function has minimal effect on blockade & reversal.

- Pt w/ neuromuscular disease is more likely to have significant neuromuscular weakness w/ gentamicin.
- Peritoneal irrigation w/ gentamicin may be assoc w/ postop weakness that does not respond to neostigmine.
- Although antibiotic-induced block can be treated w/ calcium chloride or neostigmine, this is not reliable; may be safer to continue airway & ventilation support until spontaneous recovery occurs.

■ AHA recommends use w/ ampicillin in GI/GU procedures for pts at high risk for bacterial endocarditis (30 min before procedure). (See also Coexisting Disease chapter "Infective Endocarditis".)

■ Dosing adjustment for renal failure
  ➤ GFR >50 mL/min: 60–90% of dose q8–12h
  ➤ GFR 10–50 mL/min: 30–70% of dose q12h
  ➤ GFR <10 mL/min: 20–30% q24–48h
  ➤ CAVH or CVVH: 30–70% q12h

■ Dosing for obese pts

■ Obesity (1.25–2x ideal body weight [IBW]): for dose calculation, use body weight of IBW plus (0.43 x excess body weight above IBW)

GLUCAGON

JASON WIDRICH, MD

INDICATION

■ Hypoglycemia

■ Reduce GI smooth muscle tone
  ➤ For instance, diagnostic aid during radiography or endoscopy, biliary tract pain

■ Beta-blocker overdose

DOSE

■ Hypoglycemia
  ➤ 1 mg IV, IM, SQ
  ➤ Children <20 kg: 20–30 mcg/kg up to 0.5 mg

■ Reduce GI smooth muscle tone (eg, diagnostic aid)
  ➤ 0.25–2 mg IV
  ➤ 1–2 mg IM

■ Beta-blocker overdose
  ➤ 3–10 mg bolus, 1–5 mg/h infusion

ONSET
- Diagnostic aid
  - 1 min IV
  - 5 min IM
- Hypoglycemia
  - Peak effect within 5–20 min by IM, IV, or SQ routes

KINETICS
- Half-life: 8–15 min
- Metabolized in liver & kidneys

PREPARATION
- 1 mg powder & diluent to be reconstituted to 1 mg/mL.
- Use immediately after preparation.

MECHANISM
- Polypeptide hormone made by alpha pancreatic cells
- Stimulates glycogenolysis, raising glucose level
- Provides GI tract smooth muscle relaxation, including common bile duct, small intestine, large intestine, stomach
- Increases myocardial contractility even in the presence of beta-blockade

COMMENTS
- Useful for treating hypoglycemia in pts w/o IV access
  - Administer oral carbohydrate after pt responds to therapy.
- Treatment of hypoglycemia effective only in pt w/ adequate glycogen stores
  - May not be effective in pt w/ starvation, adrenal insufficiency, or chronic hypoglycemia
- Most common adverse effects
  - Nausea/vomiting
  - Rash
  - Other allergic reaction
- Avoid in pt w/ pheochromocytoma.
  - Glucagon can stimulate catecholamine release & cause sudden increase in BP & HR.
- Avoid in pt w/ insulinoma.
  - Insulin hypersecretion can cause rebound hypoglycemia.

GLYCOPYRROLATE (ROBINUL)

JOHN TAYLOR, MD

INDICATION
- Bradycardia
- Protects against the peripheral muscarinic effects of neostigmine & pyridostigmine
- Counteracts vagal traction reflexes
- Antisialogogue

DOSE
- Adult
- Antisialogogue: 0.1–0.2 mg IV/IM/SC
- For bradycardia: 0.1–0.2 mg IV q2–3min prn
- With reversal of neuromuscular blockade, 0.2 mg for each 1 mg neostigmine or 5 mg pyridostigmine
- Pediatric
- Antisialogogue: 4–10 mcg/kg IV
- For bradycardia: 4.4 mcg/kg IV (max 0.1 mg/dose) q2–3min prn
- With reversal of neuromuscular blockade, 0.2 mg for each 1 mg neostigmine or 5 mg pyridostigmine (ie, 5–15 mcg/kg glycopyrrolate)

ONSET
- IV: <1 min
- IM: 15–30 min

KINETICS
- Duration: vagal effects 2–3 h; secretory inhibition 7 h
- Elimination: primarily renal

PREPARATION
- Injectable: 0.2 mg/mL in 1-, 2-, 5-, 20-mL vials

MECHANISM
- Blocks muscarinic acetylcholine receptors peripherally (eg, SA & AV node, secretory glands, smooth muscle)

COMMENTS
- Does not penetrate blood-brain barrier

GRANISETRON (KYTRIL)

JEREMY NUSSBAUMER, MD

INDICATION
- Antiemetic

DOSE
- Prevention of postop nausea/vomiting
- Adult: 1 mg IV over 5 min
- Pediatric (>4 years): 40 mcg/kg IV or PO

ONSET
- 4–10 min

KINETICS
- Hepatic metabolism by P450 system
- Duration: antiemetic effect lasts up to 24 h
- Elimination half-life: 3–14 h

PREPARATION
- Dilute in 20–50 mL NS.

MECHANISM
- Selective 5-HT3 (serotonin) receptor antagonist

COMMENTS
- Can lead to anxiety, constipation, abdominal pain, headache
- No dosage adjustment for hepatic or renal disease

HALOPERIDOL LACTATE (HALDOL)

J. W. BEARD, MD

INDICATION
- Psychosis
- Severe agitation/delirium

DOSE
- IM, IV: 0.5–5 mg titrated to effect, may repeat doses as needed

ONSET
- IV: <1 h

KINETICS
- Elimination half-life: 20 h

- Metabolism: hepatic
- Elimination: in urine, feces

PREPARATION
- IV: 5 mg/mL

MECHANISM
- Butyrophenone that blocks postsynaptic dopamine receptors in brain
- Also has some alpha-adrenergic & cholinergic antagonism

COMMENTS
- Causes little respiratory depression.
- Extrapyramidal symptoms (Parkinson-like symptoms, dystonia, akathisia) may occur.
  - Contraindicated in Parkinson's disease.
  - May lead to hypotension, tachycardia, or prolonged QT interval.
  - Assoc w/ torsades de pointes ventricular arrhythmias.
  - Monitor ECG QT interval & stop drug if QT prolongation occurs.
  - May be assoc w/ anticholinergic reactions.
  - Tardive dyskinesia (potentially irreversible, involuntary, dyskinetic movements) is a complication seen w/ chronic administration.
  - Neuroleptic malignant syndrome (EPS, hyperthermia, muscle rigidity, autonomic instability) is a rare complication.
  - Contraindicated in severe hepatic disease due to risk of hepatotoxicity & prolonged duration of action.
  - Haloperidol decanoate is a long-acting formulation for IM use, not to be administered IV.

HALOTHANE

ANTHONY ROMO, MD
EDMOND I EGER II, MD

INDICATION
- Induction & maintenance of GA

DOSE
- MAC (in O_2): 1.0% (infants & children); 0.75% (30–60 years); 0.6% (80 years)
- MAC-awake: 50% of MAC

ONSET
- Seconds-minutes

KINETICS
- Metabolism: 20–40% of halothane taken up
- Elimination: pulmonary (60%)
- Uptake
  - Large relative to alveolar concentration because of moderate blood/gas (2.5) & tissue/gas partition coefficients (greatest of all potent inhaled anesthetics) & because of metabolism
  - Alveolar (end-tidal) concentration differs considerably from the inspired concentration & recovery is longer than w/ other potent anesthetics
  - Rapid induction achieved by using "overpressure" (eg, 5% inspired halothane)

PREPARATION
- Clear, colorless nonflammable liquid in 125- or 250-mL amber-colored bottles (UV light degrades halothane)
- Thymol (preservative) required

MECHANISM
- Unclear
- Plausible basis: in vitro, volatile inhaled anesthetics enhance inhibitory channel (GABA, glycine, potassium) responses & block excitatory channel (glutamate, acetylcholine, sodium) responses
  - However, these effects do not necessarily translate into mechanistic effects (eg, blockade of acetylcholine receptors does not decrease MAC).

COMMENTS
- Degradation by carbon dioxide absorbents
  - Minimal at increased temperatures (eg, closed circuit)
  - Produces potential nephrotoxin ($CF_2 = CBrCl$)
- Nonpungent. Rapid inhaled induction using overpressure.
- Causes profound, dose-related muscle relaxation & enhances the effect of muscle relaxants
- Side effects
  - Higher concentrations depress heart/breathing (decrease BP, cardiac output & contractility; sustain systemic vascular resistance; increase $PaCO_2$).
  - Hypothermia

- As w/ other inhaled anesthetics, halothane decreases the set point for response to decreases in body temp.
  - More potent trigger of malignant hyperthermia than other potent inhaled agents
  - Causes nausea/vomiting
  - Enhances arrhythmogenic response to exogenous or endogenous epinephrine
- Assoc w/ two forms of hepatitis
  - Halothane hepatitis (severe)
    - Mortality: 1/35,000 anesthetics
    - Allergic response to trifluoroacetate from oxidative metabolism
    - Risk factors: multiple halothane anesthetics over a short period of time, middle-aged overweight women, familial history of predisposition to halothane toxicity
  - Halothane hepatitis (mild)
    - Incidence: common
    - Possibly from reductive metabolism
- Comparisons w/ other inhaled anesthetics
  - Advantages
    - Lowest cost
    - Absent pungency
    - Highest potency
    - Rapid inhalational induction
    - Produces muscle relaxation
  - Disadvantages
    - Slower recovery
    - Greatest biodegradation
    - Can produce halothane hepatitis & death (rarely) & mild hepatitis (common)
    - Ventricular ectopy

HEMABATE (CARBOPROST, 15-METHYL PROSTAGLANDIN F2-ALPHA)

ALISON G. CAMERON, MD

INDICATION

- Treatment of postpartum hemorrhage due to uterine atony unresponsive to conventional therapy (IV oxytocin, uterine massage, IM ergot preparations)

➤ Use of the drug has resulted in cessation of life-threatening bleeding & the avoidance of emergency surgical intervention.
■ Termination of pregnancy of 13–20 wk gestation
■ Evacuation of uterus in mgt of missed abortion or intrauterine fetal death in 2nd trimester

DOSE
■ For uterine bleeding
➤ 250 mcg IM
➤ In some cases repeat dosing is required: 250 mcg at 15- to 90-min intervals.
➤ Dose may be increased to 500 mcg if uterine contractility is judged to be inadequate after several doses of 250 mcg.
➤ Total dose should not exceed 2 mg (eight doses).
➤ Can be given intramyometrial (IMM) into the uterus if uterine hemorrhage occurs during a C-section

ONSET
■ Peak plasma levels within 30 min of IM injection

KINETICS
■ Approx half-life: 60 min (not well characterized)
■ Metabolized by lung primarily (some in liver & renal cortex); metabolites are excreted by kidneys

PREPARATION
■ 250 mcg/mL
■ Must be refrigerated at 2 to 8 degrees C

MECHANISM
■ Hemabate is a prostaglandin (cyclic fatty acid) that is oxytocic, stimulating smooth muscle contraction (eg, myometrial contractions, relieving uterine atony, providing effective hemostasis at the site of bleeding).

COMMENTS
■ Use caution in pts w/ a history of asthma, hypo- or hypertension, cardiovascular, renal, or hepatic disease, anemia, jaundice, diabetes, or epilepsy.
■ The most frequent adverse reactions observed are related to its contractile effect on smooth muscle. Most effects are short-lived & dissipate when therapy is stopped.

- ➤ Vomiting & diarrhea are most common.
- ➤ Other possible adverse reactions
  - Leukocytosis
  - Headache
  - Fever
  - Uterine rupture
  - Bronchoconstriction, pulmonary edema
- ■ Cardiovascular effects
  - ➤ Increased cardiac output
  - ➤ Increased pulmonary vascular resistance
  - ➤ Increased pulmonary artery pressure
- ■ Pulmonary effects
  - ➤ Can exacerbate airway hyperreactivity & promote broncho-spasm in asthmatics during induction of labor (oxytocin would be better choice in asthmatics)
- ■ Breastfeeding should be delayed for at least 6 hours following administration.
- ■ Called "Prostin 15" in some European & Scandinavian countries

HEPARIN

ANDREW CHUNG, MD
JASON WIDRICH, MD

INDICATION
- ■ Prophylaxis & treatment of deep venous thrombosis (DVT) & pulmonary embolism (PE)
- ■ Prevention of clotting in arterial & cardiac surgery
- ■ Diagnosis & treatment of consumptive coagulopathies (DIC)
- ■ Treatment of unstable angina & acute MI

DOSE
- ■ PE
  - ➤ 50–150 units/kg IV; keep aPTT at 1.5–2.5x control value
- ■ Cardiac surgery requiring cardiopulmonary bypass
  - ➤ 300–400 units/kg IV; keep ACT >400 sec
- ■ Acute MI
  - ➤ 60 u/kg (max 4,000) followed by 12 u/kg/h (max 1,000)
- ■ DVT
  - ➤ 80 u/kg followed by 18 u/kg/h

- DVT prophylaxis
  - ➤ 5,000 u SC 2 hours prior to surgery & q12h for 1 week postop
  - ➤ During pregnancy, 7,500–10,000 u SC q12h

ONSET
- Immediate IV, peak in 2 min
- SC injection: 20–30 min

KINETICS
- Elimination half-life: 1–6 h, increases w/ dose
- Clearance: reticuloendothelial uptake, hepatic biotransformation

PREPARATION
- Different commercial preparations vary in units of heparin per mL.
- Most common preparations: bovine lung, bovine gut mucosa, porcine

MECHANISM
- Enhances the ability of antithrombin III to inactivate coagulation enzymes, including thrombin & activated clotting factors X, XII, XI, IX
- Needs AT III & the factors to produce the anticoagulant effect

COMMENTS
- Side effects include hemorrhage, thrombocytopenia, allergic reactions, CV changes.
- Dose not cross placenta, but often held until after first trimester
- Reversed by protamine (1–1.25 mg protamine per 100 units heparin)
- Contraindicated in setting of hemorrhage, retinopathy, or diastolic blood pressure >105 mmHg
- Heparin-induced thrombocytopenia: onset is usually insidious over the course of a few days. If suspected, must be vigilant to remove all possible sources of heparin.
- Heparin resistance is often overcome by
  - ➤ Increasing heparin dose
  - ➤ Administration of FFP 5–10 cc/kg
  - ➤ Administration of AT III or cryoprecipitate
- Heparin & central neuraxial anesthesia
  - ➤ Delay heparin administration for 1 h after epidural/spinal needle placement.
- Remove epidural or intrathecal catheters 1 h before any heparin administration or 2–4 h after the last heparin dose.

HETASTARCH

WILLIAM RHOADS, MD

INDICATION
- Plasma volume expansion

DOSE
- Usual dose 500–1,000 mL up to 20 mL/kg
  - Safe use of higher doses has also been reported.

ONSET
- Within 30 min

KINETICS
- Kinetics influenced by concentration, average particle size, degree of substitution of the hetastarch
- Plasma volume expansion typically lasts 24–48 h.
- Renal excretion of small hetastarch molecules
- Larger hetastarch molecules undergo degradation by amylases or reticuloendothelial system, followed by urinary or biliary excretion.
- For severe renal failure (GFR <10 mL/min), initial dose unchanged. Subsequent dose should be reduced by up to smaller.

PREPARATION
- In U.S., prepared in 500-mL bags as
  - 6% hetastarch in 0.9% NaCl (Hespan)
  - 6% hetastarch in a balanced electrolyte solution w/ lactate buffer (Hextend)

MECHANISM
- Colloid volume expander

COMMENTS
- In large doses (>20 mL/kg), hetastarch can interfere w/ coagulation by dilution of clotting factors & by inhibition of factor VIII/von Willebrand factor.
  - Clinical coagulopathy may be less frequent w/ 6% hetastarch in lactated electrolyte solution, possibly due to calcium content.
  - Consider risk of bleeding vs risk/benefit ratio of alternate colloid therapy.

- Large volumes of Hespan (6% hetastarch in NaCl) may produce hyperchloremic metabolic acidosis.
- Serum amylase is commonly elevated w/ hetastarch therapy, but is not indicative of pancreatitis.

HYDRALAZINE

JASON LICHTENSTEIN, MD

INDICATION
- HTN

DOSE
- 2.5–10 mg IV

ONSET
- 10–20 min after IV administration

KINETICS
- Duration: 3–6 h
- Peak effect: 10–80 min after IV administration
- Elimination half-life: approx 3 h
- Hepatic metabolism
- Renal excretion up to 15%

PREPARATION
- 20 mg/mL in 1-mL vials
- Also available as tablet for PO administration

MECHANISM
- Direct-acting peripheral vasodilator
- Dilates arterioles > veins

COMMENTS
- Commonly causes tachycardia, which can be treated w/ beta-blocker therapy
- Usually causes increase in stroke volume, heart rate, cardiac output
- Decreases SVR
- Use w/ caution in pts w/ CAD, mitral valve disease, impaired renal function.
- Other adverse effects (typically w/ longer-term therapy) may include
  - Peripheral neuropathy
  - Paresthesias
  - Renal failure

➤ Hepatotoxicity
➤ Systemic lupus-like syndrome

HYDROCORTISONE (SOLU-CORTEF)

JEREMY NUSSBAUMER, MD

INDICATION
■ Treatment of adrenocorticoid insufficiency, ulcerative colitis, autoimmune diseases, allergy, inflammatory disease, asthma

DOSE
■ Surgical stress dose (in patients on chronic steroids): 50–100 mg IV q8h
■ Acute adrenal insufficiency
  ➤ Infants & young children: 1–2 mg/kg/dose bolus, then 25–150 mg/day in QID doses (IV or IM)
  ➤ Older children: same bolus, then 150–250 mg/day divided QID
  ➤ Adults: 100 mg IV bolus, then 300 mg/day divided QID or as continuous infusion. Switch to oral 50 mg q8h once stable.
■ Chronic adrenal insufficiency: Adult PO dose 20–30 mg/day

ONSET
■ 1 h

KINETICS
■ Duration: 6–8 h
  ➤ Metabolism: hepatic
  ➤ Elimination: renal

PREPARATION
■ 100 mg as powder & various other formulations

MECHANISM
■ Steroid w/ characteristic anti-inflammatory, immunosuppressive, & antiallergic actions
■ Inhibits migration of polymorphonuclear leukocytes
■ Has mineralocorticoid effect

COMMENTS
■ Use w/ caution in pts w/ hyperthyroidism, HTN, cirrhosis, osteoporosis, CHF, myasthenia gravis, PUD, DM.
■ Avoid abrupt withdrawal, which can lead to adrenocortical insufficiency.

HYDROMORPHONE (DILAUDID)

DAN BURKHARDT, MD

INDICATION
- Analgesia

DOSE
- 1–4 mg PO q4–6h prn
- 0.2–0.8 mg IV prn initially
  - Repeat & titrate to effect, maintenance q1–2h prn (or via IV PCA)
- 0.15–0.2 mg IV hydromorphone = 1 mg IV morphine
- Pediatric dose: 0.005–0.01 mg/kg IV
- Can be added to epidural infusion at 0.03 mg/mL

ONSET
- Peak onset approx 20 min

KINETICS
- Hepatic metabolism, renal excretion
- Plasma half-life: approx 2–3 h

PREPARATION
- Available in multiple strengths of tablets, liquids, suppositories & injections suitable for SC, IM, IV, epidural & IT administration

MECHANISM
- Opioid receptor agonist

COMMENTS
- Compared to morphine, hydromorphone:
  - Has similar IV pharmacokinetics
  - Has no metabolite that accumulates in renal failure
  - Does not cause histamine release
  - May have less CNS side effects in the elderly
- Dermatomal spread from continuous epidural infusion is less than morphine but more than fentanyl.
- Consider dose reduction in liver or renal failure.
- Effects common to all narcotics
  - Depresses CO_2-triggered respiratory drive in a dose-dependent fashion. Hypercarbia can also exacerbate increases in ICP. Useful in low doses to palliate the sensation of dyspnea.

➤ Crosses placenta: respiratory depression in newborn if mother has had large doses
➤ Constipation: pts on chronic narcotics should receive prophylactic treatment
➤ Nausea/vomiting: treat w/ antiemetics and/or nonnarcotic adjuncts to reduce the total opioid dose, or change opioids
➤ Modest vagotonic effect: bradycardia w/ large bolus doses
➤ Delayed gastric emptying
➤ Biliary spasm: no clinical difference between opioids
➤ Urine retention
➤ Miosis
➤ Euphoria/dysphoria, or frank delirium: more common in the elderly
➤ Myoclonus w/ extremely high doses
➤ Chest wall rigidity w/ large doses IV push
➤ Physical dependence & withdrawal after prolonged use: wean dose gently, consider adjunctive clonidine
➤ Psychiatric addiction (taking the drug for reasons other than pain relief) is very rare, especially in the acute postop setting.

HYDROXYZINE (ATARAX, VISTARIL)

JASON WIDRICH, MD

INDICATION
■ Anxiety
■ Pruritus
■ Nausea/vomiting
■ Allergies
■ Sedation

DOSE
■ IM: 25–100 mg q4–6h
■ PO: 25–200 mg q6–8h

ONSET
■ Peak effect in 15–30 min

KINETICS
■ Half-life: 2–3 h
■ Duration: 4–6 h

- Metabolism: hepatic
- Elimination: urine

PREPARATION
- PO: 25-, 50-, 100-mg tablets
- IM: 50 mg/mL

MECHANISM
- Antihistamine blocks H1 receptors; also has anticholinergic effect

COMMENTS
- Side effects include drowsiness, dry mouth.
- Enhances the sedating effect of alcohol, barbiturates, narcotics
- Do not give IV: may cause thrombosis.

INDIGO CARMINE

JOHN TAYLOR, MD

INDICATION
- Localization of ureteral orifices or sites of ureteral injury during surgery

DOSE
- 40 mg (5 cc) IV

ONSET
- Appears in urine within 10 min (average)

KINETICS
- Biologic half-life: 4–5 min
- Excreted largely by kidneys

PREPARATION
- 1 ampule contains 5 mL solution w/ 40 mg indigo carmine.

MECHANISM
- Retains blue color during passage through body
- Elimination: renal
- Metabolism: minimal

COMMENTS
- Mild pressor effect may be seen in some pts.
- Methylene blue also used for this indication.

INSULIN

JEREMY NUSSBAUMER, MD

INDICATION
- Diabetes mellitus, including treatment of DKA
- Treatment of hyperglycemia due to hyperalimentation
- Acute treatment of hyperkalemia

DOSE
- Multiple preparations available. Regular insulin is the primary topic of this chapter.
- Regular insulin may be given IV, IM or SC.
- Hyperglycemia
  - Dose will vary w/ degree of hyperglycemia as well as other therapy. Initial dose should be similar to pt's outpatient insulin regimen.
  - See also Coexisting Disease chapter "Diabetes Mellitus."
- Hyperkalemia
  - See also Critical Event chapter "Hyperkalemia" for other therapy (may include calcium, sodium bicarbonate).
  - Adult dose IV
    - Insulin 5–10 U w/
    - 50 mL 50% dextrose
  - Pediatric dose IV
    - Insulin 0.1 U/kg w/
    - Dextrose 0.5–1 g/kg
- DKA
  - See also Critical Event chapter "Diabetic Ketoacidosis."
  - Insulin bolus 0.1 U/kg then continuous infusion 0.1 U/kg/h; titrate to desired glucose

ONSET
- SC regular insulin: 0.5–1 h
- IV regular insulin: 10–20 min

KINETICS
- SC regular insulin
  - Peak: 2.5–5 h
  - Duration: 8 h

- IV regular insulin
  - Peak: 15–30 min
  - Duration: 1–2 h
- Elimination half-life
  - IV regular insulin: 5–15 min
  - SC regular insulin: 198 min
- Metabolized by liver & kidney
  - Dose reduction in renal failure
  - Give 75% of regular dose if Cr clearance 10–50 mL/min.
  - Give 25–50% of regular dose if Cr clearance <10 mL/min.

PREPARATION
- Only regular insulin should be used as IV insulin.
- Keep vial refrigerated before use.
- Suggested insulin drip preparation
  - Add 25 units regular insulin to 250 mL NS (concentration 0.1 units/mL).
  - Flush IV tubing w/ at least 50 mL of solution (due to insulin adsorption to tubing).

MECHANISM
- Insulin is a hormone produced by pancreatic islet cells.
- Actions include
  - Stimulate carbohydrate metabolism
  - Facilitate transfer of glucose to muscles
  - Facilitate conversion of glucose to glycogen

COMMENTS
- Blood glucose levels must be carefully monitored during therapy.
- Carefully check insulin dilution & preparation.
- Insulin can cause severe hypoglycemia, w/ resulting seizures & coma.
- Other signs of hypoglycemia
  - Autonomic signs
    - Sweating, tremor, tachycardia
  - Neuroglycopenic signs
    - Drowsiness, weakness, decreased concentration, anxiety, combativeness, confusion, headache
- Treatment of hypoglycemia includes
  - Decrease or stop insulin
  - Oral carbohydrate or IV dextrose
  - Glucagon (IV, IM or SC)

IPRATROPIUM BROMIDE (ATROVENT)

RENÉE J. ROBERTS, MD
IVAN ZEITZ, MD

INDICATION
- COPD
- Asthma (selected pts)

DOSE
- Adult
  - 2 inhalations qid
  - Maximum 12 inhalations in 24 h
  - 500 mcg by nebulization q6–8h
- Children 6–14 y
  - 1 or 2 inhalations tid

ONSET
- 3–15 min

KINETICS
- Peak response in 60–180 min
- Minimum absorption following inhalation
  - 90% eliminated in feces after swallowing
  - Partial hepatic metabolism
- Effect usually lasts 4 h but may last 8 h.
- Elimination half-life: 2–4 h

PREPARATION
- 18 mcg/inhalation in metered-dose inhaler
- For nebulizer use, dilute 500 mg in 2.5 cc NS.

MECHANISM
- Anticholinergic
- Dilates smooth muscles of bronchi & bronchioles
- Minimal effect on amount or viscosity of airway secretions

COMMENTS
- Relatively slow onset time compared to inhaled beta-agonist therapy
- Primarily used in long-term treatment of COPD
- Use in asthmatics less well defined
- No significant extra benefit w/ dosing above recommended frequency

- Minimal toxicity due to minimal systemic absorption
  - Unlike beta-agonist therapy, does not cause tachycardia
- Dry mouth most common adverse effect

ISOFLURANE

ANTHONY ROMO, MD
EDMOND I EGER II, MD

INDICATION
- Induction & maintenance of GA

DOSE
- MAC (O_2): 1.4% (infants & children); 1.15% (30–60 years); 1.05% (80 years)
- MAC-awake: one third of MAC
- MAC-BAR: 1.5% (opioids markedly decrease)

ONSET
- Seconds-minutes

KINETICS
- Metabolism: 0.2% of isoflurane taken up
- Elimination: pulmonary
- Uptake
  - Moderate because of moderate blood/gas (1.4) & tissue/gas partition coefficients
  - Accordingly, alveolar concentration much less than inspired concentration & recovery slower than w/ desflurane or sevoflurane
  - Induction marred by respiratory irritation at concentrations exceeding MAC

PREPARATION
- Clear, colorless nonflammable liquid in 100- or 250-mL amber-colored bottles
- No preservative required

MECHANISM
- Unclear
- Plausible basis: In vitro, volatile inhaled anesthetics enhance inhibitory channel (GABA, glycine, potassium) responses & block excitatory channel (glutamate, acetylcholine, sodium) responses.

➤ However, these effects do not necessarily translate into mechanistic effects (eg, blockade of acetylcholine receptors does not decrease MAC).

COMMENTS
■ Degradation by carbon dioxide absorbents
  ➤ None in normal (wet) absorbent, even at higher temps (eg, closed circuit)
  ➤ Degraded by desiccated absorbents to carbon monoxide (< desflurane)
■ Causes profound, dose-related muscle relaxation & enhances the effect of muscle relaxants; elimination decreases the effect of residual relaxants
■ Side effects
  ➤ Airway irritation
    • Occurs at concentrations >1.5% w/ coughing, breath-holding, laryngospasm & salivation on induction of anesthesia
    • Irritation markedly decreased by administration of small doses of opioid; is less or no problem during maintenance
    • When administered via LMA, isoflurane does not produce more evidence of respiratory irritation than other inhaled anesthetics.
  ➤ Transient tachycardia & hypertension
    • Increases in concentration >1.2%, particularly on induction of anesthesia, can cause transient (4–6 min) increases in HR & BP, especially w/ rapid increases in concentration.
    • Effect much less than seen w/ desflurane
  ➤ Higher concentrations depress heart/breathing (decrease BP, cardiac output & contractility; sustain systemic vascular resistance; increase $PaCO_2$), but no ventricular ectopy.
  ➤ Hypothermia
    • As w/ other inhaled anesthetics, isoflurane decreases the set point for response to decreases in body temp.
  ➤ Like other potent inhaled agents, can trigger malignant hyperthermia; less potent trigger than halothane.
  ➤ Causes nausea/vomiting
■ Comparisons w/ other inhaled anesthetics
  ➤ Advantages
    • Low acquisition cost
    • Resists biodegradation or degradation by normal absorbents

- • o ventricular ectopy
- • Produces muscle relaxation
- ➤ Disadvantages
  - • Moderate solubility & slower recovery than w/ desflurane or sevoflurane
  - • Respiratory irritant & transient cardiorespiratory stimulant at concentrations >1.5%
  - • Degraded by desiccated absorbents to carbon monoxide

ISOPROTERENOL

JASON WIDRICH, MD

INDICATION
- ■ Bradycardia
- ■ Sick sinus syndrome
- ■ Heart block
- ■ Mgt of shock

DOSE
- ■ IV infusion 2–20 mcg/min (0.02–0.5 mcg/kg/min)

ONSET
- ■ IV: immediate

KINETICS
- ■ Duration: 1–5 min IV
- ■ Hepatic elimination

PREPARATION
- ■ IV: 0.2 mg/mL in 1-, 5-, 10-mL ampules
- ■ Dilution of 1 mg in 250 mL produces 4-mcg/mL solution for infusion.

MECHANISM
- ■ Synthetic sympathomimetic agent that acts exclusively at beta-1 & beta-2 adrenergic receptors
- ■ Produces both positive chronotropic & inotropic effects by accelerating the discharge from cardiac pacemaker cells
- ■ Decreases SVR & PVR; could be useful agent for pt w/ pulmonary HTN who needs inotropic support
- ■ Has been shown to improve both coronary & renal blood flow

COMMENTS

- Contraindicated in arrhythmias caused by digoxin & in situations where tachycardia induced by the drug may precipitate an ischemic event
- Most commonly used after heart transplantation as a direct beta-1 agonist to increase HR & maintain CO
- Although not the treatment of choice, can be used for atropine-resistant bradycardia, third-degree heart block, or excessive beta-blockade until a pacemaker can be placed

KETAMINE

KALEB JENSON, MD

INDICATION

- Induction or maintenance of GA
- Sedation
- Analgesia

DOSE

- Induction
  - ➤ IV: 0.5–4 mg/kg (1–2 mg/kg typical)
  - ➤ IM: 4–13 mg/kg
- Maintenance
  - ➤ IV bolus: 0.5–1 mg/kg IV PRN
- IV infusion: 30–90 mcg/kg/min
- Analgesia, sedation
  - ➤ IV: 0.2–1.0 mg/kg
  - ➤ IM: 1–5 mg/kg
  - ➤ PO: 6–10 mg/kg

ONSET

- IV: 30 sec
- IM: <5 min
- PO: 10–30 min

KINETICS

- IV (1 mg/kg): 15–20 min
- IM (4–5 mg/kg): 20–30 min
- Elimination half-life: 1–2 h
- Hepatic metabolism

- Renal excretion
- Ketamine has active metabolites, yet there is little evidence of prolonged effects w/ renal failure.

PREPARATION
- 10, 25, 50, 100 mg/mL.
- Typically use 100 mg/mL for IM injections or for PO use; use or dilute to 10 mg/mL for IV administration.

MECHANISM
- NMDA receptor antagonist

COMMENTS
- Increases in HR & BP occur due to sympathomimetic actions, yet ketamine directly acts as a myocardial depressant.
- Myocardial depression is revealed in sympathetically depleted states (sepsis, shock) & can lead to hemodynamic collapse.
- Ketamine increases ICP, CBF, cerebral oxygen consumption, intraocular pressure.
- Emergence delirium: incidence likely ~50% of adults & 10% of children w/ ketamine-based anesthetics.
  ➤ Adjunctive benzodiazepine use reduces risk.
- Increased salivation.
  ➤ Pretreat w/ antisialogogue (eg, glycopyrrolate) to reduce this.
- Can cause myoclonic movements
- Rarely causes respiratory depression, unlike most IV anesthetics.
- Has bronchodilatory effects.
- Anesthesia can be induced in pts w/o an IV w/ IM ketamine & succinylcholine.

KETOPROFEN (ORUDIS)

JEREMY NUSSBAUMER, MD

INDICATION
- NSAID used in the treatment of
  ➤ Pain
  ➤ Inflammation

DOSE
- 25–75 mg PO q6–8h, max 300 mg/d

ONSET
- Approx 0.5 h

KINETICS
- Metabolized in liver
- Renal excretion
- Half-life: 1–4 h

PREPARATION
- 25-, 50-, 75-mg oral capsules
- 100-, 150-, 200-mg extended-release capsules

MECHANISM
- Inhibits the enzyme cyclooxygenase, thereby decreasing prostaglandin synthesis

COMMENTS
- Consider reducing dose in pts w/ hepatic or renal failure; may worsen renal failure.
- May increase bleeding.
- Use w/ caution in pts w/ history of GI bleeds.

KETOROLAC (TORADOL)

JASON LICHTENSTEIN, MD

INDICATION
- NSAID, predominantly used for analgesia
  - Also has anti-inflammatory & antipyretic activity

DOSE
- One-time dosing: 30 mg IV or 60 mg IM
  - Reduce dose in elderly to 15 mg IV or 30 mg IM
- 30 mg IV/IM q6h, up to 5 days
  - In elderly, use 15 mg IV/IM q6h.
- 10 mg PO q6h, up to 5 days

ONSET
- IM/IV in 30 min

KINETICS
- Duration 4–6 h
- Hepatic metabolism
- Renal excretion

PREPARATION
- 15- or 30-mg/mL vials
- 10-mg tablets

MECHANISM
- Inhibits the enzyme cyclooxygenase, thereby blocking synthesis of prostaglandins

COMMENTS
- 30 mg ketorolac is approx as potent as 12 mg morphine.
- Ketorolac has an antiplatelet effect.
    - Bleeding time increases.
    - Depending on type of surgery, some surgeons may not want increased risk of bleeding.
- Can cause bronchospasm in asthmatics, pts w/ nasal polyposis, & ASA-sensitive pts
- Contraindications
    - Active peptic ulcer disease or GI bleeding
    - Advanced renal disease
    - Pregnancy
    - Procedures where hemostasis is critical
- Risk of renal failure is increased in the pt w/ preexisting renal failure, hypotension, & hypovolemia.

LABETALOL (NORMODYNE, TRANDATE)

CHRISTINE A. WU, MD

INDICATION
- HTN

DOSE
- IV: 5–10-mg bolus q5min. May double dose if no effect; total dose limit 300 mg.

ONSET
- IV: 2–5 min

KINETICS
- Metabolism dependent on hepatic blood flow
- Duration of action: 2–4 h IV

PREPARATION
- IV: 5 mg/mL

MECHANISM
- Competitive antagonists of both alpha- & beta-adrenergic receptors

COMMENTS
- Beta:alpha blockade ratio 5–10:1
- Vasodilation not accompanied by tachycardia
- Useful for treating intraop HTN not due to inadequate anesthesia
- Consider starting with 2.5- or 5-mg dose in elderly pt because of possible exaggerated hypotension.

LIDOCAINE (XYLOCAINE)

GRETE H. PORTEOUS, MD

INDICATION
- Local anesthetic for topical anesthesia, infiltration, peripheral nerve block, spinal, epidural & IV regional anesthesia
- Antiarrhythmic agent for ventricular arrhythmias

DOSE
- Dose for regional block depends on route of administration.
  - Infiltration: 1–60 cc of 0.5–1% solution
  - Brachial plexus block: 15–20 cc of 1.5% solution
  - Epidural: 10–20 cc of 1–2% solution
  - Spinal: 25–75 mg of 0.5–2.5% solution. Use caution when adding epinephrine due to risk of transient neuro symptoms (see Technique chapter "Subarachnoid Block").
- Antiarrhythmic
  - IV bolus dose of 1 mg/kg usually leads to blood level of 1 mcg/mL.
  - Infusion of 1–4 mg/min needed to maintain blood levels
- Max dose in adults: 4.5 mg/kg (total 300 mg) w/o epinephrine, 7 mg/kg w/ epi (total 500 mg)
- Reduce dose in severe renal or hepatic disease & congestive heart failure.

ONSET
- Regional anesthesia
  - Depends on type of nerve block

➤ For local infiltration, onset in <3–5 min
➤ Onset may be faster if solution is alkalinized (see below).
■ Antiarrhythmic effect
➤ 45–90 sec

KINETICS
■ Duration
➤ Antiarrhythmic effect 10–20 min (w/ single IV bolus)
➤ Regional block: depends on type of block & presence of epinephrine
• For spinal/epidural, duration approx 45–90 min
■ Elimination half-life: 1.5–2 h.
■ Hepatic metabolism (amide local anesthetic).
■ Renal excretion of metabolites (90%) & unchanged drug (10%).
■ Therapeutic concentration for arrhythmias is 1.5–6 mcg/mL.
■ Plasma levels >4 mcg/mL assoc w/ toxicity (eg, CNS symptoms).
■ Blood level after regional block depends on type of block, dose of lidocaine, presence of epinephrine, vascularity of injection site.

PREPARATION
■ 0.5–5% solutions. Typical concentrations include
➤ Infiltration: 1–1.5%
➤ Epidural: 1–2%
➤ Topical: 4–5% cream or jelly
➤ Spinal: available as a 1.5% solution (w/ glucose) & a 5% solution (w/ glucose)
• 5% solution should be diluted with at least an equal volume of saline or CSF prior to administration.
■ Lidocaine is also a component of EMLA cream (see Drug chapter "Prilocaine").
■ Lidocaine solution has pH ~4.5.
■ Available w/ the preservative methylparaben in multidose vials (assoc w/ allergic reactions) & in methylparaben-free (MPF) single-dose vials.
■ Epinephrine 1:100,000–1:200,000 may be added to increase duration of effect. Total dose should not exceed 0.25 mg epinephrine, or 50 cc of 1:200,000 dilution. Do not add to spinal lidocaine as may increase risk of neurotoxicity.

MECHANISM
■ Local anesthetic effect
➤ Binds to open sodium channels in sensory & motor neurons & blocks propagation of nerve impulses

- Antiarrhythmic effect
  - ➤ Decreases conduction & automaticity in ventricles
  - ➤ May be more effective in ischemic myocardium
  - ➤ Little effect on atria

COMMENTS

- Major toxicity, like all local anesthetics, is neuro (confusion, agitation, tremors, seizures) & cardiovascular (dysrhythmias, hypotension, cardiovascular collapse).
- Comparison of lidocaine to other local anesthetics
  - ➤ Greater sensory & motor block than tetracaine
  - ➤ Shorter duration & less cardiotoxic than bupivacaine, slower onset than chloroprocaine
- Alkalinization speeds rate of onset & reduces pain of intradermal administration.
  - ➤ Add 1 mEq sodium bicarbonate (1 mL of 8.4% solution) to 9 mL lidocaine.
- Adverse effects w/ spinal use
  - ➤ Associated w/ transient neuro symptoms (buttock & lower extremity pain/dysesthesia), particularly in outpts & those undergoing knee arthroscopy or positioned in lithotomy. Avoided by many anesthesia providers.
  - ➤ Cauda equina syndrome has been reported w/ continuous spinal lidocaine (usually hyperbaric 5% lidocaine) administered via microcatheter.
- IV lidocaine may blunt adverse responses (ie, tachycardia, HTN, bronchospasm) to endotracheal intubation & may reduce coughing when administered prior to extubation.
- ACLS 2000 guidelines now consider lidocaine as "indeterminate" recommendation for shock-refractory ventricular fibrillation or pulseless ventricular tachycardia.

LORAZEPAM (ATIVAN)

JESSICA SAMPAT, MD

INDICATION

- Premedication
- Anxiolysis
- Status epilepticus

DOSE

- PO, IM, IV: 1–4 mg in adults, 0.02–0.08 mg/kg in children

ONSET
- IV: rapid
- IM: 20–30 min
- PO: 20–30 min

KINETICS
- Peak effect
  - IV: 15–20 min
  - IM: 45 min
  - PO: 2 h
- Duration of action: IV, IM, PO, 6–10 h
- Metabolism: hepatic
- Elimination: renal

PREPARATION
- IV: 2 or 4 mg/mL
- PO: tablets (0.5, 1, 2 mg), solution (2 mg/mL)

MECHANISM
- Benzodiazepine; interacts w/ GABA receptor in CNS to increase chloride conductance & hence inhibition in the CNS

COMMENTS
- Treat overdose w/ supportive measures & flumazenil (slow IV 0.2–1.0 mg).
- As w/ other benzodiazepines, use w/ caution in liver failure pt.

MAGNESIUM SULFATE

JEREMY NUSSBAUMER, MD

INDICATION
- Eclampsia, preeclampsia (seizure prevention)
- Hypomagnesemia
- Torsades de pointes
- Alcohol withdrawal

DOSE
- Preeclampsia, eclampsia
  - Bolus: 2–4 g (20% IV solution, over 5 min)
  - Infusion: 1–2.5 g/h (10–20 g in 1,000 cc NS or D5W)
- Torsades

➤ 1–2 g IV bolus
➤ Infusion 0.5–1 g/h IV
➤ Up to 4–6 mg of magnesium may be necessary for suppression.
■ Hypomagnesemia
➤ 1 g IV, up to 8–12 g/day in divided IV doses or by slow infusion as needed to correct magnesium level

ONSET
■ IV: immediate

KINETICS
■ Duration: 30 min
■ Metabolism: none
■ Elimination: renal
■ 1 g magnesium sulfate = 8.1 mEq

PREPARATION
■ Various, from 100 to 500 mg/mL for IV use (these should be diluted to at least 20% solution before administration)

MECHANISM
■ Cofactor for many enzymatic reactions
■ Acts on the renal tubule to maintain calcium & potassium levels
■ Multiple cardiac effects, including calcium channel blocking activity & other antiarrhythmic effects

COMMENTS
■ Administer w/ caution to pt w/ renal failure. Check serum levels to avoid overdosage.
■ Contraindicated in pts w/ heart block
■ Potentiates effects of neuromuscular blocking drugs
■ Check blood magnesium levels to guide therapy. Symptoms of toxicity vary w/ drug levels.
➤ Seizure suppression range: 4–7 mEq/L
➤ 1.5–2.5 mEq/L
  • Normal levels
➤ 3 mEq/L
  • Nausea/vomiting
➤ 4 mEq/L
  • Drowsiness, sweating, unsteady gait
➤ 5 mEq/L
  • Widened QRS & PR intervals

- ➤ 6–7 mEq/L
  - Bradycardia
  - Hypotension
- ➤ >10 mEq/L
  - Heart block, cardiac arrest
  - Muscle weakness, including respiratory muscle
  - Respiratory arrest
- ■ Calcium chloride 1 g IV q5min may temporarily reverse respiratory depression.
- ■ Dopamine or norepinephrine may be used to treat hypotension.

MANNITOL (OSMITROL)

MIMI C. LEE, MD, PHD

INDICATION
- ■ Elevated ICP
- ■ Treatment or prophylaxis of oliguria/anuria assoc w/ acute renal failure
- ■ Elevated intraocular pressure

DOSE
- ■ Adults: 0.25–1.0 g/kg IV as 20% solution over 30–60 min; may give 1.25–25 g over 5–10 min if needed acutely
- ■ Children: 0.5–1 g/kg over 30–60 min

ONSET
- ■ 15 min

KINETICS
- ■ Duration: 2–3 h
- ■ Metabolism: minimal
- ■ Excretion: renal

PREPARATION
- ■ Commercially available as 5, 10, 15, 20, 25% solutions
- ■ May need to warm mannitol solutions to dissolve crystals

MECHANISM
- ■ Causes osmotic diuresis & expansion of intravascular volume
- ■ Increases serum osmolality
- ■ Decreases ICP by decreasing cerebral edema

COMMENTS
- May lead to sudden vasodilation & hypotension
- May cause or exacerbate pulmonary edema, intracranial hemorrhage, systemic hypertension, or rebound intracranial hypertension
- Often leads to hyponatremia
- Consider monitoring serum osmolality if mannitol is given for elevated ICP.

MAO INHIBITORS: ISOCARBOXAZID (MARPLAN), PHENELZINE (NARDIL), TRANYLCYPROMINE (PARNATE)

JOHN TAYLOR, MD

INDICATION
- Atypical & refractory depression

DOSE
- Tranylcypromine: 30 mg/day
- Isocarboxazid: 20 mg/day
- Phenelzine: 45–75 mg/day

ONSET
- 1–6 wks to obtain full therapeutic effect

KINETICS
- All MAO inhibitors have relatively short half-life (hours) but have long-lasting effects because MAO inhibition is irreversible. Synthesis of new MAO may take several wks.

PREPARATION
- Tablets

MECHANISM
- Irreversibly blocks MAO, the enzyme responsible for the oxidative deamination of neurotransmitters such as serotonin, norepinephrine, dopamine.

COMMENTS
- Many potential adverse reactions, some of which can be life-threatening
  - Reactions include severe HTN, fever, seizures, coma.
  - Sympathomimetic drugs, both direct- & indirect-acting, can have exaggerated responses & cause hypertensive crisis. This includes

sympathomimetic drugs commonly used in anesthesia care, such as
- Dopamine
- Ephedrine
- Phenylephrine
- Isoproterenol
- Epinephrine

➤ Drug interactions w/ narcotics can cause fever, coma, hemodynamic instability, death.
  - This is best documented for meperidine (Demerol), but there is a theoretical risk w/ all narcotics.

■ Patients taking MAO inhibitors who receive GA are at risk for profound hypotension, in addition to the above-mentioned risk of drug interactions w/ sympathomimetics & narcotics.

■ For pts requiring GA, discontinue MAO inhibitor for at least 2 weeks prior to surgery. This must be balanced against the risk of suicide in severely depressed pts.
  ➤ Although some report uneventful anesthesia in pts on MAO inhibitors, pts should be considered at increased risk of hemodynamic instability (both HTN & hypotension) & drug interactions, especially w/ narcotics & sympathomimetic agents.
  ➤ Even w/ discontinuation of therapy for >2 weeks, pt may still be susceptible to profound hypotension, possibly related to decreased sensitivity of adrenergic receptors.

■ Considerations w/ spinal & epidural anesthesia
  ➤ Pts on MAO inhibitors are susceptible to profound hypotension from sympathetic blockade.
  ➤ Pts may then require sympathomimetic agents, w/ the potential for adverse drug interactions.

■ Considerations for pt on MAO inhibitors presenting for emergency surgery
  ➤ GA may be preferred over central neuraxial block (less effect on sympathetic tone).
  ➤ Avoid narcotics, especially meperidine.
  ➤ Consider peripheral nerve block to avoid narcotics for postop pain.
  ➤ Avoid cocaine as local anesthetic.
  ➤ Do not add epinephrine to local anesthetics.
  ➤ Small dose of benzodiazepines considered safe for premed
  ➤ Treat hypotension w/ IV fluids first to avoid use of sympathomimetic agents.

- ➤ If sympathomimetic agents are necessary, use direct-acting agents in small doses & carefully titrate to effect.
- ➤ Inhaled agents considered safe, but avoid halothane due to arrhythmogenic potential
- ➤ Monitor carefully for adverse reactions including hypotension, HTN, fever.
- ■ MAO inhibitors have potent hypotensive effects; up to 50% of pts experience dizziness. Other common side effects: dry mouth, GI upset, urinary hesitancy, headache, myoclonus.
- ■ Contraindications: uncontrolled HTN; pheochromocytoma; hepatic or renal disease; cerebrovascular defect; CHF; concurrent use of sympathomimetics, ethanol, meperidine & SSRIs, other MAO inhibitors, CNS depressants, excess caffeine, tricyclic antidepressants
- ■ Pts on MAO inhibitors are also susceptible to food interactions. Ingestion of food containing dopamine, ephedrine or tyramine (eg, fava beans, wine, some cheeses) can produce severe HTN.

MEPERIDINE (DEMEROL)

DAN BURKHARDT, MD

INDICATION
- ■ Analgesia
  - ➤ Short-term treatment of severe pain
- ■ Symptomatic control of rigors

DOSE
- ■ 12.5–50 mg IV prn rigor or pain
- ■ 25 mg via epidural for rigors secondary to regional anesthetic

ONSET
- ■ IV onset: 5 min

KINETICS
- ■ Hepatically metabolized, renally excreted
- ■ Plasma half-life: approx 2–4 h

PREPARATION
- ■ Multiple strengths of tablets, liquid, injections

MECHANISM
- ■ Opioid receptor agonist
- ■ Multiple other interactions (see comments)

COMMENTS

- Useful for treating rigors from a number of causes, including GA, amphotericin B infusion, nonhemolytic febrile transfusion reactions
- Use as an analgesic limited by multiple side effects & drug interactions
- Active metabolite normeperidine accumulates (esp in renal failure), causing CNS excitation & ultimately seizures. Effect has been seen even in healthy pts receiving >1,000 mg/day.
- Vagolytic effect can cause tachycardia.
- May directly depress myocardial contractility in high doses
- Interacts with MAO inhibitors, precipitating a potentially fatal syndrome w/ agitation, delirium, hyperthermia, convulsions
- Can precipitate histamine release (like morphine)
- No clinical difference in biliary spasm compared w/ other opioids
- Weak local anesthetic effects w/ neuraxial & subcutaneous administration
- Sometimes specifically requested by pts for its euphoric effects
- Consider dose reduction in liver or renal failure.
- Effects common to all narcotics
  - Depresses CO_2-triggered respiratory drive in a dose-dependent fashion. Hypercarbia can also exacerbate increases in ICP. Useful in low doses to palliate the sensation of dyspnea.
  - Crosses placenta: respiratory depression in newborn if mother has had large doses
  - Constipation: pts on chronic narcotics should receive prophylactic treatment
  - Nausea/vomiting: treat w/ antiemetics and/or nonnarcotic adjuncts to reduce the total opioid dose, or change opioids
  - Modest vagotonic effect: bradycardia w/ large bolus doses
  - Delayed gastric emptying
  - Biliary spasm: no clinical difference between opioids
  - Urinary retention
  - Miosis
  - Euphoria/dysphoria or frank delirium: more common in the elderly
  - Myoclonus w/ extremely high doses
  - Chest wall rigidity w/ large doses IV push
  - Physical dependence & withdrawal after prolonged use: wean dose gently, consider adjunctive clonidine
  - Psychiatric addiction (taking the drug for reasons other than pain relief) is very rare, especially in the acute postop setting.

MEPIVACAINE (CARBOCAINE, POLOCAINE)

GRETE H. PORTEOUS, MD

INDICATION
- Local anesthetic for infiltration, peripheral nerve block, epidural anesthesia
- Not for spinal use

DOSE
- Infiltration: 50–400 mg using 0.5% or 1% solution
- Brachial plexus block: 5–40 mL of 1% solution or 5–20 mL of 2% solution
- Epidural
  - ➤ 15–30 mL of 1% solution
  - ➤ 10–25 mL of 1.5% solution
  - ➤ 10–20 mL of 2% solution
- Avoid concentrations >1.5% in regional anesthesia if <3 yrs or <14 kg.
- Max dose: 5 mg/kg (max 400 mg in adults), or 7 mg/kg w/ epinephrine

ONSET
- Epidural: 5–15 min
- Major nerve block: 10–20 min

KINETICS
- Duration: typically 0.5–2 h
- For nerve block w/ epi, duration can be up to 3–5 h.
- Hepatic metabolism (amide local anesthetic)
- Renal excretion

PREPARATION
- 1%, 2% solutions.
- Multiple-dose vials contain preservative methylparaben.

MECHANISM
- Binds to open sodium channels in sensory & motor neurons & blocks propagation of nerve impulses

COMMENTS
- Major toxicity, like all local anesthetics, is neurologic (confusion, agitation, tremors, seizures) & cardiovascular (dysrhythmias, hypotension, cardiovascular collapse).

- Clinically similar to lidocaine but slightly less vasodilator effect, greater potency & duration of action.
- Use w/ caution in pt w/ liver or renal disease.

METHADONE (DOLOPHINE, METHADOSE, PHYSEPTONE)

DAN BURKHARDT, MD

INDICATION
- Analgesia
  - ➢ Severe pain (used in combination w/ a shorter-acting opioid)
- Opioid detoxification & prevention of withdrawal

DOSE
- 10–30 mg PO qd to prevent opioid withdrawal.
  - ➢ Higher dose may be necessary, depending on pt.

ONSET
- PO onset: 30–60 min
- IV onset: 10–20 min

KINETICS
- Hepatic metabolism, renal excretion
- Plasma half-life: approx 30 h

PREPARATION
- Available in multiple strengths of tablets & oral solutions, as well as IV injection (10 mg/mL)

MECHANISM
- Opioid receptor agonist

COMMENTS
- Cross-tolerance w/ other opioids can be incomplete. Convert equivalent dosage from other drugs conservatively.
- Reduce dose by approx 50% when converting from PO to IV (also a conservative estimate).
- A change in dose requires several days to demonstrate full effect.
- Metabolism is increased by carbamazepine, phenobarbital, rifampin, phenytoin, nevirapine. This could precipitate opioid withdrawal if the methadone dose is not increased.
- Effects common to all narcotics

➤ Depresses CO_2-triggered respiratory drive in a dose-dependent fashion. Hypercarbia can also exacerbate increases in ICP. Useful in low doses to palliate the sensation of dyspnea.

➤ Crosses placenta: respiratory depression in newborn if mother has had large doses

➤ Constipation: pts on chronic narcotics should receive prophylactic treatment

➤ Nausea/vomiting: treat w/ antiemetics and/or nonnarcotic adjuncts to reduce the total opioid dose, or change opioids

➤ Modest vagotonic effect: bradycardia w/ large bolus doses

➤ Delayed gastric emptying

➤ Biliary spasm: no clinical difference between opioids

➤ Urine retention

➤ Miosis

➤ Euphoria/dysphoria, or frank delirium: more common in the elderly

➤ Myoclonus w/ extremely high doses

➤ Physical dependence & withdrawal after prolonged use: wean dose gently, consider adjunctive clonidine

➤ Psychiatric addiction (taking the drug for reasons other than pain relief) is very rare, especially in the acute postop setting.

METHOHEXITAL SODIUM (BREVITAL)

JESSICA SAMPAT, MD

INDICATION
■ Induction or maintenance of GA
■ Sedation

DOSE
■ Anesthesia
  ➤ Induction
    • IV: 1–2 mg/kg
    • IM: 7–10 mg/kg
    • Rectal: 20–30 mg/kg (pediatrics)
  ➤ Maintenance
    • Infusion, 50–150 mcg/kg/min (0.2% solution) titrated to effect

ONSET
■ IV: rapid

- IM: 2–10 min
- Rectal: 5–15 min

KINETICS
- Duration of action
  - IV: 5–10 min
  - Rectal/IM: 30–90 min
- Metabolism: hepatic
- Elimination: renal

PREPARATION
- Powder for injection: 500 mg, 2.5 g, 5.0 g.
- For IV infusion, dilute to 2 mg/mL.
- For rectal administration or IV boluses, dilute to 10 mg/mL.
- For IM administration, dilute to 50 mg/mL.
- When reconstituted in D_5W or normal saline, solutions are stable for 24 h.

MECHANISM
- Ultrashort-acting barbiturate that enhances the action of GABA at GABA-A receptors

COMMENTS
- Extravascular injection may cause necrosis; intra-arterial injection may lead to gangrene.
- Contraindicated in pts w/ latent or manifest porphyria
- Reduce dose in elderly, hypovolemic pts
- Also used to induce seizure focus during brain mapping in epilepsy surgery

METHYLENE BLUE

JAMES BRANDES, MD

INDICATION
- Dye used to visualize anatomy/fistulas in surgery
- Treatment of drug-induced methemoglobinemia (not in cyanide poisoning)
- Diagnosis of amniotic membrane rupture

DOSE
- 1–2 mg/kg, injected over several min

ONSET
- Immediate IV onset

KINETICS
- Peak effect in <1 h; duration varies
- Renal excretion (75%)

PREPARATION
- 10 mg/cc in 10-cc vial
- 55-mg or 65-mg tablets

MECHANISM
- Tissue dye; renal excretion allows for visualization of ureters & urine leaks/fistulas
- Oxidation-reduction action: High concentrations reduce ferrous to ferric form of hemoglobin, & thus methemoglobin is produced. Low concentrations cause the conversion of methemoglobin into hemoglobin.

COMMENTS
- Methylene blue causes direct interference w/ light absorbance of the pulse oximeter. Oxygen saturation can fall dramatically within 30 sec & may take 3–4 min or longer to return to baseline.
- Releases cyanide from cyanomethemoglobin
- Contraindicated in pts w/ G6PD deficiency (can cause hemolysis) & in pts w/ severe renal insufficiency
- Skin stains may be removed w/ hypochlorite solution.
- Intra-amniotic injection to evaluate for membrane rupture may cause neonatal bradycardia, methemoglobinemia, hemolytic anemia, hyperbilirubinemia, & blue skin.
- Side effects include tachycardia, hypertension, chest pain.

METHYLERGONOVINE (METHERGINE)

LISA SWOR-YIM, MD

INDICATION
- Prevention & treatment of postpartum & postabortion hemorrhage caused by uterine atony or subinvolution

DOSE
- IM/IV: 0.2 mg q2–4h after delivery (max dose 1.0 mg)
  - ➤ Use IV w/ caution & only in emergencies because it may produce HTN & stroke.
- Oral: 0.2–0.4 mg q6–8h for 2–7 days

ONSET
- Oral: 5–15 min
- IM: 2–5 min
- IV: immediate

KINETICS
- Hepatic metabolism
- Half-life: 0.5–3.0 h
- Duration: usually at least 3 h

PREPARATION
- Injection: 0.2 mg/mL
- Tablet: 0.2 mg

MECHANISM
- Direct stimulation of uterine & vascular smooth muscles

COMMENTS
- Can cause uterine hypertonus.
- Do not give in uncontrolled hypertension.
- Do not routinely give IV; may cause sudden HTN & stroke.

METHYLPREDNISOLONE

IVAN ZEITZ, MD

INDICATION
- Anti-inflammatory agent
  - ➤ Asthma, acute spinal cord injury, many other conditions
- Immunosuppressant therapy
  - ➤ Organ transplant rejection, immune-mediated diseases
- Corticosteroid replacement
  - ➤ Adrenal insufficiency

DOSE
- Varies depending on indication
- May range from 10–1,500 mg/day
- For severe asthma or status asthmaticus
  - ➤ 1–2 mg/kg IV q6h
  - ➤ After acute asthma episode improves, switch to oral therapy & taper.
- Acute spinal cord injury

- ➤ Reduces motor deficit after acute spinal cord injury if given within 8 h of injury
- ➤ 30 mg/kg IV bolus followed by
- ➤ 5.4 mg/kg/h for 23 h
- Prevention of rejection w/ solid organ transplant surgery
  - ➤ Typical adult dose: 1 g IV at start of surgery

ONSET
- Time to peak IV concentration: 30 min
- Maximum clinical effects lag behind peak plasma concentrations; takes a few hours for onset.

KINETICS
- Elimination half-life: 2–3 h
- Hypothalamic-pituitary axis suppression lasts 1.25–1.5 days from single 40-mg dose.
- Hepatic metabolism
- Renal excretion of inactive metabolites

PREPARATION
- Supplied as powder, to be reconstituted

MECHANISM
- Synthetic corticosteroid
- Multiple actions, including
  - ➤ Anti-inflammatory
  - ➤ Immunosuppressive
  - ➤ Antiproliferative

COMMENTS
- Asthma & corticosteroids
  - ➤ Beneficial effects of corticosteroids in acute asthma
    - Improve response to beta agonists
    - Decrease inflammatory response
    - Decrease mucus production
    - Reduce relapse rate
  - ➤ Recommended for pts w/ moderate to severe bronchospasm, although onset may take hours
- Consider use in pts w/ refractory hypotension w/o clear cause.
- Stress-dose steroids should be given to pts on chronic steroid therapy undergoing a significant operation.
- Short-term usage unlikely to produce toxic effects, but can cause
  - ➤ CNS symptoms, including euphoria & psychosis

- ➤ Increased white blood cell count, mostly from increased release from marrow
- ➤ Arrhythmias, myocardial infarction, cardiac arrest have been reported following large doses given by rapid IV administration.
- ■ With longer course of therapy, many adverse effects can occur, including
  - ➤ Increased risk of infection
  - ➤ Delayed wound healing
  - ➤ Sodium & fluid retention
  - ➤ HTN
  - ➤ Psychosis
  - ➤ Hyperglycemia
  - ➤ Adrenal suppression
  - ➤ Cushing's syndrome
  - ➤ GI ulcers
  - ➤ Cataracts
  - ➤ Ecchymosis or easy bruising
  - ➤ Osteoporosis

METOCLOPRAMIDE (REGLAN)

EMILY REINYS, MD
JEREMY NUSSBAUMER, MD

INDICATION
- ■ Antiemetic
- ■ Accelerates gastric emptying/intestinal motility

DOSE
- ■ 10–20 mg (0.25 mg/kg) PO, IM, or IV

ONSET
- ■ IV: 1–3 min
- ■ IM: 10–15 min
- ■ PO: 30–60 min

KINETICS
- ■ Half-life: 4–7 h
- ■ Duration: 1–3 h
- ■ Urinary excretion
- ■ Elimination half-life: 5–6 h

PREPARATION
- 5-, 10-mg tablets
- 5 mg/cc for injection

MECHANISM
- Facilitates transmission at muscarinic ACh receptors (speeds gastric emptying, increases lower esophageal sphincter tone)
- Acts centrally as a dopamine antagonist (antiemetic effect)

COMMENTS
- Rapid IV injection may cause abdominal cramping.
  - Can cause CNS side effects
    - Drowsiness
    - Extrapyramidal reactions common
    - Acute dystonic reaction can also occur; may require IV antihistamine or anticholinergic therapy.
- Avoid in pts w/ Parkinson's disease (dopamine antagonism may worsen extrapyramidal symptoms).
- May facilitate gastric emptying in pts w/ diabetic gastroparesis
- In pts w/ reduced Cr clearance, dose needs to be decreased (to 50% of normal dose if Cr clearance is10–40 mL/min & to 25% of normal if Cr clearance <10 mL/min).

METOCURINE (METUBINE)

JAMES CALDWELL, MB CHB

INDICATION
- Neuromuscular block
- Facilitation of tracheal intubation
- Maintenance of surgical relaxation

DOSE
- 0.3–0.4 mg/kg IV for tracheal intubation
- 0.05–0.1 mg/kg IV to maintain surgical relaxation

ONSET
- 3–5 min

KINETICS
- Metabolism: does not occur
- Renal excretion: >95%

- Hepatic elimination: <5%
- Elimination half-life: 300 min

Duration
- Intubation dose: 60–120 min
- Maintenance dose: 30–45 min

PREPARATION
- 2 mg/mL solution in 20-mL vial

MECHANISM
- Competitive antagonist of acetylcholine at neuromuscular junction
- Semisynthetic benzylisoquinoline derivative of d-tubocurarine

COMMENTS
- Histamine release may cause hypotension.
- Acts synergistically w/ muscle relaxants that are steroid derivatives (eg, pancuronium).
- Little role in current clinical practice because of histamine release & long duration.

METOPROLOL (LOPRESSOR)

CHRISTINE A. WU, MD

INDICATION
- Antihypertensive
- Stable angina
- Initial treatment of acute MI (IV form)
- Stable heart failure

DOSE
- IV: 2.5- to 5-mg doses q2–5min.
- 100 mg/day PO BID is typical oral dose.

ONSET
- IV: 5 min
- PO: 20–30 min

KINETICS
- Complete absorption after oral administration but only 40% bioavailability due to first-pass metabolism
- Extensively metabolized by hepatic monooxygenase system

- Elimination: renal (but only 3–10% as unchanged drug)
- Dosing does not need to be adjusted in renal failure
- Half-life: 3–4 h

PREPARATION
- IV: 1 mg/mL
- PO: 25-, 50-, 100-mg tablets

MECHANISM
- B1-selective adrenergic antagonist w/o intrinsic sympathomimetic activity

COMMENTS
- Improves outcome in pts at risk for myocardial ischemia
- Abrupt withdrawal can lead to myocardial ischemia.
- Survival benefit w/ long-term beta-blocker therapy in stable heart failure
- Contraindicated in
  - Cardiogenic shock
  - Heart block greater than first degree
  - Severe bradycardia
  - Unstable or severe heart failure
  - Bronchospasm

METRONIDAZOLE (FLAGYL)

JEREMY NUSSBAUMER, MD

INDICATION
- Antibacterial & antiprotozoal antibiotic
  - Often used for activity against anaerobic bacteria
  - Used orally for treatment of pseudomembranous colitis (not discussed)

DOSE
- Adult surgical prophylaxis
  - Typical regimen: 500–1,000 mg IV 1 h before surgery followed by 500 mg IV q6h
- Anaerobic infections: 500 mg IV, PO q6–8h
- Children: 15–35 mg/kg/day PO in divided doses q8h or 30 mg/kg/day IV in divided doses q8h

ONSET
- IV: immediate; often given for a 7- to 10-day course

KINETICS
- Hepatic metabolism 30–60%
- 20% excreted unchanged in urine
- Half-life: 6–11 h
  - ➤ Up to 21 h in end-stage renal disease, 25–75 h in neonates

PREPARATION
- IV 50 mg/mL.
- Dilute in 250 mL NS or sterile water & administer over 1 h.

MECHANISM
- Complex action results in a reduction reaction, causing DNA strand breakage in susceptible organisms.

COMMENTS
- Adverse reactions
  - ➤ Disulfiram-like reaction w/ ETOH
  - ➤ Urticaria, flushing or rash secondary to hypersensitivity
  - ➤ Decreased WBC count, seizures, peripheral neuropathy have been reported w/ long-term therapy.
- Adjust dose in renal failure.
  - ➤ For GFR <10 mL/min or peritoneal dialysis, decrease dose by 50%.
  - ➤ Dose does not change w/ hemodialysis.
- Reduce dose in liver failure.
  - ➤ No consensus on degree of dose adjustment for hepatic disease
- Contraindicated in first trimester of pregnancy

MIDAZOLAM (VERSED)

RENÉE J. ROBERTS, MD
LISA SWOR-YIM, MD

INDICATION
- Conscious sedation
- Premed
- Anxiolysis
- GA induction

DOSE
- Children
  - ➤ Premed
    - PO: 0.5–1.0 mg/kg (max 20 mg)
    - IM: 0.01–0.15 mg/kg (max 10 mg)
    - IV: 0.035 mg/kg initial dose & titrate to desired effect
    - Intranasal: 0.2–0.4 mg/kg (max 15 mg)
  - ➤ Conscious sedation
    - PO: 0.2–0.4 mg/kg (max 15 mg)
    - IV: 0.05 mg/kg
- Adults
  - ➤ Premed
    - IM: 0.07–0.08 mg/kg 60 min preop
    - IV: 0.5–2.0 mg typical dose
  - ➤ Conscious sedation
    - IV: Initial: 0.5–2.0 mg, repeating doses q3–5min if needed. Reduce dose in elderly.
- GA induction: 0.1–0.4 mg/kg

ONSET
- IV: 2–4 min
- IM: 15 min

KINETICS
- Metabolism: hepatic
- Elimination half-life: approx 2 h
- Elimination: renal
- High lipid solubility

PREPARATION
- 1 mg/cc or 5 mg/cc concentrations for IV/IM use
- Syrup 2 mg/mL for PO use

MECHANISM
- Binds to BDZ receptor (alpha subunit of GABA) & causes Cl channel opening, thus hyperpolarizing postsynaptic neurons
- Potentiates GABA-mediated neural inhibition

COMMENTS
- Anterograde amnesia
- No retrograde amnesia
- Anticonvulsant

- Decreases $CMRO_2$ & cerebral blood flow & ICP
- May cause hypotension
- May cause respiratory depression
- Has no analgesic properties
- Benzodiazepines may increase risk of congenital malformations when given during pregnancy; risk probably greatest in first trimester.
- May cause neonatal depression as it does cross placenta

MILRINONE

KALEB JENSON, MD

INDICATION
- Primary indication: congestive heart failure (CHF)
- Other indications
  - ➤ Acute decompensated heart failure post-cardiac surgery
  - ➤ Pulmonary HTN: esp in presence of RV systolic or diastolic dysfunction (eg, RVH), or LV systolic dysfunction
  - ➤ In children, consider use if RV is impaired; for instance:
    - Longstanding pulmonary HTN
    - RVH w/ diastolic dysfunction (tetralogy of Fallot)
    - RV systolic dysfunction from chronic volume overload (eg, patient s/p Norwood stage I & Glenn procedure)

DOSE
- Loading dose: 50 mcg/kg IV over 10 min
- Alternative loading dose (if concern that peripheral vasodilation will cause hypotension)
  - ➤ 25 mcg/kg IV over 5 min, given at initiation of rewarming phase from CPB
- Maintenance dose: 0.375–0.75 mcg/kg/min (0.5 mcg/kg/min most common)
- Daily dose not to exceed 1.13 mg/kg
- Dose reduction for renal failure
  - ➤ Creatinine clearance (mL/min/1.73 m^2/maximum milrinone infusion rate (mcg/kg/min)
    - 5/0.2
    - 10/0.23
    - 20/0.28

- 30/0.33
- 40/0.38
- 50/0.43

ONSET
■ 5–15 min

KINETICS
■ Elimination half-life: 2.3 h
■ Most milrinone is excreted unconjugated in the urine.

PREPARATION
■ 1 mg/mL in 10-mg vial
■ Dilute to 200 mcg/cc (eg, 10 mg milrinone + 40 mL D5W or NS).

MECHANISM
■ Selective inhibitor of type III cAMP phosphodiesterase isozyme in cardiac & vascular muscle.
■ Positive inotrope, vasodilator & lusitropy w/ few chronotropic effects.
  ➤ Like nitroglycerin & nitroprusside, milrinone promotes diastolic relaxation.

COMMENTS
■ Causes dose-related cardiovascular changes
  ➤ Increase in CO
  ➤ Decrease in pulmonary capillary wedge pressure
  ➤ Decrease in pulmonary & systemic vascular resistance
  ➤ Mild to moderate HR increase
  ➤ Does not increase myocardial oxygen consumption
  ➤ Increases risk of ventricular ectopy in high-risk pts
  ➤ Shortens AV nodal conduction time; could increase SVT rates
■ Not recommended in acute MI
■ Hypotension due to decreased vascular resistance may be pronounced, especially when LVEDP is low, when used post-CPB, or in acute CHF.
  ➤ 5% of patients at low dose & 17% of those at high dose develop significant hypotension.
  ➤ For LV systolic dysfunction post-CPB, consider epinephrine rather than milrinone.
■ Comparison to amrinone
  ➤ Amrinone has faster onset (peaks at 5 min).
  ➤ Amrinone may cause thrombocytopenia.

MIVACURIUM

RENÉE J. ROBERTS, MD

INDICATION
- Neuromuscular block

DOSE
- Intubating: 0.15–0.25 mg/kg
- Maintenance: 0.1 mg/kg q15min
- Infusion: 5–8 mcg/kg/m

ONSET
- 3–5 min

KINETICS
- 10–20 min for 25% recovery
- Metabolized by plasma cholinesterase
- Metabolites excreted in urine

PREPARATION
- 2 mg/mL

MECHANISM
- Nondepolarizing neuromuscular block
- Competes w/ acetylcholine at nicotinic receptor site on motor end-plate

COMMENTS
- Slight histamine release can cause hypotension, esp if given rapidly.
- May be prolonged duration if pt has abnormal plasma cholinesterase.
- Duration may be 10–15 min if renal failure.

MORPHINE (ROXANOL, MSIR, MS CONTIN, DURAMORPH)

DAN BURKHARDT, MD

INDICATION
- Analgesia
- Anesthesia adjunct
- Adjunctive treatment of congestive heart failure

DOSE

- 10–30 mg PO q4h prn (immediate release), 30 mg PO q8–12h (sustained release)
- 1–4 mg IV initially, repeat & titrate to effect, maintenance dose q1–2h prn
- Pediatric dose: 0.025–0.05 mg/kg IV
- Preservative-free solutions: 2–5 mg epidural, 0.1–0.25 mg IT (higher dose for cardiac surgery)
- PCA
  - For postop pain, commonly administered IV as 1-mg bolus, 6-min lockout, no basal rate, 2 mg/h rescue bolus

ONSET

- IV: within 6 min
- IV peak effect: approx 20 min

KINETICS

- Hepatic metabolism, renal excretion
- Plasma half-life: approx 2–4 h

PREPARATION

- Available in multiple strengths of tablets (including sustained-release tablets), liquids, suppositories & injections suitable for SC, IM, IV, epidural & IT administration

MECHANISM

- Opioid receptor agonist

COMMENTS

- Long-acting active metabolite (morphine-6-glucuronide) can accumulate in renal failure.
- Can cause histamine release: usually manifests as a cutaneous wheal at the injection site, but can cause systemic anaphylactoid reaction. Do not give large doses IV push.
- Venodilator: reduces cardiac preload (useful in acute congestive heart failure)
- Pruritus (worse IT than IV): itching from neuraxial morphine responds well to low-dose naloxone (0.04 mg IV q15min x3 prn itch)
- Delayed respiratory depression (8–12 h) w/ epidural & IT administration; monitor appropriately
- Reduced metabolism in neonates
- Sustained-release tablets cannot be crushed for administration via a feeding tube. Doing so will result in a large bolus dose.
- Consider dose reduction in liver or renal failure.

■ Effects common to all narcotics
  ➤ Depresses CO_2-triggered respiratory drive in a dose-dependent fashion. Hypercarbia can also exacerbate increases in ICP.
  ➤ Useful in low doses to palliate the sensation of dyspnea
  ➤ Crosses placenta: respiratory depression in newborn if mother has had large doses
  ➤ Constipation: pts on chronic narcotics should receive prophylactic treatment
  ➤ Nausea/vomiting: treat w/ antiemetics and/or nonnarcotic adjuncts to reduce the total opioid dose, or change opioids
  ➤ Modest vagotonic effect: bradycardia w/ large bolus doses
  ➤ Delayed gastric emptying
  ➤ Biliary spasm: no clinical difference between opioids
  ➤ Urinary retention
  ➤ Miosis
  ➤ Euphoria/dysphoria, or frank delirium: more common in the elderly
  ➤ Myoclonus w/ extremely high doses
  ➤ Chest wall rigidity w/ large doses IV push
  ➤ Physical dependence & withdrawal after prolonged use: wean dose gently, consider adjunctive clonidine
  ➤ Psychiatric addiction (taking the drug for reasons other than pain relief) is very rare, especially in the acute postop setting.

NALBUPHINE (NUBAIN)

DAN BURKHARDT, MD

INDICATION
■ Moderate pain

DOSE
■ 5–20 mg IV q3–6h prn (max 160 mg/day)
■ IV analgesic potency similar to morphine

ONSET
■ IV peak effect: approx 3–5 min

KINETICS
■ Hepatic metabolism, excreted in feces
■ Plasma half-life: approx 5 h

PREPARATION
- 10, 20 mg/mL for injection

MECHANISM
- Synthetic opioid agonist-antagonist
- Binds to numerous opioid receptors in CNS to inhibit ascending nociceptive pathways
- Antagonizes opioid mu receptors

COMMENTS
- Has a ceiling effect: doses >30 mg IV produce no further analgesia
- Can precipitate a withdrawal syndrome in pts on chronic opioid agonists
- If used as a premed, may limit the potency of subsequent pure opioid agonists
- More cardiovascular stability than other partial agonists
- Abrupt discontinuation after prolonged use (>10 days) can precipitate withdrawal.
- Sedative effects can be reversed w/ naloxone.
- Consider dose reduction in pt w/ liver failure.

NALOXONE (NARCAN)

RENÉE J. ROBERTS, MD
MADELEINE BIBAT, MD

INDICATION
- Reversal of narcotic effect

DOSE
- Adults: 0.04–0.4 mg IV/IM/SC q3min; max 10 mg
- Pediatric: 1–10 mcg/kg IV/IM/SC q3min; max 0.4 mg

ONSET
- IV: 1–3 min
- IM/SC: 2–5 min

KINETICS
- Duration: 1 h
- Elimination half-life: 60–90 min
- Hepatic metabolism
- Renal excretion

PREPARATION
- 0.4, 1 mg/mL for injection

MECHANISM
- Pure opiate competitive antagonist
- Mu > kappa > delta opioid receptors

COMMENTS
- Repeat doses may be necessary in the presence of long-acting opiates.
- Side effects
  - Sympathetic stimulation: increased HR, HTN
  - Unmasking of postop pain
  - Pulmonary edema
  - Ventricular irritability
  - Vomiting
  - Acute withdrawal syndrome in narcotic-dependent pt
- For pt who does not have severe respiratory depression, administer in small increments (eg, 10–40 mcg) to minimize side effects.
- Naloxone is the first-line therapy to reverse opioid effects. It has a faster onset & a shorter duration of action than naltrexone, so is easier to titrate.

NALTREXONE (REVIA)

DAN BURKHARDT, MD

INDICATION
- Maintenance of opioid abstinence
- Treatment of alcohol addiction

DOSE
- 25–50 mg PO qd

ONSET
- Peak effect: approx 1 h

KINETICS
- Plasma half-life: approx 4 h for parent compound, 13 h for active metabolite (6-beta-naltrexol)
- Metabolism: hepatic
- Elimination: renal

PREPARATION
- 50-mg tablet

MECHANISM
- Competitive antagonist that binds to opioid receptors in CNS

COMMENTS
- Used to prevent relapse in pts w/ a history of opioid addiction.
- Naloxone is the first-line therapy to reverse opioid effects. It has a faster onset & a shorter duration of action than naltrexone, so it is easier to titrate.
- Consider an IV naloxone test dose before starting naltrexone if there is any possibility of recent opioid use. Naltrexone will precipitate a prolonged and difficult-to-treat withdrawal syndrome in pts physically dependent on opioids.
- Hepatotoxic at doses approx 5 times normal.

NEOSTIGMINE

RONNIE LU, MD

INDICATION
- Reversal of neuromuscular block

DOSE
- 0.04–0.07 mg/kg up to max dose 5 mg

ONSET
- 5–10 min

KINETICS
- Duration: >1 h
- Hepatic metabolism
- Renal excretion

PREPARATION
- 0.5, 1 mg/mL solution

MECHANISM
- Noncompetitive (covalent) inhibitor of acetylcholinesterase

COMMENTS
- Administer w/ glycopyrrolate 0.2 mg per 1 mg neostigmine to block muscarinic cholinergic effects.

NICARDIPINE

JEREMY NUSSBAUMER, MD

INDICATION
- Chronic stable angina
- HTN
- Migraine headache

DOSE
- PO: 20–40 mg tid
- IV: initial infusion dose 5 mg/h
  - ➤ Increase dose by 2.5 mg/hr q15min to max rate of 15 mg/h.

ONSET
- PO
  - ➤ Peak serum levels in 20–120 min
  - ➤ Decreased BP in 20 min
- IV
  - ➤ Onset within 1 min

KINETICS
- Duration: 3 h
- Elimination half-life: 45–100 min
- Extensive first-pass hepatic metabolism to inactive metabolites
- Metabolites eliminated in urine, feces

PREPARATION
- Oral tablets.
- IV preparation 2.5 mg/mL in 10-mL vial.
- For IV bolus, dilute to 1 mg/mL.
- For IV infusion, dilute 25 mg in 250 mL NS or D5W to 0.1 mg/mL.

MECHANISM
- Blocks slow calcium channels
- Produces relaxation of coronary vascular smooth muscle & increases myocardial O_2 supply

COMMENTS
- Avoid in hypotension, second- or third-degree heart block, sinus bradycardia, ventricular tachycardia, cardiogenic shock, aortic stenosis, CHF.
- Consider dose reduction in pt w/ liver failure.

- Can be used as IV infusion for BP control in pts w/ hypertensive crisis, including pre-eclampsia.
- Use w/ caution if recent use of beta-blockers.

NIFEDIPINE

EMILY REINYS, MD
JEREMY NUSSBAUMER, MD

INDICATION
- HTN
- Angina (drug of choice for Prinzmetal variant angina)
- Pulmonary HTN

DOSE
- PO capsules: initial dose 10 mg PO tid, range 10–30 mg tid
- Extended-release capsules: initial dose 30 mg PO qd, range 30–180 mg PO qd

ONSET
- Approx 20 min for capsules
- 1–2 h for extended-release form

KINETICS
- Plasma half-life: 2–5 h
- Hepatic metabolism
- Renal excretion

PREPARATION
- 10-, 20-, 30-mg capsules (short-acting) administered orally
- 30-, 60-, 90-mg tablets (extended-release)

MECHANISM
- Inhibits calcium influx into myocardial & vascular smooth muscle cells, causing coronary & systemic vasodilatation; decreases afterload, increases myocardial oxygen supply in pts w/ coronary artery spasm

COMMENTS
- Warning: Sublingual nifedipine is unsafe for treatment of HTN & should not be used! Serious adverse events, including cerebrovascular & myocardial ischemia, have been assoc w/ its use.

- Oral bioavailability may be increased two-fold in pts w/ cirrhosis.
  - ➤ Reduce dose 50–60% in pts w/ cirrhosis.
- May precipitate reflex tachycardia, severe hypotension
- Side effects may include headache, dizziness, palpitations, peripheral edema.
- Preferable to other Ca+-channel blockers for pts w/ ventricular dysfunction.
- Avoid nifedipine in pts w/
  - ➤ Hypotension
  - ➤ Second- or third-degree heart block
  - ➤ Sinus brady
  - ➤ V-tach
  - ➤ Cardiogenic shock
  - ➤ CHF
  - ➤ Use w/ caution if pt recently received beta-blocker therapy.

NIMODIPINE

MIMI C. LEE, MD, PHD

INDICATION
- Cerebral vasospasm after aneurysmal subarachnoid hemorrhage (SAH)

DOSE
- 60 mg PO/PT q4h, or 30 mg PO/PT q2h if systemic hypotension results, for first 21 days post-SAH.
- Start within first 96 hours post-SAH.

ONSET
- 1 hour to peak onset when given PO

KINETICS
- Distribution half-life: 1–2 h
- Elimination half-life: 3 h
- Metabolism: hepatic, w/ formation of inactive metabolites
- No dose alteration necessary in renal failure
- Reduce dose to 30 mg PO q4h in pts w/ liver failure

PREPARATION
- 60-mg tablets

MECHANISM
- Calcium channel blocker, reducing smooth muscle contraction
- More lipophilic & selective for cerebral vasculature than other calcium channel blockers

COMMENTS
- May cause dose-related systemic hypotension, which may reduce cerebral perfusion pressure
- Can cause GI side effects: diarrhea, nausea, vomiting, abdominal cramps

---

NITRIC OXIDE

ALISON G. CAMERON, MD

INDICATION
- Best-studied use & formal indication for the drug is neonatal respiratory failure w/ pulmonary HTN.
- Also used for
  - Pulmonary HTN after cardiac surgery or lung transplant
  - Acute respiratory distress syndrome

DOSE
- Inspired conc: 10–80 ppm
- Typical starting dose: 10–20 ppm

ONSET
- Nearly immediate

KINETICS
- Inhaled, inactivated almost immediately by binding to hemoglobin
- Systemic effects of inhaled NO rarely occur because of rapid inactivation when it binds to hemoglobin.
- Ultrashort half-life

PREPARATION
- Administration apparatus is used in conjunction w/ a ventilator or other breathing gas administration system. It includes a pressure regulator & connectors w/ specific fittings for NO gas cylinders. The apparatus also contains a device to measure the gas flow rate from the mechanical ventilator to adjust the flow of NO into the respiratory circuit to achieve the desired delivered dose.

- A complete NO delivery system includes three component medical devices: an NO administration apparatus, an NO gas analyzer, & a nitrogen dioxide gas analyzer.
- The system should include an NO administration apparatus for use as a backup system for administration of NO when the main administration apparatus cannot be used.

MECHANISM
- Naturally occurring potent vasodilator.
- Formed endogenously, also, by nitroglycerin (sodium nitroprusside & other NO donors) binding to endothelial cells & undergoing two chemical reactions to form NO.
- NO then moves out of the endothelial cell & into nearby smooth muscle cells where it activates guanylyl cyclase, promoting formation of cGMP & initiating smooth muscle relaxation.
- In pts w/ hypoxemic respiratory failure, can cause selective relaxation of the pulmonary vasculature in ventilated segments & improved arterial oxygenation. However, this improvement of oxygenation has not been demonstrated to improve pt outcome.

COMMENTS
- If pt on NO requires surgery, continue intraop to avoid rebound increase in pulmonary pressures or hypoxemia.
- In pts who have received NO for several hours or more, use caution when decreasing or stopping the drug because of serious rebound increases in pulmonary vascular resistance. This phenomenon may be secondary to decreased endogenous NO production.
- In general, inhaled NO should be initiated in centers w/ ECMO capability.
- Main contraindication is irreversible underlying cardiac or pulmonary disease.
- Side effects
  - Acute pulmonary edema
  - Methemoglobinemia
  - Tachyphylaxis
  - Possible rebound pulmonary HTN after drug discontinuation
- Special monitoring needed for methemoglobinemia & nitrogen dioxide during use
  - Methemoglobin formation more likely w/ higher NO dose.
- Expensive

NITROGLYCERIN

J. W. BEARD, MD

INDICATION
- Angina
- HTN
- Pulmonary HTN
- Congestive heart failure
- Production of uterine relaxation

DOSE
- Sublingual tablet: 0.2–0.6 mg q5min
- Translingual spray: 1 or 2 sprays under tongue q3–5min
- Paste: 0.5–2 inches of paste to skin
- IV infusion: begin at 10 mcg/min, titrate to effect up to 200 mcg/min
- IV bolus: 5–20 mcg q3–5 min

ONSET
- Sublingual tablet: 1–3 min
- Translingual spray: 2 min
- Paste: 15–60 min
- IV: immediate

KINETICS
- Peak effect
  - Sublingual tablet: 4–8 min
  - Translingual spray: 4–10 min
  - Paste: 30–120 min
  - IV: 3–5 min
- Duration of action
  - Sublingual tablet: 30–60 min
  - Translingual spray: 30–60 min
  - Paste: 2–12 h
  - IV: 3–5 min
- Half-life: 1–4 min
- Metabolism: hepatic (extensive first-pass metabolism)
- Elimination: renal

PREPARATION
- IV: 0.5, 5 mg/mL, to be diluted for IV administration
- Ointment (paste): 2%

- Tablets for sublingual use: 0.3, 0.4, 0.6 mg
- Translingual spray: 0.4 mg/spray

MECHANISM

- Relaxes smooth muscle, including vascular smooth muscle, as well as uterus
  - Decreases myocardial oxygen demand by decreasing ventricular filling pressures & SVR
  - Increases myocardial oxygen supply by dilating coronary arteries

COMMENTS

- Hemodynamic & antianginal tolerance within 24–48 h of continuous infusion
- Avoid tolerance w/ 10- to 12-hour nitrate-free period.
- Use may result in severe hypotension in preload-dependent disease states (right ventricular infarct, pericarditis, tamponade).
- Methemoglobinemia may occur w/ large doses.

NITROPRUSSIDE (NIPRIDE)

JASON LICHTENSTEIN, MD

INDICATION

- Treatment of hypertensive crisis
- Controlled hypotension
- Acute congestive heart failure

DOSE

- Start infusion at 0.3 mcg/kg/min; titrate to effect.
- Average effective dose: 3 mcg/kg/min.
- Max recommended dose: 10 mcg/kg/min.

ONSET

- 1–2 min

KINETICS

- Circulatory half-life: approx 2 min
  - Continuous infusion recommended
- Metabolism: reaction of nitroprusside w/ hemoglobin in blood yields
  - One cyanmethemoglobin molecule
  - Four cyanide ions

- Most cyanide is converted to thiocyanate by reaction w/ thiosulfate, via rhodanase enzyme system. Thiocyanate is renally excreted, w/ half-life of 3 days.
- Cyanide reacts w/ methemoglobin to form cyanmethemoglobin.
- Important: Cyanide can bind to cytochromes & interfere w/ oxidative metabolism.
- Small amount of cyanide is excreted as expired hydrogen cyanide.

➤ Nitroprusside metabolism can lead to significant (>10%) methemoglobin formation, but large doses of nitroprusside (>10 mg/kg) are required.

PREPARATION
- 50-mg vial initially dissolved in 2–3 mL dextrose in water, then further diluted in 250–1,000 mL sterile 5% dextrose solution
- Protect solution from light.
- Infusion pump highly recommended to ensure consistent delivery rate

MECHANISM
- Direct-acting nonselective peripheral vasodilator causing relaxation of arterial & venous vascular smooth muscle
- Acts via formation of nitric oxide

COMMENTS
- Nitroprusside rapidly & reliably lowers arterial BP.
  ➤ Arterial line recommended for monitoring
  ➤ Beware of excessive hypotension w/ initiation of infusion.
  ➤ BP usually returns to baseline within 2–10 min of stopping infusion.
  ➤ Tachyphylaxis can occur.
  ➤ Consider concurrent administration of longer-acting antihypertensive to reduce required dose of nitroprusside.
- Cyanide toxicity is a unique & potentially life-threatening risk of therapy.
  ➤ Administration of nitroprusside 0.5 mg/kg at rate >2 mcg/kg/min results in cyanide accumulation, overcoming body stores of thiosulfate & methemoglobin.
  ➤ Do not administer nitroprusside at dose >10 mcg/kg/min for >10 min.

➤ Clues to cyanide toxicity (may take hours to develop)
  - Increased mixed venous PO$_2$
  - Metabolic acidosis
  - Evidence of end-organ ischemia
- Mgt of cyanide toxicity
  ➤ Stop nitroprusside.
  ➤ Convert hemoglobin to methemoglobin.
    - Induce methemoglobin formation w/ sodium nitrite 4–6 mg/kg.
  ➤ Infuse thiosulfate 150–200 mg/kg.
- Thiocyanate toxicity is also a unique risk of nitroprusside therapy.
  ➤ Although less toxic than cyanide, thiocyanate can cause CNS toxicity.
  ➤ Because thiocyanate is renally cleared, toxicity is most likely in pt w/ renal failure.
  ➤ Mgt of toxicity
    - Check thiocyanate level.
    - Hemodialysis
- Contraindicated in pts w/ compensatory hypertension (eg, aortic coarctation)
- Avoid in pts w/
  ➤ Leber's optic atrophy or tobacco amblyopia
    - These pts are extremely susceptible to cyanide toxicity.
    - Increased ICP: nitroprusside can cause cerebral vasodilation w/ further rise in ICP, decrease in arterial blood pressure & reduced cerebral perfusion pressure

NITROUS OXIDE (N$_2$O)

DON TAYLOR, MD, PHD
EDMOND I EGER II, MD

INDICATION
- Induction & maintenance of GA
- Analgesia at subanesthetic concentrations

DOSE
- MAC (in O$_2$): 150% of atmosphere (infants & children); 105% (20–60 years)
- MAC-awake: two thirds of MAC

ONSET
- Seconds-minutes

KINETICS
- Metabolism: essentially inert except that it inactivates methionine synthase & thereby can affect DNA production; prolonged administration can cause neuro injury, aplastic anemia, death
- Elimination: pulmonary
- Rapid onset owing to low blood & tissue solubility (blood/gas partition coefficient of 0.47), concentration effect, absence of pungency
- Large volume uptake of nitrous oxide occurs despite low solubility because of high concentration used; leads to concentration & second gas effects.
- High concentration plus solubility relative to nitrogen (& other gases) can expand internal gas spaces (eg, air emboli, pneumothorax, bowel gas) or increase gas space pressure (eg, inner ear).
- Rapid emergence because of low solubility & high ratio of MAC-awake/MAC
- Outpouring of nitrous oxide at end of anesthesia can produce diffusion hypoxia.

PREPARATION
- Gas, from pipeline or cylinders
  - Liquid at 750 psig in cylinders color-coded blue; pressure is proportional to content only below 750 psig
  - E-cylinder holds 1,600 L when full.

MECHANISM
- Unclear
- Plausible basis: in vitro, minimally enhances inhibitory channel (GABA, glycine) responses but blocks excitatory channel (glutamate, acetylcholine) responses.
  - However, these effects do not necessarily translate into mechanistic effects (eg, blockade of acetylcholine receptors does not decrease MAC).

COMMENTS
- Degradation by carbon dioxide absorbents
  - None
- Odorless, nonirritating

- Cardiovascular effects
  - Slightly stimulates sympathetic nervous system
  - Less cardiac depression than w/ potent volatile agents
- Respiratory effects
  - Less respiratory depression than w/ potent volatile agents
  - Inhibits hypoxic & CO_2 ventilatory drive but does not increase $PaCO_2$
  - Increases in PVR are exaggerated in pts w/ pulmonary HTN.
- Nitrous oxide is an incomplete anesthetic (except at hyperbaric pressures).
- Increases muscle tone & does not potentiate effect of muscle relaxants
- Supports combustion
- Does not trigger malignant hyperthermia
- May contribute to postop nausea
- Inexpensive
- Purported to have neuroprotective effects in certain models, enhances neuronal death in others; this is highly controversial
- Comparisons w/ other inhaled anesthetics
  - Advantages
    - Absent pungency & low solubility make nitrous oxide useful as an induction adjuvant.
    - It produces most rapid recovery because of low solubility & high MAC-awake/MAC ratio.
    - Greatest resistance to biodegradation or degradation by absorbents
    - Can use at low/closed-circuit inflow rates (most economical)
    - No ventricular ectopy
    - No BP decrease
    - Does not trigger malignant hyperthermia
    - Inexpensive
  - Disadvantages
    - Increases volume or pressure in internal gas spaces
    - Limits use of higher oxygen partial pressures
    - Produces diffusion hypoxia
    - May increase muscle tone
    - Predisposes to postop nausea/vomiting more than potent inhaled anesthetics
    - Long-term administration can cause neuro injury, aplastic anemia, death.

NOREPINEPHRINE (LEVOPHED)

EMILY REINYS, MD
JEREMY NUSSBAUMER, MD

INDICATION
- Shock
- Hypotension

DOSE
- 0.1 mcg/kg IV for bolus dose
- 2–20 mcg/min as continuous infusion titrated to BP response

ONSET
- Rapid

KINETICS
- Duration: pressor action ceases 1–2 min after infusion is discontinued
- Hepatic metabolism
- Metabolites excreted in urine

PREPARATION
- 8 mcg/cc (4 mg norepinephrine base mixed in 500 cc D5W)
- Premixed ampules: 1 mg/cc

MECHANISM
- Direct alpha-1 stimulation induces intense vasoconstriction.
- Beta-1 stimulation may increase myocardial contractility (but elevated afterload & reflex bradycardia may negate any increase in cardiac output).

COMMENTS
- Decreases renal blood flow
- Increases myocardial oxygen demand; hence, may cause ischemia
- May cause ventricular arrhythmias
- Extravasation may cause tissue necrosis at site of injection

OCTREOTIDE

JAMES BRANDES, MD

INDICATION
- Symptomatic treatment in pts w/ endocrine tumors

➤ Acromegaly (growth hormone)
➤ Carcinoid
➤ Glucagonoma
➤ Gastrinoma (Zollinger-Ellison disease)
➤ Insulinoma
- Cancer therapy for tumors w/ octreotide receptors
- Variceal hemorrhage prophylaxis
- Decrease output of secretory diarrhea
  ➤ Diarrhea assoc w/ AIDS
- Decrease enteric fistula output

DOSE
- 50–200 mcg SQ bid or tid
- 50-mcg bolus IV followed by 50 mcg/h continuous infusion

ONSET
- Varies depending on delivery
- Peak SQ effect at 1–2 h

KINETICS
- Plasma half-life: 1.5 h
- Hepatic metabolism

PREPARATION
- 50-, 100-, 500-mcg/mL ampules
- 200-,1,000-mcg/mL vials for IV infusion preparation

MECHANISM
- Somatostatin analog, acts on somatostatin receptors

COMMENTS
- Side effects may include nausea, cramping, fat malabsorption, diarrhea, flatulence, glucose intolerance. These usually disappear after 2 wks of treatment.
- Long-term side effects include gallstones & biliary sludge, but usually asymptomatic.

ONDANSETRON (ZOFRAN)

LISA SWOR-YIM, MD

INDICATION
- Antiemetic, used to prevent or treat postop nausea/vomiting

DOSE
- Children <40 kg: IM, IV: 0.1 mg/kg. Can give before induction, 15 min before end of surgery, or postop.
- Adults & children >40 kg: IM, IV: 4 mg. Can give before induction, 15 min before end of surgery, or postop.
- Max dose in pts w/ hepatic impairment: 8 mg/day

ONSET
- Rapid

KINETICS
- Metabolized by hepatic P450
- Excreted by kidneys
- Half-life: 3.5–5.5 h

PREPARATION
- Injectable form: 2 mg/mL (20 mL)

MECHANISM
- Selective 5-HT3-receptor antagonist; blocks serotonin in vagal nerve terminals & in the chemoreceptor trigger zone of CNS

COMMENTS
- May not be effective in procedures w/ low risk of nausea/vomiting.
- Side effects include headache, esp at higher doses.
- Limit dose to 8 mg/day in pt w/ severe liver failure.

OXYGEN

GERALD DUBOWITZ, MB ChB

INDICATION
- Hypoxia: treatment or prevention

DOSE
- 2–6 liters per minute (Lpm) via nasal cannula provides FiO_2 ~0.25–0.28.
- Simple face mask w/ flow rate 5–10 Lpm provides FiO_2 of 0.4–0.6.
- Non-rebreather face mask w/ flow rate 15 Lpm provides FiO_2 near 1.0.
- FiO_2 depends on flow rate & minute ventilation (entrainment of air).
- Monitor SpO_2 to determine delivery rate & system.

ONSET
- Rapid; usually will see change in pulse oximeter in <1 min.
- Usually allow 20 min equilibration time before checking ABG.

KINETICS
- Stable molecule w/ indefinite half-life
- Absorbed via lungs
- Carried dissolved in blood & by hemoglobin
- Rate of utilization depends on metabolic oxygen demand; typically 3–6 mL/kg/min

PREPARATION
- Gas in (green) cylinders at 2,200 psi pressure (13,600 kPa).
  - Size E cylinder contains 640 L.
- Liquid form also at –183 degrees C.
- Air contains 21% oxygen.

MECHANISM
- Used in oxidative phosphorylation in mitochondria to produce ATP; therefore, essential to organs that utilize only this metabolic pathway (eg, brain, kidney)

COMMENTS
- Normally stable but can be partially reduced, leading to formation of toxic free radicals (superoxide, hydroxyl)
  - Free radicals affect DNA, sulfhydryl proteins, lipids
- Nervous system effects if exposure >200 kPa (2.1 atmospheres); for instance, hyperbaric oxygen chamber
  - Anxiety, nausea, twitching tonic-clonic seizure activity
  - Onset is pressure- & time-dependent.
- Pulmonary oxygen toxicity
  - Lipid peroxidation leads to disruption of alveolar/capillary membrane.
    - Irreversible changes after 7 days on 60–100%
    - More rapid in hyperbaric: pulmonary edema after about 3 h (seizures first)
    - Not evident clinically at FiO_2 <60%
  - Pulmonary absorption/collapse may also occur (especially if low V/Q ratio).
  - Pts who have lost CO_2 sensitivity rely on oxygen drive & may suffer fatal respiratory depression even at moderate O_2 concentrations.

- Retrolental fibroplasia
  - ➤ Hyperoxia implicated in retrolental fibroplasia occurring in neonates
  - ➤ Cases also reported in children who have not received O_2
  - ➤ Incidence related to PaO_2 more than FiO_2; monitoring SpO_2 critical.
- Fire/explosion hazard: oxygen does not burn but supports combustion.
  - ➤ Use lowest possible concentration during laser treatment of airway & tracheotomy using electrocautery.

PANCURONIUM

EMILY REINYS, MD

INDICATION
- Neuromuscular block

DOSE
- Intubation: 0.08–0.12 mg/kg
- Maintenance: 0.04 mg/kg initially, then 0.01 mg/kg q20–40min

ONSET
- 3–5 min

KINETICS
- Duration: 80–100 min until 25% recovery.
- Metabolic products have some neuromuscular blocking activity.
- Renal excretion primarily; 10% biliary excretion.

PREPARATION
- Premixed solution of 1–2 mg/mL

MECHANISM
- Nondepolarizing neuromuscular block
- Competes w/ acetylcholine at nicotinic receptor site on motor endplate

COMMENTS
- May cause HTN/tachycardia due to vagolytic & sympathomimetic effects.
- May cause ventricular dysrhythmias, esp w/ halothane & hypercarbia.

- Duration prolonged in renal failure.
- Pancuronium is a steroidal drug & will act synergistically w/ benzylisoquinoline muscle relaxants (eg, mivacurium).

PENICILLIN G

JEREMY NUSSBAUMER, MD

INDICATION
- Spectrum of antibacterial activity includes some gram-positive, gram-negative & anaerobic organisms.

DOSE
- Only IV use discussed in this chapter. Can also be given PO, IM.
- Adults
  - ➤ Dose varies w/ specific indication.
  - ➤ Typical dose: 1–4 million units IV q4–6h
  - ➤ Much higher doses for serious infection such as meningitis or endocarditis
    - Eg, 12–30 million units per day for endocarditis
- Infants & children
  - ➤ Dose varies by indication.
  - ➤ Typical infant dose: 30 mg/kg IV q8–12h, depending on age
  - ➤ For children >12 years, typical dose is 25,000–400,000 units/kg/day divided q4–6h.

ONSET
- Peak levels IV within 60 min

KINETICS
- Hepatic metabolism (30%)
- Renal excretion (80%)
- Elimination half-life: 20–50 min
  - ➤ Prolonged 1–10 h w/ renal failure

PREPARATION
- Powder or premixed solution

MECHANISM
- Interferes w/ bacterial cell wall synthesis during active multiplication

COMMENTS
- Reduce dose in moderate to severe renal failure.

- Adverse effects include
  - Hemolytic anemia
  - Large doses may prolong bleeding time & potentiate anti-coagulants.
  - Seizures (more common in renal failure)
  - Hyperkalemia & hypokalemia (depending on potassium- or sodium-containing Pen G)
  - Anaphylaxis
    - Pt may have cross-reactivity w/ other beta-lactam antibiotics.

PHENOBARBITAL

JEREMY NUSSBAUMER, MD

INDICATION
- Seizure disorder
- Sedation

DOSE
- Adults
  - Status epilepticus: load 300–800 mg then 120–240 mg q20min IV until seizure is controlled or a total of 1–2 g is administered
    - Max suggested rate: 60 mg/min
  - Seizure maintenance: 1–3 mg/kg/day in 3 divided doses
  - Preop sedation: 100–200 mg IM 1–1.5 h before surgery
- Children
  - Status epilepticus: 10–20 mg/kg load then 5 mg/kg q20min until seizure is controlled or a total of 40 mg/kg is administered
    - Max suggested rate: 2 mg/kg/min up to 30 mg/min
  - Seizure maintenance
    - 1–5 years: 6–8 mg/kg/day in 2 divided doses
    - 5–12 years: 4–6 mg/kg/day in 2 divided doses

ONSET
- IV: 5 min
- PO: 60 min or longer
- IM: 20–60 min

KINETICS
- Peak effect
  - IV: 30 min
  - PO: 2 h

- Metabolism: hepatic
- Elimination: 75% hepatic, 25% renal
- Duration: 10–12 h

PREPARATION
- For injection 30, 60, 65, 130 mg/mL
- PO
  - ➤ Tablets: various doses from 10 to 100 mg
  - ➤ Elixir 20 mg/mL

MECHANISM
- Barbiturate
- Hyperpolarizes neurons by enhancing chloride influx through GABA type A receptors
- Hyperpolarization of neurons raises the threshold for epileptic discharge & spread

COMMENTS
- For status epilepticus, diazepam & lorazepam are preferred therapies.
- Withdrawal can precipitate seizures, esp in epileptic pts.
- Dose should be adjusted to blood levels in pts on phenobarbital chronically.
  - ➤ Consider checking phenobarbital levels preop in pts on this drug.
- Like thiopental, phenobarbital may precipitate if given w/ acidic solutions.
- With chronic therapy, can lead to reduced duration of nondepolarizing muscle relaxant drugs
- Reduce dose in liver failure or severe renal failure.
- Use w/ caution in the elderly.
- Can produce severe hypotension
- Rapid IV administration can cause respiratory depression & apnea.

PHENTOLAMINE (REGITINE)

JOHN TAYLOR, MD

INDICATION
- Treatment of HTN assoc w/ sympathomimetic drug overdose or pheochromocytoma

- Treatment for extravasation of alpha-adrenergic drugs
- Treatment of choice for hypertensive crisis secondary to MAO inhibitors

DOSE
- Hypertensive crisis from pheochromocytoma or adrenergic overdose: 5–20 mg IV or IM (adults).
- Extravasation of adrenergic drugs: Infiltrate area w/ 1 mg/mL solution in saline, using up to a total of 0.1–0.2 mg/kg (children) or 5 mg (adult).
  - Use multiple small injections w/ a small-gauge needle.
- If used prior to pheochromocytoma surgery, as prophylaxis for HTN: 0.05–0.1 mg/kg (typical adult dose: 5 mg) IV/IM before surgery.

ONSET
- IV: immediate
- IM: within 15–20 min

KINETICS
- Half-life: 19 min
- Duration
  - IV: 15–30 min
  - IM: 30–45 min
- Metabolism: hepatic
- Elimination: renal

PREPARATION
- 5 mg/1 mL

MECHANISM
- Competitive blockade of alpha-adrenergic receptors

COMMENTS
- May be particularly useful in HTN assoc w/ elevated catecholamine levels
- Pheochromocytoma (including intraop use for pt undergoing pheochromocytoma resection)
  - Clonidine withdrawal
  - MAO inhibitor interaction
- Side effects include tachycardia, arrhythmias, prolonged hypotension.

- Can be used for prevention of skin necrosis after extravasation of potent vasoconstrictors norepinephrine, epinephrine, dopamine
  - ➤ Dilute 5–10 mg phentolamine in 10 mL NS & infiltrate in area of extravasation within 12 h.

PHENYLEPHRINE (NEO-SYNEPHRINE)

JAMES BRANDES, MD

INDICATION
- Hypotension
- Nasal vasoconstriction
- Additive to local anesthetics
- Hypoxia in the setting of right-to-left shunt

DOSE
- 50–100 mcg or 1–2 mcg/kg IV bolus
- 2–5 mg SC/IM
- Constant IV infusion: 10–200 mcg/min (0.2–5.0 mcg/kg/min)
- Spinal (w/ local anesthetics): 2–5 mg
- Epidural/regional blocks: 50 mcg/cc
- Nasal 0.5% solution, 2–3 drops

ONSET
- IV: <1 min
- SC/IM: 10 min

KINETICS
- Duration: 10–60 min
- Elimination half-life: 3–6 h
- Hepatic metabolism
- Renal excretion

PREPARATION
- 100 mcg/cc for IV bolus (10 mg phenylephrine in 100 cc NS)

MECHANISM
- Direct-acting sympathomimetic at alpha-1 receptors. Increases SVR & thus MAP & diastolic & systolic BP.

COMMENTS
- May cause a reflex bradycardia, which may decrease cardiac output

> ➤ This side effect may be useful to slow or convert PSVT (in the absence of systemic HTN) in bolus doses of 500–1,000 mcg, but this is not a first-line choice & not part of ACLS.

■ Cardiac & cerebral blood flow is preserved at the expense of renal, splanchnic, & peripheral blood flow.
  > ➤ Phenylephrine is useful to improve cerebral perfusion pressure in pts w/ increased ICP.

■ In the presence of a hypoxic event in a pt w/ a right-to-left shunt, phenylephrine may reduce the right-to-left shunt & improve systemic arterial oxygenation because pulmonary vascular resistance is increased, but not to the degree that SVR is increased.

■ Local anesthetic action is prolonged because of local vasoconstriction.
  > ➤ Risk of systemic toxicity from local anesthetic is also decreased.

■ Useful to help prepare the nose for nasotracheal intubation to ease passage of tube & decrease bleeding

■ In the setting of hypovolemia, phenylephrine is not an alternative to volume resuscitation w/ the appropriate fluid/blood products.

■ Use cautiously in pts w/ bradycardia or conduction defects.

■ Phenylephrine increases uterine vascular resistance.
  > ➤ This decreases uterine blood flow.
  > ➤ However, in the presence of severe or refractory (to volume/ephedrine) hypotension in the parturient, it may be useful.

■ Extravasation may cause tissue necrosis.
  > ➤ Treat extravasation w/ phentolamine (1 mg/cc, 5–10 cc) and/or sympathetic block of involved extremity.

■ Absolutely do not use w/ Bier block or in local anesthesia of areas w/ end arterial blood supply (digits, ears, etc).

■ Use more dilute concentrations for nasal preparation in children.

PHENYTOIN (DILANTIN)

MIMI C. LEE, MD, PHD

INDICATION

■ Seizures
■ Unlabelled or investigational uses include
  > ➤ Digoxin-induced dysrhythmias
  > ➤ Refractory ventricular tachycardia
  > ➤ Neuralgia

DOSE

- For neurosurgical prophylaxis: IV load 10–15 mg/kg up to 1,000 mg slow infusion (<50 mg/min), then 100–200 mg IV q4h maintenance
- For dysrhythmias: 50–100 mg IV slow infusion q10–15min until resolution of the dysrhythmia, or until max of 10–15 mg/kg

ONSET

- 3–5 min

KINETICS

- Duration: dose-dependent
- Elimination half-life: 24 h
- Metabolism: hepatic
- Excretion: renal; increased w/ alkalinized urine

PREPARATION

- 50 mg/mL for injection

MECHANISM

- Stabilizes cell membranes

COMMENTS

- Important: Rapid IV bolus may result in bradycardia, hypotension, respiratory arrest, CNS depression, cardiac depression.
  - ➤ Administer at rate <50 mg/min.
- May cause nystagmus, diplopia, ataxia, drowsiness, gingival hyperplasia, GI tract upset, hyperglycemia & induction of hepatic microsomal enzymes
- Tissue irritant
- May cause pain on IV delivery
- Crosses the placenta
- Adequate dosage as determined by therapeutic serum levels (7.5–20 mg/L) is highly variable between pts.

PHYSOSTIGMINE

JAMES BRANDES, MD

INDICATION

- Centrally acting anticholinergic overdose; eg:
  - ➤ Atropine
  - ➤ Scopolamine

- ➤ Antihistamine
- ➤ Tricyclic antidepressant
- ➤ Belladonna alkaloid overdose or jimson weed intoxication
- ■ Glaucoma (topical treatment)

DOSE
- ■ 10–30 mcg/kg (0.5–2.0 mg) IV/IM, may repeat in 10–30 min.
- ■ For glaucoma, an ointment is applied.

ONSET
- ■ IV: 3–8 min, peak effect in 10 min

KINETICS
- ■ Eliminated by plasma esterases
- ■ Duration of action: 30 min to 2 h

PREPARATION
- ■ 1 mg/mL injection
- ■ Ointment for ophthalmic use

MECHANISM
- ■ Cholinesterase inhibitor; increases the concentration of acetylcholine across the synapse, regardless of acetylcholine receptor type
- ■ Crosses blood-brain barrier (tertiary amine)
- ■ Also inhibits phosphodiesterase, which may account for some of the central effects by affecting other neurotransmitters

COMMENTS
- ■ Use cautiously; give slowly, titrate to effect for anticholinergic overdose.
- ■ Anticholinergic overdose manifests w/
  - ➤ Anxiety
  - ➤ Confusion
  - ➤ Seizures
  - ➤ Hyperpyrexia
  - ➤ Tachycardia
  - ➤ Vasodilation
  - ➤ Mydriasis
  - ➤ Urinary retention
- ■ Consider other interventions prior to giving this drug.
- ■ Contraindicated in pts w/ mechanical bowel obstruction/bladder outlet obstruction, or severe asthma

- Has been used for the treatment of postanesthetic shivering & reversal of the effects of sedatives & volatile anesthetics
- Overdose of physostigmine may cause cholinergic crisis w/ bronchospasm, hypersalivation, bradycardia, tremors, fasciculations, neuromuscular blockade, seizures, incontinence.
- Treat physostigmine overdose w/ atropine for muscarinic effects & possibly pralidoxime for neuromuscular & ganglionic effects.

PIPECURONIUM (ARDUAN)

JAMES CALDWELL, MB CHB
JESSICA SAMPAT, MD

INDICATION
- Neuromuscular block
- Facilitation of tracheal intubation
- Maintenance of surgical relaxation

DOSE
- 0.08–0.12 mg/kg IV for tracheal intubation
- 0.01–0.02 mg/kg IV to maintain surgical relaxation

ONSET
- 3–5 min

KINETICS
- Metabolism: <5%
- Renal excretion: >90%
- Hepatic elimination: <10%
- Elimination half-life: 110–140 min

Duration
- Intubation dose: 80–120 min
- Maintenance dose: 30–60 min

PREPARATION
- 10 mg lyophilized powder (Arduan): reconstitute w/ water or saline

MECHANISM
- Competitive antagonist of acetylcholine at neuromuscular junction
- Steroidal compound (pancuronium-like)

COMMENTS
- No cardiovascular effects
- Drug interactions: Neuromuscular blockade potentiated by aminoglycoside antibiotics, local anesthetics, loop diuretics, magnesium, lithium, hypothermia, hypokalemia, acidosis
- Has little role in current clinical practice because of long duration

---

POTASSIUM CHLORIDE

JESSICA SAMPAT, MD

INDICATION
- Hypokalemia

DOSE
- IV
  - 10–20 mEq/h
  - If critical condition, w/ close ECG monitoring, higher rates (20–40 mEq/h) & concentrations (60–80 mEq/L) may be administered.
  - Dilute with NS before use. Give by SLOW IV infusion.
  - Monitoring w/ ECG & plasma K concentrations is essential.
- PO
  - 20–200 mEq/day in divided doses

ONSET
- IV: immediate

KINETICS
- Peak effect IV is variable.
- Renal excretion
- Interactions: severe hyperkalemia may occur w/ concomitant administration of potassium-sparing diuretics, salt substitutes, ACE inhibitors.

PREPARATION
- Dilution for infusion
  - IV (piggyback, peripheral line): 10–20 mEq in 100 mL D5W, NS or LR (0.1–0.2 mEq/mL)
  - IV (piggyback, central line, cardiac monitor): 10–20 mEq in 50 mL D5W, NS or LR (0.2–0.4 mEq/mL)

➤ IV (maintenance infusion): 10–40 mEq in 1 L D5W, NS or LR (0.01–0.04 mEq/mL)
➤ IV (cardiac monitor, maintenance): 60–80 mEq in 1 L D5W, NS or LR (0.06–0.08 mEq/mL)
■ Injection: 20 mEq/10 mL, 30 mEq/15 mL, 40 mEq/20 mL, 60 mEq/30 mL, 400 mEq/200 mL
■ Tablets
➤ 8, 10 mEq capsules
➤ Extended-release preparations: 8, 10, 20 mEq

MECHANISM
■ Following absorption, potassium enters the extracellular fluid & is actively transported intracellularly, where its concentration is 40 times that of the extracellular compartment.
■ 98% of total body potassium is intracellular.
■ Total extracellular potassium content in adult is about 50 mEq.
■ Extracellular (plasma) potassium concentration is only a general guide to total body potassium stores.

COMMENTS
■ Do not use undiluted: direct injection may be instantly fatal.
■ Infuse slowly, monitoring pt continuously w/ ECG & serial serum potassium determinations.
■ Watch for ECG changes of hyperkalemia:
➤ Peaked T waves
➤ Loss of P wave
➤ QT prolongation
➤ Widening & slurring of QRS ("sine wave")
➤ Cardiac arrest
■ Watch for other signs & symptoms of hyperkalemia, which include
➤ Paresthesia of extremities
➤ Weakness
➤ Mental confusion
➤ Hypotension
■ Use cautiously in
➤ Pts w/ cardiac disease
➤ Pts on digitalis
➤ Pts w/ renal disease
➤ Pts w/ metabolic acidosis
➤ Pts w/ Addison's disease
➤ Pts w/ hyponatremia
➤ Pts w/ hypoadrenalism

- In dehydration & shock, start hydration & diuresis before replacing potassium.
- Insulin & dextrose facilitate movement of potassium into cells.

PRILOCAINE (EMLA CREAM)

GRETE H. PORTEOUS, MD

INDICATION
- Local anesthetic sold in U.S. only as topical anesthetic
  - ➤ No current commercial preparation available in the U.S. for IV use

DOSE
- 2.5 g on 20–25 cm^2. Max 2 g/10 cm^2.

ONSET
- 60 min after application under occlusive dressing

KINETICS
- Max effect 2–3 h after application
- Hepatic metabolism
- Renal excretion
- Elimination half-life: 10–150 min

PREPARATION
- EMLA (eutectic mixture of local anesthetics) cream, film or patch
  - ➤ Contains lidocaine 2.5%, prilocaine 2.5%
  - ➤ Eutectic mixture has melting point below room temperature (ie, both compounds exist as liquids).

MECHANISM
- Binds to open sodium channels in sensory & motor neurons & blocks propagation of nerve impulses

COMMENTS
- Causes local skin blanching & erythema
- Greatly increased absorption (& toxicity) if applied over broken or inflamed skin
- Major toxicity, like all local anesthetics, is neurologic (confusion, agitation, tremors, seizures) & cardiovascular (dysrhythmias, hypotension, cardiovascular collapse).
- Can cause methemoglobinemia

- Risk factors for methemoglobinemia include age <1 month; G6PD deficiency; use of sulfa drugs, antimalarials, nitrates, benzocaine.
- Treatment includes oxygen & methylene blue (1% solution, 1–2 mg/kg over 5 min).
- See also Critical Event chapter "Methemoglobinemia."
- Do not use in infants <1 mo of age.

PROCAINAMIDE

JEREMY NUSSBAUMER, MD

INDICATION
- Ventricular tachycardia
- Atrial tachyarrhythmias, including atrial fibrillation

DOSE
- Must be titrated to pt response
- Adult
  - IV load: 15–18 mg/kg over 25–30 min
  - IV maintenance: 1–4 mg/min by infusion
  - ACLS
    - Refractory V-fib: 30 mg/min up to 17 mg/kg
    - For other arrhythmias, infuse 20 mg/min until arrhythmia controlled, hypotension occurs, QRS widens by 50% or 17 mg/kg is given.
- Children
  - IV load: 10–15 mg/kg over 15 min (or 1 mg/kg q3–5min until arrhythmia controlled, with max dose 15 mg/kg over 1 h)
  - IV maintenance: 20–80 mcg/kg/min
  - Dose should not exceed 100 mg/dose or 2 g/24 h.

ONSET
- Peak levels within 20 min IV

KINETICS
- Approx 50% metabolism by liver to N-acetyl procainamide (NAPA), an active metabolite
  - NAPA undergoes renal excretion.
- Approx 40–70% renal excretion of unchanged drug
- Procainamide elimination half-life

> 2.5–8 h in adults
> 11 h in anephric pts
- NAPA elimination half-life
  > 5–9 h
  > 42 h in anephric pts

PREPARATION
- 100 mg/mL in 10-mL vial.
- Dilute in D5W.

MECHANISM
- Class IA antiarrhythmic
- Increases electrical stimulation threshold of ventricle & His-Purkinje system to depress myocardial contractility & excitability

COMMENTS
- Do not use in pt w/ torsades de pointes, heart block (complete, second or third degree).
- Use w/ caution in pt w/ AV conduction disturbances, renal disease, hepatic disease, SLE, myasthenia gravis.
- IV procainamide can cause hypotension & depression of LV function, especially in pts w/ CHF.
- Dose reduction required for renal failure.
- ECG manifestations: can widen QRS & prolong QT interval.
- Both procainamide & NAPA levels should be followed during continuous infusions.
- Long-term use
  > Can lead to bone marrow depression
  > May increase risk of death for pts w/ non-life-threatening arrhythmias

---

PROCAINE (NOVOCAIN)

GRETE H. PORTEOUS, MD

INDICATION
- Local anesthetic for infiltration, peripheral nerve block, spinal anesthesia
- Not for topical or epidural use

DOSE
- Spinal anesthesia

➤ Typical dose: 0.5–2 mL of a 10% solution (50–200 mg)
- Peripheral nerve block
  ➤ Concentrations range from 0.5% to 2%.
  ➤ Max dose: 10 mg/kg (or 1,000 mg in adults)
  ➤ Epinephrine 1:200,000 may be added for vasoconstriction.
- Infiltration
  ➤ Concentrations range from 0.25% to 0.5%.
  ➤ Max dose: 10 mg/kg (or 1,000 mg in adults)
  ➤ Epinephrine 1:200,000 may be added for vasoconstriction.

ONSET
- 2–5 min

KINETICS
- Duration: about 45–90 min for regional/spinal anesthesia
- Metabolized in plasma by hydrolysis of ester linkage by pseudo-cholinesterase (ester local anesthetic)
- Elimination half-life: typically several minutes

PREPARATION
- 1%, 2%, 10% solutions
- May be diluted to hypo- or hyperbaric 5% solutions for spinals

MECHANISM
- Binds to open sodium channels in sensory & motor neurons & blocks propagation of nerve impulses

COMMENTS
- Major toxicity, like all local anesthetics, is neurologic (confusion, agitation, tremors, seizures) & cardiovascular (dysrhythmias, hypotension, cardiovascular collapse).
  ➤ Potential for systemic toxicity is lower than other local anesthetics, due to rapid metabolism & relatively low potency.
- Like other ester local anesthetics, its metabolite PABA (para-aminobenzoic acid) is associated w/ allergic reactions.
- Short duration may be useful in outpt surgery.
- Reduce dose in elderly & pts w/ liver or renal failure.
- Compared to spinal lidocaine
  ➤ May have reduced incidence of transient neuro symptoms
  ➤ May have increased incidence of inadequate anesthesia

PROCHLORPERAZINE (COMPAZINE)

JEREMY NUSSBAUMER, MD

INDICATION
■ Antiemetic

DOSE
■ Adult
  ➤ PO: 5–10 mg tid, max 40 mg/day
  ➤ IM: 5–10 mg q3–4h, max 40 mg/day
  ➤ IV: 2.5–10 mg q3–4h prn, max 40 mg/day
  ➤ Rectal: 25 mg bid
■ Children
  ➤ PO
    • <9 kg: not recommended
    • 9–14 kg: 2.5 mg q12–24h, max 7.5 mg/day
    • 14–18 kg: 2.5 mg q8h, max 10 mg/day
    • 18–39 kg: 2.5 mg q8h, max 15 mg/day
  ➤ IM: 0.1–0.15 mg/kg/dose
  ➤ IV: not recommended

ONSET
■ PO: 30–40 min
■ IM: 10–20 min
■ Rectal: 60 min

KINETICS
■ Elimination half-life: 3–7 h
■ Hepatic metabolism

PREPARATION
■ 5 mg/mL in 2- or 10-mL vials.
■ IV administration rate should be <5 mg/min.

MECHANISM
■ Phenothiazine drug class
■ Blocks mesolimbic dopamine 1 & 2 receptors
■ Also has alpha-adrenergic antagonist & anticholinergic effects

COMMENTS
■ Can be used as tranquilizer for nonpsychotic anxiety, but other drugs may have more favorable side effect profile (eg, benzodiazepines)

- Can cause significant side effects, even at recommended doses
  - Extrapyramidal symptoms: manifestations can include Parkinson-like symptoms, dystonic reactions, or restlessness
  - Hypotension: avoid or use w/ caution in pts w/ significant cardiovascular disease
  - Lowers seizure threshold
  - Excess sedation or coma
- Adverse effects w/ long-term therapy
  - Neuroleptic malignant syndrome (NMS)
  - Tardive dyskinesia
  - Cholestatic jaundice, hepatotoxicity
  - Leukopenia, agranulocytosis
- Use w/ caution in pts w/ hepatic disease.
- Avoid use in
  - Children <2 years old or <9 kg
  - Children who may have Reye's syndrome
  - Pts w/ glaucoma
  - Pts w/ known history of tardive dyskinesia or NMS

PROMETHAZINE (PHENERGAN)

JEREMY NUSSBAUMER, MD

INDICATION
- Treatment of allergy
- Antiemetic

DOSE
- Adult
  - 12.5 mg PO/PR tid
  - 12.5–25 mg IV/IM q4h
- Children
  - 0.25–1 mg/kg IM/IV/PO/PR q4–6h

ONSET
- IV: rapid
- PO: 20 min

KINETICS
- Duration: 2–6 h
- Hepatic metabolism
- Renal excretion

PREPARATION
- IV: 25, 50 mg/mL
- Tablets & syrups for PO use
- 12.5-, 25-, 50-mg suppositories

MECHANISM
- Blocks dopamine & H1 histamine receptors to produce antiemetic & antihistaminergic effects
- Also blocks alpha-adrenergic receptors & has anticholinergic effects

COMMENTS
- Higher doses can cause sedation.
- Can cause
  - Orthostatic hypotension
  - Tachycardia
  - Extrapyramidal symptoms (eg, dystonic reactions)
    - Avoid use in pts w/ Parkinson's disease.
  - Neuroleptic malignant syndrome
  - Anticholinergic effects (eg, dry mouth, blurred vision, constipation)

PROPOFOL (DIPRIVAN)

MICHAEL H. FAHMY, MD

INDICATION
- Induction & maintenance of GA, MAC
- ICU sedation

DOSE
Usually titrated to effect, but some general guidelines are as follows:
- MAC: 25–75 mcg/kg/min
- ICU sedation: 5–50 mcg/kg/min
- Induction of GA: 1.5–2.5 mg/kg
- Maintenance of GA: 100–200 mcg/kg/min

ONSET
- 30–60 sec

KINETICS
- Metabolism: hepatic
- Elimination: renal

PREPARATION
- Propofol is formulated in an isotonic soybean fat emulsion.
- Concentration is 10 mg/mL at pH 4.5–6.6.

MECHANISM
- Sedative-hypnotic agent; presumed action is enhancement of the effect of GABA on GABA type A receptors.

COMMENTS
- Current formulation promotes bacterial growth. Use strict aseptic technique when handling. Used vials should be discarded approx 5 h after first use.
- Adjust dose for age: elderly pts require significantly less propofol than younger pts.
- Can cause pain on injection
- Cardiac effects such as hypotension more common in following conditions. Reduce dose accordingly.
  - Elderly
  - Hypovolemic pt
  - Pt w/ limited cardiovascular reserve

PROPRANOLOL (INDERAL)

CHRISTINE A. WU, MD

INDICATION
- HTN
- Angina
- Arrhythmias (eg, atrial arrhythmias, AV nodal reentrant tachycardias)
- Migraine prophylaxis
- Thyrotoxicosis
- Suppression of exercise-induced tachycardia
- Hypertrophic cardiomyopathy

DOSE
- Adults: typically 0.25–0.5 mg IV boluses titrated to effect, max dose 0.1 mg/kg.
- Pediatrics: 0.01–0.1 mg/kg/dose titrated to effect, max dose 1 mg.
- 40–80 mg/day PO as antihypertensive or antiangina treatment is typical, titrated to effect.

ONSET
- IV: 2–10 minutes

KINETICS
- Duration: 1–6 h IV
- Onset: rapid
- High lipid solubility, readily penetrates CNS
- Metabolism: hepatic
- Elimination: renal
- Half-life 4 h; however, typical PO dosing is QD or bid

PREPARATION
- IV: 1 mg/mL

MECHANISM
- Nonselective beta blocker

COMMENTS
- Like atenolol, beta blockade from propranolol may be given perioperatively to improve cardiac outcome in at-risk pts.
- Abrupt withdrawal can lead to angina in pts w/ coronary artery disease.
- Avoid in pts w/ second- or third-degree heart block.
- Has negative inotropic effects
- May cause bronchospasm

PROSTACYCLIN (PGI2, EPOPROSTENOL, FLOLAN)

ALISON G. CAMERON, MD

INDICATION
- Pulmonary hypertension (PH)
- Primary PH
- PH/scleroderma spectrum of diseases (PH/SSD)

DOSE
- Start at 2 ng/kg/min IV.
- Increase by 2 ng/kg/min q15min until dose-limiting effect occurs or therapeutic dose reached (9-11 ng/kg/min in most studies).
  - ➤ For chronic use, pt will eventually need long-term indwelling central line.

ONSET
- Several minutes
- Steady state reached within 15 min w/ infusion

KINETICS
- Half-life: 3-5 min
- Hydrolyzed in plasma to inactive metabolites
- Cardiovascular effects diminish within 5 min of stopping infusion.
- Platelet aggregation effects last for 2 h.

PREPARATION
- Flolan supplied as powder in 0.5- or 1.5-mg vials
- Must be reconstituted in 50 mL sterile diluent supplied w/ product

MECHANISM
- Prostacyclin is a naturally occurring prostaglandin.
  - Synthesized by vascular endothelial cells as vasoactive mediator
  - Works in concert w/ nitric oxide (NO) to prevent intravascular thrombosis
- Potent vasodilator & inhibitor of platelet aggregation
- Cardiac effects
  - Increases cardiac index
  - Decreases pulmonary vascular resistance
  - Decreases systemic vascular resistance
  - Increases HR

COMMENTS
- Chronic administration in pts w/ PH may result in improved outcome.
- Abrupt withdrawal can cause rebound PH.
- Contraindications
  - Pt w/ CHF from severe LV systolic dysfunction
  - Pt who develops pulmonary edema during initial dosing
- Most common dose-limiting effects
  - Hypotension
  - Nausea/vomiting
  - Headache
- Other adverse reactions
  - Facial flushing (very common)

- ➤ Hyperglycemia
- ➤ GI symptoms
- ➤ Tachycardia
- ➤ Myocardial ischemia (related to tachycardia & decrease in diastolic BP)
- ➤ Vagal-like reaction w/ bradycardia (uncommon)

PROTAMINE

RENÉE J. ROBERTS, MD

INDICATION
- ■ To reverse anticoagulation from heparin

DOSE
- ■ Give peripherally & slowly (5 mg/min).
- ■ 1–1.5 mg IV per 100 U of heparin
  - ➤ If 1 h has elapsed since heparin was given, use half the dose of protamine.
  - ➤ If 2 or more h have elapsed since heparin was given, use 1/4 the dose of protamine.
- ■ Check ACT or PTT for normalization of coag status.

ONSET
- ■ Rapid

KINETICS
- ■ Heparin:protamine complexes are removed by the reticuloendothelial system.
- ■ Degradation via circulatory protease, carboxypeptidase

PREPARATION
- ■ 10 mg/mL

MECHANISM
- ■ Polycationic base that binds heparin (a polyanionic acid) directly

COMMENTS
- ■ Increased risk for protamine reactions include:
  - ➤ NPH insulin use

- ➤ Prior protamine
- ➤ Seafood allergy
- ➤ Men s/p vasectomy
- ➤ Rapid injection
- ■ Three types of reactions:
  - ➤ Type I: systemic hypotension, flushing, edema, bronchospasm
    - • Also has elevated PVR PAP, low SVR & CO
    - • From NO and H2 receptor activation, causing histamine release from MAST cells
  - ➤ Type IIa: true anaphylaxis
    - • From IgE binding to MAST cells & releasing His
    - • Risks for this reaction listed above
    - • Decreased arterial & RAP & LAP, +/− bronchospasm
  - ➤ Type IIb: immediate anaphylactoid reactions
    - • Mediated by complement activation & w/ secondary release of H2 & vasoactive substances
    - • Skin edema, flushing, decreased SVR, bronchospasm
  - ➤ Type IIc: delayed anaphylactoid reaction
    - • Noncardiogenic pulmonary edema occurring 1 or more h after administration
  - ➤ Type III: severe pulmonary HTN w/ severe decrease in SVR, decreased LAP, RV distention
    - • Arises from catastrophic complement activation & thromboxane production

PYRIDOSTIGMINE

RONNIE LU, MD

INDICATION
- ■ Reversal of neuromuscular block

DOSE
- ■ 0.4 mg/kg up to max dose 20 mg

ONSET
- ■ 10–15 min

KINETICS
- ■ Duration: >2 h

- Hepatic metabolism
- Renal excretion

PREPARATION
- 5 mg/mL solution

MECHANISM
- Noncompetitive (covalent) inhibitor of acetylcholinesterase

COMMENTS
- Administer w/ glycopyrrolate 0.05 mg per 1 mg of pyridostigmine to block muscarinic cholinergic effects.

RANITIDINE (ZANTAC)

DAN WAJSMAN, MD

INDICATION
- Prophylaxis & treatment of gastric & duodenal ulcers
- Prophylaxis of aspiration pneumonitis
- GERD

DOSE
- 50 mg IV q6–8h

ONSET
- <30 min

KINETICS
- Duration: 6–8 h
- Elimination half-life: 2–2.5 h
- Hepatic metabolism
- Renal excretion

PREPARATION
- 50 mg/mL

MECHANISM
- Histamine H2-receptor antagonist

COMMENTS
- Not recommended for routine prophylaxis of aspiration pneumonitis, but may be of use in those w/ high risk for aspiration (morbid obesity, parturients, GERD symptoms)

REMIFENTANIL (ULTIVA)

ANNE NOONEY, MD
DHANESH K. GUPTA, MD

INDICATION
- Anesthesia adjunct

DOSE
- Important: all doses should be titrated to effect depending on a variety of factors, including
  - Pt age
  - Body weight
  - Pt's physical status
  - Coexisting disease
  - Other CNS depressant drug administration
  - Surgery or procedure performed
- IV infusion: 0.025–2.0 mcg/kg/min
- IV bolus: 0.25–1 mcg/kg

ONSET
- <1 min

KINETICS
- Peak effect in 1–3 min
- Duration: 3–10 min
- Elimination half-life: 8–20 min
- Context-sensitive half-time is constant (3–5 min) for any infusion duration.
- Metabolism: tissue & blood nonspecific esterases

PREPARATION
- Lyophilized powder in 1-, 2-, or 5-mg vials
- Reconstituted from powder, to be used within 24 h
- Usual concentrations 10–20 mcg/mL for sedation, 50 mcg/mL for GA

MECHANISM
- Mu opioid receptor agonist

COMMENTS

- Unique among opioids in allowing complete recovery from profound opioid effect within 5–15 min, w/o residual effects on respiratory drive
  - May be useful for procedures w/ high intraop stimulus but little postop pain
  - Administer agent for postop analgesia prior to stopping remifentanil.
  - Can cause a withdrawal response of tachycardia & hyperalgesia
  - Naloxone usually not necessary, since recovery from opioid effects is rapid
- Important respiratory effects
  - Like other opioids, will cause respiratory depression & hypoventilation, which can ultimately lead to apnea & respiratory arrest
  - Like other potent opioids, can cause significant chest wall rigidity & difficulty w/ ventilation, requiring muscle relaxant administration. This is very common w/ rapid IV administration of large doses.
  - Do not give as bolus for postop pain.
- Important cardiac effects
  - In general, minimal effects on hemodynamic status
  - Like other potent opioids, can cause significant bradycardia & hypotension
    - Can occur within 1 min of starting infusion & can lead to asystole
  - When used in combination w/ other sedative meds (eg, benzodiazepines, barbiturates), hypotension can be more pronounced.
- No dose reduction required for renal or liver failure
- Reduce dose in elderly or debilitated pt.
- Does not release histamine

REOPRO (ABCIXIMAB)

DHANESH K. GUPTA, MD

INDICATION

- Adjuvant for anticoagulation for non-Q wave MI, unstable angina, vascular stenting/angioplasty

DOSE
- 0.25 mg/kg IV loading dose over 10–60 min
- 0.125 mcg/kg/min (max 10 mcg/min) infusion for 12–48 h

ONSET
- <5 min

KINETICS
- Unclear metabolism & excretion.
- Active form binds irreversibly to platelets.

PREPARATION
- 2 mg/mL solution

MECHANISM
- Inhibitor of platelet glycoprotein IIb/IIIa receptor, effective when >80% receptors are blocked

COMMENTS
- Most often administered concomitantly w/ heparin.
- Platelet function does not recover for days after discontinuation of infusion.
- No clinical measure of effect except prolonged bleeding.
- Antiplatelet action is reversible w/ transfusion of platelets (>10 mL/kg of platelets).

ROCURONIUM

MANUEL PARDO, JR., MD

INDICATION
- Neuromuscular block
- Facilitation of tracheal intubation
- Maintenance of surgical relaxation

DOSE
- Intubation: 0.6–1.2 mg/kg
- Maintenance: 0.1–0.2 mg/kg q15–25min
- Infusion: 10–12 mcg/kg/min

ONSET
- 1–2 min

KINETICS

- Duration 30–60 min for intubating dose, 15–25 min for maintenance dose
- 70% hepatic elimination, 30% renal excretion

PREPARATION

- 10 mg/mL

MECHANISM

- Nondepolarizing neuromuscular block
- Competes w/ acetylcholine at nicotinic receptor site on motor endplate

COMMENTS

Because of rapid onset, used as an alternative to succinylcholine for rapid sequence intubation in doses up to 1.2 mg/kg

- No dose adjustment required for renal failure
- Liver failure will prolong duration of action up to 50%. Reduce dose accordingly.

Acid pH of rocuronium may cause precipitation w/ basic solutions (eg, barbiturates).

ROPIVACAINE

MICHAEL H. FAHMY, MD

INDICATION

- Local or regional anesthesia
- Postsurgical analgesia

DOSE

- Varies depending on type of block

see Kinetics section for details

ONSET

- 10–30 min for regional block
- 1–15 min for local or field block

KINETICS

- Dose required, onset, duration vary w/ pt & clinical situation, but general guidelines include
  - ➤ Local infiltration for surgery: 0.5% conc, 2–6 h duration

- ➤ Local infiltration for postop analgesia: 0.2–0.5% conc, 2–6 h duration
- ➤ Peripheral nerve block: 0.5–0.75% conc, 5–10 h duration
- ➤ Epidural block: 0.5% conc, 2–4 h duration
- ➤ Epidural block: 0.75% conc, 3–5 h duration
- ➤ Epidural block: 1% conc, 4–6 h duration
- ➤ OB epidural labor analgesia: 0.2%, 0.5–1.5 h duration
- ■ Hepatic metabolism, renal excretion of metabolites

PREPARATION
- ■ 0.2%, 0.5%, 0.75%, 1% solutions

MECHANISM
- ■ Amide-type local anesthetic
- ■ Increases threshold for electrical excitation at level of sodium channel, blocking nerve conduction

COMMENTS
- ■ Addition of epinephrine does not prolong block or reduce chance of systemic absorption, unlike many other local anesthetics.
- ■ As with all local anesthetics, ropivacaine can cause CNS & cardiovascular toxicity (see Critical Event chapter "Local Anesthetic Toxicity").
  - ➤ Systemic concentration will depend on total dose, route of administration, vascularity of injection site, pt's medical condition.
- ■ Comparison to bupivacaine
  - ➤ Ropivacaine may have decreased potential for cardiac & CNS toxicity.
  - ➤ Ropivacaine may have less motor block for equivalent level of sensory block.
- ■ Consider dose reduction in pt w/ liver disease, esp for repeat dosing or continuous infusion.
- ■ Relatively few clinical studies of use in pediatric pts

SCOPOLAMINE (HYOSCINE)

J. W. BEARD, MD

INDICATION
- ■ Production of amnesia
- ■ Antisialogogue
- ■ Antiemetic

DOSE
- IV, IM, SC: 0.3–0.65 mg q4–6h
- Transdermal: 2.5-cm^2 patch (apply to skin behind ear)

ONSET
- IV: 5–10 min
- Transdermal: 4 h

KINETICS
- Duration: IV 2 h, transdermal 72 h
- Metabolism: hepatic
- Elimination: in urine

PREPARATION
- 0.4 mg/mL IV injectable
- 1.5-mg disc transdermal

MECHANISM
- Anticholinergic; crosses blood-brain barrier & hence has CNS effects

COMMENTS
- Patch should be applied the night before surgery for nausea prophylaxis
- May induce tachycardia & may be used to treat bradyarrhythmias at doses >1 mg
- May induce paradoxical bradycardia at doses <0.1 mg secondary to CNS activity
- Can cause central anticholinergic syndrome including drowsiness, altered mental status

SEVOFLURANE

ANTHONY ROMO, MD
EDMOND I EGER II, MD

INDICATION
- Induction & maintenance of GA

DOSE
- MAC (in O_2): 2.5% (infants & children); 1.85% (30–60 years); 1.5% (80 years)
- MAC-awake: one third of MAC
- MAC-BAR: 3.5% (opioids markedly decrease)

ONSET

- Seconds-minutes

KINETICS

- Metabolism by hepatic P450 (2E1 isoform): 3–5% of sevoflurane taken up
- Elimination: pulmonary (95–97%)
- Uptake
  - ➤ Small relative to alveolar concentration because of small blood/gas (0.65) & tissue/gas partition coefficients (less than all potent inhaled anesthetics except desflurane) & recovery shorter than w/ isoflurane or halothane
  - ➤ Rapid (eg, "one-breath") induction w/ "overpressure" (eg, 8% sevoflurane)
  - ➤ In 1- to 5-year-old children, recovery assoc w/ agitation (minimized by use of opioids or ketorolac)

PREPARATION

- Clear, colorless nonflammable liquid in 250-mL plastic-lined amber-colored bottles
- Water (preservative) required to prevent degradation to highly acidic compounds

MECHANISM

- Unclear
- Plausible basis: in vitro, volatile inhaled anesthetics enhance inhibitory channel (GABA, glycine, potassium) responses & block excitatory channel (glutamate, acetylcholine, sodium) responses
  - ➤ However, these effects do not necessarily translate into mechanistic effects (eg, blockade of acetylcholine receptors does not decrease MAC).

COMMENTS

- Degradation by carbon dioxide absorbents
  - ➤ Appreciable at increased temperatures (eg, closed circuit)
  - ➤ Produces potential nephrotoxin compound A, leading to the U.S. package label warning not to use sevoflurane at <1 L/min inflow & not 1 L/min for >2 MAC-hours
  - ➤ Degradation by desiccated absorbents sufficient to slow induction of anesthesia
- Premier agent for inhaled induction of anesthesia because of low solubility, absent pungency, absent cardiac stimulation

- Causes profound, dose-related muscle relaxation & enhances the effect of muscle relaxants
- Side effects
  - Higher concentrations cause cardiorespiratory depression (decreased blood pressure & systemic vascular resistance but w/ sustained cardiac output; increased $PaCO_2$), but no ventricular ectopy
  - Can cause (rarely) slow heart rate & asystole (esp in pts w/ torsades de pointes)
  - Can cause convulsions in rare pts
  - Hypothermia
    - As w/ other inhaled anesthetics, sevoflurane decreases the set point for response to decreases in body temp.
  - Like other potent inhaled agents, sevoflurane can trigger malignant hyperthermia; less potent trigger than halothane.
  - Nausea/vomiting
- Comparisons w/ other inhaled anesthetics
  - Advantages
    - Absent pungency
    - Low solubility
    - Rapid inhalational induction & recovery
    - No cardiovascular stimulation
    - No ventricular ectopy
    - Produces muscle relaxation
  - Disadvantages
    - Substantial biodegradation
    - Recovery slower than w/ desflurane
    - Postop agitation in preschool children
    - Can cause profound slowing of HR & asystole (rare)
    - Can cause convulsions (rare)
    - High acquisition cost
    - Should not use at inflow rates <1 L/min
    - Degraded by absorbents to potential nephrotoxin

SODIUM BICARBONATE

JEREMY NUSSBAUMER, MD

INDICATION
- Mgt of metabolic acidosis

- Alkalinization of urine
- Treatment of hyperkalemia

DOSE
- Metabolic acidosis
  - Bicarb deficit in mEq = $0.6 \times$ body wt in kg $\times$ base deficit
  - Do not correct entire deficit in first hour.
- Urine alkalinization
  - Children: PO 1–10 mEq/kg/day divided q4–6h
  - Adults: initial 48 mEq then 12–24 mEq q4h
- Hyperkalemia
  - Consider initial dose of 1 mEq per kg body weight.
  - Follow ECG closely.
  - See also Critical Event chapter "Hyperkalemia."

ONSET
- Minutes

KINETICS
- Duration: 8 min-2 h.
- Initial dose of exogenous bicarbonate is distributed in vascular space, then equilibrates w/ bone & intracellular buffers.
- Kidneys involved in bicarbonate metabolism.

PREPARATION
- Injection forms available
  - 4% (40 mg/mL = 2.4 mEq/5 mL)
  - 4.2% (42 mg/mL = 5 mEq/10 mL)
  - 7.5% (75 mg/mL = 8.92 mEq/10 mL)
  - 8.4% (84 mg/mL = 10 mEq/10 mL)

MECHANISM
- Dissociates to provide bicarbonate ion, which neutralizes hydrogen ion & raises blood/urinary pH
- Raises serum bicarbonate, forms water & CO_2

COMMENTS
- Caution in treating anion gap metabolic acidosis.
  - Control the underlying cause of the acidosis (eg, hypoperfusion causing lactic acidosis).
  - In lactic acidosis, sodium bicarbonate administration can cause intracellular acidosis, which could adversely affect pt outcome.

➤ Must have means to ventilate CO_2 produced by acid neutralization, or pH will drop from respiratory acidosis.

➤ Administer only enough sodium bicarbonate to improve hemodynamic stability, or to raise pH >7.20.

■ Therapy can lead to hypocalcaemia, hypokalemia, hypernatremia, metabolic alkalosis.

➤ 1 g $NaHCO_3$ provides 12 mEq Na, or 50 mL of 8.4% solution provides 1,150 mg Na.

➤ Do not administer to pt w/ metabolic or respiratory alkalosis, hypocalcemia, or hypernatremia.

■ Do not add to calcium-containing solution, because precipitation will occur.

■ No longer recommended in ACLS guidelines as routine therapy during cardiac arrest.

■ Raising urine pH may promote clearance of acidic drugs or substances.

SODIUM CITRATE (BICITRA, SHOHL'S SOLUTION)

JESSICA SAMPAT, MD

INDICATION
■ Nonparticulate antacid
■ Systemic or urine alkalinization

DOSE
■ Antacid: 15–30 mL PO
■ Systemic alkalinization: 10–30 mL PO diluted w/ 10–90 mL water after meals & at bedtime

ONSET
■ Immediate (for gastric acid neutralization)

KINETICS
■ Peak effect: few minutes
■ Duration of action: 1–2 h

PREPARATION
■ Bicitra & Shohl's solution contain mixture of sodium citrate & citric acid.
■ Protect solution from excessive heat.

MECHANISM
- Nonparticulate acid-neutralizing buffer.
- Alkalinizing activity depends on oxidation to bicarbonate in the body.
- Each mL of sodium citrate contains 1 mEq sodium & is equivalent to 1 mEq bicarbonate.
- Produces a rapid rise in the pH value of gastric acid.

COMMENTS
- Commonly used as premed in pts at risk for aspiration pneumonitis
  - 30 mL of 0.3 molar sodium citrate raises gastric pH >2.5 in most pts.
  - Most effective when given within 45 min before anesthesia induction
- Also used to treat metabolic acidosis from renal tubular acidosis
- Contraindications & cautions w/ repeated dosing are related to high sodium content.
  - Contraindicated in pts w/ renal impairment or those on sodium-restricted diets
  - Use cautiously in pts w/ cardiac failure, HTN, peripheral & pulmonary edema, toxemia of pregnancy.

SUCCINYLCHOLINE (ANECTINE, QUELICIN)

EMILY REINYS, MD

INDICATION
- Muscle relaxant

DOSE
- 1–1.5 mg/kg IV for intubation (use higher dose if pt is given defasciculating dose of nondepolarizing muscle relaxant)
- Repeat boluses (10 mg) or IV infusion (1 g in 500 mL) titrated to effect for some surgical procedures
- 2.5–4 mg/kg IM

ONSET
- IV: 30–60 sec
- IM: 1.5–3 min

KINETICS
- Duration: <10 min (typically)
- Metabolized by pseudocholinesterase (in plasma)

PREPARATION
- Premixed 20 mg/mL solution in 10-mL ampule

MECHANISM
- Agonist at nicotinic ACh receptors at neuromuscular junction, causing prolonged depolarization of muscle endplate & thus muscle relaxation

COMMENTS
- Fasciculations & myalgia may be prevented by pretreatment w/ small dose of nondepolarizing muscle relaxant
- Life-threatening K+ elevation in pts w/ burn injury, massive trauma, myopathies, prolonged immobilization, paraplegia, denervation of skeletal muscle
- Potential trigger of malignant hyperthermia
- Prolonged paralysis in pts w/ atypical pseudocholinesterase
- May increase vagal tone, particularly w/ repeated doses

SUFENTANIL

KALEB JENSON, MD

INDICATION
- Analgesia
- Anesthesia adjunct

DOSE
- Important: all opioid doses should be titrated to effect depending on a variety of factors, including
  - Pt age
  - Body weight
  - Physical status of pt
  - Coexisting disease
  - Other CNS depressant drug administration
  - Surgery or procedure performed
- As supplement to GA, dose requirement will vary w/ stress of surgery & other anesthetic agents.
- IV
  - Cardiac surgery: 8–30 mcg/kg. Inadequate for use as a sole anesthetic. Anticipate need for postop mechanical ventilation.
  - Adjunct to GA, low dose: 1–2 mcg/kg

➤ Adjunct to GA, moderate dose: 2–8 mcg/kg, plus maintenance dose of 10–50 mcg as necessary. Some attenuation of stress response to surgery.
■ Intrathecal: 5–15 mcg
■ Epidural
➤ Labor analgesia: 10–20 mcg mixed w/ 0.125% bupivacaine or 0.2% ropivacaine. For infusion, can combine local anesthetic w/ 0.5 mcg/mL sufentanil.

ONSET
■ IV: 1–3 min
■ Intrathecal: 2–5 min
■ Epidural: 7–8 min

KINETICS
■ IV duration (typical maintenance dose): 35 min
■ Epidural duration: 4 h
■ Intrathecal duration: 2–4 h
■ Elimination half-life: 164 min
■ Hepatic & small intestine metabolism

PREPARATION
■ 50 mcg/cc in 2- or 5-cc vial

MECHANISM
■ Mu opioid receptor agonist

COMMENTS
■ Sufentanil is 10 times more potent than fentanyl.
■ Does not release histamine.
■ Important respiratory effects
➤ Like other opioids, will cause respiratory depression & hypoventilation, which can ultimately lead to apnea & respiratory arrest.
➤ Like other potent opioids, can cause significant chest wall rigidity & difficulty w/ ventilation, requiring muscle relaxant administration. This is very common w/ rapid IV administration of large dose.
■ Important cardiac effects
➤ In general, sufentanil has minimal effects on hemodynamic status & has been widely used for cardiac surgery.

- ➤ Like other potent opioids, can cause significant bradycardia & hypotension.
- ➤ When used in combination w/ other sedative meds (eg, benzodiazepines, barbiturates), hypotension can be more pronounced.
- Consider dose reduction in elderly or debilitated pts, or those w/ liver failure.
- Compared to fentanyl, sufentanil has shorter duration & slightly faster onset.
- Opioids not considered suitable for use as a sole anesthetic because of breakthrough hypertension, inadequate anesthesia, high incidence of recall, muscle rigidity, postop respiratory depression.

TERBUTALINE (BRETHINE, BRICANYL)

IVAN ZEITZ, MD

INDICATION
- Bronchospasm
- Preterm labor

DOSE
- Bronchospasm
  - ➤ Adult dose: 0.25 mg IM/SQ, may repeat after 15 min
  - ➤ Pediatric dose: 0.005–0.01 mg/kg SC up to 0.3 mg/dose; may repeat q15min up to 3 doses
- Preterm labor: 25–10 mcg/min IV; may increase q20min up to 30 mcg/min

ONSET
- 15 min SQ/IM

KINETICS
- SQ/IM peak effect within 30–60 min, lasts 90 min to 4 h
- Metabolism: hepatic
- Elimination: renal

PREPARATION
- 1 mg/cc solution

MECHANISM
- Synthetic sympathomimetic amine; B2 > B1 effect causing relaxation of bronchial smooth muscle

COMMENTS
- Cardiac toxicity (arrhythmias, tachycardia) is dose-limiting.

TETRACAINE

JAMES BRANDES, MD

INDICATION
- Regional/spinal/topical anesthesia

DOSE
- Spinal: 5–20 mg (in children 1 mg/kg)
- Regional: 0.5–1.0 mg/kg (usually combined w/ intermediate- or short-acting agent)
- Max dose w/o vasoconstrictor 1.5 mg/kg, w/ vasoconstrictor (epinephrine or phenylephrine) 2.5 mg/kg

ONSET
- Regional block: 15–20 min
- Spinal: ~10 min

KINETICS
- Duration: ~3 h for spinal anesthesia
- Hepatic & plasma metabolism

PREPARATION
- 20 mg powder for reconstitution
- 1% in 10% dextrose
- 0.2 or 0.3% in 6% dextrose for pediatric/neonatal spinal

MECHANISM
- Blocks sodium channels in nerves

COMMENTS
- It is an ester.
- PABA is a metabolite, so pts w/ allergy to suntan lotion should not receive tetracaine.
- Standard cautions as w/ other local anesthetics related to pt characteristics & anesthetic technique.

THAM ACETATE

DONAL RYAN, MD

INDICATION
- Acidosis: as an alternative to $NaHCO_3$ (eg, respiratory acidosis, hypernatremia)

DOSE
- Assumes standard strength of 0.3 mol/L
- 1 mL/kg times base deficit (mEq/L) IV
- Give 25–50% as a loading dose over 5–10 min & remainder over 1 h, or start empirically w/ 3 mL/kg IV over 5–10 min
- Max: 5 mL/kg in 20 min, 15 mL/kg in 1 h, 45 mL/kg in 1 day

ONSET
- Immediate

KINETICS
- >80% renal excretion of protonated form

PREPARATION
- THAM acetate solution (0.3 mol/L), pH 8.6. May be administered peripherally or centrally.

MECHANISM
- Surrogate buffer system; proton acceptor w/ pKa of 7.8

COMMENTS
- May cause hypokalemia, hypocalcemia, hypoglycemia, respiratory depression, osmotic diuresis
- In neonates, give w/ 5% dextrose.
- Avoid or use w/ caution in pts w/ renal failure: increased risk for hyperkalemia.

THIOPENTAL SODIUM (PENTOTHAL)

MADELEINE BIBAT, MD

INDICATION
- Induction of anesthesia
- Anticonvulsant

DOSE

- For induction: 3–5 mg/kg IV for adults, 5–6 mg/kg for children
- For convulsions: 75–125 mg IV in adults, repeated as needed. For children, 2–3 mg/kg IV, repeated as needed.
- 25 mg/kg rectally in children

ONSET

- 30–60 sec

KINETICS

- Duration: 10–60 min
- Elimination half-life: 15 h
- Hepatic metabolism
- Renal excretion

PREPARATION

- Reconstitute 500 mg w/ 20 cc 0.9% sodium chloride for a 2.5% solution, pH 10.5.

MECHANISM

- Enhances the ability of GABA to activate GABA-A receptors

COMMENTS

- Avoid in pts w/ acute intermittent porphyria: may cause elevated porphyrins & lead to neuro disturbances.
- Preferred induction agent in pts w/ hyperthyroidism (decreases T4 to T3 conversion)
- Cardiac effects such as hypotension more pronounced in following conditions. Reduce dose accordingly.
  - ➣ Hypovolemia
  - ➣ Elderly pt
  - ➣ Pt w/ limited cardiac reserve (eg, critically ill pt in ICU)

TRIAMCINOLONE (AZMACORT, KENALOG, NASACORT)

ANDREW GRAY, MD, PHD

INDICATION

- Asthma
- Pain assoc w/ radiculopathy
  - ➣ Often used topically or systemically for other conditions requiring steroid treatment (dermatoses, allergic rhinitis, etc)

DOSE
- Typical adult dose for asthma: 4 inhalations (400 mcg) twice daily
- For epidural steroid injection in an adult: 50–80 mg epidural at interspace near affected nerve root

ONSET
- For asthma, relief of symptoms may occur as soon as 1 wk after initiation of therapy.
- Following epidural injection, pain relief onset & duration are highly variable. Pain relief may last from days to months after injection. Some pts do not experience relief of symptoms.

KINETICS
- Inhaled: Max benefit may not be observed for 2 wks or more after initiation of therapy.
- Injected
  - Suspension slowly absorbed from injection site
  - Repeat injection may be performed 1–6 wks after initial injection for pts who have partial improvement or recurrence of symptoms.

PREPARATION
- Inhalation: Triamcinolone acetonide inhalation aerosol
- For epidural injection
  - Triamcinolone diacetate & acetonide are relatively insoluble & are therefore prepared as a sterile suspension.
  - Although commercial preparations of triamcinolone contain benzyl alcohol, evidence regarding toxicity is lacking.
  - Often administered w/ preservative-free saline & local anesthetic

MECHANISM
- Both the inhaled & epidural routes of administration provide local anti-inflammatory effects w/o major systemic effects.

COMMENTS
- Inhaled steroids are not effective for treatment of acute exacerbation of asthma.
- Adverse reactions are uncommon but similar to those observed w/ other corticosteroids.
- Diabetic pts often have increased insulin requirements for days after epidural steroid injection.
- Pts w/ duration of radicular symptoms >6 mo or prior laminectomy are less likely to respond to epidural steroid injection.

- Most practitioners do not inject after dural puncture because of the possible risk of arachnoiditis.
- Soluble steroid preparations should not be used for epidural injection because they are rapidly absorbed & may cause seizures.
- Pts w/ recent signs of overt nerve compression (bowel/bladder dysfunction or foot drop) need prompt neurosurgical evaluation rather than triamcinolone injection.

TRIMETHAPHAN (ARFONAD)

DORRE NICHOLAU, PHD, MD

INDICATION
- Deliberate hypotension
- Use in anesthesia may include:
  - ➤ Dissecting aortic aneurysms
  - ➤ Intraop deliberate hypotension
  - ➤ Hypertensive crisis
  - ➤ Autonomic hyperreflexia

DOSE
- Begin infusion at 10–20 mcg/kg/min (0.5–5 mg/min).
- Recommend arterial line monitoring
- Dose >1 g likely to result in persistent ganglionic blockade, direct vasodilation, histamine release, neuromuscular blockade

ONSET
- Immediate

KINETICS
- Hydrolyzed by pseudocholinesterase
- Duration: minutes

PREPARATION
- Available in 10-mL 500-mg ampules (50 mg/mL)
- For infusion, dilute 500 mg in 500 cc D_5W or Ringer's

MECHANISM
- Ganglionic blocking agent
- Selective nondepolarizing blockade of neurotransmission at autonomic ganglia

COMMENTS
- Rapid onset
- Tachyphylaxis limits use.
- Cardiac effects
  - Lowers BP w/o reflex tachycardia
  - Reduces dP/dT
  - Decreases both arteriolar & venous tone, decreasing both resistance & capacitance
- Neuro effects
  - Pupils become fixed and dilated, obscuring neuro exam.
  - Possible alteration of cerebral vascular autoregulation
  - May increase ICP, so not recommended for neurosurgical pts
  - Recommended doses do not produce nicotinic neuromuscular blockade.
- Adverse effects can include:
  - Dry mouth
  - Visual changes
  - Paralytic ileus
  - Urinary retention
  - Bronchospasm from histamine release
  - Respiratory arrest w/ dose >5 mg/min
  - Neuromuscular blockade w/ high doses. Can also prolong effects of nondepolarizing neuromuscular blockers & succinylcholine.

VANCOMYCIN

MICHAEL H. FAHMY, MD

INDICATION
- Tricyclic glycopeptide antibiotic for the treatment of serious gram-positive infections

DOSE
- Usual dose for pt w/ normal renal function is 2 g/day, divided q6h or q12h.
- For pts w/ impaired renal function, give 15 mg/kg loading dose. For maintenance, approximate creatinine clearance to vancomycin dose is:
  - Creatinine clearance 100 mL/min: 1.5 g/24 h
  - Creatinine clearance 80 mL/min: 1.2 g/24 h
  - Creatinine clearance 60 mL/min: 900 mg/24 h

➤ Creatinine clearance 40 mL/min: 600 mg/24 h
➤ Creatinine clearance 20 mL/min: 300 mg/24 h
➤ Anuric pt: 1 g q7–10 days
➤ Renal failure pt on hemodialysis: 500 mg q48–96h

ONSET
■ Peak plasma levels at end of infusion

KINETICS
■ Mean elimination half-life: 4–6 h
■ 70–90% renal excretion of unchanged drug

PREPARATION
■ 500-mg, 1-g vials
■ Reconstitute to 5 mg/mL or more dilute
  ➤ eg, 500 mg in 100 mL, or 1 g in 200 mL

MECHANISM
■ Interferes w/ microbial cell wall synthesis
■ Alters bacterial cell membrane permeability & RNA synthesis

COMMENTS
■ Important: NEVER infuse vancomycin over <1 h, as this can lead to hypotension, flushing, erythema, urticaria, & pruritus ("red man syndrome").
■ If possible, infuse at least 1 hour prior to onset of anesthesia. Infusion-related events may be more common w/ concomitant administration of anesthetic agents.

VASOPRESSIN

BRANDON GINIECZKI, MD

INDICATION
■ Shock-refractory ventricular fibrillation (VF)
■ Refractory vasodilatory shock
■ Treatment of central (neurogenic) diabetes insipidus (DI)

DOSE
■ VF: 40 units × 1 IV
■ Vasodilatory shock: 0.02–0.1 units/min IV infusion
■ DI: 5–10 units IM q8–12h

ONSET
- IV pressor effect in 30–60 sec
- Antidiuretic effect in 2–6 h

KINETICS
- Half-life: 10–35 min
- Duration of pressor effect after bolus: 30–60 min
- Metabolized in liver, kidney

PREPARATION
- 20 units/mL
- Infusion: 40 units in 250 cc NS

MECHANISM
- Vasoconstriction from nonadrenergic stimulation of V1 receptors in vascular smooth muscle
- Vasodilation of cerebral vasculature from nitric oxide-mediated pathway
- Antidiuresis mediated by V2 receptors in renal collecting ducts
  - Increases cortical & medullary collecting duct permeability to H_2O
  - Maximizes concentrating ability of kidney

COMMENTS
- Recommended in ACLS 2000 guidelines as alternate to epinephrine in adult w/ shock-refractory VF
- Avoid in awake pt w/ coronary disease. Can cause coronary constriction, angina & reduced cardiac output.
- Causes significant peripheral vasoconstriction
- May cause uterine contractions, bowel peristalsis & abdominal cramps, increased mesenteric vascular resistance & reduced portal venous blood flow
- Potential adverse effects
  - Tremor
  - Sweating
  - Vertigo
  - Water intoxication. Symptoms may include altered mental status, headache.
  - Hyponatremia
  - Metabolic acidosis
  - Nausea, vomiting
  - Allergic reactions including urticaria & anaphylaxis
- For antidiuretic effect, other agents (eg, desmopressin) often chosen because of longer duration & improved side effect profile

VECURONIUM

RONNIE LU, MD

INDICATION
- Neuromuscular block

DOSE
- Intubation: 0.08–0.12 mg/kg
- Maintenance: 0.04–0.05 mg/kg, then 0.01 mg/kg q15–20min
- Infusion: 0.05–0.10 mcg/kg/min

ONSET
- 3–5 min

KINETICS
- Duration: 20–35 min
- Minimal hepatic metabolism
- Biliary excretion (75%)
- Renal excretion (25%)

PREPARATION
- 10 mg lyophilized powder

MECHANISM
- Nondepolarizing neuromuscular block
- Competes w/ acetylcholine at nicotinic receptor site on motor endplate

COMMENTS
- Long-term use in the ICU in pts w/ renal failure may cause prolonged muscle relaxation secondary to active metabolites.
- Renal failure may prolong duration of action.
- Liver failure may prolong duration of action.

VERAPAMIL

DAN WAJSMAN, MD

INDICATION
- Antihypertensive
- Antiarrhythmic, paroxysmal SVT

- Antianginal
- Hypertrophic cardiomyopathy

DOSE
- 5–10 mg IV over 2 min; may repeat in 30 min (adult)
- 100–200 mcg/kg IV (pediatric)

ONSET
- 3–5 min IV

KINETICS
- Duration: 10–20 min for hemodynamic effect, 2 h for antiarrhythmic effect
- Liver metabolism: w/ continued dosing, consider dose reduction in pts w/ liver failure
- Renal excretion

PREPARATION
- 2.5 mg/mL

MECHANISM
- Calcium channel blocker
- Modulates calcium influx in arterial smooth muscle, conductile & contractile myocardium

COMMENTS
- More potent negative inotrope than diltiazem & other calcium channel blockers
- Slows AV node conduction & prolongs refractory period
- Most common uses in anesthesia may be for SVT, or pt w/ hypertrophic cardiomyopathy
- For SVT, would preferentially use adenosine, short-acting beta blocker, or diltiazem, because these agents have less negative inotropy
- Avoid in pt w/
  - Wide complex tachycardia unless known to be supraventricular. Can cause worsening hypotension or VF in pts w/ ventricular tachycardia.
  - Second- and third-degree heart block
  - Severe congestive heart failure from LV systolic dysfunction
  - Accessory bypass tracts (eg, WPW)
- Use caution in pts receiving beta-blockers (synergistic reduction of LV contractility) .

WAFARIN SODIUM (COUMADIN)

DHANESH K. GUPTA, MD

INDICATION
- Chronic anticoagulation (deep vein thrombosis, pulmonary embolism, atrial fibrillation, etc)

DOSE
- Adults: 2–10 mg PO qHS
- Children: 0.05–0.34 mg/kg/day

ONSET
- 1–3 days

KINETICS
- Liver metabolism, urine excretion

PREPARATION
- Tablets

MECHANISM
- Inhibits vitamin K-dependent coagulation factor synthesis (II, VII, IX, X, protein C & S)

COMMENTS
- Monitor INR to determine adequate dosage.
- Overdose is treated w/ vitamin K or w/ FFP transfusion.
- Initial administration must be w/ concomitant heparin to prevent skin necrosis from initial prothrombotic state (protein C & S deficiency).
- Adjust dose for increased or decreased vitamin K intake, or w/ hepatic disease, which may interfere w/ vitamin K absorption or synthesis of vitamin K-dependent clotting factors.
- Stop at least 3 days prior to elective surgery, & obtain INR prior to surgery.